Critical Care Nursing of the Surgical Patient

Critical Care Nursing of the Surgical Patient

Maureen E. Shekleton, D.N.Sc., R.N.

Assistant Professor, Medical-Surgical Nursing,
College of Nursing, The University of Illinois at Chicago;
Associate Faculty, Rush University College of Nursing,
Chicago, Illinois

Kim Litwack Ph.D., R.N.

Unit Leader, Post Anesthesia Recovery,
Rush Presbyterian-St. Luke's Medical Center;
Associate Professor, Rush University College of Nursing,
Chicago, Illinois

1991

W. B. SAUNDERS COMPANY

Harcourt Brace Jovanovich, Inc.
Philadelphia, London, Toronto, Montreal, Sydney, Tokyo

W. B. SAUNDERS COMPANY
Harcourt Brace Jovanovich, Inc.
The Curtis Center
Independence Square West
Philadelphia, PA 19106

Library of Congress Cataloging-in-Publication Data

Critical care nursing of the surgical patient/[edited by] Maureen
  Shekleton. Kim Litwack.
     p.   cm.
  Includes bibliographical references.
  ISBN 0-7216-3090-1
  1. Surgical nursing. 2. Intensive care nursing. I. Shekleton.
Maureen E. II. Litwack, Kim.
  [DNLM: 1. Critical Care—nursing. 2. Surgical Nursing. WY 161
  C9343]
  RD99.C75   1991
  610.73'677—dc20
  DNLM/DLC   90-8560
  for Library of Congress   CIP

Acquisitions Editor: Michael Brown
Developmental Editor: Robin Richman

Critical Care Nursing of the Surgical Patient   ISBN   0-7216-3090-1

Printed in the United States of America.

Last digit is the print number: 9   8   7   6   5   4   3   2   1

Contributors

MARY BALLOU, Ph.D.
Associate Professor Counseling Psychology, Northeastern University, Boston, Massachusetts.
The Concept of Crisis and Crisis Intervention

LINDA BERNARD, M.S., R.N.
Assistant Professor, Rush University College of Nursing, Chicago, Illinois; Associate Unit Leader, Surgical Intensive Care, Rush Presbyterian-St. Luke's Medical Center, Chicago, Illinois.
Thoracic Surgery

SALLY A. BROZENEC, M.S., R.N.
Practitioner-Teacher, Rush University College of Nursing, Practitioner-Teacher, Rush Presbyterian-St. Luke's Medical Center, Department of OR/Surgical Nursing, Chicago, Illinois.
Gastrointestinal Surgery

SYLVIA ELSON CANFIELD, M.S., R.N.
Oncology Clinical Nurse Specialist, Mercy Medical Center, Cedar Rapids, Iowa.
Alterations in Body Defenses

JANET M. DELGADO, M.N., CNRN
Doctoral Candidate, Medical-Surgical Nursing, University of Illinois, College of Nursing, Chicago, Illinois; Staff Nurse, Rush Presbyterian-St. Luke's Medical Center, Chicago, Illinois.
Altered Levels of Consciousness and Mentation; Neurosurgical Procedures

EDWARD J. GOODEMOTE, D.N.Sc., R.N.
Director of Nursing, Lakeland Regional Medical Center, Lakeland, Florida.
Alterations in Rest and Sleep Patterns

LINDA HAGGERTY, M.S., R.N.
Practitioner-Teacher, Rush University College of Nursing, Chicago, Illinois; Transplant Clinical Specialist, Rush Presbyterian-St. Luke's Medical Center, Chicago, Illinois.
Transplantation

JOYCE K. KEITHLEY, D.N.Sc., R.N.

Associate Professor, Rush University College of Nursing; Chairperson, Department of O.R. and Surgical Nursing, Rush Presbyterian-St. Luke's Medical Center, Chicago, Illinois.

Alterations in Nutrition

DEBORAH GOLDENBERG KLEIN, M.S.N., R.N., CCRN, C.S.

Clinical Instructor, Acute and Critical Care Nursing, Frances Payne Bolton School of Nursing, Case Western Reserve University, Cleveland, Ohio; Clinical Nurse Specialist, Trauma/Critical Care Nursing, MetroHealth Medical Center, Cleveland, Ohio.

Thermal Injury

JANE K. KRAY, M.S., C.R.N.A.

Partner, Tri-County Anesthesia Associates, Ltd., Private Practice CRNA Corporation.

Alterations in Fluid Volume, Composition, Distribution and Acid-Base Balance

CLINTON E. LAMBERT, Jr., M.S.N., C.S.

Assistant to the Dean, School of Nursing, Kent State University, Kent, Ohio; Private Practitioner, Psychiatric-Mental Health Nursing.

Behavioral Responses to the Critical Care Environment

VICKIE A. LAMBERT, D.N.Sc., F.A.A.N.

Associate Dean, Frances Payne Bolton School of Nursing, Case Western Reserve University, Cleveland, Ohio.

Behavioral Responses to the Critical Care Environment

JAN LITWACK, Ed.S., R.N.

Counselor, Northeastern University Counseling and Testing Center, Boston, Massachusetts.

The Concept of Crisis and Crisis Intervention; Death and Dying

LAWRENCE LITWACK, Ed.D.

Professor and Chairperson, Department of Counseling Psychology, Rehabilitation and Special Education, Northeastern University, Boston, Massachusetts.

Coping with Critical Illness

SHARON DOLCE MANSON, M.S., R.N.

Instructor, Rush University College of Nursing, Chicago, Illinois; Joint Practice Bone Marrow Transplant Center-Rush Presbyterian-St. Luke's Medical Center, Chicago, Illinois.

Alterations in Body Defenses

JULIE R. MARSHALL, M.S., R.N.

Associate Faculty, Rush University College of Nursing, Chicago, Illinois; Cardiovascular Clinical Specialist, Elmhurst Memorial Hospital, Elmhurst, Illinois.

Cardiac Surgery

LISA SIGG MENDELSON, M.S., R.N.

Instructor, Rush University College of Nursing, Chicago, Illinois; Practitioner-Teacher, Ambulatory Surgery Unit, Rush Presbyterian-St. Luke's Medical Center, Chicago, Illinois.

Alterations in Thermoregulation

JO ANN O'REILLY, M.A., M.A.R.S.

Assistant Professor, College of Health Sciences, Rush University College of Nursing, Chicago, Illinois; Coordinator of Geriatric Pastoral Services, Rush Presbyterian-St. Luke's Medical Center, Chicago, Illinois.

Death and Dying

SANDRA OWENS-JONES, M.S., R.N.

Chicago, Illinois.

Alterations in Oxygenation Processes

ANGIE ZAHAROPOULOS PATRAS, M.S., R.N.

Continuing Education Coordinator, Department of OR/Surgical Nursing, Rush University College of Nursing, Chicago, Illinois.

Gastrointestinal Surgery

CAROLE TEMMING, M.S.N., D.MIN., R.N.

Assistant Professor, Rush University College of Nursing, Chicago, Illinois; Assistant Professor and Associate Coordinator of Pastoral Services, Rush Presbyterian-St. Luke's Medical Center, Chicago, Illinois.

Death and Dying

JILL SCHOERGER WALSH, M.S., R.N.

Lecturer, Marcella Niehoff School of Nursing, Loyola University of Chicago; Clinical Nurse Specialist, Emergency Medical Services, Loyola University Medical Center, Maywood, Illinois.

Trauma

CYNTHIA A. WONG, M.D.

Clinical Associate of Anesthesia, Northwestern University Medical School; Staff Anesthesiologist, Northwestern Memorial Hospital, Chicago, Illinois.

Physiologic Responses to Anesthesia

Preface

Critical Care Nursing of the Surgical Patient has been written primarily as a reference text for the surgical intensive care staff nurse. Graduate students, nursing faculty members, and staff development personnel will also find the text useful as a reference for orientation programs, critical care courses, and inservice programs. The bibliographies provided at the ends of chapters give the reader some useful additional references for further study.

Not all surgical patients require intensive nursing care. Critical care of a surgical patient may be warranted due to the extent of the surgical procedure itself, the anesthetic risk, the presence of an underlying pathological condition which adds further risk to the patient's condition, or when any of the usual responses to surgery are exaggerated, extreme, or abnormal in some way. Because there are many possible reasons for which a surgical patient may be admitted to a critical care unit, this book has been organized using two complementary frameworks. In the first sections physiologic and psychologic responses to surgery, critical illness, and the critical care environment are discussed within a nursing process framework. In the last section the relevant pre-, intra-, and post-operative aspects of surgical procedures and treatments which most often accompany or precipitate critical illness are addressed.

The book is organized into four sections. Presented in the first section is an overview of the surgical experience as a stressor which elicits responses to which the body must adapt in order to regain and maintain homeostasis. This section is intended to serve as a general introduction to the effects of surgery and anesthesia which will apply to all surgical patients regardless of the underlying pathophysiology being treated.

Examined in section two are psychosocial responses to critical illness in the surgical patient. Responses of the family are also addressed. The "high tech" environment of critical care makes attending to the psychosocial and spiritual dimensions of patient care very important if "high touch" nursing care is to counter the negative aspects of the environment. The concepts of crisis, coping and adaptation, and death and dying are discussed within the context of critical illness. A chapter on behavioral responses to the critical care environment deals with the behaviors that a critical care unit nurse might have to manage. The concepts of crisis and coping are inherently related to one another and are the basis for many of the behaviors exhibited by the critically ill patient; therefore, there is some necessary overlap between these chapters. This overlap allows the reader to refer to an individual chapter without reading the entire section.

The focus of section three is on the physiologic responses to critical illness in the surgical patient. The expected physiologic responses to surgery, critical illness, and the critical care environment are presented conceptually.

Discussed in section four are the surgical procedures and treatments which most often necessitate intensive nursing care. This section is organized so that the relevant pre-, intra-, and post-operative nursing care for surgical procedures performed on the various body systems is addressed. There are also chapters on the surgical aspects of trauma and burns. Transplantation is presented within one chapter rather than as a part of those chapters organized by body system.

Nursing diagnoses relevant to the surgical critical care patient are addressed throughout the book. Like all other clinical practice disciplines, nursing uses the clinical problem solving method which incorporates the steps of assessment and diagnosis and the planning, delivery, and subsequent evaluation of care. The term *diagnosis* is used here to refer to the recognition and labeling of a pattern within the data derived from assessment. Breu, Dracup & Walden (1987) state that "while involvement with medical diagnoses and treatment is essential in critical care, the focus of nursing has evolved to be distinct from that of medicine" (p. 606). As editors of this text we agree with that statement, viewing nursing, as defined in the A.N.A. Social Policy Statement (1980), as the diagnosis and treatment of the human responses to actual or potential health problems. These human responses are the phenomena of concern to nurses while the health problem and its medical management are the concern of physicians.

Many of the responses which critical care nurses diagnose and treat are physiologic in nature (Roberts, 1988). We acknowledge the controversy which exists currently within nursing regarding the appropriateness of physiologic diagnoses within a nursing diagnostic taxonomy. Kim (1984) and Cassmeyer (1989) have summarized the issues related to the use of physiologic nursing diagnoses. We believe that physiologic diagnoses do have a place in a nursing diagnostic taxonomy for the following reasons.

The nature and scope of nursing practice are not static but, rather, reflect the dynamic nature of science, health care, and the ever changing needs of society. While the nature and scope of practice cannot, therefore, be defined solely by the content of that practice, the content does help to define and delineate that practice. Incorporation of the biophysical with the psychosociocultural and spiritual domains is necessary if a holistic perspective is to be achieved in practice. Dismissing diagnoses that are physiologic in nature or that require collaborative or interdependent nursing interventions would result in a scope of practice that is too narrowly circumscribed to reflect actual, present day practice let alone future practice as multidisciplinary, collaborative models grow and care becomes increasingly complex (Drew, 1988).

As long as different disciplines use a shared knowledge base and have similar missions, their respective roles will overlap. This is reflected by the following statement from the A.N.A. Social Policy Statement (A.N.A., 1980), "All of the health care professions interact, share the same mission, have access to the same published scientific knowledge, and in some degree overlap in their activities" (p. 16). Critical care nurses are in a prime position to see how the scientific base of both nursing and medical practice overlap, especially within the physiologic domain. It is the application of the underlying knowledge base that differentiates the practice of one discipline from that of another. Physicians establish and treat disease while nurses treat the responses to the functional changes brought about by the pathophysiology which characterizes that disease process (Cassmeyer, 1989). These two applications of the same biologic science base are obviously related and it is, therefore, a fact of clinical life that nurses must collaborate with members of other health care disciplines (Kim, 1985). The complexity of patient problems and responses also mandates a need for collaborative patient care management (Roberts, 1988).

Collaboration does not preclude independent thought or action on the part of the nurse. This becomes apparent if one examines the clinical judgment process. Diers (1985) describes clinical judgment as an artful and scientific process whereby clinical decisions about diagnosis and treatment are made based on the available assessment data and diagnostic resources, using theories and knowledge which enable the clinician to predict outcome with a given probability. Tanner (1983) describes the process as one of identifying alternatives, gathering information to reduce uncertainty about the alternatives and selecting the most likely diagnosis or optimal treatment plan. This process, the author continues, requires consideration of the probabilistic relationships between assessment and diagnosis and between diagnosis and management strategies. Clinical judgment, then, requires more than mere application of knowledge to a particular phenomenon—it requires that the clinician move from the observed to the conceptual, consider multiple explanations for the occurrence of the phenomenon and the most appropriate treatment related to each explanation, and estimate the probability of success for each. The clinician is required to reason inductively and to sort out competing hypotheses. This thought process is required even when the interventions are prescribed within a medical regimen including standing orders. This is consistent with Kim's (1984) definition of an interdependent nursing intervention as "that which the nurse makes on the basis of independent judgment and decision making to carry out medical orders or to implement the medical regimen" (p. 60). Roberts' (1988) definition, while stated slightly differently, concurs that "expert judgment" by the nurse and consultation with the physician are required for an interdependent intervention.

Physiologic diagnoses do not only require interdependent interventions. Dougherty (1985), as one example that is extremely relevant to critical care nursing, has demonstrated through research that the majority of nursing interventions for the diagnosis of decreased cardiac output are independent in nature. Jacoby (1985) states that while nurses do diagnose and treat independently physiologic dysfunction, more often potential physiologic alterations are diagnosed and treated independently. This is certainly the case in critical care where monitoring functions comprise a major portion of nursing activities. The phenomenon of *deterioration* has only recently begun to be described (Smith, 1988) but represents the almost subliminal recognition of the worsening of a patient's condition. This is one example of the application of the skills of clinical judgment within a monitoring situation.

We believe that the format of this text will facilitate the development of the skills inherent to clinical judgment. These skills are very important in critical care nursing practice and will become more so as the ever expanding technology allows the accumulation of greater amounts and types of clinical data. The ability to integrate and synthesize these data rapidly as a basis for action is at the core of critical care nursing practice. The high level of clinical judgment which is necessary in this practice has served to help establish critical care as a vital and evolving specialty within the discipline of nursing. Even more important is the fact that the skill with which clinical judgment is exercised in actual practice is the basis for evaluation of that practice and the core of our contract with society as a professional practice discipline.

REFERENCES

A.N.A. (1980). *Nursing: A social policy statement.* Kansas City, Mo.; American Nurses' Association.

Breu, C., Dracup, K., & Walden, J. (1987). Integration of nursing diagnoses in the critical care nursing literature. *Heart Lung, 16*(6), 605–616.

Carnevali, D. (1984) The diagnostic reasoning process. In Carnevali, D., Mitchell, P., Woods, N., Tanner, C. *Diagnostic reasoning in nursing* (pp. 25–56). Philadelphia, Pa.; J. B. Lippincott Co.

Carpenito, L. J. (1987). Nursing diagnosis in critical care: Impact on practice. *Heart Lung, 16* (6), 595–600.

Cassmeyer, V. L. (1989). Using physiology and pathophysiology in the nursing diagnostic process. *J. Adv. Med. Surg. Nsg., 1* (3), 1–10.

Diers, D. (1985). Preparation of practitioners, clinical specialists and clinicians. *J. of Prof. Nsg.,* Jan.–Feb., 41–47.

Dougherty, C. (1985). The nursing diagnosis of decreased cardiac output. *Nsg. Clin. of No. Am., 20* (4), 787–800.

Drew, B. J. (1988). Devaluation of biological knowledge. *Image, 20* (1), 25–27.

Jacoby, M. (1986). The dilemma of physiological problems: Eliminating the double standard. *A.J.N., 85,* 281 & 285.

Kim, M. (1984). Physiologic nursing diagnosis: its role and place in nursing taxonomy. In Kim, M. J., McFarland, G., & McLane, A. (Eds). *Classification of nursing diagnoses: Proceedings of the Fifth National Conference* (pp. 60–62), St. Louis; C. V. Mosby.

Kim, M. (1985). Without collaboration, what's left? *A.J.N., 85,* 281 & 285.

Roberts, S. L. (1988). Physiologic nursing diagnoses are necessary and appropriate for critical care. *Focus on Critical Care., 15*(5), 42–49.

Smith, S. K. (1988). An analysis of the phenomenon of deterioration in the critically ill. *Image, 20* (1), 12–15.

Tanner, C. (1983). Research on Clinical Judgment. In Holzemer, W. (Ed.). *Review of research in nursing education* (pp. 2–32), Thoroughfare, N. J.; Slack.

Wake, M. (1987). Symposium: Nursing diagnosis in critical care. *Heart Lung. 16* (6), 593–594.

Contents

SECTION I

Overview of the Surgical Experience

1 General Responses to Surgery

Maureen E. Shekleton, D.N.Sc., R.N.

Many compensatory and adaptive responses occur as the body attempts to maintain homeostasis after surgery. This major insult to the body tissues evokes the stress response and all of its sequelae, in addition to the direct effects of the surgical destruction and manipulation of tissue and the anesthesia. The direct effects of surgery will be the focus of this chapter; the stress response and the effects of anesthesia will be discussed in more detail in other chapters.

Not all surgical patients require intensive nursing care. Critical care of a surgical patient may be warranted because of the extent of the surgical procedure itself, the anesthetic risk, the presence of an underlying pathological condition that adds further risk to the patient's condition, or when any of the responses to surgery are exaggerated, extreme, or abnormal in some way. The human responses to surgery that are the phenomena of concern to the nurse are varied, and these should be anticipated in any patient who has had surgery. The responses include alterations in comfort; fluid volume, distribution, and composition; nutrition; elimination patterns; respiratory function and oxygenation; body temperature; thought processes; communication and sensory–perceptual abilities; and impaired physical mobility and tissue integrity. Also, depending on the type of surgery, there will be associated knowledge deficits and underlying pathologic conditions, as well as the diagnoses of anxiety and the potential for infection and injury. Many of these responses are discussed in detail in subsequent chapters. The nursing diagnoses discussed in this chapter include alteration in fluid volume, distribution, and composition; impaired skin and tissue integrity; alteration in respiratory function; alteration in elimination patterns; and knowledge deficit: preoperative information. These diagnoses are discussed in terms of the direct effects of surgery and the presence of a wound regardless of the patient's underlying condition or the type or extent of the surgical procedure.

ALTERATION IN FLUID VOLUME, DISTRIBUTION AND COMPOSITION

The signs and symptoms of various alterations of fluid volume and composition are discussed in detail in chapter 9. Disruption of body fluid homeostasis in the surgical patient can occur anywhere in the spectrum between dehydration and overhydration and may be accompanied by a variety of electrolyte and acid–base disorders. Restoration and maintenance of normal body fluid volume and composition is a priority in the care of the critically ill surgical patient. Attainment of this goal may be difficult and will depend on the preoperative status of the patient, the extent of the operative procedure, and the adequacy of the adaptive physiologic response to surgery.

Before surgery the patient may already have a significant disruption in body fluid homeostasis due to effects of the disease process and/or treatment. Bleeding, evaporation of fluid from the organs as they are exposed to the environment, and inadequate fluid replacement during surgery may result in significant fluid loss. Overhydration may be the result of administration of an excessive amount or too rapid an infusion of intravenous (IV) fluid. During the postoperative period, wound drainage and gastrointestinal (GI) suction as well as inappropriate fluid and electrolyte replacement may also disrupt body fluid homeostasis. Underlying all of these imposed conditions is the metabolic response that surgical stress evokes.

Retention of water is markedly increased after surgery, and dilution resulting from water retention may cause hyponatremia, decreased serum osmolality, and signs of water excess or intoxication. Water retention can be attributed to several factors. The usual regulation of antidiuretic hormone (ADH) secretion through osmoreceptor control is overridden by the effects of stress, which causes extremely potent direct stimulation of the posterior pituitary. The posterior pituitary gland is responsible for the secretion of ADH, and elevated levels of this hormone may persist for 2 to 4 days after uncomplicated surgery (Groer & Shekleton, 1989).

Water retention can also be attributed to the effects of stimulation of the sympathetic nervous system and the adrenal medulla. The subsequent release of epinephrine and norepinephrine causes vasoconstriction and decreased renal blood flow. In response, the juxtaglomerular cells are stimulated to release renin, which catalyzes the conversion of a plasma protein polypeptide—angiotensinogen—into a peptide, angiotensin I. A converting enzyme changes angiotensin I into angiotensin II, which stimulates the zona glomerulosa of the adrenal cortex to release the mineralocorticoid aldosterone. Aldosterone causes resorption of sodium and, subsequently, water in the renal tubule. The subsequent water resorption is osmotic in nature, while sodium resorption occurs actively through a pump mechanism linked to the excretion of potassium.

Aldosterone secretion is also stimulated by adrenocorticotropic hormone (ACTH) and elevated plasma potassium levels. ACTH is secreted in response to trauma and stress and causes the adrenal cortex to secrete glucocorticoids as well as aldosterone. Increased blood glucose levels and glycosuria may result from the glycogenolysis and gluconeogenesis that occur in response to the adrenal hormones. The glucocorticoids also cause increased protein catabolism, which leads to a loss of nitrogen and potassium from the catabolized tissue (Marcinek, 1977). Initially, serum K^+ levels will increase as the potassium released from the catabolized cells enters the extracellular fluid. Eventually, however, negative nitrogen and potassium balances develop. The negative nitrogen balance is the result of direct tissue damage, protein catabolism and the effects of starvation discussed in detail in chapter 8. The serum K^+ level will fall after the initial slight increase. Urinary excretion of potassium increases in the presence of aldosterone as resorption of Na^+ in the distal tubule is accomplished in exchange for K^+. If excessive losses of potassium due to vomiting, diarrhea, gastric suction, or draining fistulas occur before or after surgery without adequate replacement therapy, hypokalemia may become quite severe (Groer & Shekleton, 1989).

Water is also endogenously formed as tissue catabolism increases to meet the body's caloric requirements. Approximately 1 ml of sodium-free water is formed with each gram of tissue oxidized. Metabolic processes accelerate in order to facilitate tissue repair, which in turn increases the utilization of energy. Abrams and Cerra (1985) report that research has demonstrated that the resting metabolic expenditure may increase up to 100% in the presence of major burns, sepsis, or severe trauma. Because the surgical patient is usually fasting, substrates for the production of energy must be supplied endogenously.

Accelerated metabolic processes and the inflammatory response to tissue trauma cause the body temperature to rise 24 to 48 hours after surgery. This results in greater than normal amounts of fluid being lost via the skin and lungs. Fluid sequestration around the damaged tissue may be significant enough to produce a third space, (see chapter 9) which will contribute to extracellular fluid depletion. All possible water losses and gains must be considered when calculating requirements for replacement fluids.

Acid–base disorders can develop as a result of fluid and electrolyte disorders and conditions that accompany surgery and the primary disease. For example, respiratory acidosis may occur as a result of hypoventilation due to the pattern of shallow, tidal breathing that occurs in the immediate postoperative period. Respiratory alkalosis may develop if hyperventilation due to either anxiety or mechanical ventilation occurs. Hypokalemia causes H^+ to substitute for K^+ on the Na^+–K^+ renal pump and a state of metabolic alkalosis will ensue as excess H^+ is lost (Groer & Shekleton, 1989). If liver function is impaired, metabolic acidosis can develop, as the oxidation of glucose for wound healing causes lactate formation and the Cori cycle in the liver is responsible for the recycling of lactate to glucose (Goodson & Hunt, 1985).

The duration of the metabolic response to surgery depends on the extent of the injury and the presence of complications. The development of shock, sepsis, or organ failure will further complicate the restoration and maintenance of body fluid homeostasis in the surgical patient. Nursing responsibilities include monitoring the patient's response to surgery, administering the appropriate replacement fluids and electrolytes, and monitoring the patient's response to that replacement therapy.

IMPAIRED SKIN AND TISSUE INTEGRITY

A wound can be the result of surgery, trauma, burns, pressure, or any other condition that creates a disruption in the continuity of the skin and the underlying subcutaneous tissue, fascia, and muscles. If the edges of the wound are approximately equal to one another and there is little or no tissue loss, the wound will heal by *primary intention*. An example of such a wound is a clean surgical incision or a simple laceration. If there is a great deal of tissue destruction or loss and the wound remains open to heal by granulation, the wound is said to heal by *secondary intention*. Examples of this type of wound include burns, pressure ulcers, stasis ulcers, or surgeries in which extensive resection is necessary. Wound healing by *tertiary intention* is said to occur when the wound is left open initially while infection is treated and closed surgically at a later time (Sieggreen, 1987).

The process by which a wound heals is a complex series of interacting events that allows closure of the wound with the formation of new tissue. There are three major stages or phases that occur in the process of wound healing: the inflammatory phase, the proliferative or regenerative phase, and the differentiation or remodeling phase. While all wounds heal through the same process, the duration of each phase will vary depending on whether healing is occurring through primary, secondary, or tertiary intention (Stotts, 1986).

The inflammatory process begins when the injury occurs and is absolutely essential if healing is to occur. The central role of inflammation in wound healing is depicted in Figure 1–1. Hemostatic, vascular, and cellular responses are stimulated at this point, as well as epithelialization. The initial response, vasoconstriction, lasts about 5 to 10 minutes, and causes a state of hypoxia and acidosis around the wound. Vessels retract and a fibrin plug is formed as coagulation is stimulated. The interaction of thrombin and platelets that occurs in clotting causes the release of locally acting growth factors that stimulate cell growth and movement. Initial vasoconstriction is followed by vasodilation, which is thought to occur in response to substances such as histamine, the kinins, and the prostaglandins released at the wound site. As blood flow and capillary permeability increase and the lymph channels be-

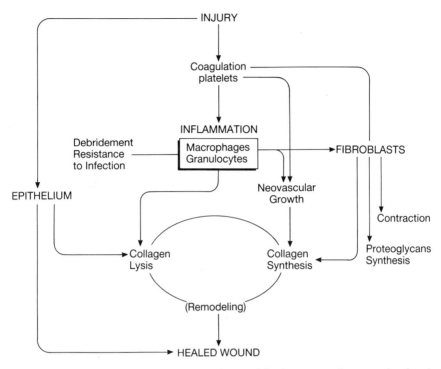

Figure 1–1. A general flow diagram of wound healing. Note the central role of inflammation in the process. From *The Surgical Wound* (p. 5) by P. Dineen, Ed., 1981, Philadelphia: Lea & Febiger. Reprinted by permission.)

come blocked with fibrin, the classic signs of inflammation—heat, redness, and swelling (edema)—become apparent.

During this phase, the complement system is activated and leukocytes are chemotactically drawn to the wound. The activity of polymorphonuclear granulocytes predominates at first and assists in controlling bacterial growth. Although polymorphonuclear granulocytes help resist infection, they are not critical to the repair process. The mononuclear granulocytes, however, give rise to macrophages, which help debride the wound and release factors that stimulate angiogenesis and the growth of fibroblasts. Experimental evidence suggests that in the absence of macrophages, healing will occur but will be impaired. It is believed that macrophages are critical to the body's recognition of injury (Goodson & Hunt, 1985).

Epithelialization also occurs during this phase, forming a watertight seal. This will occur within 24 to 48 hours in a sutured wound but will take longer in a wound healing by secondary intention. Epithelial cells reproduce by mitosis from the wound edges and nearby appendages (hair follicles and apocrine gland ducts) and migrate toward the middle of the wound until the wound edges are joined. Healthy tissue shows an 80% growth rate by the third day after injury (Sieggreen, 1987).

The proliferative phase of wound healing begins 2 to 4 days after injury, and is characterized by fibroblast activity and collagen synthesis, angiogenesis and the growth of granulation tissue, and contraction. Proteoglycans and collagen, the support matrix of the newly synthesized tissue, are produced by the fibroblasts, cells without which no healing could occur. Fibroblast growth at the wound site is stimulated by macrophage- and platelet-derived growth factors. Collagen synthesis begins on the ribosomes of the fibroblast. The amino acids proline and lysine are incorporated into the structure and must be hydroxylated, which requires iron, vitamin C (ascorbic acid), alpha-keto-glutarate, and molecular oxygen as cofactors. Collagen synthesis will be limited by the absence or deficiency of any of these cofactors, resulting in a wound that lacks tensile strength and is at greater risk of dehiscence (Goodson & Hunt, 1985; Sieggreen, 1987). The newly formed collagen fibers bond together through a cross-linkage pattern that becomes increasingly more organized, and therefore stronger, over time. Collagen synthesis occurs most actively for approximately 2 to 3 weeks, with the peak occurring at the end of the first week after injury (Sieggreen, 1987). Tensile strength in the healing wound builds more slowly, however, with attainment of just over 70% of the original strength at 8 weeks after injury in the wound that is healing normally under optimal conditions (Stotts, 1986).

Granulation tissue has a characteristic red appearance due to the presence of newly formed capillary buds. These newly formed capillaries arise from existing blood vessels in response to stimulation from the macrophages. Production of angiogenesis factor(s), plasminogen activator, and mitogenesis factor by the macrophages is, in turn, thought to be stimulated by hypoxic wound gradients (Whitney, 1989). This angiogenesis allows the formation of a vascular bed from which new tissue can be nourished. Vitamin C is also needed for angiogenesis.

Contraction, the inward migration of normal tissue, also occurs during the proliferative phase. Myofibroblasts are cells that have contractile properties and form from fibroblasts and help to allow this type of closure. Contraction is an important mechanism in wounds involving extensive tissue loss and, in combination with the formation of granulation tissue and epithelialization, may allow complete closure of the wound.

The remodeling or differentation phase of repair begins at about 3 weeks after the injury and can continue for months and even up to 2 years. Maturation of the scar tissue occurs during this phase as a result of the balance between collagen formation and lysis. The bonds between collagen fibers continue to tighten and tensile strength is increased. The visible scar will shrink in size and fade in color from a dark red to a silvery white during this phase.

There are many factors that influence the process of wound healing; disruption of any of the phases described above will result in impaired healing. Mechanisms that can result in impaired wound healing include suppression of the inflammatory response, substrate deficiencies, infection, and structural abnormalities. Any or all of these mechanisms might be operating in the critically ill patient.

As stated above, inflammation has a critical role in the process of wound healing. Suppression of the inflammatory response prevents the process from beginning. It is through this mechanism that diabetes mellitus and pharmacologic therapy with steroids or antineoplastic agents inhibit wound healing. The function of white blood cells is adversely affected by hyperglycemia and insulin deficiency. Steroids not only suppress inflammation (probably by preventing or "quieting" the activation of macrophages) but cause protein depletion as well (Goodson & Hunt, 1985). Neonates and elderly patients are also at risk for impaired wound healing because of age-related altered immune function (Stotts, 1986).

Substrate deficiencies can occur because of the unavailability of nutrients and depletion of body stores or failure of delivery of substrates. The effects of critical illness and surgery on nutritional status are discussed in detail in chapter 8. A list of nutrients necessary for wound healing is shown in Table 1–1. Critically ill patients are at risk for deficiencies in these nutrients because of decreased intake and absorption and increased metabolism and loss. They also are more likely to experience low perfusion states such as decreased cardiac output, alteration in tissue perfusion, shock, fluid volume deficit, or hypothermia, in which substrates, including oxygen, may not be delivered to the wound site. The elderly are at risk because in that age group there is an increased incidence of disease conditions that reduce tissue perfusion, as well as because of limited body stores and the overall decrease in physiologic functioning that accompanies the aging process (Stotts, 1986). Actively growing children, especially adolescents, may experience deficiencies due to the increased metabolic rate and the subsequent need for substrates required for anabolic processes. Neonates have limited stores of glycogen and fat (Stotts, 1986). Adipose tissue is poorly perfused, causing difficulty with healing. Smoking reduces the amount of oxygen delivered to the wound, because the carbon monoxide formed by smoking has a greater hemoglobin affinity than oxygen. (Oxygen is necessary for the formation of collagen by fibroblasts, thus contributing to scar strength [Whitney, 1989].) Additionally, smoking alters platelet function, leading to increased platelet adhesiveness, which in turn may lead to a state of hypercoagulability in which microthrombi can form, with the potential for reducing tissue perfusion (Schumann, 1979).

The surgical incision represents a breach in the first line of the body's defenses against infection, the skin. The potential for infection may be increased in the critically ill patient because of impairment of the immune system (either as a result of disease or treatment), vascular insufficiency, increased exposure (especially if the operating time is prolonged), multiple puncture sites for drains and intravascular lines, preexisting infection in a site not related to the surgical incision, poor nutritional status, and, most likely, the presence of a urinary drainage catheter (Baron, 1983; O'Byrne, 1979).

Table 1–1 Nutrients Affecting Wound Healing

Nutrient	Specific Component	Contribution to Wound Healing
Proteins	Amino acids	Needed for neovascularization, lymphocyte formation, fibroblast proliferation, collagen synthesis, and wound remodeling. Required for certain cell-mediated responses, including phagocytosis and intracellular killing of bacteria.
	Albumin	Prevents wound edema secondary to low serum oncotic pressure.
Carbohydrates	Glucose	Needed for energy requirement of leukocytes and fibroblasts to function in inhibiting activities of wound infection.
Fats	Essential unsaturated fatty acids a. Linoleic b. Linolenic c. Arachidonic	Serve as building blocks for prostaglandins, which regulate cellular metabolism, inflammation, and circulation. Are constituents of triglycerides and fatty acids contained in cellular and subcellular membranes.
Vitamins	Ascorbic acid	Hydroxylates proline and lysine in collagen synthesis. Enhances capillary formation and decreases capillary fragility. Is a necessary component of complement that functions in immune reactions and increases defenses to infection.
	B complex	Serve as cofactors of enzyme systems.
	Pyridoxine, pantothenic and folic acids	Required for antibody formation and white-blood-cell function.
	A	Enhances epithelialization of cell membranes. Enhances rate of collagen synthesis and cross linking of newly formed collagen. Antagonizes the inhibitory effects of glucocorticoids on cell membranes.
	D	Necessary for absorption, transport, and metabolism of calcium. Indirectly affects phosphorus metabolism.

Table 1–1   *(Continued)*

Nutrient	Specific Component	Contribution to Wound Healing
	E	No special role known; may be important if there is a fatty acid deficiency.
	K	Needed for synthesis of prothrombin and clotting factors VII, IX, and X. Required for synthesis of calcium-binding protein.
Minerals	Zinc	Stabilizes cell membranes. Needed for cell mitosis and cell proliferation in wound repair.
	Iron	Needed for hydroxylation of proline and lysine in collagen synthesis. Enhances bactericidal activity of leukocytes. Secondarily, deficiency may cause decrease in oxygen transport to wound.
	Copper	Is an integral part of the enzyme lysyloxidase, which catalyzes formation of stable collagen cross links.

From "Preoperative Measures to Promote Wound Healing," by D. Schumann, 1979. *Nursing Clinics of North America, 14*(4), p. 696. Copyright 1979 by W. B. Saunders Company. Reprinted by permission.

Operations performed as emergency measures carry an increased risk of postoperative wound infection (Burke, 1981). Wounds with extensive tissue loss and healing by secondary intention are more likely to become infected than those healing by primary intention (Baron, 1983). Traumatic injuries and burns are more likely to become infected than other wounds because of the introduction of organisms at the time of injury and the greater likelihood of additional tissue damage. The incidence of wound infection has been found to increase as the length of hospitalization increases (Stotts, 1986).

Structural abnormalities, including disordered collagen synthesis, can also impair wound healing. Conditions that put pressure on the suture line (edema, inadequate drainage at the operative site or abdominal distention, improper suture technique or material, premature removal of sutures, and use of improper dressing material) can disrupt the normal healing process. Abnormal collagen synthesis can result in hypertrophic scarring or keloid formation. These types of scars cause cosmetic disfigurement and may cause functional impairment of the tissue as well.

Assessment of the wound can provide information about the cause of impaired wound healing. Guidelines for wound assessment are shown in Table 1–2.

Table 1–2 Guidelines for Wound Assessment

1. Examine wound for approximation of suture line; epithelialization occurs within 48 to 72 hours postoperatively. Protein-calorie malnutrition and vitamin C and zinc deficiencies delay epithelialization.

2. Observe for edema at wound edges; tight sutures and torn skin may occur. Hypoalbuminemia causes a third-space shift.

3. Check for bleeding in and around wound edges. A vitamin K deficiency will interfere with normal clotting times.

4. Assess for presence of "healing ridge" during proliferation phase; it should be present by Day 5 to 8. Absence of healing ridge occurs in protein-calorie malnutrition and vitamin deficiency and forewarns of dehiscence.

5. Observe wounds healing by secondary intention for the presence of granulation tissue; assess tissue integrity and color. Pallor may be caused by decreased iron; protein-calorie malnutrition alters all stages of healing.

6. Inspect wound for signs of infection: erythema, drainage, odor, pain, induration, suture tension. Protein-calorie malnutrition decreases immunocompetence and increases the risk of colonization.

From "Malnutrition and Wound Healing" by M. E. Young, 1988, *Heart and Lung, 17*(1), pp. 60–69. Reprinted by permission.

There are many pathologic consequences of impaired wound healing. Delayed wound closure and failure to heal will prolong hospitalization and the period of discomfort, and will increase the risk of infection for the patient. If the wound remains open and/or draining or if there is abnormal or excessive scarring, the patient may experience a disturbance in body image, ineffective coping, or self-care deficit. Dehiscence, or the reopening of the wound after initial closure, may occur as a result of impaired wound healing. Loss of function may also occur.

Localized wound infection always has the potential for becoming generalized, which would result in the development of sepsis. In an already critically ill patient this development is very grave. Possible sequelae of sepsis include development of the adult respiratory distress syndrome (ARDS) and multiple organ system failure, both of which carry a high mortality rate despite aggressive supportive therapy (Bell, Coalson, Smith, & Johanson, 1983). ARDS is discussed in detail in chapter 7.

Multiple-organ-failure (MOF) syndrome follows 7 to 22% of emergency operations and between 30 to 50% of operations for intraabdominal sepsis (Carrico, Meakins, Marshall, Fry, & Maier, 1986). The mortality rate varies between 30 and 100%, rising as the number of involved organs increases (Carrico et al., 1986). It is, in fact, a principal cause of death after severe trauma or major operative procedures (Fry, Pearlstein, Fulton, & Polk, 1980).

The syndrome seems to be initiated by a massive insult to the body, such as multiple trauma or overwhelming sepsis, and is characterized by sequential organ failure (Abrams & Cerra, 1985; Carrico et al., 1986). The pathogenesis is hypothesized to be due to posttraumatic activation of inflammatory mediators, which cause vascular endothelial injury, permeability edema, and disruption of mitochondrial function, which is manifested clinically as organ dysfunction (Goris, teBoekhorst, Nuytinck, & Gimbrere, 1985; Nuytinck, Goris, Redl, Schlag, & van Munster, 1986; Carrico et al., 1986). Carrico et al. (1986) describe the clinical stages that are seen as the syndrome progressively worsens. These stages are summarized in Table 1–3. Treatment consists of providing support for the failing organ systems and identifying and treating the source of sepsis if that is the cause.

Optimal wound healing requires that both local and systemic factors that promote healing be considered. Stotts (1986) identifies the goals of care for each. At the local level, the goals are to provide a moist environment, as wounds epithelialize faster in a moist than in a dry environment; to minimize contamination, exudate, and necrotic tissue; and to provide local treatments

Table 1–3 Stages of Multiple-Organ-Failure Syndrome

Indicators	Stage I	Stage II	Stage III	Stage IV
1. General appearance	No obvious signs	"Ill," metastable	Obviously unstable	Terminal illness
2. Cardiovascular function	Increased volume requirements	Hyperdynamic; volume dependent	Shock, decreased cardiac output, edema	Ionotropes, volume "overload"
3. Respiratory function	Mild respiratory alkalosis	Tachypnea, hypocapnia, hypoxia	Severe hypoxia	Hypercapnia. barotrauma
4. Renal function	Limited responsiveness	Fixed output, mimimal azotemia	Azotemia	Oliguria
5. Metabolism	Increased insulin requirement	Severe catabolism	Metabolic acidosis, hyperglycemia	Severe acidosis, increased oxygen consumption
6. Hepatic function	?	Chemical jaundice	Clinical jaundice	Encephalopathy
7. Hematology	?	Decreased platelet count, increased or decreased white-cell count	Coagulopathy	Immature cells, coagulopathy
8. Central nervous system	Confusion	Variable	Some response	Coma

From "Multiple Organ Failure Syndrome" by C. J. Carrico et al., 1986, *Archives of Surgery, 121,* pp. 196–208. Copyright 1986 by American Medical Association. Adapted by permission.

(e.g., ointments, irrigations, packing, etc.) as indicated. At the systemic level, the goals include providing adequate perfusion, optimal oxygenation, sufficient nutrients, and systemic therapy (e.g., antibiotics or vitamin A) as indicated.

The patient must, therefore, receive adequate nutritional support, and aseptic technique must be followed during invasive procedures and while caring for the wound, drainage tubes, intravascular access sites, and indwelling urinary drainage catheters. The effects of steroid therapy can be countered and a healing effect promoted with the use of both systemic and topical vitamin A. It is important to note, however, that the desired therapeutic effect, for which steroid therapy is being used, will also be lessened (Goodson & Hunt, 1985; Sieggreen, 1987).

Dressings that promote an optimal local environment for the wound should be used; the choice of a dressing will depend on the purpose it will serve (Sieggreen, 1987). The dressing may be used simply to protect the wound from trauma and contamination, it may be used to apply medication to the area, or it may be used to help debride wound exudate and necrotic tissue and facilitate the formation of granulation tissue. An example of the latter use are the wet to damp or dry dressings that are sometimes used in large, open wounds.

Antibiotic therapy becomes necessary when a wound infection develops, but it can also be used to prevent infection when there is a high probability that the patient's own defense mechanisms will be incapable of responding to microbial contamination. An example is the transplant patient, whose immune response will be intentionally weakened by treatment. The important point is that when preventive antibiotic therapy is used there is a period of time when its administration is most effective. The major tissue response to bacterial contamination occurs within 3 hours after that contamination; it is during this period that the patient's own natural antibacterial mechanisms can be augmented through antibiotic therapy (Burke, 1981).

ALTERATION IN RESPIRATORY FUNCTION

There are unavoidable changes in pulmonary function that are direct results of anesthesia and surgery (Brown, 1987; Risser, 1980). These changes are discussed in detail later in this chapter and in chapter 2. These changes can lead to pulmonary complications such as atelectasis, pneumonia, acute respiratory failure, and embolism, which are the most frequent causes of postoperative morbidity (Bartlett, Brennan, Gazzaniga, & Hanson, 1973; Pontoppidan, 1980; VanDeWater, 1980). Possible consequences of such complications include physical discomfort, prolonged hospitalization, the beginning of permanent lung damage, and even death. Factors that have been identified as predisposing to the development of postoperative pulmonary complications include the site of operation, age, during of anesthesia, smoking, obesity, and preexisting bronchopulmonary disease and/or impaired pulmonary function (Brown, 1987).

The greatest incidence of pulmonary complications comes after upper abdominal surgery. The next highest incidence of pulmonary complications comes after thoracic and lower abdominal surgery. Peripheral and limb surgery have the lowest incidences of pulmonary complications (Benbow, 1971). A variety of studies have demonstrated that the closer a surgical incision is to the diaphragm, the more severe is the reduction of pulmonary function (Churchill & McNeil, 1927; Beecher, 1933; Anscombe, 1957; Anscombe & McNeil, 1927; Beecher, 1922; Anscombe, 1957; Anscombe & Buxton, 1958; Egbert, Laver, & Bendixen, 1962; Latimer, Dickman, Day, Gunn, & Schmidt, 1971).

The incidence of postoperative pulmonary complications also increases with age (Brown, 1987). Such complications occur most frequently in patients over 60 years of age (Benbow, 1971). This is most probably related to the physiologic effects of aging on the respiratory system, which include decreases in the static lung volumes, maximal expiratory flow, elastic recoil, the PaO_2, and the activity of upper airway reflexes (Tisi, 1979).

As the duration of anesthesia lengthens, the incidence of postoperative pulmonary complications also increases. Latimer et al. (1971) found that all patients for whom the anesthesia time was 3.5 hours or longer had some degree of atelectasis. Of those patients in whom the most severe atelectasis developed, 29% had experienced an anesthesia time of 3.5 hours or longer. This has implications for critically ill patients who have undergone lengthy surgical procedures; the most notable example is the liver transplant patient, since that procedure may be 15 to 20 hours in length.

It is well accepted that a higher incidence of pulmonary complications occurs in patients who smoke. The increased incidence of pulmonary complications occurs secondarily to the chronic bronchitic and emphysemic changes that develop in the lungs and bronchi of smokers and that impair the mechanics of ventilation. Additionally, smoking impairs the phagocytic ability of the alveolar macrophage; this predisposes the patient who smokes to an increased risk of pulmonary infection (Newhouse & Bienstock, 1983).

Obesity contributes to the development of pulmonary complications through an ineffective breathing pattern that is caused by interference with the mechanics of breathing (Brown, 1987). Obesity creates a restrictive defect in which lung expansion is limited because of increased mass loading. The pathologic consequences of a restrictive disorder include a reduction in functional lung volume, a decrease in compliance and in increase in elastance, and subsequently, an increase in the work of breathing (Hopp & Williams, 1987). Obese patients with the *obesity hypoventilation syndrome* will demonstrate an even greater impairment of pulmonary function and, therefore, are at increased risk for the development of postoperative pulmonary complications. This syndrome is characterized by hypoventilation, hypoxemia, hypercapnia, and increased pulmonary artery pressure leading to hypertrophy and eventual failure of the right side of the heart (cor pulmonale) (Groer & Shekleton, 1989).

As in the obese patient, it can be inferred that patients with preexisting pulmonary impairment have a higher probability of postoperative pulmonary complications developing than do patients who have normal pulmonary function. All of the patients studied by Latimer et al. (1971) who had preexisting pulmonary disease developed pulmonary complications. Impaired pulmonary function may be manifested clinically by abnormal pulmonary function tests, which reflect the adequacy of ventilation; abnormal arterial blood gas values, which reflect the adequacy of exchange; abnormal breath sounds, which reflect the adequacy of airway clearance; and/or changes in other parameters of respiratory function such as rate, depth, ease, and rhythm of breathing.

Responses to pulmonary impairment diagnosed and treated by nurses include ineffective breathing pattern, ineffective airway clearance, and impaired gas exchange. Patients in whom these responses are identified preoperatively must be considered at high risk for the development of postoperative pulmonary complications and should, in fact, be treated preoperatively to minimize these responses. Examples of conditions related to ineffective breathing pattern, defined as a state in which the inspiratory and expiratory pattern does not provide adequate ventilation, include those characterized by chronic air-flow limitation (emphysema, bronchitis, and asthma) (Lareau & Larson, 1987), decreased lung expansion (Hopp & Williams, 1987), neuromuscular dysfunction, malnutrition (Openbrier & Covey, 1987), and respiratory muscle fatigue (Larson & Kim, 1987). Examples of conditions related to ineffective airway clearance, defined as a state in which an individual is unable to clear secretions or obstructions from the respiratory tract to maintain airway patency, include infection (Hanley & Tyler, 1987), chronic air-flow limitation (Kim & Larson, 1987), neuromuscular dysfunction (Hoffman, 1987), and the presence of an artificial airway (Shekleton & Nield, 1987). Impaired gas exchange, defined as a state in which there is an imbalance between oxygen uptake and carbon dioxide elimination at the alveolar-capillary membrane level, can be the result of disruption of the normal ventilation–perfusion ratio (V/Q) or a reduction in the functional capacity of the alveolar-capillary membrane space (Groer & Shekleton, 1989). Both ineffective breathing pattern and ineffective airway clearance, if allowed to progress untreated, may lead to impaired gas exchange because of the subsequent disruption in the V/Q relationship that will eventually develop. Examples of conditions in which the functional area of the alveolar-capillary membrane space is reduced include pulmonary edema (cardiogenic and noncardiogenic), granulomatous and fibrotic processes, cancer, and oxygen toxicity.

Atelectasis is a condition characterized by collapse of the alveoli due to inadequate expansion of the lung tissue. It is considered to be the most common postsurgical pulmonary complication (Tisi, 1979; O'Donohue, 1985a, 1985b; VanDeWater, 1980). The postoperative course of atelectasis is one of gradual and progressive alveolar collapse, reflected by decreases in total lung capacity, functional residual capacity, residual volume and compliance, and subsequently, an increase in the work of breathing. If the collapsed alveoli continue to be perfused with arterial blood with low oxygen and high carbon dioxide concentrations, a physiologic shunt ensues, disrupting the normal ventilation–perfusion ratio, which results in venous admixture and its sequela of arterial hypoxemia (Groer & Shekleton, 1989).

The pattern in most postoperative patients is that these changes become maximal within 48 to 72 hours after surgery and then revert to normal over the next 7 to 10 days (Bartlett, Gazzaniga, & Geraghty, 1973; Alexander, Horton, Millar, Parikh, & Spence, 1972; Alexander, Spence, Parikh, & Stuart, 1973). In some patients, however, these changes do not return to normal but progressively worsen, and atelectasis becomes clinically significant with x-ray changes, tachypnea, fever, hypoxemia, and other physical findings. Pneumonia may be superimposed on this process if the atelectatic areas become infected. The average incidence of clinically significant atelectasis is reported to range between 19 and 22% in patients who have undergone an abdominal surgical procedure and between 26 and 32% in patients who have undergone a thoracic surgical procedure. These figures vary depending on hospital size and number of procedures performed on a monthly basis (O'Donohue, 1985b).

The causes of atelectasis include airway obstruction and what has been termed inspiratory failure or inspiratory insufficiency (Shekleton, 1982). The potential for the development of atelectasis due to either cause or a combination of both exists because of the presence of ineffective breathing pattern and ineffective airway clearance in the postoperative patient. The pattern of ventilation and the difficulty that the surgical patient might experience with the expectoration of respiratory tract secretions are the responses to surgery diagnosed and treated by nurses. If treatment is inadequate or ineffective and clinically significant atelectasis develops, the response diagnosed and treated by the nurse is impaired gas exchange.

The ineffective breathing pattern seen in the postoperative patient is characterized by shallow breathing and the reduction of diaphragmatic movement, which promote ventilation at a constant and reduced tidal volume with no periodic deep breaths or sighs (Latimer et al., 1971). During normal tidal respiration, when the lungs return to a resting position at the end of expiration, some alveoli collapse and there is a decrease in lung compliance assumed to reflect this collapse. Lung volumes and compliance will continue to decrease during ventilation at a constant tidal volume since the pressures and volumes associated with tidal respiration are insufficient to reexpand the already collapsed alveoli and prevent the collapse of others. Higher than normal pressures and volumes are required to reexpand the collapsed alveoli. In normal respiration very deep breaths or sighs provide such pressures and volumes, promoting expansion of the alveoli with the reversal of the atelectatic changes described above. Caro, Butler, and DuBois (1960) and

Ferris and Pollard (1960) demonstrated that the normal pattern of tidal respiration punctuated by periodic deep breaths is essential to maintain alveolar inflation. They found that in persons who had normal tidal volume and alveolar ventilation who were prevented from taking deep breaths, functional residual capacity and residual volume decreased and transpulmonary shunting occurred within 1 hour. Deep breaths reversed these changes. Bendixen, Bullwinkel, Hedley-White, and Lauer (1964) demonstrated similar findings in anesthetized persons.

This ineffective breathing pattern is generally thought to be the primary mechanism in the development of atelectasis in the postsurgical patient, and its occurrence has been attributed to a number of factors, including "splinting" due to incisional pain, relative immobility, tightly applied bandages, and the general depression of respiration caused by the use of narcotic, sedative, and anesthetic agents (Shekleton, 1982). Speculation about another possible cause for this pattern of ventilation has been reported recently in the literature. There is some preliminary experimental support for the postulate of Ford and Guenter (1984) that reflex inhibition of inspiratory muscle activity via intraabdominal afferent nerves may occur as a direct effect of upper abdominal surgery.

Retained secretions can lead to airway obstruction through mucus-plug formation, and can increase the potential for infection because the retained secretions serve as a suitable medium for the growth of bacteria. Ineffective airway clearance after surgery is the result of many interacting factors. After surgery the expectoration of respiratory tract secretions becomes more difficult than it is normally because of increased viscosity of the secretions, inhibition of ciliary action, pain, and depression of the cough mechanism. The mucous membranes of the mouth, nasopharynx, and respiratory tract become very dry and mucus secretion is reduced because of the anticholinergic drugs that are administered preoperatively to promote smooth muscle relaxation and minimize secretions. Endotracheal intubation bypasses the normal humidifying mechanisms of the upper airway and can cause mechanical damage to the cilia. Mucociliary transport will be adversely affected by the lack of humidity, ciliary damage, and the reduction of ciliary movement due to direct action of drugs and anesthetic agents on the cilia. Depression of the cough mechanism is a result of the combination of direct drug action and the altered level of consciousness (Groer & Shekleton, 1989).

Nursing measures that may be instituted postoperatively to treat ineffective breathing pattern and ineffective airway clearance include coughing and deep breathing exercises, turning the patient or assisting the patient to turn frequently, early ambulation, the administration of various forms of respiratory therapy, the judicious use of analgesics to enhance performance of these activities, and the provision of adequate environmental humidity and systemic hydration to thin secretions. Bartlett et al. (1973) concluded that the ideal respiratory maneuver for preventing and reversing atelectatic changes is one that "emphasizes maximal alveolar inflation and maintenance of a normal function residual capacity" (p. 1018). Such a maneuver requires a high alveolar inflating pressure which is exerted over a long period with the largest possible inhaled volume. Deep breathing provides higher transpulmonary pressures and greater volumes than those seen during normal or tidal respiration. Deep breathing with emphasis on sustained maximal inspiration will promote expansion of all alveoli throughout the lung.

Various devices such as blow bottles, rebreathing tubes, intermittent positive pressure breathing, continuous positive airway pressure, positive expiratory pressure, and incentive spirometry have been used to enhance patients' performance of deep breathing exercises. There are conflicting reports and an ongoing debate in the literature about the relative efficacy of some of these devices in promoting postoperative ventilatory function (Belman & Mittman, 1981; Bartlett, 1982; O'Donohue, 1985a). Comparison of the results of studies in which these devices were evaluated is difficult because of differences in the samples and definitions of pulmonary complications used across studies (Pontoppidan, 1980). A general conclusion that can be drawn is that deep breathing exercises alone are as effective in promoting postoperative ventilatory function as other techniques if deep breathing exercises are done frequently and consistently. Lederer, VanDeWater, and Indech (1980) state that hourly coaching in deep breathing exercises is more important than any device used to encourage deep breathing.

The nurse at the bedside has the primary responsibility for helping the patient overcome the effects of an ineffective breathing pattern by performing coughing and deep breathing exercises. The emphasis should be on sustained maximal inspiration and use of the abdominal muscles to allow diaphragmatic breathing. Specifically, the patient should inhale slowly and deeply through the nose with the mouth closed while expanding the abdomen, hold the breath for 3 to 5 seconds, and then slowly exhale through the mouth while contracting the abdomen. This should be repeated three to five times, and a deep breath should be taken immediately, followed by a low-pitched, hollow-sounding cough from the chest area. During these exercises, which should be repeated on an hourly basis, the incision should be supported by the hands, a pillow, or a folded blanket. One institution has reported giving their surgical patients a teddy bear to be held and used as a splint and which the patients take home with them.

Ineffective airway clearance will be helped by the exercises described above, but for patients who have large amounts of thick, tenacious secretions, chest physical therapy (CPT) and suctioning may be required to assist in the removal of secretions. Based on a review of the research literature, Kiriloff, Owens, Rogers, and Mazzocco (1985) drew the following conclusions about the efficacy of CPT treatments in acutely ill patients. Generally, CPT has been shown to promote positive outcomes in patients with large amounts of secretions and in those with lobar atelectasis. The authors also conclude that the efficacy of CPT has not been demonstrated in patients with exacerbations of chronic bronchitis, pneumonia without large amounts of secretions, and status asthmaticus. Also reviewed were studies in which the component activities of CPT were evaluated; the authors concluded that there are no data that demonstrate a beneficial effect of vibration and percussion, but that postural drainage and directed coughing were efficacious treatments. They also noted that CPT has been associated with the occurrence of bronchoconstriction and hypoxemia in acutely ill patients. Chest physical therapy may be contraindicated in some critically ill patients, such as those with increased intracranial pressure or severe cardiac disease.

Suctioning is associated with the risks of hypoxemia, microatelectasis, laryngospasm, tracheal tissue damage, and arrhythmias and death in the acutely ill patient (Shekleton & Nield, 1987). Given the serious nature of these potential consequences, suctioning protocols should be based on research findings that indicate the safest, least traumatic suctioning technique. The ideal suctioning technique is one in which the maximum removal of secretions is achieved with a minimum of tissue damage and hypoxemia. An overview of the literature on the topic of suctioning has been provided by Shekleton and Nield (1987).

If gas exchange is impaired, positioning can be used to promote gas exchange and facilitate the drainage of secretions. Because of the gravity-dependent nature of perfusion and ventilation in the lungs, with positioning blood flow can be increased in well-ventilated areas of the lungs and decreased in poorly ventilated areas. The outcome will be a better match of ventilation and perfusion (Tyler, 1984; Grosmaire, 1983).

It has been noted that hypoxemia often accompanies many of the procedures intended to promote airway clearance. Hypoxemia constitutes a serious threat to homeostasis in the critically ill patient, and should be prevented. Pulse oximetry is easy to use and provides a noninvasive and inexpensive means of monitoring the patient's oxygenation status. The oxygen saturation level can be monitored during procedures known to produce hypoxemia and, if the patient becomes desaturated to dangerous levels, the procedure could be terminated or altered.

ALTERATION IN ELIMINATION PATTERNS

Elimination patterns of both the bowel and the bladder will be disrupted by surgery because of changes in intake of food and liquids, the effects of anesthetic and narcotic agents, and the hormonal and metabolic responses of the body to surgery that were described in an earlier section of this chapter. Most critically ill patients will have a urinary drainage catheter in place in order to monitor fluid output accurately. The presence of an indwelling catheter increases the potential for infection. Some patients will come to the surgical intensive care unit without a urinary drainage catheter in place and will need to be monitored for the development of urinary retention or the inability to void after surgery. This may be the result of position, pain, decreased awareness of the sensation to void due to narcotic and anesthetic agents, or anxiety. Innervation of the bladder may be directly affected by the surgical procedure or by edema. The patient will be oliguric immediately after surgery but should be expected to void within the first 6 to 8 hours after surgery. A distended bladder is palpable immediately above the symphysis pubis. Retention with overflow will cause the patient to void small amounts of urine at frequent intervals. Voiding can be facilitated by running water, pouring water over the perineal area, assisting the patient to use a commode, and offering the bedpan at frequent intervals. Catheterization may be necessary if these measures are unsuccessful (Phipps, Long, & Woods, 1983).

A urinary output of less than 400 ml in a 24-hour period may indicate the onset of *acute renal failure* (ARF). In the critically ill surgical patient, the cause will most likely be acute tubular necrosis secondary to ischemia. Any condition accompanied by hypotension and reduced perfusion of the kidneys has the potential to cause ischemic injury. The response of the kidney to a reduction in blood flow is vasoconstriction, which further compounds the problem. Causes of hypotension most likely to be seen in the surgical patient include volume depletion, decreased cardiac output, or shock. Trauma involving a severe crush injury or burns are both conditions in which large amounts of myoglobin are released. The resulting tubular obstruction is a pathogenetic mechanism which can precipitate ARF (Groer & Shekleton, 1989).

The severity of ARF can be quite variable but, regardless of severity, it is usually reversible. Complete anuria is seldom seen and after 10 to 12 days the initial, oliguric phase is followed by a diuretic phase in which 4 to 5 liters per day of urine may be excreted (Groer & Shekleton, 1989).

Because of the loss of renal function, the patient will experience alterations in fluid volume and composition. During the oliguric phase these alterations can include fluid overload, hyperkalemia, hyperphosphatemia, hyponatremia, and acidosis. Blood urea nitrogen (BUN) and plasma creatinine levels will be high. Nausea and vomiting, due to the accumulation of metabolic wastes and any electrolyte imbalance, may complicate care. During the diuretic phase there is an inability to conserve fluid and electrolytes and the patient will be at risk for fluid deficit and the loss of sodium and potassium (Phipps et al., 1983). Dialysis will be necessary until renal function returns.

After surgery, bowel elimination may be altered in a number of ways. Peristalsis will be decreased because of the effects of anesthesia and narcotics, because of the neuroendocrine response to surgery and physical manipulation of the bowel, and potentially, as a result of hypokalemia. The patient may experience constipation or abdominal distention due to the accumulation of gas in the bowels. Distention exerts pressure against the diaphragm and can impede its movement, leading to decreased expansion of the lungs, hypoventilation, and atelectasis. It also exerts pressure against the incision, possibly impairing the normal healing process.

If distention progresses and peristalsis ceases, a *paralytic ileus* is suspected. Pain and an absence of bowel sounds are associated with distention. The effect is that of an acute intestinal obstruction. The gut will be distended by accumulated gas, and the increased intraluminal pressure will cause tissue edema and a decrease in mucosal blood flow. Normal absorptive functions are impaired and large amounts of fluid and electrolytes can become sequestered as isotonic fluid moves from the plasma and intestinal spaces into the gut. The major effects of a net increase in secretion over absorption include hypovolemia, hyponatremia, hypochloremia, and acidosis. Ischemia causes increased permeability of the mucosa, and plasma proteins leak into the gut while toxins and bacteria from the gut leak into the blood (Groer & Shekleton, 1989). This sequence of events is depicted in Figure 1–2. Potentially lethal complications of paralytic ileus include hypovolemic shock, perforated bowel and peritonitis, gangrene, and sepsis. Intake is limited to the parenteral route and intestinal decompression is necessary until normal bowel tone and peristalsis return.

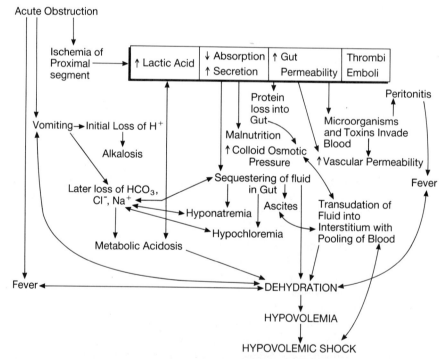

Figure 1–2. Pathophysiology of acute intestinal obstruction. End results of numerous pathophysiologic mechanisms that are perpetuated by acute intestinal obstruction are vascular dehydration, hypovolemia, septicemia, and shock. Reproduced by permission from M. E. Groer and M. E. Shekleton, *Basic Pathophysiology: A Holistic Approach,* 3rd ed. St. Louis, 1989, The C. V. Mosby Co.

Vomiting is another abnormal pattern of elimination that may develop in response to surgery. It is usually accompanied by the uncomfortable sensation of nausea. Initiation of the vomiting pathway (Figure 1–3) and stimulation of the medullary vomiting center in the postoperative patient can be the result of drugs, anesthetic agents, pain, gas accumulation in the stomach and intestines, anxiety, electrolyte imbalance, or premature intake of liquids or food. Treatment consists of administration of antiemetic drugs, keeping the patient NPO, and use of gastric decompression and drainage.

Vomiting can put a strain on the incision line, tires the patient, and is very distressing for both the patient and family (Phipps et al., 1983). It also increases the potential for aspiration that is already present because of the depression of the cough and gag reflexes secondary to anesthesia, narcotics, and a decreased level of consciousness. Vomiting and gastric suction cause a loss of gastric secretions, which are the most acidic of all the gastrointestinal tract secretions. Loss of gastric secretions is most often associated with metabolic alkalosis and potassium, sodium, chloride, and magnesium deficits (Table 1–4). If excessive loss occurs, a fluid volume deficit may develop (Groer & Shekleton, 1989).

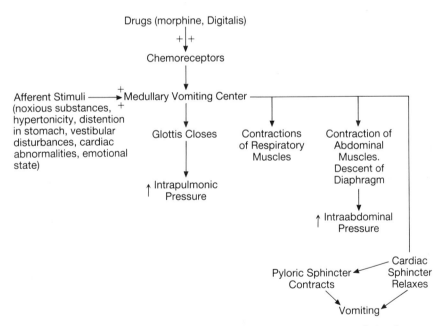

Figure 1–3.   Vomiting pathway. Medullary vomiting center causes a chain of events that acts to increase intraabdominal pressure, increase intrapulmonic pressure (thus compressing esophagus), and relax cardiac sphincter while pylorus contracts. Thus, chyme moves in antiperistalsic direction. Reproduced by permission from M. E. Groer and M. E. Shekleton, *Basic Pathophysiology: A Holistic Approach,* 3rd ed. St. Louis, 1989, The C. V. Mosby Co.

Table 1–4 Electrolyte Concentration of Body Excretions and Secretions (mEq/liter)

Source	Sodium	Chloride	Potassium	Bicarbonates
Sweat	15–80	15–80	>5	0
Saliva	20–80	20–40	10–20	20–60
Gastric juice	20–100	20–160	5–10	0
Bile	150–250	40–80	5–10	20–40
Pancreatic juices	120–250	10–60	5–10	80–120
Ileum (mean)	129	116	11	29
Cecum (mean)	80	48	21	22

Reproduced by permission from M. E. Groer and M. E. Shekleton, *Basic Pathophysiology: A Holistic Approach,* 3rd ed. St. Louis, 1989, The C. V. Mosby Co.

Abnormal elimination of intestinal secretions can occur because of the presence of a fistula, drains, intestinal suction, or diarrhea. Intestinal secretions are alkalotic and contain a relatively large amount of potassium (Table 1–4) and loss can cause metabolic acidosis and sodium, potassium, and bicarbonate deficits.

KNOWLEDGE DEFICIT: PREOPERATIVE INFORMATION

While many surgical patients are not in the intensive care unit preoperatively, some institutions do have mechanisms in place for the critical care nurse to meet with the patient and family during the preoperative period. Preoperative teaching is an essential component of nursing care that can help the patient to become an informed and active participant in postoperative care. It involves teaching–learning activities directed toward physically and emotionally preparing the patient and family for all facets of the operative experience. The goals of preoperative teaching include familiarizing the patient and family with postoperative routines and procedures, increasing the patient's motivation to cooperate with and participate in postoperative care, decreasing anxiety by reducing the "unknown" and giving the patient some control over the situation, and reducing the risk of complications.

If possible, the patient and family can be shown the critical care unit, and unit policies and procedures can be explained at that time. It is sometimes helpful for the patient to meet with other patients who have had the same type of surgery; many institutions provide support groups for patients and families. Other preoperative information should include specifics on the surgical procedure and postoperative care, instruction on and demonstration of coughing and deep breathing exercises, and techniques to minimize the discomfort of moving. Anxiety-reducing techniques may need to be taught as well.

The amount and type of preoperative information to impart must be carefully determined based on an assessment of the patient's and family's learning needs and level of preoperative anxiety. Denial can be operating as a protective mechanism at this time and needs to be acknowledged as such by the nurse. Much of the information will need to be repeated and reinforced during the postoperative period because of the stress imposed by critical illness. It is important that the critical care nurse demonstrate an openness to listening and responding to the emotional needs of the patient and family despite the severity of the physical needs.

SUMMARY

Surgery can have profound effects on the physiologic function of a relatively healthy individual. In the critically ill patient these effects can have even more serious consequences. The critical care nurse is in a key position to identify potential problems and to treat them if they occur. Many of the direct effects of surgery can be minimized and potential complications prevented through aggressive nursing vigilance and care—hallmarks of the critical care environment.

BIBLIOGRAPHY

Abrams, J. H., & Cerra, F. B. (1985). Homeostatic response to operation & stress. In R. Condon & J. J. DeCosse (Eds.), *Surgical care II* (pp. 299–310). Philadelphia: Lea & Febiger.

Alexander, J., Horton, P., Millar, W., Parikh, R., & Spence, A. (1972). The effect of upper abdominal surgery on the relationship of airway closing point to end tidal position. *Clinical Science, 43,* 137–141.

Alexander, J., Spence, A., Parikh, R., & Stuart, P. (1973). The role of airway closure in postoperative hypoxaemia. *British Journal of Anaesthia, 45,* 34–40.

Anscombe, A. R. (1957). *Pulmonary complications of abdominal surgery.* London: Lloyd-Duke Ltd.

Anscombe, A., & Buxton, R. (1958). Effects of abdominal operation on total lung capacity and its subdivisions. *British Medical Journal, 2,* 84–87.

Baron, M. C. (1983). The skin & wound healing. *Topics in Clinical Nursing, 5*(2), 11–22.

Bartlett, R. H. (1982). Postoperative pulmonary prophylaxis: Breathe deeply and read carefully. *Chest, 81*(1), 1–3.

Bartlett, R., Brennan, M., Gazzaniga, A., & Hanson, E. (1973). Studies on the pathogenesis and prevention of postoperative pulmonary complications. *Surgery, Gynecology and Obstetrics, 137,* 925–944.

Bartlett, R., Gazzaniga, A., & Geraghty, T. (1973). Respiratory maneuvers to prevent postoperative pulmonary complications. *Journal of the American Medical Association, 224,* 1017–1021.

Beecher, H. (1933). Effect of laparotomy on lung volume, demonstration of a new type of pulmonary collapse. *Journal of Clinical Investigation, 12,* 651.

Bell, R. C., Coalson, J. J., Smith, J. D., & Johanson, W. G. (1983). Multiple organ system failure & infection in adult respiratory distress syndrome. *Annals of Internal Medicine, 99*(3), 293–298.

Belman, M., & Mittman, C. (1981). Incentive spirometry: The answer is blowing in the wind. *Chest, 79*(3), 254–255.

Benbow, B. (1971). Insidious postoperative pulmonary complications. *AORN Journal, 14,* 52–56.

Bendixen, H., Bullwinkel, B., Hedley-White, J., & Laver, M. (1964). Atelectasis & shunting during spontaneous ventilation in anesthetized patients. *Anesthesiology, 25,* 297–301.

Brown, L. K. (1987). Surgical considerations: Effects of surgery on lung function; preoperative preparation. In A. Miller (Ed.), *Pulmonary function tests: A guide for the house officer* (pp. 213–226). New York: Grune & Stratton.

Burke, J. F. (1981). Risk factors predisposing to wound infection and means of their prevention. In P. Dineen & G. Hildick-Smith (Eds.), *The Surgical Wound* (pp. 132–145). Philadelphia: Lea & Febiger.

Caro, C., Butler, J., & Dubois, A. (1960). Some effects of restriction of chest cage expansion on pulmonary function in man: An experimental study. *Journal of Clinical Investigation, 39,* 573.

Carrico, C. J., Meakins, J. L., Marshall, J. C., Fry, D., & Maier, R. V. (1986). Multiple-organ-failure syndrome. *Archives of Surgery, 121,* 196–208.

Churchill, E., & McNeil, D. (1927). The reduction in vital capacity following operation. *Surgery, Gynecology and Obstetrics, 44,* 483–488.

Dineen, P., & Hildick-Smith, G. (Eds.) (1981). *The surgical wound.* Philadelphia: Lea & Febiger.

Egbert, L., Laver, M., & Bendixen, H. (1962). The effect of site of operation and type of anesthesia upon the ability to cough in the postoperative period. *Surgery, Gynecology and Obstetrics, 115,* 295–298.

Ferris, B., & Pollard, D. (1960). Effect of deep and quiet breathing on pulmonary compliance in man. *Journal of Clinical Investigation, 39,* 143.

Ford, G. T., & Guenter, C. A. (1984). Toward prevention of postoperative pulmonary complications. *American Review of Respiratory Disease, 130,* 4–5.

Fry, D. E., Pearlstein, L., Fulton, R. L., & Polk, H. C. (1980). Multiple system organ failure. *Archives of Surgery, 115,* 136–140.

Goodson, W. H., & Hunt, T. K. (1985). Wound healing. In R. Condon & J. J. DeCosse (Eds.), *Surgical care II* (pp. 313–322). Philadelphia: Lea & Febiger.

Goris, R. J., teBoekhorst, T. P., Nuytinck, J. K., & Gimbrere, J. S. (1985). Multiple-organ failure. *Archives of Surgery, 120,* 1109–1115.

Groer, M. E., & Shekleton, M. E. (1989). *Basic pathophysiology: A holistic approach,* 3rd ed. St. Louis: C. V. Mosby.

Grosmaire, E. (1983). Use of patient positioning to improve PaO_2: A review. *Heart and Lung, 12*(6), 650–653.

Hanley, M., & Tyler, M. (1987). Ineffective airway clearance related to airway infection. *Nursing Clinics of North America, 22*(1), 135–150.

Hoffman, L. (1987). Ineffective airway clearance related to neuromuscular dysfunction. *Nursing Clinics of North America, 22*(1), 151–166.

Hopp, L., & Williams, M. (1987). Ineffective breathing pattern related to decreased lung expansion. *Nursing Clinics of North America, 22*(1), 193–206.

Kim, M., & Larson, J. (1987). Ineffective airway clearance & ineffective breathing patterns: Theoretical and research base for nursing diagnosis. *Nursing Clinics of North America, 22*(1), 125–134.

Kiriloff, L. Owens, G., Rogers, R., & Mazzocco, M. (1985). Does chest physical therapy work? *Chest, 88*(3), 436–444.

Lareau, S., & Larson, J. (1987). Ineffective breathing pattern related to airflow limitation. *Nursing Clinics of North America, 22*(1), 179–192.

Larson, J., & Kim, M. (1987). Ineffective breathing pattern related to respiratory muscle fatigue. *Nursing Clinics of North America, 22*(1), 207–224.

Latimer, R., Dickman, M. W., Day, W., Gunn, M., & Schmidt, C. (1971). Ventilatory patterns and pulmonary complications after upper abdominal surgery determined by preoperative and postoperative computerized spirometry and blood gas analysis. *American Journal of Surgery, 122,* 622–632.

Lederer, D. H., VanDeWater, J. M., & Indech, R. B. (1980). Which deep breathing device should the postoperative patient use? *Chest, 79*(5), 610–613.

Marcinek, M. (1977). Stress in the surgical patient. *American Journal of Nursing, 77*(11), 1809–1811.

Newhouse, M. T., & Bienstock, J. (1983). Respiratory tract defense mechanisms. In G. P. Baum & E. Wolinsky (Eds.), *Textbook of pulmonary diseases* (pp. 3–24). Boston: Little, Brown.

Nuytinck, J. K., Goris, R. J., Redl, H., Schlag, G., & van Munster, P. J. (1986). Posttraumatic complications & inflammatory mediators. *Archives of Surgery, 121,* 886–890.

O'Byrne, C. (1979), Clinical detection & management of postoperative wound sepsis. *Nursing Clinics of North America, 14*(4), 727–742.

O'Donohue, W. J. (1985a). Prevention and treatment of postoperative atelectasis. *Chest, 87*(1), 1–2.

O'Donohue, W. J. (1985b). National survey of the usage of lung expansion modalities for the prevention and treatment of postoperative atelectasis following abdominal and thoracic surgery. *Chest, 87*(1), 76–80.

Openbrier, D., & Covey, M. (1987). Ineffective breathing pattern related to malnutrition. *Nursing Clinics of North America, 22*(1), 225–247.

Phipps, W., Long, B. & Woods, N. (1983). *Medical surgical nursing: Concepts and clinical practice* (2nd ed.). St. Louis: C. V. Mosby.

Pontoppidan, H. (1980). Mechanical aids to lung expansion in non-intubated surgical patients. *American Review of Respiratory Diseases, 122,* 109–19.

Risser, N. (1980). Preoperative and postoperative care to prevent postoperative pulmonary complications. *Heart and Lung, 9*(1), 57–67.

Schumann, D. (1979). Preoperative measures to promote wound healing. *Nursing Clinics of North America, 14*(4), 683–699.

Shekleton, M. (1982). *The effect of preoperative instruction in coughing and deep breathing exercises on postoperative ventilatory function.* Ann Arbor: University Microfilms Inc.

Shekleton, M., & Nield, M. (1987). Ineffective airway clearance related to artificial airway. *Nursing Clinics of North America, 22*(1), 167–178.

Sieggreen, M. Y. (1987). Healing of physical wounds. *Nursing Clinics of North America, 22*(2), 439–447.

Stotts, N. (1986). Impaired wound healing. In V. K. Carrieri, A. M. Lindsey, & C. M. West (Eds.), *Pathophysiological phenomena in nursing: Human responses of illness* (pp. 343–366). Philadelphia: W. B. Saunders.

Tisi, G. (1979). Preoperative evaluation of pulmonary function: Validity, indications, & benefits. *American Review of Respiratory Diseases, 119,* 293–310.

Tyler, M. (1984). The respiratory effects of body positioning and immobilization. *Respiratory Care, 29*(5), 472–483.

VanDeWater, J. M. (1980). Preoperative and postoperative techniques in the prevention of pulmonary complications. *Surgical Clinics of North America, 60*(6), 1339–1348.

Whitney, J. D. (1989). Physiologic effects of tissue oxygenation on wound healing. *Heart and Lung, 18*(5), 466–474.

Young, M. E. (1988). Malnutrition and wound healing. *Heart and Lung, 17*(1), 60–69.

ADDITIONAL READINGS

Besst, J. A., & Wallace, H. L. (1979). Wound healing—Intraoperative factors. *Nursing Clinics of North America, 14*(4), 701–712.

Bruno, P. (1979). The nature of wound healing. *Nursing Clinics of North America, 14*(4), 667–682.

Cooper, D. M., & Schumann, D. (1979). Postsurgical nursing intervention as an adjunct to wound healing. *Nursing Clinics of North America, 14*(4), 713–726.

Physiologic Responses to Anesthesia

2

Cynthia A. Wong, M.D.

Anesthetic considerations play a part in both the preoperative and the postoperative care of the critical care patient. Patients who are in the critical care unit prior to surgery are often unstable. It is to their benefit to be stabilized as much as possible before undergoing surgery since anesthesia and surgery can have major physiologic effects on the human organism. Furthermore, transportation from the critical care unit to the operating room poses an additional hazard to unstable patients. Postoperatively, residual anesthetic effects, as well as effects from the surgery itself, may have major influences on the cardiovascular, respiratory, and central nervous systems. These residual effects must be taken into account when caring for the patient immediately after surgery.

In this chapter preanesthetic care of the critically ill patient is reviewed. Postanesthesia care will then be discussed according to organ systems.

PREANESTHESIA CARE IN THE ICU

The preanesthesia care of the critically ill patient is somewhat more involved, but essentially the same, as for any other surgical patient. Patients are kept NPO for 6 to 8 hours before surgery because of the potential for aspiration during and after the induction of anesthesia. This includes nasogastric feedings and particulate antacids. Patients undergoing emergency surgery are especially at risk for gastric retention, as are patients in pain, recent trauma patients, and patients receiving narcotics (Gibbs & Modell, 1986). The anesthesiologist may prescribe preoperative histamine-2 blockers, metroclopramide, or clear antacids for patients who may have a full stomach. If a nasogastric tube is in place, it should be suctioned and clamped prior to transport. The anesthesia team will suction residual gastric contents upon arrival in the operating room and then remove the nasogastric tube before the induction of anesthesia, since its presence during induction may serve to wick gastric contents into the oropharynx by interfering with the competency of the gastroesophageal sphincter. Maintenance intravenous fluids should be adjusted for the NPO status so patients do not arrive in the operating room in a hypovolemic state.

Several routine laboratory tests aid in administration of a safe anesthetic, although obtaining all laboratory results in an emergency situation may not be possible. Critically ill patients are likely to be receiving intravenous fluids and medications and to have drains and pathologic processes, all of which can contribute to deranged and frequently changing electrolyte values. Blood-cell counts are often iatrogenically low because of frequent phlebotomy. Patients on antibiotics for several days may have abnormal coagulation function. Medications commonly given to ICU patients may affect many body systems, and abnormalities may be reflected in routine laboratory values. In addition, critically ill patients often receive medications with low therapeutic indexes, e.g., theophylline, digoxin, and quinidine. Recent blood levels of these medications are helpful in the perianesthetic management of these patients, since anesthetics may potentiate or interfere with the action of these drugs. Finally, the availability of any blood and blood products must be checked prior to surgery.

While the administration of medication preoperatively depends on many factors and should be determined on an individual basis, most medications should be continued up to the time of surgery. Oral medications may be administered with small amounts of water (30 ml). This is important for a stable anesthetic experience. For example, patients whose hypertension is not well controlled, or who have not taken their antihypertensive medications, are at increased risk for wide fluctuations of blood pressure (both hypertension and hypotension) during anesthesia (Roizen, 1986). Antianginal medications should also be continued up to the time of surgery, as the preanesthetic period is stressful for patients. Perioperative myocardial ischemia is associated with a higher rate of perioperative myocardial infarction in coronary artery bypass and should be avoided if possible (Slogoff & Keats, 1985). Digoxin given for congestive heart failure is usually withheld the morning of surgery as its therapeutic index is low and intraoperative potassium shifts may lead to toxicity. However, digoxin given to control the rapid rate of a supraventricular tachycardia is often given on the morning of surgery at the discretion of the anesthesiologist. Oral hypoglycemics are usually withheld on the morning of surgery to prevent intraoperative hypoglycemia. Insulin-dependent diabetics should receive a fraction, usually one half, of their normal daily insulin dose on the morning of surgery. Insulin should not be given unless intravenous glucose is being infused. Hyperglycemia is then controlled with further insulin, as needed, in the perioperative period. Occasionally, the anesthesiologist may wish to start an insulin infusion prior to surgery (Ammon, 1987).

Hyperalimentation may be discontinued before surgery because it is inconvenient and potentially dangerous to have a hyperosmolar solution infusing during surgery. If hyperalimention is discontinued, a glucose-containing solution should replace it for several hours to prevent hypoglycemia.

Most patients are frightened to be undergoing surgery and anesthesia. A critically ill patient is probably more anxious than most, as the surgical procedure is often emergent, leaving the patient and family emotionally unprepared. Family support is not optimal because visiting hours are usually restricted in critical care units. In addition, because of hemodynamic, respiratory, and central nervous system pathology, the anesthesiologist may not be able to prescribe the usual preoperative sedation. For these reasons, empathy and supportive care from the critical care staff are essential for the well-being of the preoperative patient. Studies have shown that a well-conducted preanesthesia visit from the anesthetist is more important in allaying anxiety than is sedation (Stoelting, 1986). Preoperative teaching by the nursing staff is imperative and should begin as soon as possible.

Transportation of the unstable patient to and from the operating room must be carefully orchestrated. This is a hazardous period for the patient. Communication between the nursing, surgical, and anesthesia staff can facilitate safe transport.

It is easier and safer to transfer the patient in the bed, rather than on a cart. Oxygen should be available, as well as an ambu bag and mask. Electrocardiographic (ECG) monitoring is usually appropriate, and if the patient has an arterial line, a continuous pressure tracing should also be monitored. Resuscitation equipment should accompany unstable patients being transported over long distances.

Critically ill patients invariably have multiple peripheral and central lines, invasive monitors, and vasoactive infusions, which cannot be discontinued during transport. Attention to details may make the anesthesia team's job easier and more efficient, and thus safer for the patient. Peripheral intravenous cannula sites can be labeled as to cannula size and date of placement. If no drugs are being infused through a line, it may be disconnected at the extension site and connected to a heparin flush syringe. Vasoactive drug lines must have their needles securely taped to injection ports or secured by a Luer-lok to stopcocks and be appropriately labeled. IV poles at the head and foot of the bed aid in keeping lines less tangled, eliminating the need for a separate IV pole and the potential for disconnecting lines under tension. Finally, both the operating room and critical care staff should be notified ahead of time and be prepared for the arrival of the patient, so no delay occurs in the monitoring and care of the patient during transfer.

POSTANESTHESIA CARE IN THE ICU

Anesthesia and its physiologic effects cannot be terminated precisely at the end of surgery. Therefore, anesthesia will affect multiple organ systems for variable periods after surgery. Recovery rooms, with nurses specially skilled in recognizing and treating immediate postsurgical and postanesthesia complications, were set up to monitor postoperative patients. However, the critically ill postsurgical patient often bypasses the recovery room and is taken directly to the surgical intensive care unit. Therefore, surgical critical care nurses also need to be able to recognize postanesthesia effects and complications. Table 2–1 lists commonly used anesthetic agents with indications for postoperative care. In the following section postanesthesia considerations are reviewed according to organ system, with emphasis on the critically ill.

Central Nervous System

General anesthesia, by definition, must primarily affect the central nervous system (CNS), causing loss of consciousness. Not only primary anesthetics but many supplemental drugs used in anesthesia may adversely affect central

Table 2–1   Comparison of Selected Anesthetic Agents

Name	Method of Administration	Advantages	Disadvantages	Special Postoperative Care
Enflurane (Ethrane)	Inhalation	Rapid induction and recovery; some muscle relaxation on its own; nonflammable	Circulatory and respiratory depression (dose dependent); expensive; shivering on emergence; vasodilator	Monitor vital signs frequently; oxygen therapy
Halothane (Fluothane)	Inhalation	Rapid induction; low incidence of postoperative nausea or vomiting; nonirritating; nonflammable	Shivering on emergence; circulatory and respiratory depressant	Monitor vital signs closely; oxygen therapy
Isoflurane (Forane)	Inhalation	Smooth and rapid induction; good muscle relaxant; nonirritating; cardiovascular stability	Expensive	Hypotension may occur; oxygen therapy
Nitrous oxide	Inhalation	Rapid induction and recovery; nonirritating; nonflammable but supports combustion	Possible hypoxia with excessive amounts	Monitor for signs of hypoxia; oxygen therapy

Table 2–1 *(Continued)*

Name	Method of Adminis- tration	Advantages	Disadvantages	Special Postoperative Care
Droperidol and fentanyl (Innovar)	IV	Rapid smooth induction and recovery; nontoxic to liver, kidneys, and heart; less analgesia required postoperatively	Hypoventilation; hypotension and skeletal muscle rigidity may occur	Monitor for depressed respiratory rate or depth; decrease postoperative narcotics to one-third to one-fourth of usual dose
Fentanyl (Sublimaze)	IV or IM	Abolition of the stress response; very potent analgesic	Respiratory depressant; muscle rigidity and bradycardia may occur	Monitor for decreased respiratory rate and depth and decreased blood pressure
Ketamine	IV or IM	Profound analgesia with no loss of consciousness; amnesia for surgical event	Unpleasant dreams in early postoperative period and sometimes later; does not block visceral pain	Maintain quiet environment postoperatively
Sufentanil citrate (Sufenta)	IV	Rapid onset, producing hypnosis and anesthesia without use of additional agents; inhibits sympathetic response to surgical stress	Respiratory depression and skeletal muscle rigidity	Monitor for muscle rigidity of chest wall and respiratory depression; have naloxone available to reverse respiratory depression
Procaine Cocaine Tetracaine Dibucaine Lidocaine Carbocaine Bupivacaine Chloroprocaine	Tissue injection (local); spray	No loss of consciousness	CNS stimulation or seizures; cardiac depression; absorbed into bloodstream	Monitor for excitability, twitching, pulse or blood pressure changes, pallor, respiratory difficulty

Reproduced by permission from Judith L. Greig: Intraoperative nursing. In Wilma J. Phipps, Barbara Long, and Nancy Fugate Woods, (Eds.), 1987. *Medical-Surgical Nursing,* 3rd ed., St. Louis: The C. V. Mosby Co.

nervous system function in the postoperative period. Somnolence, lethargy, disorientation, agitation, and amnesia are common findings, no matter what anesthetic technique is used. Adverse and prolonged central nervous system effects are more common in the elderly. During this time, the nursing diagnosis of the potential for injury must be considered.

Most patients are amnesic for a period after general anesthesia. They may seem awake and respond appropriately to commands, but they do not remember this period. Therefore, patients often ask the same question repeatedly, not remembering that they have asked before. Benzodiazepines, anticholinergics, ketamine, volatile anesthetics, and nitrous oxide all cause amnesia.

Anticholinergics are often given both preoperatively and intraoperatively. They have several beneficial actions, including drying of secretions, sedation and amnesia, and protection against bradycardia. However, an undesirable effect is central nervous system (CNS) toxicity. Symptoms include restlessness, agitation, somnolence, seizures, and coma. Scopolamine is the worst offender, although atropine can also cause toxicity. Glycopyrrolate does not cross the blood–brain barrier and does not cause CNS toxicity. Elderly patients are at the highest risk for CNS toxicity. The symptoms may be reversed by administering physostigmine, 1 to 2 mg intravenously. Atropine, or glycopyrrolate, must be on hand when physostigmine is given, as bradycardia may occur (Stoelting, 1986).

Ketamine produces a so-called dissociative or catalepsy-like state of anesthesia. Emergence from ketamine anesthesia can be associated with psychic sensations characterized by weird dreams or illusions, alterations in mood or body image, floating sensations, and occasionally frank delirium. Benzodiazepines, given before emergence from ketamine, attenuate the emergence phenomena (White, Way, & Trevor, 1982). The analgesic effects of ketamine far outlast its anesthetic effect, and therefore, analgesics may not be necessary for some time.

Other drugs used during anesthesia, including narcotics, droperidol, and chlorpromazine, may cause postoperative CNS depression. The CNS depression of many of these agents is potentiated when given with other depressants.

Toxic blood levels of local anesthetics used for regional anesthesia initially cause central nervous system excitation, manifested by tinnitus, light-headedness, visual and auditory disturbances, restlessness, and seizures. This is followed by CNS depression, and then coma.

Finally, many common postsurgical physiologic and electrolyte derangements produce CNS manifestations, such as disorientation and lethargy. These include hypoxia, hypercarbia, hypocalcemia, and hyponatremia. Urinary distention, gastric distention, and pain may cause agitation and hypertension. These causes must be ruled out before attributing CNS symptoms to residual anesthetic effects.

Cardiovascular System

Almost all anesthetic agents and adjuncts have direct or indirect effects on the cardiovascular system. These may or may not be desirable, but must be taken into account when caring for a patient who has received these drugs (Kaplan, 1987).

Commonly, patients are returned to the surgical intensive care unit emerging from an anesthetic and are neither fully anesthetized nor fully awake. They are often hypertensive from pain, agitation, or vasoconstriction secondary to hypothermia. Hypoxia, hypercarbia, fluid overload, and urinary or gastric distention may also cause hypertension. Hypertension and tachycardia are usually not desirable, especially in patients with coronary heart disease and increased intracranial pressure. In patients with coronary heart disease, hypertension and tachycardia increase myocardial oxygen demand, which can lead to myocardial ischemia. The mortality from a perioperative myocardial infarction is 50 to 70%, much higher than the mortality from an infarction not related to surgery and anesthesia (Tinker & Roberts, 1986). Postoperative hypertension should be treated expeditiously but cautiously. Residual anesthetic agents may decrease the amount of sedative or antihypertensive agents required. As patients warm, they will vasodilate and become normotensive or even hypotensive. In addition, postoperative patients are at increased risk for hypovolemia secondary to bleeding and third-spacing or sequestration of fluids outside the vascular compartment (see chapter 9). Hypertensive, hypovolemic patients are at especially increased risk for sudden hypotension.

The volatile anesthetic agents (halothane, enflurane, and isoflurane) are direct myocardial depressants; therefore, the myocardium may not respond appropriately to stress in the immediate postoperative period. Decreased cardiac output and tissue oxygen delivery will result. They also blunt baroreceptor reflexes. Although narcotics and benzodiazepines by themselves are usually not considered cardiac depressants, when used in combination, they exert a more depressant effect (Reeves, Flezzani, & Igor, 1987). In addition, volatile anesthetics (especially isoflurane) are vasodilators, and may contribute to hypotension in the immediate postoperative period.

Ketamine is a sympathetic nervous system stimulant. It causes hypertension and tachycardia in patients with intact sympathetic nervous systems. However, ketamine is a direct myocardial depressant. Hypotension may ensue when ketamine is administered to critically ill patients who are unable to mount a sympathetic response. The sympathomimetic effects of ketamine may be decreased when administered with a benzodiazepine (White et al., 1982).

Patients may be at increased risk for dysrhythmias in the postoperative period, especially patients undergoing open heart surgery. The reasons for the increased risk include direct or indirect actions of drugs administered

intraoperatively, hypoxia, hypercarbia, metabolic alkalosis and acidosis, myocardial ischemia, electrolyte abnormalities, hypothermia, direct manipulation
of the heart, and altered central nervous system autonomic output secondary
to drugs or CNS pathology. The volatile anesthetics tend to be intrinsically
antiarrhythmic, but Halothane potentiates the dysrhythmogenic effects of
both endogenous and exogenous catecholamines. Opioids, given in large
bolus doses cause bradycardia, although this is unlikely to be a factor in the
postoperative period. Anticholinesterases, given to reverse neuromuscular
blockade, cause bradycardia. This is prevented by the concomitant administration of anticholinergics. Local anesthetics, when inadvertently injected intravascularly (for example, topping off an epidural catheter that has migrated
intravascularly), may cause life-threatening dysrhythmias. Vasoactive drugs
often administered to critically ill patients, including dopamine, dobutamine,
isoproterenol, and theophylline, may potentiate dysrhythmias.

Respiratory System

Anesthesia and mechanical ventilation affect the respiratory system in a number of ways causing alterations in central control, musculoskeletal mechanics,
and lung physiology. Extubated patients who are lethargic may not be able to
consistently maintain an airway. They may seem awake and responsive when
stimulated by an endotracheal tube or transportation, but once settled in the
critical care unit and unstimulated, they may develop airway obstruction.
There is also the potential for aspiration.

Anesthetic agents alter the body's normal protective reflex responses to
hypoxia and hypercarbia. Trace amounts of volatile anesthetics may be ex-
haled for hours after general anesthesia and severely attenuate the chemore-
ceptor response to hypoxia. Volatile anesthetics also blunt the central-brain-
stem response to hypercarbia and base-line carbon dioxide levels are higher
(Pavlin, 1986). Patients with chronic obstructive pulmonary disease (COPD)
are especially at risk for postoperative hypercarbia. Narcotics also attenuate
the body's normal response to hypercarbia; some carbon dioxide retention is
the norm. Narcotics are often used in very high doses as a primary anesthetic,
necessitating postanesthesia mechanical ventilation because of their prolonged respiratory depressant effects.

Anesthetics and vasoactive drugs often administered to critically ill patients can alter pulmonary blood flow. This may lead to an altered pulmonary
ventilation–perfusion relationship and may contribute to hypoxia.

Most patients receiving general anesthesia for major surgical procedures
receive muscle relaxants as an adjuvant to anesthesia. This allows for better
exposure of the operative area (organs and tissues) and the use of less anesthetic. After elective surgery in healthy patients, the effects of nondepolarizing
muscle relaxants are usually reversed by administering cholinesterase inhibi-
tors. However, these drugs have side effects (bradycardia, bronchospasm)

that may further compromise unstable patients. Patients are often returned to the ICU still paralyzed, requiring mechanical ventilation at least until the muscle paralysis has worn off. It is important to keep paralyzed and partially paralyzed patients well sedated, as it is a terrifying experience for a patient to be awake and not be able to move. Conversely, in patients whose paralysis has been reversed and who have been extubated, the differential diagnosis of respiratory distress must include inadequate reversal. These patients often display uncoordinated movements.

Prolonged mechanical ventilation during anesthesia may adversely affect postoperative lung function. Mucociliary transport is impaired. Factors contributing to this include volatile anesthetics, inspiration of dry gases, high inspired oxygen concentration, endotracheal tube cuffs, and positive pressure ventilation (Pavlin, 1986). Patients kept immobile in one position for prolonged periods may have increased lung water in dependent parts of the lung. Functional residual capacity (FRC), the volume of the lung at end-expiration, is decreased during anesthesia and this decrease persists into the postoperative period. The supine position, muscle paralysis, and increased lung water also contribute to decreased FRC, and can lead to impaired oxygenation. Impaired gas exchange also occurs as a result of disruption of the normal ventilation–perfusion ratio as dead space increases because of mechanical ventilation, and perfusion of nondependent areas of the lung is decreased. Positive-end-expiratory pressure is often used to increase FRC (Benumof, 1986). Endotracheal tubes may exacerbate obstructive or reactive airway disease in patients with COPD or asthma.

All of the above factors may contribute to ineffective airway clearance and an ineffective breathing pattern, which contribute to an increased risk of postoperative pulmonary complications. Should these complications occur, impaired gas exchange will result. Therefore, good pulmonary hygiene, including endotracheal tube suctioning, turning, chest physical therapy, coughing, deep breathing, and use of incentive spirometry, are important in the postoperative period.

Finally, patients brought to the ICU after surgery should routinely have a chest roentgenogram. The roentgenogram should be checked for endotracheal tube placement, and the presence of any pulmonary pathologic processes.

Metabolic and Endocrine Systems

Anesthesia is associated with multiple changes in the metabolic and endocrine systems, however it is often difficult to separate anesthetic- from surgery-induced effects. These direct and indirect metabolic and endocrine effects may persist into the postoperative period.

Anesthesia and surgery are often associated with hypothermia. Hypothermia is intentional for patients placed on cardiopulmonary bypass, otherwise it is usually unintentional. It is always unintentional during the postoperative period. Anesthetics may contribute to hypothermia by several mechanisms. They increase surface blood flow (volatile agents), depress central thermoregulatory structures, depress metabolic rate, abolish shivering (muscle relaxants), and depress normal behavioral responses (putting on more clothes and seeking a warmer environment). In addition, inhalation of room temperature, nonhumidified gases, cold operating rooms, and the use of cold irrigating and intravenous solutions and blood products, all contribute to hypothermia. Patients with core temperatures below 33°C are at increased risk for dysrhythmias, CNS changes, and decreased cardiac output.

Postoperative effects of hypothermia include vasoconstriction, shivering, and delayed drug clearance. Vasoconstriction leads to initial hypertension, followed by hypotension with rewarming. Shivering greatly increases oxygen consumption in a patient who already has some impairment of oxygen delivery. Patients with coronary artery disease are especially at risk. Delayed drug clearance prolongs the elimination of anesthetic drugs. Patients should be treated with warming blankets, increased ambient temperature, heated and humidified inhaled gases, and warmed intravenous fluids and blood products (Morley-Forster, 1986). Discussion of hypothermia is continued in chapter 12.

Hypocalcemia secondary to the rapid administration of citrated blood products, especially in patients with liver disease, may be seen in the postoperative period. It is manifested by hypotension secondary to decreased cardiac output and should be treated with calcium chloride administered intravenously. Other electrolyte abnormalities, hyperglycemia, metabolic and respiratory acidosis, and alkalosis are common in the postoperative period and should be treated because they can lead to CNS, respiratory, or cardiovascular complications. Patients with adrenocortical suppression require continued supplemental administration of steroids postoperatively.

Renal System

General anesthesia temporarily depresses renal function as measured by urine output, glomerular filtration rate, renal blood flow, and electrolyte excretion. The anesthesia-induced depression of renal function may be caused by direct or indirect effects. The indirect effects are probably more important. For example, intraoperative hypotension may cause stimulation of the sympathetic and endocrine systems (catecholamines, antidiuretic hormone, renin–angiotensin, and aldosterone), which in turn, affect renal function. Anesthetic agents may directly affect renal tubular function. No currently used anesthetic agent causes nephrotoxicity (Mazze, 1986).

Therefore, in the postoperative period, patients may have impaired renal function, including a decreased ability to maintain osmotic and electrolyte homeostasis and excrete drugs (see chapter 1). This is normally a temporary aberration, however, sicker, hemodynamically unstable patients may have prolonged impairment.

Hepatic and Gastrointestinal System

Minor reversible changes in liver function are common in the immediate postoperative period. The cause remains unclear; however, a variety of contributing factors may have a role. All types of general and regional anesthesia are associated with a decrease in hepatic blood flow. Transient hypotension, hypoxia, the general stress of surgery, calorie deprivation, and drug toxicity may all have a role (Maze & Baden, 1986). Patients with preexisting liver disease are at risk for worsening liver function postoperatively.

Usually these changes have little clinical significance. However, significant postoperative jaundice is not uncommon after major surgical procedures. It can occur from a variety of causes. Halothane is the only anesthetic agent that has been consistently associated with hepatic toxicity. The mechanisms remain unclear.

Hepatic drug metabolism may be affected in the perioperative period. Several drugs commonly administered to critically ill patients may cause induction (e.g., diphenylhydantoin, phenobarbital, volatile anesthetics) or inhibition (cimetidine) of drug-metabolizing systems in the liver (Baden & Rice, 1986). Drugs, including anesthetics, may compete with each other for hepatic enzyme systems. Consequently, serum drug levels and half-lives of drugs that are dependent on liver metabolism may be altered.

Narcotic anesthetics may cause a temporary ileus secondary to increased gastrointestinal sphincter tone. The ileus associated with general anesthesia is temporary and resolves shortly after surgery.

Neuromuscular System

The neuromuscular system is intentionally depressed during anesthesia by the use of muscle relaxants. Postoperative residual neuromuscular depression adversely affects respiratory mechanics, as discussed above.

SUMMARY

The preoperative and postoperative care of the surgical critical care patient involves special considerations because of anesthesia. The preoperative care is essentially the same as for any surgical patient, but may be more involved. Unique considerations have been identified. The postoperative effects of anesthesia on major organ systems are likely to be more dramatic and detrimental in the unstable critically ill patient, and therefore must be recognized and treated before further complications ensue.

BIBLIOGRAPHY

Ammon, J. (1987). Perioperative management of the diabetic patient. In *Annual Refresher Course Lectures* (p. 272). Park Ridge, IL: American Society of Anesthesiologists.

Baden, J., & Rice, S. (1986). Metabolism and toxicity of inhaled anesthetics. In R. Miller (Ed.), *Anesthesia*, 2nd ed. (pp. 701–744). New York: Churchill-Livingstone.

Benumof, J. (1986). Respiratory physiology and respiratory function during anesthesia. In R. Miller (Ed.), *Anesthesia*, 2nd ed. (pp. 1115–1164). New York: Churchill-Livingstone.

Gibbs, C., & Modell, J. (1986). Aspiration pneumonitis. In R. Miller (Ed.), *Anesthesia*, 2nd ed. (pp. 2023–2052). New York: Churchill-Livingstone.

Kaplan, J. (Ed.) (1987). *Cardiac Anesthesia*. Orlando, FL: Grune & Stratton.

Maze, M., & Baden, J. (1986). Anesthesia for patients with liver disease. In R. Miller (Ed.), *Anesthesia*, 2nd ed. (pp. 1165–1180). New York: Churchill-Livingstone.

Mazze, R. (1986). Renal physiology and the effects of anesthesia. In R. Miller (Ed.), *Anesthesia*, 2nd ed. (pp. 1223–1248). New York: Churchill-Livingstone.

Miller, R. (1986). *Anesthesia*, 2nd ed. New York: Churchill-Livingstone.

Morley-Forster, P. (1986). Unintentional hypothermia in the operating room. *Canadian Anesthesia Society Journal, 33*(4), 516–527.

Pavlin, E. (1986). Respiratory pharmacology of inhaled anesthetic agents. In R. Miller (Ed.), *Anesthesia*, 2nd ed. (pp. 667–700). New York: Churchill-Livingstone.

Reeves, J., Flezzani, P., & Igor, K. (1987). Pharmacology of intravenous anesthetic induction drugs. In J. Kaplan (Ed.), *Cardiac Anesthesia*, 2nd ed. (pp. 125–150). Orlando, FL: Grune & Stratton.

Roizen, M. (1986). Anesthetic implications of concurrent diseases. In R. Miller (Ed.), *Anesthesia*, 2nd ed. (pp. 255–358). New York: Churchill-Livingstone.

Slogoff, S., & Keats, A. (1985). Does perioperative myocardial ischemia lead to postoperative myocardial infarction? *Anesthesiology, 62,* 107–114.

Stoelting, R. (1986). Psychological preparation and preoperative medication. In R. Miller (Ed.), *Anesthesia*, 2nd ed. (pp. 381–408). New York: Churchill-Livingstone.

Tinker, J., & Roberts, S. (1986). Anesthesia risk. In R. Miller (Ed.), *Anesthesia*, 2nd ed. (pp. 359–380). New York: Churchill-Livingstone.

White, P., Way, W., & Trevor, A. (1982). Ketamine: Its pharmacology and therapeutic uses. *Anesthesiology, 56,* 119–136.

Psychosocial Responses to Critical Illness in the Surgical Patient

3 The Concept of Crisis and Crisis Intervention

Mary Ballou, Ph.D.
Jan Litwack, Ed.S., R.N.

"The core of the crisis in critical care is the confrontation with the threat to one's body; loss of functions, disfigurement, even death" (Slaikeu, 1984, p. 206). Patients admitted to any critical care unit are in the midst of a multi-faceted crisis situation. It is imperative for the critical care nurse to understand this crisis situation conceptually and theoretically in order to assess and intervene appropriately in the critical care environment.

In the critical care environment, the nurse is dealing with situational crises as opposed to maturational crises. By definition, a situational crisis is a stressful event that threatens biological, psychological, and/or social integrity, and it has the ability to affect one or many members of a family or support group (Aguilera & Messick, 1986). In contrast, a maturational crisis is a normal process of growth and development that results in periods of great social, physical, and psychological change (Aguilera & Messick, 1986).

In this chapter we will explore situational crisis theory, with the goal of applying crisis theory and intervention to the critical care environment. Using the Fink-Ballou model, nursing assessment, diagnosis, and interventions appropriate to the critically ill patient are presented.

CRISIS THEORY

Crisis theory is based on the concept that individuals strive to maintain a homeostatic balance in their lives. The goal is to respond to internal and external threats to this balance in a way that maintains system equilibrium and results in minimal conflict within the system (Caplan, 1964). When individuals are faced with events for which their coping mechanisms are inadequate, crisis occurs. Disequilibrium in the system by itself does not result in crisis. Crisis results when the disequilibrium overwhelms the individual's ability to restore homeostasis, or to cope.

The significant concept is an individual's perception of the threat, not how others might judge the seriousness of the event. Internal threats may be pathologies, physiologic disequilibrium and physical change, and psychological coping abilities. External threats may include a significant loss or threat of loss, role disruption, trauma, or a challenge to the individual that places overwhelming demands on attempts to maintain equilibrium.

There are a number of variables that influence the likelihood of an event becoming a crisis. These include the intensity of the event, the number of events occurring simultaneously or sequentially, the psychological strength of the individual, the physiologic state of the individual, and the adequacy of social support systems.

In the critical care environment, it is most likely that patients and families will experience a state of crisis. Predisposing factors include a vulnerable physiologic state, life-threatening situations, separation from family and significant others, disruption of daily activities and roles, and uncertainty about outcome and role resumption. For some, the intensity is compounded by the sudden nature of hospitalization, trauma, or lack of previous related experiences. Some patients are further compromised by losing their ability to talk because of endotracheal intubation, to write because of multiple IVs and debilitation, and to move about freely because of attachment to monitors, ventilators, drains, and intravenous lines. Individuals in critical care environments are in new, unfamiliar situations, and have little or no opportunity to gain control over themselves, their environment, and/or their destiny.

During this period of overwhelming disequilibrium, the individual in crisis is quite susceptible to the influence of others. The time, the intensity, the need, and the susceptibility necessitate that crisis intervention be immediate, proximate, and short-term in nature. The goal of this intervention is to assist the individual to return to his or her homeostatic balance. The goal is not the same as psychotherapy, which could be used to restructure the personality or resolve longstanding conflict or disorders. Neither is the goal simply problem solving, for crisis is much more than a problem.

Although a physiologic crisis may require surgical, pharmacologic, and medical intervention, the critical care nurse, in addition to supporting and implementing physiologic therapies, can assist the patient in reaching psychological stability as well. The goal is to help the patient to adapt to the crisis situation in healthy ways, by focusing on the particular precipitating events and the problems within them. The existing strengths and motivation of the patient must be mobilized to deal with the problems at hand. The approach should be empathic, pragmatic, reality-oriented, and creative. In addition to the adaptive resolution of the immediate crisis, the individual may develop new problem-solving mechanisms or insights into personal coping styles that may help to prevent or minimize crisis situations in the future.

It is important, at this time, to emphasize that crisis is a natural, normal process. The crisis situation is a process that can be viewed through a developmental or stage model. Each stage has unique internal events for the patient in crisis and specific interventions for the crisis worker, who in this case is the critical care nurse. As with any model, it is important to remember that stages may not occur in a chronological order and that each stage may be entered more than once. It is critical to determine which stage of the crisis process the patient is in, for different interventions are needed for each stage. The competent critical care nurse already has the training and skill needed for most interventions in crisis management. A staging model that allows for the identification, organization, and validation of skills and resources for intervention is the Fink-Ballou model, which is explained below.

FINK-BALLOU MODEL

Fink-Ballou (Ballou, Litwack, & Romanielleo, 1986) use a four-stage model to describe the individual response to crisis. These four stages include

1. Shock—the period of initial psychological impact.
2. Defensive retreat—the period during which the individual defends against the full implications of the crisis.
3. Acknowledgment—the period during which the individual faces the realities of the crisis.
4. Adaptation and change—the period during which the individual actually begins to cope with the situation in a constructive manner.

Each stage is discussed in greater detail below.

Shock

Shock occurs when the psychological alarm sounds and when various aspects of psychological functioning become frozen. As a result of the overwhelming anxiety, coping mechanisms fail. As in physiologic shock, in which cardiac output is inadequate to meet the demands of the system, the physiologic coping mechanisms (compensatory mechanisms) have failed. As the threat to the system becomes overwhelming, the individual experiences disorganization in thinking, with decreasing ability to plan, to reason, or to understand. With the cognitive confusion and the inability to think, there is often a perception of an inadequate self.

The individual in the shock stage of crisis may display panic, anxiety and fear, and feelings of helplessness or powerlessness. We shall see later that anxiety, fear, and powerlessness are the nursing diagnostic categories for the individual (and family) experiencing crisis.

Defensive Retreat

In the same manner that physiologic threat is addressed with compensatory mechanisms, so are psychological threats. Out of fear of losing control, falling apart, or being overwhelmed, the individual engages in a number of defensive strategies. These strategies may be viewed as psychological compensatory mechanisms. The reality of the event and/or its impact is avoided through mechanisms such as wishful thinking, fantasizing, denial, or repression. There is a sense of emotional relief experienced as the distance from the threat increases. The avoidance mechanisms are actually reinforced by the decrease of anxiety that occurs. During this stage, thinking becomes rigid and there is much resistance to change or to anyone who attempts to enforce reality. Upsetting this precarious balance is seen as a threat, and anger usually ensues.

There are a number of implications for the critical care nurse in working with patients in this stage. It is important to recognize that the use of defensive mechanisms is vitally important for protection and the minimization of threat to the individual. These defensive strategies enable the individual in crisis to maintain some sense of balance.

Acknowledgment

Eventually, defensive strategies no longer protect the individual from reality, and the temporary sense of balance is upset. The individual realizes that old ways of being or doing are no longer successful. Distress increases as defenses weaken and it is no longer possible to escape the impact of the events.

Feelings during this period are varied and complex. There is depression, as in mourning, with a deep sense of loss and often bitterness. With the renewed threat, fear, anxiety, and powerlessness may again be felt. On the cognitive level, there is confusion as defensive thinking breaks down and perceptions of reality are altered. Past losses are reviewed and a sense of worthlessness may be felt. Suicide and psychotic breaks may occur during this stage. Things are recognized, either slowly or rapidly, for what they are, and the need for a plan of action begins to emerge. The need to restore equilibrium begins to take hold and the individual gains motivation to cope with the situation.

Adaptation and Change

Coping processes are dependent on many factors. Some of these factors include the motivation of the individual, general beliefs of the individual, a sense of trust, and the internal and external resources available to the individual. In this stage, the individual develops new perceptions of self with a renewed sense of self-worth. The individual begins to explore and test resources in terms of limitations and expectations of reality. Thinking is reorganized and problem solving is initiated. New satisfactions are experienced, and with this, a gradual lessening of depression and anxiety. The individual gains personal strength as feelings of fear and powerlessness dissipate.

CRISIS INTERVENTION STRATEGIES

Before moving to specific interventions for each stage of the Fink-Ballou model, there are some generic strategies of crisis intervention. These strategies include

- providing psychological first aid to the patient and significant others,
- keeping the patient alive,
- helping to keep options open,
- helping to decrease losses,
- allowing for crisis behavior (recognizing that crisis is normal), and
- assisting the individual to live in the present

Individuals aided by a practitioner skilled in intervention strategies have the probability of learning healthy, adaptive coping, and are able to survive and recover more quickly and fully, take care of themselves and regain feelings of power, learn to experience and manage intense, painful feelings, master crises intellectually and interpret the experience realistically, and cope with life more effectively by their own standards (Aguilera & Messick, 1986; Fink, 1967; Rapoport, 1962).

At this time, interventions specific to the stages of the Fink–Ballou model shall be presented. Although specific to the stages of shock, defensive retreat, acknowledgment, and adaptation and change, we shall later see how interventions identified in the Fink-Ballou model can be related to the nursing diagnoses of fear, anxiety, and powerlessness.

In the stage of shock, the first and usually briefest stage of the crisis model, the nurse can

- establish a relationship with the patient and family and maintain ongoing contact, which is a concept basic to primary nursing.
- offer support and acceptance through empathic understanding and reflection of feelings.
- encourage the patient and family to acknowledge and express feelings generated by the situation.
- gather information about the situation by supporting discussion about the recent events.
- begin to assess the dimensions and extent of the situation.
- mobilize medical resources as necessary.

- take control in decision making for the patient's protection, safety, and comfort.
- identify and mobilize environmental and interpersonal support systems as necessary.

It is critical during this stage that the nurse not direct the patient toward problem solving alternatives. Because of the overwhelming emotional response and the subsequent disorganized thinking, this would serve only to further frustrate, confuse, and alienate the patient. Empathy—the ability to have and demonstrate understanding, acceptance, and genuine concern—is far more essential. Overt external decision making for the patient may be necessary, for the individual is frequently physiologically and psychologically overwhelmed.

In defensive retreat, the second stage of the process in the crisis model, the nurse can

- paraphrase and summarize the affective content of the patient's and family's messages.
- acknowledge, but not support or reinforce, wishful thinking, fantasies, denials, or repressions.
- avoid direct confrontation with unrealistic thinking but may gently ask for explanations of the consequences of intended actions.
- be available and communicate, "I am here, I care, and if or when you are ready, I will help." This helps to increase the individual's level of trust.
- point out, in specific terms, behaviors that are seen as confusing, inconsistent, or incongruent with previously stated perceptions of reality.
- intervene when self-destructive behavior occurs.

This stage is characterized by needed denial, and is a normal part of the crisis process. Nurses should neither confront nor agree with the magical thinking. Instead, they should see this as an important and necessary rest period that follows being overwhelmed and precedes the genuine engagement with the crisis seen in the next stage.

In acknowledgment, the third stage of the crisis process, the nurse can

- seek to understand the patient's experience, which may include both past unresolved conflicts and current issues.
- monitor established environmental and interpersonal support systems.
- allow the expression of dependency during periods of depression, worthlessness, and failure.
- be sensitive to the patient's readiness, encouraging exploration of feelings and an awareness of those feelings.

- assist in the clarification of events and identification of core issues.
- help identify multidimensional implications.
- begin the initial stage of problem solving (i.e., gathering information).
- mobilize various professional and community resources.
- reinforce strengths and coping potential.

The central goals of the acknowledgment stage are to be with the person emotionally and to communicate reality-based hope. It is also important for nurses to be aware that suicide attempts and psychotic breaks can occur in this phase because feelings of anxiety, fear, and powerlessness are so great in the face of ineffective coping abilities.

In adaptation and change, the fourth stage in the model, the nurse can

- continue empathic communication while confronting unrealistic alternatives and unsound advice.
- assist in continuing the problem-solving process (i.e., exploring tentative plans, anticipating problems, choosing and implementing a plan of action, and evaluating outcomes).
- support movement toward newly established goals and affirm the individual's sense of worth and personal growth.
- initiate discussion of the crisis, new skills, and understandings that have been gained as a result of the crisis.
- collaborate with the individual in recognizing autonomy and strengths.
- maintain psychosocial communication until goals are completed and referrals are made to the appropriate resources.

In this final phase, crisis resolution is occurring. Homeostasis is being regained and the rehabilitation process has begun. The individual develops new perceptions of self and a renewed sense of self-worth.

ASSESSMENT OF THE POTENTIAL FOR CRISIS

The assessment of the individual in crisis and assessment for the potential for crisis may be difficult for the critical care nurse, whose energies are focused on physiologic concerns. Although it is difficult to manage both, a skilled practitioner is able to interweave both physiologic and psychological caring in providing for patients.

Previously identified in this chapter are potential crisis events that a patient in the critical care unit may face, including a vulnerable physiologic condition, threat of death, loss of control, physical change and/or disfigurement, and significant losses or threats of loss. Other threats include separation from family and significant others, exposure to unfamiliar environmental stimuli, confinement to bed and to monitors, and the experience of pain, sleep deprivation, and discomfort. The highly technological environment of the critical care unit may cause a sense of depersonalization and may serve as a precipitant of crisis in and of itself. It is the rare individual and/or family who would not perceive the critical care environment and the reason for being there as a crisis.

The assessment of patients in various stages of crisis requires the study of psychological status through both verbal and nonverbal communication. Data from a variety of patient interactions and interactions of family and significant others can facilitate a deeper understanding of the crisis situation. Although numerous potential threats that individuals and families may face are identified throughout this chapter, it is the perception of the threat by the individual patient or family that determines the reality and intensity of the crisis.

Insight into a patient's and/or family's perception of the threat may be gained through subjective and/or objective data. Subjectively, the nurse may hear comments such as

"I just can't take it anymore. I don't know what to do."
"I've done everything I could and was supposed to do. It hasn't done any good. What else could I have done?"
"That's my mother in that bed. She can't die. You have to make her better. I need her. I can't live without her."

Objectively, the nurse may identify unclear thinking, ineffective problem solving, lack of action, excessive concern, anxiety, panic, fear, and powerlessness. Assigning a label of anxiety, fear, or powerlessness becomes the basis for nursing diagnoses specific to crisis.

Anxiety is defined as a vague, uneasy feeling, the source of which is often nonspecific or unknown to the individual. It is the anticipation of danger or of an unpleasant event. Anxiety is a perceived threat that has no identifiable source.

For the patient and family facing a critical care hospitalization, there are a number of events that may evoke an anxiety response. Although the identification of events does provide a source of the anxiety response, the events are nonspecific and vague. The feelings of anxiety may come from a threat to self-concept, threat of death, threat to or change in health or socioeconomic status, threat to or change in role functioning, threat to or change in environment, or a threat to or change in interaction patterns and unmet needs (Doenges and Moorhouse, 1985).

The patient experiencing anxiety may report feelings of tension, helplessness, hopelessness, shakiness, apprehension, uncertainty, fear, worry, and distress. These subjective signs of anxiety may be revealed either overtly or covertly:

"I have a feeling that something's not right."
"I feel shaky, nervous, I can't eat. Something's wrong, but I'm not sure what. I'm worried about everything."

Objective signs of anxiety are nonspecific and may simply reveal or suggest someone in distress. Objective signs may include

- sympathetic stimulation—tachycardia, hypertension, peripheral vasoconstriction, pupil dilation,
- increased wariness—glancing about,
- restlessness—insomnia,
- poor eye contact,
- trembling,
- voice quivering, and
- diaphoresis.

Again, the objective signs are nonspecific and may be the presenting picture of a patient in pain, in hypoxic distress, or in shock. Further exploration of the signs and symptoms is mandatory. Data obtained from patient interactions, family interactions, and situational events will facilitate a deeper understanding of the patient in crisis.

Reflecting back to the Fink–Ballou crisis model, the individual experiencing anxiety may be in any of three stages—shock, acknowledgment or adaptation and change. In the shock phase, the anxiety level is high and overwhelming. In defensive retreat, the individual "retreats" from the crisis in an attempt to minimize the anxiety. The individual protects against the intensity of anxiety. In acknowledgment, the level of anxiety increases once again as the individual begins to recognize the reality of the situation. Medium levels of anxiety may serve as motivators for action. If the anxiety becomes overwhelming, the individual may attempt suicide or may experience psychotic break (ICU psychosis). In adaptation and change, there is a gradual lowering of anxiety concomitant with a gradual increase in satisfying experiences. In many respects, anxiety is the key concept underlying the crisis model.

Fear is a feeling of dread related to an identifiable source validated by the person (North America Nursing Diagnosis Association [NANDA]). Fear has an object, an identifiable cause. It is the reaction to a real threat of injury—physical or psychological—or death. (Anxiety, in contrast, has no identifiable source and is a threat to the individual only from within.) For the patient and family facing a critical care hospitalization, there are many threats against the self, including

- environmental stimuli (electrocardiographic [ECG] monitors, ventilators),
- invasive procedures (surgery, intravenous therapy, dialysis),
- knowledge deficits (an issue for informed consent),
- inability to communicate (because of intubation, trauma, language barrier),
- physiologic demands (pain, hunger, hypoxema, hypoperfusion),
- threat of death (perceived or actual).

Subjectively, the individual in fear may report feeling tense, nervous, terrified, frightened, panicky, or afraid. All are descriptors of fear, and differ only in their intensity. It is frequently subjective descriptors given by patients and families that lead the nurse to the diagnosis of fear.

Again, objective signs of fear are nonspecific. The individual in fear may withdraw, or may act defensive (fight-or-flight reaction). Examination of patient and family interactions, as well as the realization that the critical care environment has many threats, may lead the nurse to explore fear as a potential or actual diagnosis:

> Dr. Jacobson had just presented to Mrs. Baker the need for surgery for her husband, who was dying from an infection for which no antibiotic seemed to be effective. Dr. Jacobson wanted to do an exploratory laparotomy in an attempt to identify the source of infection. Mrs. Baker listened carefully, but when it came time to sign the consent form, she sat paralyzed, unable to place the pen to the paper. She started to speak, but dissolved into tears. "I'm afraid. I'm scared he's going to die, that I'll never see him again. I'll be alone. I'll have no one."

Reflecting back to the Fink-Ballou model, fear too has its place. The intensity of fear parallels the intensity of anxiety in the model. In the shock stage, the individual is overwhelmed with fear. The individual's very existence is threatened. Acute medical intervention is required and the possibility of death may be quite real and imminent. In defensive retreat, the individual attempts to regain strength by denying the reality of the threats. In acknowledgment, fears are confronted, but serve as motivators for action or as sources of depression. Either the individual is able to reorganize thinking and activities, or the threats again overwhelm and lead to disorganization. In adaptation and change, the intensity of fear lessens as the individual gains strength and control over destiny, environment, and self.

Powerlessness is the last nursing diagnosis specific to the individual in crisis. Powerlessness is defined as the perception that one's action will not significantly affect an outcome—a perceived lack of control over a current situation or immediate happening (NANDA). In the critical care environment, there are many factors that may contribute to feelings of powerlessness:

- medical control as opposed to self-control over decision making,
- mechanical as opposed to physiologic control (ventilators, pacemakers, dialysis, intravenous therapy, catheterization),
- institutional control as opposed to self-control in social interactions (visiting hours, restrictions on who may visit).

Subjective characteristics of powerlessness identifiable by nurses are as follows. The individual (or family) experiencing loss of control may verbalize exactly that, "Nothing I'm doing makes any difference." Effort is extended without positive outcome. Patients (and families) may report feelings of depression, exhaustion, and frustration. Anger is frequently expressed in words or actions.

Objective signs of powerlessness are nonspecific and relate more to the feelings of depression, frustration, exhaustion, and anger that may be experienced. If the individual perceiving a lack of control reacts with depression, there may be signs of withdrawal, crying, silence, and verbal outbursts of anger. Frustration may be identified by anger, lack of initiative, passivity, and dependence. Exhaustion is readily identified by lack of energy, passivity, dependence, and withdrawal. Anger may be in the form of acting out behavior, verbal abuse and outbursts, depression, and withdrawal:

> "Nothing I'm doing works. I watched my diet, took all my medications, and went to dialysis just like I was supposed to. I did everything they told me to do. It isn't fair. What else could I have done? What else can I do?"

Powerlessness, too, can be related to the Fink-Ballou crisis model, particularly in the shock stage. In this stage, the individual is absolutely overwhelmed and has no control over the situation. Events have overwhelmed the ability of the individual to meet the physiologic and/or psychological stressors being faced. In defensive retreat, the individual once again regains control by denying the crisis events. It is the ability of the individual to regain control that becomes comforting and reassuring. In acknowledgment, the individual may again feel powerlessness in the realization of crisis events. Crisis necessitates change. The individual must mobilize resources, both internal and external, to address the reality of the situation. In adaptation and change, the individual begins to regain control. The individual begins to test problem-solving strategies and to engage in decision making to regain self-control over present and future events.

INTERVENTION STRATEGIES

Intervention strategies specific to each of the four stages of the Fink-Ballou crisis model have been identified above. Here we will identify the goals of the interventions, and further interventions specific to these goals. Goals related to crisis management in the critically ill patient are as follows:

1. Anxiety is reduced to a manageable level.
2. Fears are replaced by knowledge.
3. Control and choice replace powerlessness.

Additional nursing interventions, specific to these goals, include:

> Teaching—about the critical care environment, patient status, equipment, intensive care unit routines, resources, problem solving, and decision making.

Reinforcement of individual/family strengths—in coping, in problem solving, and in utilization of internal and external resources.

Allowing for control—by providing the patient/family opportunities, when feasible, to make decisions and to have choices, and helping them to keep options open.

Not overwhelming individual/family abilities—by allowing for individual pacing and, when necessary, for "timeouts" for both the patient and the family/significant others.

Providing for physiologic and psychological comfort—meeting the needs for nutrition, rest and sleep, social interaction, touch, privacy, and pain relief.

It is also important to apply the intervention strategies applicable to the stage of the crisis model being experienced by the patient. These strategies were discussed above. Interventions specific to coping, which also relate to crisis resolution, are discussed in chapter 4.

EVALUATION

Evaluation, although the last step in the nursing process, is actually ongoing when dealing with individuals and families in crisis. The nurse must consider the goals of crisis intervention discussed above, and must determine whether the goals were or were not achieved. The nurse must continually monitor for improvement or worsening of the crisis situation, for effectiveness of interventions, for alleviation of precipitating factors, and for the responses for the patient and/or family.

Just as the crisis situation erupts from a patient and/or family's perception of being overwhelmed, resolution of the crisis state must also be acknowledged by the patient and/or family. This acknowledgment must be assessed as part of the evaluation process.

PREVENTION

Heretofore, the role of the nurse in crisis intervention has been discussed. Prevention of a crisis state is equally important. Although hospitalization in a critical care environment is stressful, the surgical critical care nurse may be able to strengthen the coping mechanisms of the individual and/or family and thus thwart the development of a crisis situation, through preoperative visits, teaching and anticipatory guidance, listening to concerns, and provision of emotional support.

SUMMARY

It is important for critical care nurses to understand and intervene in the psychological dimension of crisis just as they do in the physiologic dimensions. The whole person is in crisis and in need of assistance. The Fink-Ballou model offers a conceptual and practical approach to crisis. It is a model attendant to the abundant crisis literature and to the physical dimensions of crisis. Additionally, there is empirical evidence that practicing crisis workers agree with the model (Ballou, Brad, & Boyer, 1987).

The 1980s is a decade in which physiologic and psychological interactions are being acknowledged and investigated in medicine and psychology. This chapter presents interdisciplinary conceptualizations and interventions for dealing with crisis in critical care nursing. Detailed in chapter 4 are further strategies designed to prevent crisis and to enable the critical care nurse to assist the patient and family to cope with the crisis situation.

BIBLIOGRAPHY

Aguilera, D., & Messick, J. (1986). *Crisis intervention.* St. Louis: C. V. Mosby.

Ballou, M., Brad, M., & Boyer, M. (1987). Practicing professionals' validation of the Fink–Ballou model of crisis intervention. *Psychotherapy, 24*(3), 31–38.

Ballou, M., Litwack, J., & Romaniello, J. (1986). *Fink–Ballou crisis intervention training manual.* Unpublished manuscript.

Caplan, G., (1964). *Principles of preventive psychiatry.* New York: Basic Books.

Doenges, M., & Moorhouse, M. (1985). *Nurse's pocket guide: Nursing diagnoses with interventions.* Philadelphia: F. A. Davis.

Fink, S. (1967). Crisis: motivation. *Archives of Physical Medicine and Rehabilitation, 48*(11), 592–597.

Rapoport, L. (1962). The state of crisis: Some theoretical considerations. *The Social Science Review, 36,* 211–217.

Slaikeu, K. (1984). *Crisis intervention: A handbook for practice and research.* Boston: Allyn & Bacon.

ADDITIONAL READINGS

Baldwin, B. (1979). Crisis intervention: An overview of theory and practice. *Professional Psychology, 8,* 43–52.

Baldwin, B. (1980). Styles of crisis interventions: Toward a convergent model. *Professional Psychology, 10*(2), 113–120.

Erikson, E. (1963). *Childhood and society.* New York: Norton.

Ewing, D. (1978). *Crisis intervention as psychotherapy.* New York: Oxford University Press.

Fink, S., Beak, J., & Taddeo, K. (1971). Organizational crisis and change. *Journal of Applied Behavioral Science, 7,* 15–37.

Kendal, P., Williams, L., Pechacek, T., Graham, L., Shisslak, C., & Herzoff, N. (1979). Cognitive–behavioral and patient education interventions in cardiac catheterization procedures: The Palo Alto Medical Psychology Project. *Journal of Consulting and Clinical Psychology, 47*(1), 49–58.

Klein, D. C., & Lindemann, E. (1961). Preventive intervention in individual and family crisis situations. In G. Caplan (Ed.). *Prevention of mental disorders in children.* New York: Basic Books.

Kubler-Ross, E. (1969). *On death and dying.* New York: MacMillan.

Kuenzi, S. H., & Fenton, M. V. (1975). Crisis intervention in acute care areas. *American Journal of Nursing, 75,* 830–834.

Lewis, M., Gottesman, D., & Gutstein, S. (1979). The course and duration of crisis. *Journal of Consulting and Clinical Psychology, 47*(1), 128–134.

Lindemann, E. (1944). Symptomatology and management of acute grief. *Psychiatry, 101,* 141–148.

Murgatory, S. (1983). Training for crisis counseling. *British Journal of Guidance & Counseling, 11*(2), 131–144.

Sandoval, H. (1985). Crisis counseling: Conceptualizations and general principles. *School Psychology Review, 14*(3), 257–265.

Selye, H. (1974). *Stress without distress,* Philadelphia: J. B. Lippincott.

Smith, L. (1978). A review of crisis intervention theory. *Social Casework, 59,* 369–405.

Taplin, J. (1971). Crisis theory: Critique and reformulation. *Community Mental Health Journal, 7*(1), 13–23.

Williams, J. R. & Rice, D. G. (1977). The intensive care unit. *Social Work in Health Care, 2,* 391–398.

Wise, D. J. (1975). Crisis intervention before cardiac surgery. *American Journal of Nursing, 75,* 1316–1318.

4 Coping with Critical Illness

Kim Litwack, N.D., Ph.D., R.N.
Lawrence Litwack, Ed.D.

In the previous chapter, material was presented related to the theory and practice of crisis intervention. This intervention deals with the physical and psychological needs of the individual at a critical point in life. In this chapter, we move beyond the point of crisis to coping with life events that contributed to the crisis in the first place.

We shall examine what coping means, how it may be assessed, and the various nursing interventions that may be used to encourage coping. With particular reference to critical care nursing, and using many of the principles of the nursing process, we will use case examples to illustrate the various types of effective and ineffective coping strategies used by families and clients that the critical care nurse will see on a regular basis in a critical care unit.

DEFINITIONS OF COPING

Some general definitions help to set the stage for an examination of coping. Pearlin and Schooler (1978) state, "By coping we refer to the things people do to avoid being harmed by life strains." They go on to say that coping "represents . . . concrete efforts to deal with the life strains they encounter in their different roles" (p. 5). They identify three different types of coping:

1. "Responses that modify the situation," such as negotiation in marriage, discipline of children by parents, and giving and receiving of advice.
2. "Responses that . . . control the meaning of a problem," such as neutralizing responses, selective shutting out, and positive comparisons.

3. Responses that help to manage stress after it has occurred, such as "denial, passive acceptance, withdrawal, magical thinking, hopefulness, avoidance of worry, [and] relaxation."

They discuss several specific mechanisms for coping that include "emotional discharge vs controlled reflectiveness, . . . passive forebearance vs self-assertion, . . . potency vs helpless resignation, . . . optimistic faith" (Pearlin & Schooler, 1978, pp. 6–7).

Coping has also been described as enhancing the adjustment between the individual and the environment, or as attempts to meet the demands of the environment to prevent the inception or continuance of negative consequences. For the purposes of this book, it seems most appropriate to use the definition by Lazarus and Folkman (1984), who describe coping as "constantly changing cognitive and behavioral efforts to manage specific external and/or internal demands that are appraised as taxing or exceeding the resources of the person" (p. 141). This definition focuses on coping strategies that consist of a number of simultaneous or sequential adjustments, and excludes habitual or automatic adjustments to the stresses of daily living.

In a review of the literature, several different styles of coping have been identified. To provide a framework for discussion in this chapter, it is useful to briefly describe these coping methods.

Problem-focused coping consists of direct actions on the environment or on the self to remove or alter circumstances determined to be threatening (Thoits, 1986). The two subcategories are behavioral and cognitive problem-focused coping. The former refers to a method that directly alters situational circumstances that are perceived as threatening. Through this, an individual may consciously avoid or leave the situation, replace particularly threatening aspects with aspects that elicit pleasurable reactions, or construct new solutions to the existing stressors. Avoiding or manipulating the situation itself reduces threat and at least temporarily reduces distress.

The latter refers to cognitive manipulation of the stressors. The individual may reinterpret existing circumstances so that they seem less threatening to the self, and therefore produce less intensely undesirable feelings. This method may be particularly appropriate when the situation is uncontrollable, such as in cases of permanent injury or bereavement, or when the individual lacks the power or the resources necessary to escape or modify the situation. A variation of this method is to remove attention from existing stressful cues.

Emotion-focused coping consists of actions or thoughts designed to control the undesirable feelings that result from stressful circumstances. As Thoits (1986) describes, "If situational features cannot be changed easily in these behavioral or cognitive ways, or if emotional responses are too intense for effective problem solving, an alternative is to engage in emotion-focused coping" (p. 418).

Here again, the two subcategories are behavioral and cognitive emotion-focused coping. The former refers to a process by which an individual can act directly on the physiologic sensations that accompany an undesirable emotional state with stimulants or depressants. One can also resort to the behavioral manipulation of expressive gestures—i.e., if I act positively, I may start to feel positive. The latter refers to techniques such as biofeedback, which can alter physiologic sensations cognitively. A variation of this occurs when an individual reinterprets his or her existing undesirable state by substituting another label for that state, i.e., negative or socially inappropriate feelings can be relabeled with more desirable designations.

Pearlin and Schooler (1978) have added a third broad description of coping, which they call *perception-focused coping*. They describe this as a cognitive attempt to alter the meaning of situational stressful difficulties so that they are perceived as less threatening.

ASSESSMENT OF COPING PATTERNS

The assessment of coping patterns of individuals is at best a difficult task. The critical care nurse has both advantages and disadvantages in such an assessment process. On the positive side, the nurse is typically operating as part of a one-to-one or a one-to-two staffing ratio, which allows for intensive interaction in the nurse–patient relationship. On the negative side, patients in a critical care unit may be in such a state of crisis that coping strategies are not readily apparent. Additionally, the nurse may become heavily involved with the physiologic management of the patient, unable or neglecting to attend to the psychosocial needs of either the patient or family.

It is important, however, for the nurse who is committed to providing comprehensive nursing care to develop a sensitivity to the coping strategies of patients, family members, and significant others. Frequently, these coping strategies affect the psychological intensity of the stressors found in critical care settings.

The critical care nurse has the ability to gather a variety of data as part of the assessment process. These data facilitate the nurse's ability to understand more fully the dynamics of the situation, as well as the ability to use more effectively the skills and knowledge of other members of the health care team, as that may become necessary.

Subjective data may be obtained from several sources. The first is through self-report by the patient, family member, or significant other. When nurses develop the sensitivity to "listen with the third ear," they are able to gain a deeper understanding of what the individual is experiencing and how well the individual feels he or she is coping with the stressors in the given situation.

A second source of data is information gained through structured questioning of patients and their significant others. Significant others may be able to provide information when the patient is unable to because of the severity of illness, language barriers, and/or limited interaction.

What follows are examples of patient- and family-focused questions that may be useful to the nurse in completing an assessment of coping strategies.

- What is it that scares you?
- Is anything scaring you now?
- When you feel tense at home, what helps you relax?
- Have you ever felt powerless before?
- What helps you feel that you're back in control?
- What do you wish would happen?
- If this could turn out any way you wanted, what do you want to happen?
- What would help you to feel better?
- Who in your family are you closest to now?

In addition to verbal information provided by patients and families, behavioral, or nonverbal, information may provide the nurse with major clues. For example:

> Mrs. Greer visits her son, who is dependent on a ventilator, every day. She has learned how to suction him, to manage his ventilator, and to regulate his tube feedings. However, when it comes to setting a date for a trial home visit, Mrs. Greer becomes hesitant and refuses to name a date.

> Jennifer is admitted to your ICU in acute renal failure. It appears that she is rejecting her kidney transplant. She refuses to answer your questions, refuses to have an IV started, and remains curled up under the covers.

> Every time Mrs. Cutter comes to visit her husband, she stands in the doorway of the ICU, crying, unable to move closer to her husband's bed. She never misses visiting hours, but appears unable to interact with her husband.

Each of the case examples presented gives the critical care nurse clues about the present level of coping of the patient and/or family. Using behavioral cues and verbal statements, the nurse can begin to make a judgment as to the nature of that coping and to the degree of its effectiveness.

Additional data may be obtained from several other excellent sources. Other members of the health care team who come into contact with the patient may provide insights into the individual's or family's behavior and feelings, both of which provide signals about the effectiveness or ineffectiveness of the coping behaviors being used. Other members of the health care team who may be useful in gathering and/or providing insight include social workers and clergy.

Assigning a label of effective coping or ineffective coping means the nurse has attached a meaning to the data obtained in assessment, and now has the opportunity to formulate a care plan consistent with that judgment. Currently found in the literature are four nursing diagnostic categories that relate to the concept of coping:

- Coping: Ineffective Individual
- Coping: Family—Potential for Growth
- Coping: Ineffective Family—Compromised
- Coping: Ineffective Family—Disabling

Each shall be identified in terms of definition, cause, and defining characteristics, and will be followed by a case example illustrating the particular diagnostic category. Appropriate nursing interventions shall also be presented and discussed as they relate to critical care nursing.

Coping: Ineffective Individual

This category is defined as the impairment of adaptive behaviors and problem-solving abilities of an individual in meeting life's roles and stressors. The cause may be one or more of the following with relevant examples:

situational crisis—hospitalization, diagnosis of critical illness;
personal vulnerability—intubation, technology-dependence;
little or no exercise—confinement in bed, restraints;
inadequate support systems—limited vising hours, separation from
loved ones;
poor nutrition—NPO, parenteral nutrition;
sensory–perceptual alterations—ICU psychosis;
multiple life changes—hospitalization, dependency, poor or uncertain
prognosis;
unmet personal expectations—poor prognosis, unsuccessful medical
interventions; and
inadequate coping skills—undeveloped or nonexistent.

The defining characteristics of individuals within this group include subjective and objective signs and symptoms. Subjectively, the patient may verbalize an inability to cope or may ask for help. The individual may complain of headaches, lack of appetite, fatigue, insomnia, or an irritable bowel. The individual may express feelings of worry, anxiety, fear, or depression, and overtly may react in anger or frustration, or by withdrawal. Objectively, it may be noted that the individual lacks problem-solving skills, demonstrates destructive behavior toward self and others, changes usual communication patterns, and/or becomes verbally manipulative or abusive.

After having two myocardial infarctions and a diagnostic cardiac catheterization, Mr. Smith has been scheduled for a coronary artery bypass graft. During a preoperative visit, the nurse finds Mr. Smith packing his suitcase. Mr. Smith states, "I'm leaving. I don't need the surgery. I'm fine. I can go back to work tomorrow. Get out and leave me alone."

In acknowledging Mr. Smith's remarks, the nurse asks him to stop packing, and to sit and talk for a minute. She asks about his history of infarctions, the catheterization, and acknowledges that both may be very frightening events. Mr. Smith begins to share his fears—of death, of losing his job, of being dependent, and of not knowing. He asks for help.

Coping: Family—Potential for Growth

This category is defined as one in which the family member or significant other has effectively managed adaptive tasks involved with the patient's health situation, and is demonstrating both a readiness and willingness for health-enhancing activities for self and the patient. As far as the cause is concerned, the patient and/or significant other's basic needs are sufficiently satisfied and adaptive tasks effectively addressed to enable individual goals and personal needs to surface and be met.

The defining characteristics of this category include both subjective and objective data. Subjectively, family members and significant others attempt to describe the positive and negative impacts of the crisis situation on their personal values, priorities, goals, and relationships, e.g., "The family crisis has brought us closer together as a family to meet each other's needs." Individuals express interest in contacting others on an individual or group basis who have experienced a similar situation, e.g., Alanon, Reach for Recovery, Ostomy groups, and Critical Care Support Groups.

Objectively, family members are moving toward health-promoting lifestyles that support and monitor growth processes. They may get involved, when appropriate, in treatment programs, and generally choose experiences that promote individual and family wellness. Overall, there seems to be clear evidence that family members, significant others, and the patient are collectively meeting the demands of the situation in a positive fashion, with the goal of treatment, rehabilitation, and the restoration of health to the extent possible.

Mrs. Evans has been dying in your ICU of sepsis, disseminated intravascular coagulation, and renal failure. She has been unresponsive for several days. Her family has been actively involved throughout her hospitalization, and are aware of her prognosis. They ask you to help set up a meeting between the medical and nursing team and themselves.

Coping: Ineffective Family—Compromised

This category is defined as one in which a usually supportive family member or significant other is providing insufficient, ineffective, or compromised support. In terms of cause, there seem to be inadequate levels of understanding by significant others. A significant other may be preoccupied by trying to handle personal concerns, and is thus unable to perceive or act effectively to meet the needs of the patient. There may be at least temporary family disorganization, as well as changes in the roles played by family members. Other situational or developmental crises the significant other may be facing tend to get in the way of helpful interaction. The patient in turn is unable to provide much support for family members or significant others. There may also be a prolonged disease or progression of disability that has exhausted the supportive capacity of family members and/or significant others.

The defining characteristics of this category include both subjective and objective data. Subjectively, the patient expresses a concern about the response or lack of response by a significant other to the patient's health problem. At the same time, significant others reflect a preoccupation with personal reactions to the patient's illness or disability or to other crises in their lives. In addition, they may describe an inadequate understanding of the situation that interferes with their providing effective support to the patient.

Objectively, family members and others may have attempted to provide support to the patient with unsatisfactory results. Significant individuals may withdraw or restrict themselves to limited communication with the patient at a time when the patient needs support. In an alternative scenario, family members or others may display disproportionate behaviors that are either too much and interfere with the patient's need for autonomy, or too little in relation to the patient's expressed needs.

> Wayne Stevens has been a patient in your ICU for several weeks, status post craniotomy. Although he has intact motor function, at times he moves very slowly. He is able to feed himself. During visiting hours one evening, his wife arrives and finds him eating dinner, again moving slowly. She becomes angry, asking why he is not being helped, and proceeds to take over feeding her husband.

Coping: Ineffective Family—Disabling

This category is defined as one in which the behavior(s) of family members or significant others disables both their capacities and the patient's capacities to deal effectively with the challenge essential for personal and family adaptation to the health situation present. In terms of cause, there may be highly ambivalent family relationships. Significant individuals may have chronically unexpressed feelings of guilt, anxiety, hostility, etc. Arbitrary handling by health team members of a family's resistance to treatment may solidify defensiveness of key individuals, as it fails to deal adequately with underlying feelings. There may be a discrepancy in the coping styles being used by various individuals, including the patient, to deal with the tasks at hand. The discrepancy may result in individuals working at cross purposes.

Additionally, family members may become so overwhelmed that they are unable to cope effectively with the situation at hand. Diagnosis, prognosis, hospitalization, and uncertainty may be too many stressors at any given time. Fear, loss of control, and anxiety may overwhelm a family's ability to support the patient and/or each other.

The defining characteristics of this category include minimal subjective and extensive objective data. Subjectively, key individuals may express despair and disappointment at family members' reactions to the situation at hand. There may be a perceived lack of involvement by significant others.

Objectively, the critical care nurse may see a variety of behaviors by the patient, family members, and/or significant others. These may include a combination of the following: intolerance, abandonment, rejection, desertion, psychosomatic tendencies, agitation, depression, aggression, neglect of self/family, neglect of the patient in regard to needs and/or treatment, distortion of reality or denial regarding diagnosis and/or prognosis, and dependency and/or inability to act.

> Sharon Jacobs is an 18-year-old patient on your unit following her involvement in a motor vehicle accident. She has adult respiratory distress syndrome (ARDS), is on high levels of positive end expiratory pressure (PEEP) and has required multiple chest tubes for pneumothoraces. Her mother has not left your ICU waiting room for three days. She is there for every visiting hour, and never leaves the waiting room, constantly expecting a change in Sharon's condition. She has gotten little uninterrupted sleep, has been eating food from the vending machine, and seems to be alone in her vigil. After missing a 6 P.M. visiting hour, you go to the waiting room and find her sitting on the couch crying. "I can't go in there anymore. I have to, but I can't. Help me."

INTERVENTION STRATEGIES

Once the assessment and diagnostic phases are completed, it is appropriate to move to the planning and implementation stages. It is at this point that the critical care nurse begins to develop a plan of action to help the patient and significant others cope more effectively with the stressors brought about by the health situation.

Generally, one may use a cognitive or an affective approach. Cognitively, the nurse may use both information-giving and teaching techniques. These actions are based on the premise that the individual's coping skills would be enhanced by increasing the level of understanding, providing new information and explanations, and/or providing teaching for all concerned. Affectively, the nurse may concentrate on empathic understanding and enhanced listening skills with the patient and significant others in order to become more aware of the emotional levels present, and to be able to provide increased support when necessary.

Thoits (1986), in discussing techniques of coping assistance, states

"significant others can suggest techniques of stress-management or can participate directly in those efforts, thereby facilitating and strengthening a person's own coping attempts. These actions can alter threatening aspects of the situation, threatening emotional reactions to the situation, or both. In essence, this approach suggests that support works like coping by changing or eliminating the primary sources of threat to the individual. By implication . . . damaged self-esteem, mastery, and identity are thus restored indirectly, rather than directly. That is, support works through the mechanisms of behavioral or cognitive operations on the individual's stressors; self-regard is bolstered as a result." (p. 419)

Pearlin and Schooler (1978) describe a range of coping responses that individuals may use in dealing with the stressors of life. These include the following:

1. Responses that modify the situation and are focused on changing the source of the stress. These include negotiation, optimistic action, self-reliance, and exercise of personal power rather than helpless resignation.
2. Responses that control the meaning of the problem in order to neutralize the threat cognitively. These include positive comparisons, selective ignoring, and/or substitution of rewards.
3. Responses that help the individual manage stress after it has occurred without being overwhelmed by it. These include emotional discharge or venting of feelings, self-assertion of personal needs, and/or passive avoidance of stressors.

Schlossberg (1984), referring to the work of Lazarus, states that

"Lazarus classifies coping in two major ways: instrumental behavior that intends to change the situation and palliative behavior that intends to help minimize individual distress. Whether the individual wants to change the situation or reduce his or her distress, he or she can choose from among four coping modes: information seeking, direct action, inhibition of action, and intrapsychic behavior. The first three seem self-explanatory; the last one (intrapsychic) refers to the thoughts an individual employs to resolve the issue he or she faces. These thoughts, which include denial, wishful thinking, and distortion, enable the individual to carry on." (p. 94)

Schlossberg also reports on a study by Cohen (1980), who looked at ways people coped with surgery. Fifty-nine hernia, gallbladder, and thyroid patients were studied the night before surgery and rated on a continuum from avoidance (avoid information and knowledge about surgery and outcome) to vigilance (seek out information about surgery). Recovery was measured on a

number of levels. Contrary to expectations, neither age nor life change score
was a factor in recovery, but the coping strategy of denial was. In this kind of
situation dependency, passivity, and lack of knowledge seem to be the best
coping mechanisms; too much knowledge can lead to panic. Furthermore,
trying to be in charge of a situation that the individual is unable to control can
lead to frustration (Schlossberg, 1984, pp. 95–96). The Cohen study has interesting implications for the principles of informed consent and health teaching.

It is important for the nurse to take an active role in providing interventions for the individual and family in need. These interventions include

1. Providing continuity through primary nursing or at least stable as-
   signments, through sharing of information, and through consistency of approach by all staff, which requires sharing of information about the plan of care with other nurses and members of
   other disciplines.
2. Teaching about the critical care environment, patient status, and
   reality of the situation.
3. Reinforcement of family/individual strengths in coping, in care giving, and in decision making.
4. Not overwhelming family/individual strengths via continually assessing readiness and the need for intervention and information.
5. Identification of sources of hope, including reality-based sources
   of possibilities as differentiated from wishes, which are not
   grounded in reality.
6. Providing comfort measures, including support of physiologic
   needs for rest and sleep, nutrition, absence of pain, and psychological needs for control, love, and belonging.
7. Allowing for control within the critical care environment in light
   of the patient's prognosis and status, and allowing for active decision making when feasible.

In order to allow greater specificity regarding nursing interventions in critical
care situations, it is helpful to return to the four diagnostic categories described earlier. Each has several suggested priorities of nursing care designed
to facilitate the coping status of the patient and his or her significant others.
The interventions suggested for the first category (Coping: Ineffective Individual) include determining the degree of psychological and physical impairment for the patient; assessing the coping skills of the patient and significant
others who have an impact on the patient; assisting the patient to deal with
the current health situation, including both the physical and psychosocial
needs; providing support through empathic listening and interaction; and
promoting wellness, facilitating rehabilitation, making referrals and consultations, and teaching when appropriate.

The interventions suggested for the second category (Coping: Family—Potential for Growth) include the following: assessing the situation and adaptive skills being used by the patient, family members, and significant others; assisting those concerned to develop their potential for growth in the situation; and promoting understanding through effective teaching. Effective teaching includes working directly with the individuals involved, as well as referring them to appropriate support sources in and out of the medical setting. Finally, the nurse needs to provide ongoing support for family members and reinforce effective coping strategies already being employed.

Interventions for the third category (Coping: Ineffective Family—Compromised) include the following actions: assessing the causative and/or contributory factors that may be affecting individuals; assisting individuals in the reactivation or development of effective coping skills in order to deal with the present health situation; and promoting concepts of wellness through effective health teaching. Again, the latter involves both information giving and appropriate referral when indicated.

The last diagnostic category (Coping: Ineffective Family—Disabling) has the following indicated nursing interventions: assessing the constellation of factors that may be contributing to ineffective patient or family behaviors; providing assistance to family members to help them deal more effectively with the present situation, which may require collaboration with other members of the health care team; incorporating principles of effective health teaching in order to promote wellness; and assisting the family in contacting and using appropriate support resources.

EVALUATION

The final stage of the nursing process is the evaluation phase, i.e., determining how effective the nursing intervention has been in meeting the covert and expressed needs of the situation. In the final analysis, evaluation may perhaps be done most effectively by a combination of observation, reflection, validation, reassessment, listening, and communication with other members of the health care team. Through direct observation, the critical care nurse is in an excellent position to observe the patient's coping behaviors, as well as the quality of interaction with family members and significant others. This helps in determining not only what exists (assessment and diagnosis), but also what has possibly changed as interventions are tried and/or the dynamics of the situation change.

Through active listening to the patient and significant others, the nurse may gain insight into their current thoughts and feelings. Demonstrated empathic understanding will help individuals express fears, raise questions, and seek support when they are experiencing feelings that seem to be overwhelming their coping skills. Finally, interaction with other members of the health care team will assist the critical care nurse not only in being alert to the unmet needs, but also in using the myriad of support personnel and groups available within and outside of the medical setting.

Key to the evaluation phase is continued reassessment. It is important to note that patients and family members may move between diagnostic categories, that is, successful coping may be replaced with ineffective or unsuccessful coping over time, with changes in prognosis, and as hopes are lost. As intervention strategies differ, it is important continually to reevaluate the current state of functioning of individuals and families.

Lastly, it is important to emphasize the value of documentation. Documentation organizes data and provides for continuity. It becomes a mechanism to note change over time. Documentation is the last step in the nursing process, and is an integral part of care.

BIBLIOGRAPHY

Cohen, F. (1980). Coping with surgery: Information, psychologic preparation and recovery. In L. W. Poon (Ed.) *Aging in the 1980's: Psychologic issues.* (pp. 69–81). Washington, DC: American Psychological Association.

Lazarus, R. S., & Folkman, S. (1984). *Stress, appraisal, and coping.* New York: Springer.

Pearlin, L. I., & Schooler, C. (1978). The structure of coping. *Journal of Health and Social Behavior, 19,* 2–21.

Schlossberg, N. K. (1984). *Counseling adults in transition.* New York: Springer.

Thoits, P. A. (1986). Social support as coping assistance. *Journal of Consulting and Clinical Psychology, 54*(4), 416–423.

ADDITIONAL READINGS

Jennings, C. (1986). Children's understanding of death and dying. *Focus on Critical Care, 13*(2), 41–45.

Leske, J. (1986). Needs of relatives of critically ill patients: A follow-up. *Heart and Lung, 15*(2), 189–193.

Nyamathi, A., & Van Servellen, G. (1989). Maladaptive coping in the critically ill population with acquired immunodeficiency syndrome: Nursing assessment and treatment. *Heart and Lung, 18*(2): 113–120.

Raffin, T., Shurkin, J., & Sinkler, W. (1989). *Intensive care: facing the critical choices.* New York: W. H. Freeman.

Schoenhofer, S. (1989). Affectional touch in critical care nursing: A descriptive study. *Heart and Lung, 18*(2), 146–154.

Slade, M. (1986, October 13). Handling crises, big or little. *The New York Times,* p. 4C.

5 Behavioral Responses to the Critical Care Environment

Vickie A. Lambert, D.N.Sc., F.A.A.N.
Clinton E. Lambert, Jr., M.S.N., C.S.

Patients enter the environment of the surgical intensive care unit (SICU) when health status warrants continuous observation and intense delivery of health care. Patients entering the SICU often find themselves attached to various monitoring and drainage devices, in pain, and hearing the unfamiliar sounds of various pieces of mechanical equipment. Such a scenario does not exemplify the peace and quiet traditionally associated with the environment needed for recovery from a serious illness. Instead, as research has shown (Helton, Gordon, & Nunnery, 1980; Katz, Agle, & DePalma, 1972; Taylor, 1971; Kornfeld, Heller, Frank, & Mosowitz, 1974; Ballard, 1981), the environment of critical care units tends to incite stress responses on the part of the patient. Dealing with the stress of the acute health care situation that has placed the individual in the critical care unit is, in and of itself, very stressful without the added burden of dealing with the stressors of the environment.

The nurse is the one health care provider who is continuously attending to the needs of the critically ill surgical patient. Therefore, the nurse is in the best position to deal with the patient's responses to the stressors of the immediate surroundings. This chapter will address what the nurse must consider when assessing needs, diagnosing signs and symptoms, prescribing care, intervening, and evaluating the results of the prescribed interventions in regard to the patient's behavioral responses to the stressful environment.

HUMAN STRESS RESPONSE

In order to understand what constitutes appropriate assessment, diagnosis, and intervention with regard to a patient's behavioral response to the critical care environment, a nurse first must have an understanding of the human stress response. Dealing with the ramifications of a critical care environment is highly stressful and the stress experienced by the patient is compounded by his or her decreased psychological resilience and increased physical incapacitation.

Stress, as defined by Lazarus, Averill, and Opton (1974), is the psychobiologic appraisal of stimuli that are highly relevant to one's welfare, whether this relevance be positive or negative. According to Lambert and Lambert (in press) the stress process is composed of two basic components: situational factors and personal factors. Situational factors include environmental and personal events that place adaptive requirements on an individual and external adaptive mechanisms that aid the individual in dealing with the stressful event. Environmental and personal events include such things as strange noises, unrecognizable health care providers, or illness, while external adaptive mechanisms include such things as the presence of a significant other or social support system. Personal factors include the person's physical capabilities, personality structure, and prior experiences in dealing with stressful events.

Situational factors and personal factors coexist, and are continually interacting. When the balance between the demands placed on the individual by an event and the available personal and external resources for dealing with the event is disrupted, the event, such as being a patient in a critical care unit, is perceived as stressful by the individual. By comparison, adaptation to the event occurs when the personal and external resources are sufficiently available and mobilized to meet the demands of the event.

When the individual encounters a situation, potential stressors are sensed by receptor organs (i.e., visual, auditory, olfactory, gustatory, enteroceptive, thermal, touch, and proprioceptive) and impulses are sent to the cerebral cortex (cortical pathway), directly to the thalamus without passing through the cortex (thalamic pathway), or to both areas (West, 1985) (Figure 5–1). Neural impulses that travel by way of the cortical pathway are processed to memory. If logical or symbolic analogy concludes that the stimulus is a stressful event, signals are passed to the limbic system, where unpleasant emotions are generated; to the ascending reticular activating system, which increases the level of cortical arousal; and to the hypothalamus, which activates neural and hormonal responses (Figure 5–2). Stimuli traveling by way of the cortical pathway result in a conscious awareness of stress. By comparison, neural impulses that travel by way of the thalamic pathway and go directly to the sensory receptors of the thalamus and hypothalamus (Figure 5–3) do not stimulate conscious awareness of stress. The existence of the thalamic pathway helps to explain why some critical care patients do not report the presence of stress-related feelings when they are manifesting physical and/or behavioral responses to stress.

Both cortical and thalamic stimulation activate the hypothalamus, which in turn produces increased neuromuscular tone via activation of the gamma motor neurons, stimulation of the sympathetic nervous system, discharge of

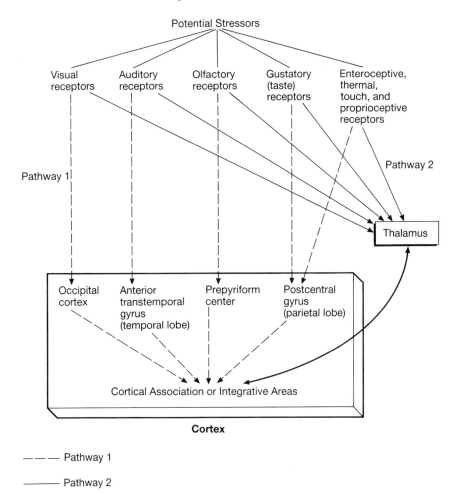

Figure 5–1.   Activation of neuroanatomic pathways of the stress reaction. From "Stressors and Stress in Critical Care" by J. Harris, 1984, *Critical Care Nurse, 4*(1), p. 86. Copyright 1984 by Cahners Publishing Co. Reprinted with permission.

releasing and inhibiting factors to the anterior pituitary, and release of antidiuretic hormone from the posterior pituitary gland (West, 1985). As shown in Figures 5–4 and 5–5, activation of the sympathetic nervous system and pituitary gland produces a myriad of responses. These responses prepare the body for "fight or flight," but can result in dysfunction or disease if maintained for long periods (Harris, 1984). For example, mineralocorticoid-induced electrolyte changes are a preparation for volume loss. If volume loss does not occur, the hypervolemia, hypokalemia, and catabolism that occur can prove detrimental. The enhancement of clotting mechanisms is beneficial in the event of an injury, however, thrombi and/or emboli can also result. Increases in blood pressure and volume and vasoconstriction are responses

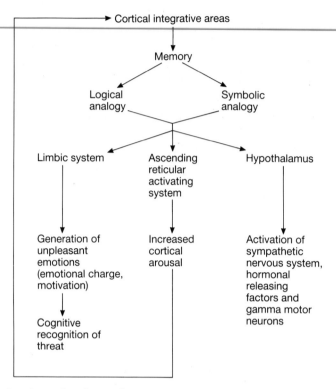

Figure 5–2. Cortical pathway of stress activation. From "Stressors and Stress in Critical Care" by J. Harris, 1984, *Critical Care Nurse, 4*(1), p. 86. Copyright 1984 by Cahners Publishing Co. Reprinted with permission.

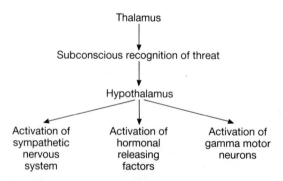

Figure 5–3. Thalamic pathway of stress activation. From "Stressors and Stress in Critical Care" by J. Harris, 1984, *Critical Care Nurse, 4*(1), p. 86. Copyright 1984 by Cahners Publishing Co. Reprinted with permission.

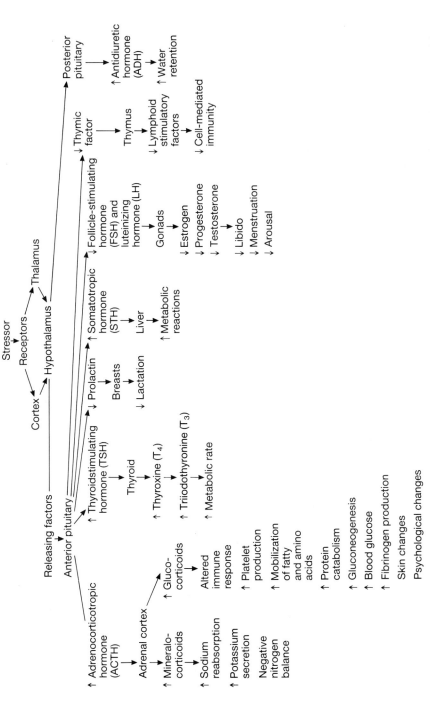

Figure 5–4. The endocrine response to a stressor. From "Stressors and Stress in Critical Care" by J. Harris, 1984, *Critical Care Nurse, 4*(1), p. 88. Copyright 1984 by Cahners Publishing Co. Reprinted with permission.

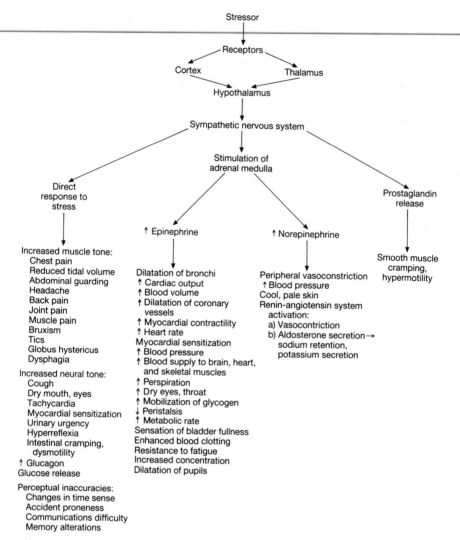

Figure 5–5. Sympathetic nervous system activation during stress.

to anticipated blood loss. If blood loss does not occur, local vasoconstriction and hypertension can cause tissue damage. An increase in serum fatty acids proves helpful as a source of energy, but prolonged hyperlipidemia can lead to arteriosclerosis. Even suppression of reproductive function that occurs as a result of the stress response can become a social liability if continued over a long period. Thus it is important that the nurse be cognizant of the human stress response and how it may influence the welfare of the already compromised patient in the critical care setting.

ASSESSMENT

In order to diagnose and prescribe appropriate treatment for the patient responding to the critical care environment, a thorough assessment of the patient must be carried out. Both objective and subjective data are necessary in order to attain a thorough understanding of how the patient is reacting to his or her surroundings and to validate the nurse's conclusions about the patient.

Objective Data

As previously discussed, an individual's reaction to a stressful situation, such as his or her presence in a critical care unit, incites a multitude of both physiologic and psychosocial responses. Some of the more prevalent responses that occur and that should be closely monitored by the nurse are listed in Table 5–1.

Any one of the responses listed in Table 5–1 could be due to a change in the patient's illness or disease state. Therefore, it is imperative that the nurse, by way of a process of differential diagnosis, determine if these responses are the result of a change in illness state, the patient's response to the SICU environment, or both.

Subjective Data

To validate much of the objective patient data, the nurse must also obtain subjective data. If the critical care nurse does not verify perceptions with the patient, he or she is practicing in a robotic, nontherapeutic manner. Nursing assessment that includes consultation with the patient is more likely to yield correct diagnoses and effective nursing prescriptions and interventions.

Subjective data that are found most prevalently in a patient in the SICU environment include description of fears about the environment, expressions about having difficulty sleeping, expressions about feeling restless, expressions about having difficulty remembering what the nurse or physician has told the patient about the illness or related therapies, expressions about having difficulty carrying on a conversation with health care providers and signif-

Table 5–1   Responses to Stressful Situations: Objective Data

Physiologic

Increase in blood pressure

Cool, pale skin

Increased perspiration

Increased dryness in the eyes and throat

Increased rate and depth of respirations

Dilated pupils

Rapid shifts in body temperature

Diarrhea

Urinary urgency

Enuresis

Decreased appetite

Rapid, extreme shifts in menstrual flow for women in childbearing years

Increased muscle tension (rigidity)

Fatigue

Muscle tremors

Restlessness

Chest pain

Headaches

Difficulty swallowing

Hyperactive reflexes

Distortion in auditory, visual, olfactory, gustatory, tactile, and kinesthetic sensory perception (i.e., failure to respond to verbal stimuli; holding objects too close or at a distance for viewing; squinting; double vision; decreased sensitivity to odors and taste; paresthesia, hyperesthesia, or anesthesia; vertigo; and inability to sit or stand)

Psychosocial

Decreased attention span

Decreased ability to follow directions

Increased acting out behavior

Increased question asking

Constant seeking of reassurance

Frequent shifts in topics of conversation

Focusing on the presence of mechanical equipment and medical procedures

Frequent, inappropriate requests for pain medications

Behavior not consistent with developmental age level

Avoidance in focusing on feelings

Inappropriate dependency

Easy arousal

Frequent awakening

Gross disorientation

Paranoia

Psychosis

icant others, expressions of low self-worth, expressions about feeling powerless, expressions about feeling depressed, and expressions of self-blame for
the illness. Several of these subjective data items (i.e., expressions about difficulty sleeping, restlessness, memory, and conversation) also could be the
result of changes in the patient's physical health status. Therefore, like the
objective data, subjective data must be closely analyzed and submitted to the
process of differential diagnosis.

RELATED NURSING DIAGNOSES

Once sufficient objective and subjective data have been gathered in regard to
the patient's response to the critical care environment, the nurse must use
clinical judgment to identify the relevant diagnoses. The diagnoses made
most commonly as a result of the examination of the data include ineffective
individual coping, sensory–perceptual alteration, sleep pattern disturbance,
powerlessness, and social isolation.

Ineffective Individual Coping

Ineffective individual coping is the person's inability to engage in adaptive
behaviors to meet life's demands, such as dealing with the critical care environment. The objective and subjective data indicative of a diagnosis of ineffective individual coping are likely to include any number of the responses listed
in Table 5–1 and above. In other words, the signs and symptoms of ineffective
coping coincide with those of the human response to stress. The objective
and subjective data manifested may begin with some of the less dramatic
responses, such as headaches, increased pulse, perspiration, inappropriate
verbal statements and behaviors, and decreased attention span and progress
to more major ones, such as gross disorientation, paranoia, and psychosis.
The factors that most likely contribute to a diagnosis of ineffective individual
coping include the catastrophic illness that has placed the individual in the
critical care environment, the critical care environment itself, and separation
from family or significant others as a result of being hospitalized. However,
before a diagnosis of ineffective individual coping can be made, the nurse
must, by way of the process of differential diagnosis, rule out other diagnoses,
such as powerlessness, sensory–perceptual alteration, alteration in thought
processes, and dysfunctional anxiety (Kelly, 1985). Ineffective coping is discussed in greater detail in chapter 4.

Sensory–Perceptual Alteration

Sensory–perceptual alteration, another common diagnosis related to the patient's response to the critical care environment, is the interruption or change
in reception and/or interpretation of stimuli by receptors for hearing, sight,
smell, taste, touch, and body position and motion. The objective and subjective data indicative of a diagnosis of sensory–perceptual alteration for the

critical care patient are likely to be a distortion in auditory, visual, olfactory, gustatory, tactile, and kinesthetic sensory perception; decreased appetite; headaches; decreased attention span; and expressions about having difficulty remembering things or carrying on a conversation. Factors that most likely contribute to such a diagnosis include continuous exposure to excessive noise, such as mechanical equipment and conversation of staff (Hansell, 1984); constant lighting conditions; a reduction in meaningful sensory stimuli; impaired communication; sleep deprivation; general immobility and the restriction of head and neck motion due to the presence of a subclavian catheter, intravenous catheter, or intracranial pressure monitoring lines or the presence of an endotracheal tube; inflammation or obstruction of the nasal or oral passages due to the presence of drainage and breathing tubes or an oxygen cannula; the presence of various anesthesia states due to general, local, or regional anesthetics; and response to medications such as narcotics, analgesics, tranquilizers, sedatives, muscle relaxants, or antihistamines (Table 5–2). Before a diagnosis of sensory–perceptual alterations can be made, the nurse must examine all of the existing data and rule out, by way of differential diagnosis, other diagnoses such as impaired physical mobility, impairment of skin integrity, and alteration in tissue perfusion (Kelly, 1985).

A severe form of sensory–perceptual alteration experienced by an estimated 12.5 to 38% of conscious patients in the critical care setting is frequently referred to as "ICU psychosis" (Easton & Mackenzie, 1988). This syndrome is described as a "global clouding of consciousness, resulting from a potentially reversible impairment of the ability to maintain attention and cognitive processes" (Ballard, 1981, p. 89). The patient's ability to think, perceive, and remember decreases, as does his or her ability to be oriented to time, place, and person. Disorientation, confusion, illusions, delusions, and hallucinations may be experienced. Intensive care psychosis typically manifests itself on the third to the seventh day of the critical care unit stay and subsides within 48 hours after discharge from the unit (Laynet & Yudofsky, 1971). Research has suggested that the critical care environment is the most important causal factor of the resulting psychosis (Kornfeld et al., 1974), since patients generally have a two- to three-day lucid period in which the critical care environment is experienced before the psychosis begins. The highest incidence of ICU psychosis reportedly occurs in the SICU (Easton & MacKenzie, 1988). ICU psychosis compromises the patient's recuperative powers, since the individual is directing his or her energies toward coping with the stressors of the ICU environment rather than toward the healing process (Fisher & Moxham, 1984).

A sensory–perceptual alteration can have detrimental effects on the quality of life experienced by the patient in the critical care unit. Alterations, even minor ones, may lead to a major loss in communication, which could impede the nurse's ability to evaluate the patient's response to therapy and present a threat to the safety and well-being of the individual. The nursing diagnosis, potential for injury, may also be appropriate in this situation. In addition, lack

Table 5–2 Potential Psychological Side Effects of Pharmacologic Agents Commonly Used in Critical Care Areas

Name	Effect
Aminocaproic acid	Acute delirium, hallucinations
Anticonvulsants	Tactile, auditory, and visual hallucinations, delirium, agitation, paranoia, confusion
Antihistamines	Anxiety, hallucinations, delirium
Atropine and anticholinergics	Confusion, memory loss, delirium, auditory and visual hallucinations, paranoia
Barbiturates	Visual hallucinations, depression
Cephalosporins	Confusion, disorientation, paranoia
Corticosteroids	Depression, confusion, paranoia, hallucinations
Digitalis glycosides	Nightmares, confusion, delusions, hallucinations, paranoia
Diazepam	Hallucinations, depression
Lidocaine	Disorientation, hallucinations, paranoia
Methyldopa	Hallucinations, paranoia, nightmares
Morphine	Transient hallucinations, disorientation, visual disturbances
Penicillin G	Hallucinations, disorientation, confusion, agitation
Albuterol	Hallucinations, paranoia

From "Sensory–Perceptual Alterations: Delirium in the Intensive Care Unit" by C. Easton and F. Mackenzie, 1988, *Heart and Lung, 17*(3), p. 231. Copyright 1988 by C. V. Mosby. Reprinted with permission.

of knowledge and understanding about sensory–perceptual alterations that a patient may be experiencing can greatly increase the stress response of family members. Unless family members are provided with adequate information about a sensory–perceptual alteration that their loved one may be experiencing, they may fear that a life-threatening change in health status has occurred.

Sleep Pattern Disturbance

Sleep pattern disturbance, a third type of diagnosis common in the patient who is responding to the critical care environment, is the failure to achieve required rest and/or sleep resulting in adverse physical, mental, and emotional changes. Rarely does the critically ill surgical patient sleep more than a few hours at a time; this is due to routine external interruptions such as monitoring of vital signs, suctioning, and positioning. It is not uncommon for the critically ill patient to demonstrate signs and symptoms of sleep pattern disturbance after 2 to 5 days in the intensive care unit. Since sleep serves to maintain and rebuild one's physiologic and psychological function, sleep pattern disturbance will produce stress and its concomitant responses. In a study of patients undergoing open heart surgery, Kornfeld, Zimbert, & Malm (1965) found that sleep pattern disturbance with the added stress of surgery was a major contributing factor in the occurrence of ineffective individual coping (ICU psychosis). Ballard (1981), in a study of postoperative surgical intensive care patients, supported the findings of Kornfeld and associates (1965) by finding sleep pattern disturbances to be a significantly stressful aspect of the environment. Fortunately, studies suggest that patients recover from sleep pattern disturbances after one night of uninterrupted sleep (Helton et al., 1980; Kornfeld, 1972). The recovery usually occurs after transfer from the critical care unit to a less intense hospital environment.

The objective and subjective data indicative of a diagnosis of sleep pattern disturbance for the SICU patient are likely to include enuresis, fatigue, restlessness, distortions in sensory perception, decreased attention span, decreased ability to follow directions, easy arousal, frequent awakening, paranoia, gross disorientation, expressions about having difficulty sleeping, and expressions about feeling restless. Factors that most likely contribute to a diagnosis of sleep pattern disturbance include postoperative pain; being placed in unfamiliar surroundings, such as the SICU; environmental noises; interruptions in sleep patterns due to the administration of required treatments; and the emotional response to the stress of illness and its related treatments. The effect of the critical care environment on usual sleep patterns is discussed in depth in chapter 10. As with the preceding diagnoses, before a diagnosis of sleep pattern disturbance can be made, the nurse must rule out through the process of differential diagnosis other diagnoses such as fear, impaired gas exchange, dysfunctional anxiety, ineffective individual coping, and pain (Kelly, 1985).

Powerlessness

Powerlessness, the perception that one's own action will not effect change in self or the environment, is another common diagnosis for patients who are in the critical care environment. According to Lambert and Lambert (1981), an individual who is in an acute state of physical illness, such as the patient in the critical care setting, is a prime candidate for the diagnosis of powerlessness. Powerlessness is discussed in relation to a model of crisis in chapter 3.

The subjective and objective data indicative of a diagnosis of powerlessness are likely to include increased acting out behavior; increased question asking; frequent shifts in topics of conversation; focusing on the presence of mechanical equipment and medical procedures; inappropriate dependency; and expressions about low self-worth, feelings of powerlessness, and depression. Factors that most likely contribute to the occurrence of powerlessness in the critically ill patient include the presence of the major illness that placed the individual in the critical care unit and impaired physical mobility due to the illness and related treatments. In a study of postoperative critically ill patients, Ballard (1981) found that physical immobility due to the illness and related treatments was the most stressful element of the surgical intensive care environment. The immobilization, as stated by the patients in the study, was primarily due to attachment to some type of therapeutic equipment. Before a diagnosis of powerlessness justifiably can be made, the nurse must rule out, by way of the process of differential diagnosis, the following diagnoses: alteration in thought processes, dysfunctional grieving, anxiety, disturbance in self-concept, fear, knowledge deficit, and ineffective individual coping (Kelly, 1985).

The experience of ill health can bring with it numerous occasions for experiencing powerlessness. Patients who seek assistance from health care providers in maintaining or restoring health have surrendered some degree of control over their lives. When hospitalization in a critical care environment occurs, the degree of lost control is compounded.

The patient's family may experience the same sense of powerlessness as does the patient in the critical care environment. Family members often feel that there is nothing that they can do to assist the patient during the critical care stay, and that they and the patient are at the "mercy" of critical care providers. Lack of familiarity with the treatments prescribed, terminology used, and equipment present in the critical care unit only compound the family's feeling of lack of control (Johnson, 1986; Leske, 1986). Family members will manifest many of the same signs and symptoms of powerlessness as the patient.

Social Isolation

Social isolation, the fifth and final diagnosis frequently manifested by the patient in the critical care environment, is the lack of interpersonal contact or involvement with other individuals or groups who provide support or socialization. Isolation or separation from interpersonal contact and involvement with significant others can prevent successful adjustment to health problems, since relationships with others contributes to one's identity, self-esteem, and general well-being (Northouse, 1982; Lambert, 1985; Lambert & Lambert, 1985).

The subjective and objective data indicative of a diagnosis of social isolation are likely to include constant seeking of reassurance; frequent, inappropriate requests for pain medication; behavior not consistent with developmental age; expressions about feeling depressed; and expression of self-blame for the illness. Factors that most likely contribute to the occurrence of social isolation in the critically ill surgical patient include being separated from one's spouse or significant other and not being able to be with family and friends. Often these separations are imposed by the policies of the critical care unit regarding visitation times. Ballard (1981) found that being separated from one's spouse and being able to see family and friends for only a few minutes each day were two highly stressful situations for patients in a surgical intensive care unit. Before a diagnosis of social isolation can be made, the nurse must rule out, through the process of differential diagnosis, the diagnoses of ineffective individual coping, dysfunctional grieving, powerlessness, and disturbance in self-concept (Kelly, 1985).

PLANNING AND INTERVENTIONS

Once nursing diagnoses are made, the nurse moves on to plan and carry out the appropriate interventions. Most interventions involve compassionate and prudent nursing care; however, some may require changes in the physical design and/or policies and procedures of the nursing unit. The nursing interventions for the five diagnoses related to a patient's behavioral response to the critical care environment (ineffective individual coping, sensory–perceptual alteration, sleep pattern disturbance, powerlessness, and social isolation) are presented below.

Ineffective Individual Coping

Ineffective individual coping, as stated previously, is the person's inability to engage in adaptive behaviors to meet life's demands, such as dealing with the critical care environment. To assist the individual in coping with the demands of the critical care environment the nurse will find it helpful to

1. provide continuity of care by assigning the same nursing staff to the patient. Such continuity lessens the number of new adjustments required by the patient.
2. use discretion when emergency care is being provided to patients undergoing an acute episode. Blocking emergency procedures from the sight of adjacent patients assists in decreasing unnecessary stressful input.
3. allow the patient's significant others reasonable visitation privileges. Availability of social support systems can greatly enhance one's ability to cope effectively with a stressful situation.
4. respond to all questions in a compassionate manner no matter how trite the question may seem. The critically ill patient's memory and ability to communicate verbally may be impaired temporarily because of the illness and related treatments.
5. tell the patient what is being done during a therapeutic procedure. Since most activities and procedures carried out in the criti-

cal care unit are completely foreign to the patient, when they occur they can be very stress provoking.

Sensory–Perceptual Alteration

Sensory–perceptual alteration is the interruption or change in reception and/or interpretation of stimuli by receptors for hearing, sight, smell, taste, touch, and body position and motion. To assist the critically ill surgical patient in preventing the occurrence of or in dealing with the existence of a sensory–perceptual alteration, the nurse will find it helpful to

1. alter sensory monotony by eliminating continuous low-level noises such as the buzzing of a faulty fluorescent light. Such sound can become almost hypnotic after hours of exposure.
2. eliminate as much noise as possible, such as unnecessary staff conversation and machinery that is noisy because of faulty functioning. Lower the sound level of monitor alarms and noise.
3. provide early mobility according to the patient's ability. Simply sitting on the side of the bed or in a chair for a few minutes can place an entirely different perspective on one's perception of the surroundings.
4. orient the patient consistently to time, place, person, and current events through the use of clocks, calendars, windows, radios with earphones, and television. Studies have shown that patients in windowless environments experience organic delirium twice as frequently as patients in units with windows (Wilson, 1972).
5. explain environmental sights and sounds to the patient. Since the patient may be recovering from anesthesia or be responding to sense-altering medications, his perceptions of the surroundings may be highly altered.
6. provide the patient with any prescribed sensory devices, such as a hearing aid or eyeglasses. When one cannot hear or see effectively without a prescribed sensory device, undoubtedly sensory–perceptual alterations will occur.
7. maintain the integrity of the nasal and oral mucosa by cleansing and providing tissue lubrication as needed.
8. provide family members with information concerning any sensory alteration that they observe the patient to be experiencing.
9. acknowledge the reality of sensory–perceptual alterations to the patient and family and provide reassurance as to the temporary nature of such alterations. Providing information as to the origins and incidence of ICU psychosis may ease the family's anxiety and promote their participation in care and in reassuring the patient that cognitive capacity has not been permanently affected.

Sleep Pattern Disturbance

Sleep pattern disturbance is the failure to achieve required rest and/or sleep, which results in adverse physical, mental, and emotional changes. To assist the critically ill surgical patient in acquiring adequate rest, the nurse may find it helpful to

1. minimize the visual and auditory presence of monitoring equipment by situating it away from or behind the patient's bed.
2. design nursing protocols that permit the greatest number of completed sleep cycles. If a patient must be awakened, the interruptions should be brief, comprehensive, and well coordinated.
3. lower the lights in the patient's room or sleeping area of the critical care unit at night to maintain day–night/waking–sleep cycles. Since one's sleep cycles are governed by the sun rising and setting, such an activity will assist in maintaining the patient's normal sleep behavior.
4. be sure that the patient is receiving adequate medication for postoperative pain and that other measures intended to promote comfort and reduce anxiety are included in the plan of care. In many situations the patient may not be sleeping because of pain and/or anxiety.
5. familiarize the patient with the surroundings. Lack of familiarity with surroundings can contribute to sleeplessness.

Powerlessness

Powerlessness is the perception that one's own action will not effect change in self or the environment. Interventions directed toward powerlessness and that are specific to the stage of crisis being experienced are discussed in chapter 3. To assist the critically ill patient in dealing with feelings of powerlessness the nurse may find it advantageous to

1. provide early mobility according to the patient's capabilities. Remove restrictive devices when possible, such as monitoring equipment, which can minimize activity because of the monitor's cables. Simply being able to move about to some degree can assist the individual in feeling that he or she has some sense of control over self and the environment.
2. involve the patient in decision making about care. Having input into such activities as when daily hygiene needs are carried out, what type of food or fluids will be served (if the patient is on oral intake), and when ambulation activities will take place can enhance the individual's sense of control.
3. keep the patient and family members informed of what type of therapeutic and diagnostic procedures are going to be carried out

and what purpose is served by the equipment in the environment (Norris & Grove, 1986). Knowledge assists one in having some control over one's surroundings. Research has suggested that an education–orientation program for family members, which addresses aspects of the critical care environment, may be an effective means for reducing the stress response in families visiting their significant other who is hospitalized in the intensive care unit (Chaves & Faber, 1987).

4. encourage the patient and family members to verbalize feelings, to examine the reality of those feelings, and to identify ways to cope. Suppressing feelings of low self-worth, lack of control, and depression only prolongs and perpetuates a sense of powerlessness.

Social Isolation

Social isolation is the lack of interpersonal contact or involvement with other individuals or groups who provide support or socialization. To assist the critically ill surgical patient in dealing with feelings of social isolation the nurse may find it beneficial to

1. encourage cognitive functioning. Having the individual involved in some form of mental activity, such as watching television or conversing with health care providers, family, and friends can enhance his or her interaction with the environment.
2. provide reasonable visitation privileges to significant others. Availability of social support systems enhances one's ability to interact appropriately with the environment.

EVALUATION

Once the nursing interventions have been planned and carried out, evaluation of the effectiveness of the interventions must be made. The specific outcome criteria that the nurse needs to examine in relation to each of the five diagnoses are listed below.

Ineffective Individual Coping

To determine whether the interventions carried out were successful in assisting the patient in the ability to cope effectively, the nurse will find it helpful to look for

1. a decrease or cessation of the physiologic responses to stress, such as a decrease in pulse rate, cessation of diarrhea, or increased restfulness. (For a complete list of the physiologic stress responses, refer to Table 5–1.)

2. a decrease or cessation of the psychosocial responses to stress, such as increased attention span, expressions of self-worth, and lack of paranoid feelings. (For a complete list of the psychosocial stress responses, refer to Table 5–1.)

Sensory–Perceptual Alteration

To determine whether the interventions carried out were successful in assisting the patient in dealing with sensory–perceptual alterations, the nurse will find it helpful to look for

1. correct auditory, visual, olfactory, gustatory, tactile, and kinesthetic sensory perceptions,
2. an increase in appetite,
3. a lack of headaches,
4. increased attention span,
5. increased ability to remember things,
6. ability to carry on a coherent conversation.

Sleep Pattern Disturbance

To determine whether the interventions carried out were successful in assisting the patient with sleep pattern disturbance, the nurse will find it helpful to look for

1. cessation in enuresis, fatigue, and restlessness;
2. correct sensory perception;
3. increased attention span;
4. increased ability to follow directions;
5. lack of frequent awakening;
6. cessation of paranoid feelings;
7. orientation as to time, place, person, and current events;
8. expressions of feeling rested.

Powerlessness

To determine whether the interventions carried out were successful in assisting the patient and family in dealing with a sense of powerlessness, the nurse will find it helpful to look for

1. cessation of acting out behavior,
2. appropriate question asking,
3. appropriate level of dependency,
4. acceptance of the presence of mechanical equipment in the environment and of necessary medical procedures,
5. expressions of self-worth, of feeling in control, and of general well-being.

Social Isolation

To determine whether the interventions carried out were successful in assisting the patient to deal with feelings of social isolation, the nurse will find it helpful to look for

1. expressions of feeling in control,
2. appropriate requests for pain medication,
3. behavior consistent with developmental age level,
4. expressions of general well-being.

SUMMARY

The surgical patient who is subjected to a critical care environment must deal with a new and very stressful situation. In order to provide comprehensive psychosocial care to the patient, the nurse must be skilled in assessing objective and subjective data, making a diagnosis, prescribing care, intervening, and evaluating the results of the prescribed care. Each of these salient points has been addressed in relation to the potential behavioral responses by a critically ill surgical patient to the critical care environment.

BIBLIOGRAPHY

Ballard, K. (1981). Identification of environmental stressors for patients in a surgical intensive care unit. *Issues in Mental Health Nursing, 3,* 98–108.

Chaves, C., & Faber, L. (1987). Effect of an education-orientation program on family members who visit their significant other in the intensive care unit. *Heart and Lung, 16*(1), 92–99.

Easton, C., & Mackenzie, F. (1988). Sensory–perceptual alterations: Delirium in the intensive care unit. *Heart and Lung, 17*(3), 229–237.

Fisher, M., & Moxham, P. (1984). ICU syndrome. *Critical Care Nurse, 4*(3), 39–46.

Hansell, H. N. (1984). The behavioral effects of noise on man: The patient with intensive care unit psychosis. *Heart and Lung, 13,* 59–65.

Harris, J. (1984). Stressors and stress in critical care. *Critical Care Nurse, 4*(1), 84–97.

Helton, M., Gordon, S., & Nunnery, S. (1980). The correlation between sleep deprivation and the intensive care unit syndrome. *Heart and Lung, 9*(3), 464–468.

Johnson, S. (1986). 10 ways to help the family of a critically ill patient. *Nursing '86, 16*(1), 50–53.

Katz, N., Agle, D., & DePalma, R. (1972). Delirium in surgical patients under intensive care. *Archives of Surgery, 104*(3), 310–313.

Kelly, M. (1985). *Nursing diagnosis source book: Guideline for clinical application.* Norwalk, CT: Appleton-Century-Crofts.

Kornfeld, D. (1972). The hospital environment: Its impact on the patient. *Advances in Psychosomatic Medicine, 8,* 252–270.

Kornfeld, D., Heller, S., Frank, K., & Moskowitz, R. (1974). Personality and psychological factors in post-cardiotomy delirium. *Archives of General Psychiatry, 31,* 249–253.

Kornfeld, D., Zimbert, S., & Malm, J. (1965). Psychiatric complications of open-heart surgery. *New England Journal of Medicine, 273,* 287–292.

Lambert, V. (1985). Study of factors associated with psychological well-being in rheumatoid arthritic women. *Image: The Journal of Nursing Scholarship, 17*(2), 50–53.

Lambert, V., & Lambert, C. (1981). Role theory and the concept, powerlessness. *Journal of Psychosocial Nursing and Mental Health Services, 19*(9), 11–14.

Lambert, V., & Lambert, C. (1985). The relationship between social support and psychological well-being in rheumatoid arthritic women from two ethnic groups. *Health Care for Women International, 6*(5 & 6), 405–414.

Lambert, V., & Lambert, C. (in press). Theories of stress and adaptation. In L. Burrell (Ed.). *Adult Nursing.* Norwalk, CT: Appleton-Lange.

Laynet, O., & Yudofsky, S. (1971). Postoperative psychosis in cardiotomy patient. *New England Journal of Medicine, 248,* 518–520.

Lazarus, R., Averill, J., & Opton, E. (1974). The psychology of coping: Issues of research and assessment. In G. Coelho, D. Hamburg, and J. Adams (Eds.). *Coping and adaptation.* New York: Basic Books.

Leske, J. (1986). Needs of relatives of critically ill patients: A followup. *Heart and Lung, 15*(2), 189–193.

Norris, L., & Grove, S. (1986). Investigation of selected psychosocial needs of family members of critically ill adult patients. *Heart and Lung, 15*(2), 194–199.

Northouse, L. (1982). Coping with the mastectomy crisis. *Topics in Clinical Nursing, 4,* 57–65.

Taylor, D. (1971). Problems of patients in an intensive care unit: The aetiology and prevention of the intensive care syndrome. *International Journal of Nursing Studies, 8,* 47–57.

West, J. (Ed.). (1985). *Best and Taylor's physiological basis of medical practice.* Baltimore: Williams & Wilkins.

Wilson, L. (1972). Intensive care delirium? The effect of outside deprivation in a windowless unit. *Archives of Internal Medicine, 130,* 225–226.

ADDITIONAL READING

MacKenzie, T., & Popkin, M. (1980). Stress response syndrome occurring after delirium. *American Journal of Psychiatry, 137,* 1433–1435.

6 Death and Dying

Jan Litwack, Ed.S., R.N.
Kim Litwack, N.D., Ph.D., R.N.
Carole Temming, D.Min.
Joanne O'Reilly, M.A.

In one sense, including a chapter on death and dying may seem somewhat extraneous—after all, the primary focus of nursing is on restoration to a state of wellness. Although death and dying are as much a part of life as is birth, it is not unusual to attempt to deny its existence. To surgical nurses working every day with a wide variety of surgical procedures, issues related to death and dying receive minimal consideration. Their skill, professional judgment, and technology all focus on the maintenance of functions and the restoration of a homestatic state of health. Again, the denial of death may be present: "Patients do not die, at least not while I'm on duty."

In the past 20 years we have seen increased awareness of death. More material has appeared in the literature and more has been verbalized by professional and lay people alike. However, such discussions generally remain superficial and/or academic, with deeper fears unexplored. Most Americans remain in a denial state most of the time—except in times of heightened stressors, such as impending surgery.

It is beyond the scope of this chapter to explore the developmental views of death. Suffice it to say that each of us, depending on our age, personality, and life experiences, has at some point thought about and/or confronted the idea of our own death. Seldom do we dwell on such thoughts—after all, we intend to live forever. However, the possibility or actuality of impending surgery may well evoke the thoughts/fears of death. The necessary informed consent for surgical procedures heightens patients' feelings of vulnerability or, at the very least, brings it to their awareness. This sense of vulnerability comes from relinquishing total control of one's life to the physician, surgeon, anesthesiologist, and nurses. Such feelings of loss of control are directly related to the fears of loss of life.

When individuals are asked what concerns them most about dying and death, the areas identified most often include the fear of pain, the fear of losing control of their lives, the fear of the unknown, the fear of being a burden, the fear of mutilation, and the loss of self. Impending surgery tends to heighten these fears of impotency—of loss of personal power. Additional fears that surface include the fear of not behaving properly, the fear of not waking up, and the fear of being alone.

FEARS ABOUT DEATH AND THE SURGICAL INTENSIVE CARE UNIT

The surgical intensive care unit tends to feed the fears of both patients and significant others. For patients expecting to have a "routine surgical procedure," the arrival or regaining consciousness in SICU is another stress for an already physically stressed person. Intensive care is a very serious place; it is usually viewed/experienced as a place for individuals in crisis. Significant others frequently have ambivalent feelings about the SICU. On one hand, the patient is receiving more complete and comprehensive direct care. On the other hand, the patient's situation is probably more serious, and thus there is an increased possibility of death.

It should be noted that 70 to 80% of patients admitted to the ICU leave the ICU alive. The emphasis of care is on intensive monitoring and stabilization. Many patients admitted to the SICU require only 24 to 48 hours of postoperative monitoring. Death in this population is unexpected (Raffin, Shurkin, & Sinkler, 1989).

It is possible, however, to identify patient characteristics indicative of a poor prognosis, including advanced age, patients in cardiogenic shock, and those with sepsis, carcinoma, acute renal failure, pneumonia, and multisystem failure. These patients are unlikely to survive their ICU stay. Death in this population is often expected and predictable (Rozenbaum & Shenkman, 1988; Taffet, Teasdale, & Luchi, 1988; Lawrence & Clark, 1987).

Basically, for the patient and significant others, the presence in SICU creates a crisis situation for all concerned. This adds to the physical crisis situation for the patient. Recall from chapter 3 the discussion of crisis theory. Crisis refers to situations perceived as hazards, threats, and/or challenges for which we have no coping mechanisms. The key lies in the lack of coping mechanisms. The old ways of dealing with problems do not work. In the various stages of crisis and loss, there are cognitive as well as emotional responses to the perceived threats to homeostasis.

As described by Kubler-Ross (1969), SICU nurses will most often see the early stages of shock, denial, anger, and generally, the acknowledgment of one's condition manifested by sadness. It is important to remember that different cultures and ethnic groups express emotions in different ways. Of all the emotions, anger is perhaps the most difficult for caretakers to deal with in a useful way. From a therapeutic point of view, to allow and encourage anger is helpful; anger in response to loss is normal, it may be helpful, and it certainly needs venting. Do not personalize such anger. Its expression provides some feeling of control for the patient/significant others, and allows for movement through the crisis stages. Such anger may be expressed directly, reflecting the sense of hurt and loss, or indirectly about events/people in the SICU that seemingly do not relate to the significant event.

Patients immediately taken to SICU are generally not fully aware of the state of their condition upon arrival. The usual nursing activity is to provide what is physiologically necessary. After the patient is admitted and stabilized, significant others frequently become the concern for SICU staff members. Each individual present may now be in a crisis situation, depending on age, personality, and life experiences. Thus, some individuals may be denying the severity of the patient's condition, while others may be expressing anger or using other protective defense mechanisms as means for dealing with ever-increasing anxiety.

Because of the intensive medical procedures being carried out, visitors are often kept waiting. As they wait they experience spoken or unspoken fears about the patient. It is important to remember that these emotional responses are normal. In the face of a threat of death all of us react in some way, and generally will seek out the caretakers within the environment for information and reassurance. Thus, SICU nurses will be sought out, pressured, and feel intruded upon as significant others try to cope with what is happening to the patient.

Since SICU nurses are heavily involved in stabilizing the patient, using all available technology and resources, their energies justifiably are directed toward the patient. Such technology is another frightening aspect for family members/significant others. The kinds of lifesaving procedures used, taken for granted by skilled SICU nurses, are additional stressors for others to witness.

Should the condition of the patient deteriorate, the availability and use of life-prolonging/support equipment becomes another serious issue, raising questions related to quality of life and the right to die. With all life-maintaining procedures, unexpected complications do arise. As in a medical ICU, the goals are restoration and rehabilitation; yet patients do not always recover. There are times when, after all that can be done has been done, a dignified death must take precedence.

Ethical issues related to both living and dying may present. Health care workers practice under the tenet that preservation of life is paramount. However, increasingly, in light of advances in technology, our ability to preserve life may prove to be at the expense of dignity and the family's wishes.

Questions that may be raised include

1. When, if ever, is it ethically right to place Do Not Resuscitate orders on a chart?

2. When, if ever, is it right to withdraw extraordinary life support from a patient?

3. When, if ever, is it ethically right to withhold or withdraw ordinary care (food, oxygen, antibiotics) from a patient? (Raffin et al., 1989)

Ideally, the answers to these questions will be the result of conversations between the patient, family and members of the health care team. The ability to have such conversations is dependent upon a relationship built on mutual respect and a history of honesty in communication.

THE LIVING WILL

The Living Will is designed to allow individuals the opportunity to indicate their desire that no excessive medical interventions be instituted in the event of their deterioration. Although the Living Will is only legally binding in states whose legislature has passed approval, most physicians and family members will use the Living Will as a means to indicate patient preference. The family generally retains ultimate control. Both the family and/or the physician may use the Living Will as a component of the decision-making process when addressing issues such as not resuscitating or withdrawing/withholding care.

COMMUNICATION WITH FAMILY MEMBERS

Patients in the SICU, as well as significant others, often ask questions related to dying. Sometimes such questions are straightforward; sometimes they are more abstract and require some decoding by the caretakers. Because of the inevitable uncertainties, forthright concrete answers are useful within the limits of the situation. When people are in a crisis situation, the ability to process information may be diminished.

It is important to be clear and to avoid jargon, which may be misinterpreted. Honesty and respect for all concerned will generally be viewed as caring. The old adage of treating patients as if they were members of your family is a guide for communication. False reassurances are basically dishonest communications and often create unrealistic expectations.

As significant others gather and want to talk to nurses (who usually are the most available and knowledgeable health care givers), the conflicts of time and work are real. Nurses often feel the conflicting pulls of patient care and the needs of significant others. This is the kind of situation in which other members of the health delivery team—e.g., clergy, social workers, etc.—can often be helpful to the family in lessening stress and anxiety by allowing the venting of emotions and removing some of the fear of the unknown.

When communicating patient status information to a family, it is important for the health care team to identify who is going to talk to the family about what. Family members frequently look to the physician for initial prognosis data (i.e., the surgery is over, the course was stable, the patient will be in the ICU overnight) and will look to the nurses for the hour by hour status (i.e., what is the blood pressure? Did he sleep? Is she off the breathing machine yet?).

If the prognosis deteriorates, suddenly or expectedly, it is usually the responsibility of the physician (often by default, as opposed to preference) to communicate with the family. Again, involvement of support services (clergy, social workers) may be helpful at this time.

As patients regain consciousness and become more aware of their surroundings in SICU, their concerns about their status and vulnerability surface. The awareness of monitors and the inability to move or speak heightens the fears and increases the anxiety about their life situation. Questions may or may not be asked. Either way, nurses must be alert to the patient's emotional responses. Here again, cross-cultural perspective is necessary and helpful. When persons are familiar only with their own culture/class, certain expectations regarding behavior occur. When an individual's behavior fails to match these known cultural expectations, it is often seen as deviant. When behavior is difficult to understand, culture is an excellent place to start looking for reasons.

TERMINAL CARE

Almost all hospitals and certain units experience the deaths of patients. Perhaps more than any other unit, a SICU is not set up to allow for dying with dignity. The aims and functions of the SICU are to handle acute problems after surgery. When patients are dying, usually this precipitates heroics marked by an increased intensity to prolong life. In the SICU, patients tend not to die peacefully and at their own pace.

In September 1989, the U.S. Supreme Court began to consider issues related to an individual's constitutional right to die. There is considerable evidence that passive euthanasia—the withdrawing and withholding of certain measures so that one's existence is not merely extended—has been used and has become almost routine. Yet dilemmas ensue for both patients and families. In an SICU, decisions are most often not made by the patient. Unless there are written requests by patients, families are often torn as to what should be done. Usually, they will seek the advice of the attending physician; often nurses are also consulted.

Life and death judgments involve religious, moral, and social ethics. These kinds of decisions involve and are affected by the rights and obligations of all concerned. Issues evolve from beliefs in the sanctity and the quality of life. Questions arise as to whether biological life is sacrosanct. Life at any cost often produces dissonance, a disconnection with traditional views. Joseph Fletcher (1975, p. 69) raises four ethical questions for consideration:

1. Which do we prefer—quantity or quality of life?
2. May death sometimes be a friend rather than an enemy?
3. May we humans assume any initiative in dying?
4. What are those situations in which we may let the dying go and not keep a patient going?

CARE FOR THE CARE GIVERS

The goal of intensive care is to preserve life. Intensive care nurses should take satisfaction and pride in their contribution to this goal. However, when the outcome of the admission of a patient is death, the care giver may experience feelings for which there is little outlet.

If the death is expected, the nurse may experience a relief, for both the patient and the family. The health care team is prepared for the death and it is handled matter-of-factly.

However, if the death is sudden and unexpected, feelings of anger, concern about "missing something," not acting fast enough, sadness, and frustration may present. Staff need time to express these feelings, but may have limited opportunity to do so if energies are focused toward the family and/or the next patient being admitted.

As ICUs admit sicker, more physiologically challenged patients, these issues will increase in frequency and intensity. Intensive care nurses are challenged by physiologic instability, challenged to stabilize, to heal. Patients who "do not heal" are often overwhelming, exhausting, and frustrating, and may be the cause of nurses' leaving intensive care nursing.

Care givers need to take care of themselves too.

SUMMARY

There are no definitive answers to the above issues and questions. Perhaps the best summation rests on these cornerstones:

1. Good nursing care involves the critical element of a caring nurse–patient relationship. This ability to interact with patients and family members is of utmost importance in the SICU, and is what separates the technician from the professional nurse.
2. It is important for SICU nurses to become aware of their personal attitudes toward death and dying in order to achieve a balance between hospital expectations and patient wishes.

BIBLIOGRAPHY

Fletcher, J. (1975). In M. Kohl (Ed.). *Beneficient euthanasia.* Chapter 4, pp. 69–91. Buffalo, NY: Prometheus Books.

Kubler-Ross, E. (1969). *On death and dying.* New York: Macmillan.

Lawrence, V., & Clark, G. (1987). Cancer and resuscitation: Does the diagnosis affect the decision? *Archives of Internal Medicine, 147*(9): 1637–1640.

Raffin, T., Shurkin, J., & Sinkler, W. (1989). *Intensive care: Facing the critical choices.* New York: W.H. Freeman.

Rando, T. (1984). *Grief, dying and death: Clinical interventions for care givers.* Champaign, Illinois: Research Press.

Rozenbaum, E., & Shenkman, L. (1988). Predicting outcome of inhospital cardiopulmonary resuscitation. *Critical Care Medicine, 16*(6): 583–586.

Taffet, G., Teasdale, T., & Luchi, R. (1988). In-hospital cardiopulmonary resuscitation. *Journal of the American Medical Association, 260*(14): 2069–2072.

ADDITIONAL READINGS

Bachman, C. (1964). *Ministering to the grief sufferer.* Englewood Cliffs, NJ: Prentice Hall.

Dempsey, D. (1975). *The way we die: An investigation of death and dying in America today.* New York: McGraw-Hill.

Doyle, P. (1980). *Grief counseling and sudden death: A manual and guide.* Springfield, IL: Charles C. Thomas.

Feifel, H. (1977). *New meaning of death.* New York: McGraw-Hill.

Kohl, M. (1975). *Beneficient euthanasia.* Buffalo, NY: Prometheus Books.

Morrio, S. (1972). *Grief and how to live with it.* New York: Grosset & Dunlap.

Pacholski, R. (1986). *Researching death: Selected essays in death education and counseling.* Lakewood, Ohio: Forum for Death Education and Counseling.

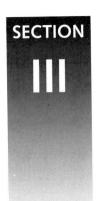

SECTION III

Physiologic Responses to Critical Illness in the Surgical Patient

7 Alterations in Oxygenation Processes

Sandra Owens-Jones, M.S., R.N.
Maureen Shekleton, D.N.Sc., R.N.

Organ and tissue function depend on a supply of oxygen adequate for the maintenance of life. Cellular uptake of oxygen results in the generation of adenosine triphosphate (ATP) which is an energy source for metabolic functions. Healing of the surgical wound depends on appropriate oxygen gradients to stimulate collagen synthesis, angiogenesis, and epithelialization for tissue repair and an adequate supply of oxygen for phagocytic leukocytosis to prevent wound infection (Whitney, 1989).

Impaired oxygenation results when the supply and/or utilization of oxygen are insufficient to meet either normal or increased requirements of the body tissues for oxygen. Lack of an adequate supply of oxygen or the inability to use oxygen can lead to functional impairment and/or death of the cell. Impaired oxygenation in the surgical patient can cause impaired wound healing, predispose the patient to the development of infection, and cause dysfunction of organ systems that are oxygen dependent, such as the brain, kidneys, and heart. Impaired oxygenation can be life threatening. Patients with preexisting cardiopulmonary problems are at highest risk for impaired oxygenation during the intraoperative and postoperative periods. Assessment of oxygenation status and identification of alterations in oxygenation are therefore essential to the care of the surgical patient.

In this chapter we present information on the causes and effects of inadequate cellular oxygenation. The nursing process is used as an organizing framework for discussion of the identification and management of patient responses to surgery that can disrupt the balance between cellular oxygenation supply and demand.

OVERVIEW

Effective oxygenation depends on a balance existing between the supply of and the demand for oxygen at the cellular level. Delivery of an adequate supply of oxygen to the cells depends on the processes of ventilation, exchange, and perfusion while demand is determined by the rate of utilization of oxygen by the cell (or the cellular rate of oxygen consumption).

Ventilation refers to the mechanics of inspiration to deliver oxygen to the alveoli and expiration to expel carbon dioxide from the lungs. Ventilation depends on neurogenic and chemical factors, the respiratory muscles, compliance of lung tissue, and the patency and resistance of the chest wall and airways.

Exchange refers to the diffusion of oxygen from the alveoli into the blood and subsequently into the body tissues, replacing carbon dioxide, which is removed in the same way. Exchange depends on the integrity, thickness, and surface area of the membranes across which the exchange is to occur, the relative pressure gradients and solubility of gases on each side of the membrane, the affinity between oxygen and hemoglobin, and at the alveolar capillary membrane, the relative distribution of ventilation and perfusion.

Perfusion refers to the flow of blood that allows the transport of oxygen and carbon dioxide between the alveoli and body tissues. Perfusion depends on the pump (heart), intact blood vessels, maintenance of pressure and flow within the vessels, and the oxygen-carrying capacity of the blood.

Utilization refers to the process by which the cell makes use of oxygen to form ATP. Utilization depends on intact cellular enzyme systems and mitochondrial mechanisms for oxidative phosphorylation. The rate of utilization depends on the metabolic requirements of the cell.

The effects of surgery, preexisting pathologic conditions and the stress of critical illness all have the potential for affecting these oxygenation processes in the critically ill surgical patient. Disruption of these processes to the extent that an imbalance between oxygen supply and demand occurs will cause impaired oxygenation. Responses to disruption of the processes that supply oxygen to the tissues are shown in Figure 7–1. The resulting tissue hypoxia can lead to other responses that will require nursing intervention. The rate of utilization or demand for oxygen can be affected directly by stress and surgery as well as by pathologic conditions such as infection, fever, endocrine disease, or any condition that causes a hypermetabolic state and increases demand beyond the ability to meet the demand.

Hypoxia is the term applied to the condition that exists when oxygenation at the cellular level is impaired or inadequate. Tissue hypoxia is the response that occurs when the requirement for oxygen (demand) exceeds the supply being delivered to and used by the cells. Tissue hypoxia related to an inadequate cellular supply of oxygen can be the result of poor perfusion of the tissue with blood (stagnant or ischemic hypoxia), a reduction in the ox-

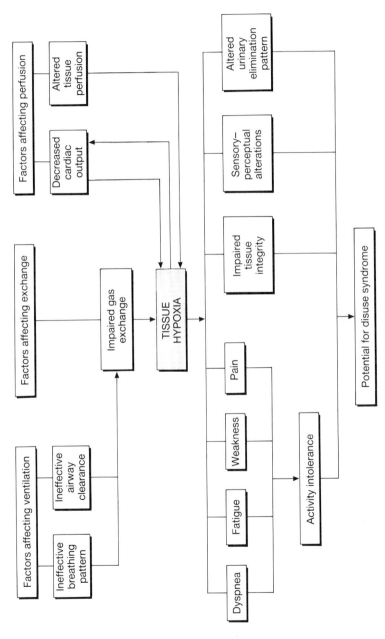

Figure 7–1. Central role of hypoxia as a sequel to physiologic responses to alterations in the oxygenation processes of ventilation, exchange, and perfusion as a cause of other physiologic responses that are in the domain of nursing practice. Reproduced by permission from *Basic Pathophysiology: A Holistic Approach*, 3rd ed. (p. 575) by M. E. Groer and M. E. Shekleton, 1989, St. Louis: The C. V. Mosby Co.

ygen-carrying capacity of the blood due to inadequate amounts of either blood or hemoglobin (anemic hypoxia), or a reduction in the arterial oxygen concentration (hypoxemic hypoxia). Tissue hypoxia related to the cellular demand for oxygen can be the result of inability of the cell to use the oxygen being delivered to it (histotoxic hypoxia) or metabolic requirements for oxygen that are increased beyond the body's ability to meet those requirements. When these conditions exist, the goals of nursing care include preventing the development or minimizing the effects of hypoxia.

The physiologic effects of hypoxia are depicted in Figure 7–2, and include a shift to anaerobic metabolism and the production of lactic acid, decreased ATP production, loss of cell volume and composition control, a shift in the pH of the body fluids to an acidotic state, and eventual cell death if oxygen does not become available before irreversible changes occur. As functional impairment or death of the hypoxic cells within the affected organ systems and body tissues occurs, hypoxia becomes clinically detectable (Groer & Shekleton, 1989).

ASSESSMENT AND DIAGNOSIS

Preoperative evaluation of oxygenation status is an integral part of surgical treatment. It allows identification of a base line, which can be used for comparison during the postoperative period to monitor changes in condition as well as the effectiveness of therapeutic interventions, and the identification of patients who are at risk for perioperative oxygenation problems. If high-risk

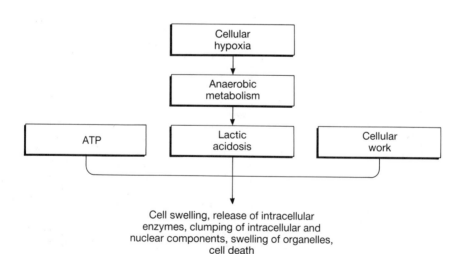

Figure 7–2. Results of prolonged cellular hypoxia. From *Physiology and Pathophysiology of the Body Fluids,* (p. 139) by M. Groer, 1981, St. Louis: The C. V. Mosby Co. Reproduced with permission of M. Groer.

patients are identified preoperatively, therapeutic measures can be implemented during both the preoperative and intraoperative periods in order to minimize postoperative complications, and postoperative assessment can be focused on anticipated problems that may require prompt identification and treatment.

Delivery of an adequate supply of oxygen to the cells through the processes of ventilation, perfusion, and exchange depends primarily on an intact cardiopulmonary system. Diagnostic tests that are routinely performed during the preoperative period in order to assess cardiopulmonary function include the chest radiograph and the electrocardiogram (ECG). Additional diagnostic tests are indicated when the patient's history suggests impaired cardiopulmonary function. Pulmonary function testing, arterial blood-gas analysis or lung scanning may be indicated in a patient suspected of having pulmonary impairment. Cardiac function may be further evaluated with exercise stress testing, echocardiography, cardiac radionuclide scanning, or cardiac catheterization and coronary angiography.

Patients who have preexisting cardiopulmonary disorders or who are having surgery in these systems have an increased risk of developing oxygenation problems, since these systems are directly affected by surgery and anesthesia (see Section I). General and cardiopulmonary risk factors related to the development of postoperative oxygenation problems are summarized in Table 7–1. In addition to the cardiac factors listed in Table 7–1, patients who are classified according to the New York Heart Association Functional Classification System (Table 7–2) as being in Class III or IV are at risk for complications because they have little or no cardiac reserve with which to handle the stress of anesthesia and surgery.

Tissue hypoxia cannot be measured directly. Assessment of oxygenation status will, therefore, focus on indicators of the adequacy of the processes of ventilation, exchange, and perfusion and on identification of clinical manifestations (signs and symptoms) that reflect functional impairment or death of cells due to hypoxia.

Clinical Manifestations of Hypoxia

Different tissues and organ systems respond to hypoxia in specific ways. The cells of the central nervous system are particularly sensitive to hypoxia, as oxygen is rapidly used by cerebral tissue. Change in behavior such as increased restlessness or uncooperativeness, inability to concentrate, dizziness or syncope, agitation, apprehension or any change in the level of consciousness from mild lethargy, disorientation, or confusion to unconsciousness may be indicative of the physiologic dysfunction caused by hypoxia, although other possible causes of cerebral dysfunction must be ruled out.

Renal tubular absorption is dependent on renal oxygen consumption and will be altered under hypoxic conditions. Renal ischemia can cause acute tubular necrosis and, subsequently, renal failure. A decrease in urinary output

Table 7–1   Risk Factors for Postoperative Oxygenation Complications

General	Cardiac	Pulmonary
Obesity (>20% above IBW)	Recent myocardial infarction (less than 6 months before surgery)	Chronic obstructive lung disease
Age greater than 65 years	Heart failure Jugular venous distention Third heart sound Pulmonary congestion	Abnormal spirogram studies MBC (MVV) < 50% predicted FEV_1 < 2 liters FEV_1/FVC < 50% predicted
History of smoking	Abnormal ECG Heart rhythm other than sinus Atrial and ventricular arrhythmias Evidence of acute ischemia or infarction	Abnormal blood gases pCO_2 > 45 mm Hg pO_2 < 50 mm Hg
Upper abdominal or thoracic surgery	Aortic stenosis/mitral-valve disease	Post-balloon occlusion PA pressure > 30 mm Hg
Emergency surgery	Severe coronary atherosclerotic disease Three-vessel disease	
Prolonged anesthesia time (>3 hours)	Severe ventricular dysfunction Ejection fraction <20–25% Hypokalemia	

IBW = ideal body weight
MBC = maximum breathing capacity; MVV = maximum voluntary ventilation; FEV_1 = forced expiratory volume in 1 second; FVC = forced vital capacity; PA = pulmonary artery.
Data in the "Cardiac" column from Goldman et. al. (1977); (1978); and Goldman, Wolf, and Braunwald (1988). Data in the "Pulmonary" column from Harmon and Lillington (1979) and Tisi (1979).

Table 7–2 New York Heart Association Functional and Therapeutic Classification of Heart Disease

Class I: Patients with cardiac disease who have no limitations. Ordinary physical activity does not cause undue fatigue, palpitations, dyspnea, or anginal pain.

Class II: Slight limitation of physical activity. The patient is comfortable at rest, but ordinary activity may result in fatigue, palpitations, dyspnea, or anginal pain.

Class III: Marked limitation of physical activity. The patient is comfortable at rest but less than ordinary activity causes fatigue, palpitations, dyspnea, or anginal pain.

Class IV: The patient is unable to carry on any physical activity without discomfort. Symptoms of cardiac insufficiency or of the anginal syndrome may be present even at rest. If any physical activity is undertaken, discomfort is increased.

Data from Criteria Committee of the New York Heart Association (1986). Nomenclature and criteria for diagnosis of diseases of the heart and great vessels.

may be indicative of this complication and, therefore, intake and output must be monitored closely.

Hypoxia causes vasoconstriction of the precapillary vessels in the pulmonary capillary bed, which increases pulmonary vascular resistance and therefore the workload of the right side of the heart. The myocardium has a lower capacity for anaerobic energy production than any other tissue. ATP production is limited because myocardial glycogen stores are depleted rapidly and the anaerobic enzyme content of myocardial tissue is minimal. The conduction tissue has a high oxygen consumption rate and the development of dysrhythmias reflects its sensitivity to hypoxia. Tachycardia will occur early, with bradycardia developing if the hypoxia continues.

Cyanosis, a bluish grey discoloration of the lips, nailbeds, and mucous membranes, which occurs because of the presence of reduced hemoglobin, is a very unreliable and late sign of hypoxia. Its perception is questionable depending on the lighting, skin thickness, and pigmentation and the examiner's powers of observation. Cyanosis becomes apparent when 5 g of hemoglobin per 100 ml of blood has been reduced to deoxyhemoglobin in the presence of a normal amount of hemoglobin. This is equivalent to a PaO_2 of 50 mm Hg or less and an oxygen saturation level of 75%. A person with a hemoglobin deficiency may be extremely hypoxic before cyanosis becomes apparent, while a person with an increased hemoglobin content might appear cyanotic even without tissue hypoxia. It is likely that many critically ill surgical patients may experience a deficiency of hemoglobin because of bleeding.

Dyspnea is the subjective sensation of difficult or uncomfortable breathing (Carrieri & Janson-Bjerklie, 1986). It may be described as air hunger or the inability to get enough air. The term dyspnea is used to describe responses on a continuum between the subjective report of difficult breathing to a visible, extremely exaggerated respiratory effort characterized by use of the accessory muscles of respiration, flaring of the nares, and an extreme increase in the rate of respiration. Dyspnea is not so much a reflection of the state of tissue oxygenation but, rather, is a symptom reflecting the conscious perception of the need for respiration and the body's inability to meet that need (Groer & Shekleton, 1989). Conditions surrounding the occurrence of dyspnea need to be determined, as they will provide information about the possible cause. For example, does dyspnea occur at rest or with exertion? Is it brought on by a change in position (orthopnea)? Does it occur only at night (paroxysmal nocturnal dyspnea)? or Did it begin suddenly or worsen over time?

Fatigue, weakness, and activity intolerance can also be reflections of tissue hypoxia as a result of the inadequate energy production that occurs. Assessment should include questions regarding the severity and the impact of these symptoms on activities of daily living.

Ischemic pain may also be a manifestation of tissue hypoxia. Pain is thought to be the result of neural stimulation by the acidic end products of anaerobic metabolism, removal of which is a problem because of impaired perfusion. Effects of stagnant or ischemic hypoxia may also include abnormal sensations such as numbness or tingling as nerve endings are affected.

Chest pain that is ischemic in nature must be differentiated from other types of chest pain. While ischemic pain signals a problem with the supply of oxygen, chest pain may be a symptom of many other conditions that have the potential of disrupting normal oxygenation processes. The cause of chest pain must be determined in order to provide effective treatment. Assessment should include a complete description of the onset, duration, location, character, frequency, precipitating and alleviating factors, and any associated symptoms.

Chest pain caused by ischemic heart disease (angina pectoris) is often described as crushing, burning, squeezing, choking, pressing, or a heavy or constricting sensation. The pain is often located in the anterior midthoracic region and is substernal in origin, although it may radiate to the arms, jaw, shoulders, or teeth. The more severe the attack, the greater the radiation to the left arm, particularly to the ulnar aspect. Precipitating factors include heavy meals, physical exertion, cold weather, and emotional excitement. The pain of angina can be relieved with rest or nitroglycerin. In contrast, the pain of myocardial infarction, which may occur while the patient is at rest, is unrelieved by rest or nitrates, is of longer duration, and may be accompanied by shortness of breath and/or hypotension. Morphine sulfate administration is often required for relief. Changes on the electrocardiogram include Q-wave development in transmural infarction and ST–T-wave changes in subendocardial infarction (Braunwald, 1984; Burden, 1984). Associated manifestations may include diaphoresis, tachycardia, nausea and vomiting, weakness, dizziness, and a feeling of impending doom.

Chest pain caused by pericarditis may be pleuritic or substernal in origin. Since the pericardium is insensitive to pain, the pain associated with pericarditis is believed to be due to inflammation of the adjacent parietal pleura (Braunwald, 1984). Pericardial pain that is pleuritic in nature is described as being sharp and knife-like. The pain is usually located on the left side of the chest and is often referred to the neck or flank, and the duration of the pain is much longer than anginal pain, sometimes lasting for hours. Substernal pericardial pain may be dull and oppressive, resembling the pain of myocardial infarction; however, the aggravating and relieving factors are the same as those seen in pleuritic pericardial pain. The presence of a pericardial friction rub, fever, leukocytosis, acute enlargement of the cardiac silhouette on chest roentgenography and ST-segment elevation without QRS changes on the ECG provide additional evidence of a pericardial cause.

Chest pain can also be caused by many other conditions, including pneumonia, dissecting aneurysm, pulmonary embolism, gastrointestinal disease, musculoskeletal disorders, and anxiety. A summary of the differentiating features of chest pain due to a variety of causes is presented in Table 7–3.

Assessment of Oxygenation Processes

The adequacy of ventilation and exchange can be examined most reliably through arterial blood-gas analysis. Arterial blood-gas analysis also allows evaluation of the response to treatment and the course of cardiopulmonary complications in addition to assessment of the acid–base status of the body (see chapter 9). The partial pressure of oxygen in the arterial blood reflects the adequacy of exchange, while the partial pressure of carbon dioxide in the arterial blood reflects the adequacy of alveolar ventilation.

Instability of the body-fluid pH can be experienced during or after surgery and information about the arterial-blood pH, which affects the exchange of oxygen at the tissue level, can also be obtained from the arterial blood-gas analysis. Because of the Bohr effect, the affinity of hemoglobin for oxygen is greater at an increased pH and is less at a decreased pH. This effect serves to promote the release of oxygen in the tissues where pH tends to be low. When affinity is low, the oxygen-carrying capacity of hemoglobin is decreased but release of oxygen to the tissues is facilitated. Other conditions besides decreased pH that cause decreased affinity or a shift to the right of the oxyhemoglobin dissociation curve include increased pCO_2, increased temperature and increased amounts of 2,3 diphosphoglycerate (2,3-DPG), an organic phosphate produced by glycolysis, which binds hemoglobin in the red blood cell. When the affinity between hemoglobin and oxygen is increased, release of oxygen to the tissues is inhibited. Other conditions besides increased pH that cause increased affinity or a shift to the left of the oxyhemoglobin dissociation curve include decreased pCO_2, decreased temperature, and decreased levels of 2,3-DPG. The amount of 2,3-DPG is reduced in stored blood; therefore, surgical patients who have received transfusions with stored blood are at risk for tissue hypoxia through this mechanism. Conditions associated with surgery that alter pH are discussed in chapter 9 and conditions that affect the body temperature are discussed in chapter 12.

Table 7–3 Assessment of Chest Pain

Condition	Location	Quality	Severity
Angina	Retrosternal region; radiates to neck, jaw, epigastrium, shoulders or arms—left common	Pressure, burning, squeezing, heaviness, indigestion	Moderate to severe
Intermediate syndrome or coronary insufficiency	Same as angina	Same as angina	Increasingly severe
Myocardial infarction	Substernal, and may radiate like angina	Heaviness, pressure, burning, constriction	Severe, sometimes mild (in 25% of patients)
Pericarditis	Usually begins over sternum and may radiate to neck and down left arm	Sharp, stabbing knife-like	Moderate to severe
Dissecting aortic aneurysm	Anterior chest; radiates to thoracic area of back; may be abdominal; pain shifts in chest	Tearing	Excruciating, tearing knife-like
Mitral-valve prolapse syndrome	Substernal; sometimes radiates to the left arm, back, jaw	Stabbing, sharp	Variable, generally mild, can become severe
Pulmonary embolism (most pulmonary emboli do not produce chest pain)	Substernal "anginal"	Not pleuritic unless infarction exists	Can be severe
Pulmonary hypertension	Substernal	Pressure; oppressive	Variable

Course	Aggravating or Relieving Factors	Associated Symptoms or Signs
<10 minutes	Aggravated by exercise, cold weather, emotional stress, or after meals; relieved by rest or nitroglycerin; atypical (Prinzmetal's) angina may be unrelated to activity and caused by coronary artery spasm	S_4, paradoxical split S_2 during pain
>10 minutes	Same as angina, with gradually decreasing tolerance for exertion	Same as angina
Sudden onset, 30 minutes or longer but variable; usually goes away in hours	Unrelieved	Shortness of breath, sweating, weakness, nausea, vomiting, severe anxiety
Lasts many hours to days	Aggravated by coughing, deep breathing, rotating chest or supine position; relieved by sitting up and leaning forward	Pericardial friction rub, syncope, cardiac tamponade, pulsus paradoxus (Kussmaul sign)
Sudden onset, lasts for hours	Unrelated to anything	Lower blood pressure in one arm, absent pulses, paralysis, murmur of aortic insufficiency, pulsus paradoxus, stridor: myocardial infarction can occur
Episodes are paroxysmal, may be prolonged	Not related to exertion, not relieved by nitroglycerin or rest	Variable palpitations, dizziness, syncope, dyspnea
Sudden onset; minutes to 1 hour	May be aggravated by breathing	Fever, tachypnea, tachycardia, hypotension, elevated jugular venous pressure, right ventricular lift, accentuated P_2, occasional murmur of tricuspid insufficiency and right ventricular S_4, with infarction usually in the presence of congestive heart failure, rales, pleural rub, hemoptysis, clinical phlebitis present in minority of cases
	Aggravated by effort	Pain usually associated with dyspnea; right ventricular lift, accentuated P_2

Table 7–3   *(Continued)*

Condition	Location	Quality	Severity
Spontaneous pneumothorax	Unilateral	Sharp, well localized	
Pneumonia with pleurisy	Localized over area of consolidation	Pleuritic, well localized	Moderate
Gastrointestinal disorders	Lower substernal area, epigastric, right or left upper quadrant	Burning, colic-like aching	
Musculoskeletal disorders	Variable	Aching	
Neurologic disorders (herpes zoster)	Dermatomal in distribution		
Anxiety states	Usually localized to a point	Sharp burning, commonly location of pain moves from place to place	Mild to moderate

From *Comprehensive Cardiac Care,* 6th ed. (pp. 54, 55) by K. G. Andreoli, D. P. Zipes, A. G. Wallace, M. R. Kinney, and V. Fowkes (Eds.), 1987, St. Louis: C. V. Mosby. Copyright 1987 by C. V. Mosby. Reprinted with permission.

The oxygen-carrying capacity of the blood can be further assessed by examining the percentage of hemoglobin bound with oxygen. A value for arterial O_2 saturation can be obtained through arterial blood-gas analysis or noninvasively using a pulse oximeter. It must be noted that the accuracy of pulse oximetry will be reduced in states of decreased tissue perfusion such as hypotension, shock, or intense vasoconstriction due to hypothermia or vasopressor therapy or in conditions characterized by increased levels of carboxyhemoglobin or methemoglobin (Szaflarski & Cohen, 1989).

The nonlinear S shape of the oxyhemoglobin dissociation curve with the flat upper right side allows the saturation of hemoglobin with oxygen to remain high even at relatively low partial pressures of oxygen. For example, with a pH of 7.4 and a PaO_2 of 60 mm Hg, the oxygen saturation would be approximately 89 to 90%. While O_2 saturation is independent of the hemoglobin concentration, the actual amount of oxygen to be delivered to the cells depends on the oxygen content in volume/percent that is related to hemoglobin concentration. At the same arterial O_2 saturation level, an anemic patient will have less oxygen delivered to the tissues than a normal patient while a polycythemic patient will have more.

Course	Aggravating or Relieving Factors	Associated Symptoms or Signs
Sudden onset, lasts many hours	Painful breathing	Dyspnea, hyperresonance, and decreased breath and voice sounds over involved lung
	Painful breathing	Dyspnea, cough, fever, dull to flat percussion, bronchial breathing, rales, occasional pleural rub
	Precipitated by recumbency or meals	Nausea, regurgitation, food intolerance, melena, hematemesis, jaundice
Short or long duration Prolonged period of time	Aggravated by movement, history of muscle exertion	Tender to pressure or movement
Unassociated with external events		Rash appears in area of discomfort with herpes
Varies; usually very brief	Situational anger	Sighing respirations, often chest-wall tenderness

Mixed venous oxygen saturation ($S\bar{v}O_2$) can also be monitored as an indicator of the relation between oxygen delivery and oxygen demand. Determinants of mixed venous oxygen saturation include the arterial oxygen saturation (SaO_2) (an indicator of oxygen exchange or transfer at the alveolocapillary membrane), oxygen consumption ($\dot{V}O_2$) (an indicator of the utilization of oxygen by the peripheral tissues), and the cardiac output and hemoglobin (Hgb) (indicators of oxygen delivery to the tissues) in the following relationship:

$$S\bar{v}O_2 \approx SaO_2 - \frac{\dot{V}O_2}{CO \times Hgb}$$

The normal $S\bar{v}O_2$ lies in a range between 68 and 77%. Mixed venous oxygen saturation will be decreased when exchange or transport of oxygen is impaired (e.g., states of low tissue perfusion or hypoxemia) or when peripheral utilization of oxygen is increased (e.g., shivering, seizures, or hyperthermia). It will be increased when there is an increase in oxygen delivery in excess of demand, such as in states in which oxygen transfer or delivery is increased and/or peripheral utilization of oxygen decreases (Shively, 1988). Examples of such states include the hyperdynamic phase of sepsis, hypothermia, metabolic cell failure, cirrhosis, and pharmacologic paralysis (Leasa & Sibbald, 1988).

The adequacy of the ventilatory process can be further assessed by examining the respiratory rate and pattern, measuring end tidal (expired) levels of carbon dioxide, the work of breathing, and the ratio of dead space to tidal volume (V_D/V_T). Respiratory rate and pattern can be examined using the techniques of inspection and palpation, however, new, noninvasive, computerized monitoring systems employing inductive plethysmography are available. Information about respiratory rate, tidal volume, duty cycle, inspiratory flow, and the degree of synchrony between chest wall and abdominal movement can be obtained through this type of monitoring. Computerized monitoring systems are also available on newer ventilators, which provide information on pressures and volumes in the respiratory system. Bedside estimation of the work of breathing in ventilated patients has recently been described and may have relevance for determining when a patient is ready to begin the weaning process (Marini, 1988; Marini, Roussos, Tobin, MacIntyre, Belman, & Moxham, 1988; Capps & Schade, 1988).

Ineffective breathing pattern is commonly seen after surgery (see chapter 1). A rapid, shallow breathing pattern increases dead space and the work of breathing. A sustained increase in the respiratory workload may contribute to the development of respiratory muscle fatigue (Capps & Schade, 1988). Respiratory muscle weakness and fatigue are postulated to be related to the development of ventilatory failure in pathologic conditions in which the respiratory muscles are affected (Macklem & Roussos, 1977; Larson & Kim, 1987; Shekleton, 1987). Physical signs of inspiratory muscle fatigue (in the characteristic order of appearance) include tachypnea, decreased tidal volume, the development of asynchronous breathing patterns, including abdominal paradox (an inward movement of the abdomen on inspiration) and respiratory alternans (alternating abdominal and thoracic respiration), increased pCO_2 (which is a late sign), and bradypnea and decreased minute ventilation (which immediately preceded respiratory arrest in laboratory animals) (Cohen, Zagelbaum, Gross, Roussos, & Macklem, 1982).

Measurement of pressures and volumes within the cardiovascular system, evaluation of the cardiac rate and rhythm through the ECG, and determination of the presence and pattern of pulses throughout the body provide information on the adequacy of perfusion and oxygen transport. Cardiac rate and rhythm disturbances are often associated with underlying heart disease and poor cardiac reserve (Goldman et al., 1978).

A variety of causes may contribute to the development of postoperative dysrhythmias and conduction defects. Although such alterations may be benign in the normal heart, disturbances in rhythm can increase postoperative morbidity and mortality in the presence of underlying heart disease (Davis, 1983). Postsurgical complications such as acute myocardial infarction, bleeding, hypovolemia, hypoxemia, acid–base disturbances, hypokalemia and other electrolyte disorders, pneumonia, infection, and fever can precipitate the development of various tachyarrhythmias and bradyarrhythmias. In the presence of massive infarction, severe coronary artery disease, cardiomyopathy, or valvular lesions, disturbances in rhythm can severely compromise cardiac function and lead to a decline in cardiac output and the development of cardiogenic shock. Assessment of the type, frequency, hemodynamic effects, and cause of dysrhythmias is necessary. Antidysrhythmic therapy should be continued until the day of surgery and be resumed as soon as possible during the postoperative period.

Tachyarrhythmias increase myocardial oxygen requirements by increasing the cardiac workload and decrease oxygen supply by decreasing coronary perfusion. The presence of unstable tachyarrhythmias may necessitate intravenous antiarrhythmic management during surgery.

Because anesthesia may further depress automaticity and ventricular rate, perioperative morbidity and mortality is increased in patients with heart block (Wolf & Braunwald, 1984). Patients with complete heart block should have a pacemaker inserted before surgery. Patients with a history of bifascicular block who also have Mobitz Type II second-degree atrioventricular (AV) block and patients with unexplained syncope, transient third-degree AV block or sick sinus syndrome should have a temporary pacemaker inserted before surgery since the risk to progression to complete heart block is enhanced in these patients. Patients with asymptomatic bifascicular heart block, first degree AV block and Mobitz Type I second degree AV block do not require presurgical pacemaker insertion but equipment for emergency insertion should be available (Rose, Corman, & Mason, 1979; Wolf & Braunwald, 1984).

Arterial insufficiency is reflected by changes in the arterial pulse and the presence of cool, mottled skin. Peripheral pulses should be palpated bilaterally for their presence, regularity, quality, and amplitude. Pulsus alternans, beat-to-beat variation in the amplitude of the pulse, is a finding in left ventricular failure. Pulsus paradoxus, decrease of more than 10 mm Hg in systolic blood pressure during inspiration, is due to pooling of blood in the pulmonary vasculature and increased intrathoracic pressure during inspiration, and occurs in cardiac tamponade, obstructive lung disease, and constrictive pericarditis. The presence of edema may reduce local tissue perfusion, leading to pallor and decreased skin temperature as well.

Information about central venous pressure and right ventricular function can be obtained indirectly by examining the neck veins. Venous pressure is elevated when the vertical distance between the highest point of pulsation and the sternal angle is greater than 3 to 4 cm. Jugular venous distention (JVD) is a finding in patients with right heart failure, circulatory overload, constrictive pericarditis, and tricuspid stenosis. In patients with obstructive lung disease, venous pressure may appear elevated on expiration. In order to assess venous pressure further, a catheter can be inserted into the vena cava or right atrium. Central venous pressure monitoring allows evaluation of the function of the right side of the heart. It is a reliable indicator of fluid volume status in patients without significant heart or lung disease.

Hemodynamic monitoring is helpful in assessing left and right ventricular function. High-risk or critically ill surgical patients may require hemodynamic monitoring before, during, or after surgery. Insertion of pulmonary artery and intraarterial lines is necessary for the patient who develops complications such as persistent hypotension, moderate or severe heart failure, pulmonary edema, cardiogenic shock, tachyarrhythmias or bradyarrhythmias that compromise cardiac output, mitral regurgitation, ventricular septal defect, or cardiac tamponade (Sobel & Braunwald, 1984). Hemodynamic monitoring allows evaluation of the pressures within the cardiopulmonary system (Figure 7–3). Such pressure measurements are useful for determining heart function, managing fluid balance, and assessing the effectiveness of therapeutic interventions. Fluid status can be most accurately determined with the pulmonary artery catheter. In addition, differentiation between the causes of hypotension and decreased cardiac output (for example, myocardial dysfunction versus hypovolemia) can be accomplished with hemodynamic monitoring. The hemodynamic findings seen in potential oxygenation complications of the postoperative course are summarized in Table 7–4 and discussed in subsequent sections of this chapter.

Responses to treatment and disease in the surgical patient that can lead to tissue hypoxia include impaired gas exchange, altered tissue perfusion, and decreased cardiac output. Each of these nursing diagnoses will be covered below.

IMPAIRED GAS EXCHANGE

Impaired gas exchange is defined as the state in which an individual experiences decreased transfer of oxygen and carbon dioxide between the alveoli of the lungs, the vascular system, and the body tissues. The defining characteristics associated with impaired gas exchange include abnormal arterial blood-gas values reflecting decreased oxygen tension (hypoxemia) or carbon dioxide tensions outside the normal range (hypercapnia or hypocapnia). Acute respiratory failure, the most extreme manifestations of impaired gas exchange, exists when the PaO_2 is less than 50 mm Hg, the $PaCO_2$ is greater than 50 mm Hg, and there is an acid pH in conjunction with acute and severe dyspnea and signs of tissue hypoxia (Gray & Rogers, 1983; Kirby & Taylor, 1986; Bone, George, & Hudson, 1987).

Related Factors

Causes of low arterial oxygen levels (hypoxemia) include ventilation–perfusion inequality, shunting of blood, alveolar hypoventilation, and impaired diffusion. Alterations in arterial carbon dioxide levels are the result of alterations in ventilation. Alveolar hypoventilation (or ventilation at a level

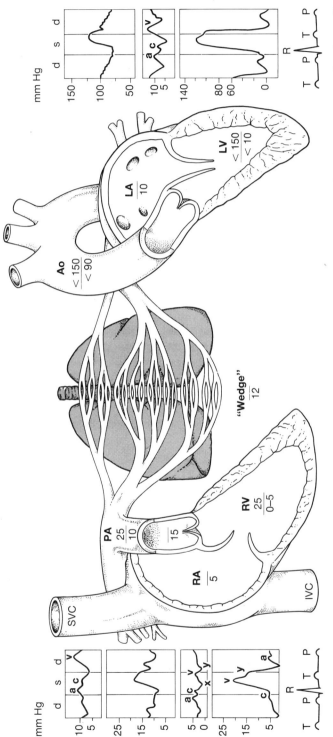

Figure 7-3. Summary of pressures within atria and ventricles. Note similarity of diastolic pressures within communicating chambers of pulmonary artery, left atrium, and left ventricle. During diastolic phase of contraction, this pressure may be transmitted to pulmonary capillary bed and may be measured using flow-directed balloon-tipped catheter. Reproduced by permission from *Congestive Heart Failure* by C. Michaelson, ed., St. Louis, 1983, The C. V. Mosby Co. SVC = superior vena cava; IVC = inferior vena cava; RA = right atrium; RV = right ventricle; "Wedge" = pulmonary capillary wedge pressure; Ao = aorta; LA = left atrium; LV = left ventricle.

Table 7–4 Normal and Abnormal Hemodynamic Values*

Pressures	Normal	Uncomplicated Myocardial Infarction	Left Ventricular Failure	Hypovolemia
Right atrium	0–8 mm Hg; O_2 saturation of right atrium, 60%	N	N	↓
Right ventricular, systolic	25 mm Hg; O_2 saturation of right ventricle, 60%	N	↑	<20↓
Right ventricular, diastolic	0–6 mm Hg	N	N	↓
Pulmonary artery, systolic	15–30 mm Hg; O_2 saturation of pulmonary artery 60%	May be slightly↑	>30 mm Hg	↓
Pulmonary artery, diastolic	12 mm Hg (range 6–15 mm Hg)	N	>18 mm Hg	<6↓
Pulmonary artery, mean	10–18 mm Hg	N	↑	↓
Pulmonary capillary wedge pressure	4–12 mm Hg	<18 mm Hg	>18 mm Hg; ↑ to 30 mm Hg in pulmonary edema	<6↓
Cardiac output	4–8 liters/min	N	↓	↓
Cardiac index	2.5–4 liters/min/m²	N	2.0–2.5	↓
Systemic vascular resistance	900–1500 dyn/sec/cm⁵	N	1500	
Mean blood pressure	70–105 mm Hg	↑ with autonomic stimulation; ↓ with vagal stimulation	Initially slightly ↑	↓

N = within normal limits; ↑=increased; ↑↑=greatly increased; ↓=decreased
CO = cardiac output
MAP = mean arterial pressure
RA = right atrium

*Calculations: mean blood pressure = $\dfrac{2\,(\text{diastolic}) + \text{systolic}}{3}$

systemic vascular resistance = $\dfrac{\overline{MAP} - \overline{RA}}{CO} \times 80$

Right Ventricular Failure	Cardiac Tamponade	Pulmonary Embolism	Cardiogenic Shock	Ventricular Septal Defect	Mitral Regurgitation
↑>12 Y descent preserved	↑>12 Y descent absent	↑	↑	N Right atrial oxygen saturation, 55%	
N	N	↑↑	↑>30	↑↑60	
↑>12	12–16	↑>12	↑	N	
N	N	↑↑	↑>30	↑↑60 Pulmonary artery oxygen saturation ↑75%	↑
N	12–16	N	↑>18	↑↑	↑
N	Slightly ↑	↑	↑	↑↑	↑
≤12	12–16	≤12	↑>18	↑↑May have tall V waves	↑Giant V waves
↓	↓	↓	↓	↓	↓
↓	↓	↓	↓1.8	↓1.9	↓
↑	↑	↑	>1500	>1500	↑
↓	↓	↓	↓	↓	↓

Data from Buchbinder and Ganz (1976); Gore et. al. (1985); and Daily and Schroeder (1981).

insufficient to meet metabolic demands) results in a rise in arterial pCO_2 while alveolar hyperventilation (or ventilation in excess of metabolic requirements) will cause a decrease in arterial pCO_2.

A reduction in ventilation (hypoventilation) causes impaired gas exchange because with a decrease in the movement of air in and out of the lungs there is a decrease in the alveolar partial pressure of oxygen and retention of carbon dioxide that is reflected by an increase in the arterial partial pressure of carbon dioxide. Eventually, hypoventilation leads to hypoxemia, hypercapnia, and respiratory acidosis. Hypoventilation can be a physiologic response to either decreased respiratory drive due to altered sensitivity and function of the respiratory center or decreased ventilatory response through impairment of the mechanics of ventilation (Groer & Shekleton, 1989). The respiratory center can be depressed by sedatives, narcotics, and certain analgesics and anesthetics as well as by cerebral ischemia. The mechanics of respiration are impaired in disorders that affect the respiratory muscles and movement of the chest wall (obstructive and restrictive pulmonary disorders) and in conditions characterized by pulmonary surfactant deficiency.

Alveolar hyperventilation leads to respiratory alkalosis because of the excessive loss of carbon dioxide through the lungs. As a result of this loss, less carbon dioxide is available to combine with water and form carbonic acid. Subsequently, the hydrogen ion concentration decreases and the arterial pH rises. Hyperventilation can occur in response to anxiety; as a compensatory homeostatic mechanism in the presence of metabolic acidosis, fever, or any condition that increases the body's metabolic rate; and as a result of mechanical overventilation. Increased respiratory drive due to infection, high fever, salicylate poisoning and central nervous system trauma, lesions, or bleeding can also cause alveolar hyperventilation.

In the normal lungs, the distribution of blood flow and ventilation is uneven across the lung fields. Because pulmonary blood flow (perfusion) and alveolar ventilation are not uniformly proportionate to one another there will be some degree of inequality in the ventilation–perfusion relationship that exists in the normal lung. If ventilation and perfusion are relatively equal, the relationship is expressed by a ratio between 0.8 and 1.0. When the ratio is above or below this value, ventilation–perfusion (V/Q) inequality or mismatch exists. Preexisting lung disease or a response to surgery that disrupts either ventilation or pulmonary blood flow can cause ventilation–perfusion imbalance, which may ultimately lead to impaired gas exchange. If the ventilation of alveoli is relatively greater than the surrounding blood flow, a high ventilation–perfusion ratio exists, and the effect is that of increased dead space (or wasted ventilation). This can occur in response to decreased perfusion (as in the case of pulmonary embolism or increased pulmonary vascular resistance) or overventilation such as occurs with a rapid, shallow breathing pattern. Perfusion in excess of ventilation results in a low ventilation–perfusion ratio and shunting, or flow of blood that does not participate in gas exchange, occurs. Shunting is the major pathogenetic mechanism of hypoxemia in pulmonary edema, pneumonia, and atelectasis (Dantzker, 1986). A true (or absolute) shunt can be differentiated from ventilation–perfusion abnormality (shunt effect) by a lack of response to increased concentrations of inspired oxygen, especially as the degree of shunting increases.

Impaired gas exchange is the ultimate response to acute, diffuse lung injury, as is seen in the adult respiratory distress syndrome (ARDS) and gastric aspiration injury. The pathophysiologic and clinical pictures are very similar in these two conditions, the difference between the two being the initiating event. Gastric aspiration in the surgical patient most commonly occurs during induction of anesthesia and intubation. Aspiration injury can lead to the development of ARDS. ARDS is not a disease in itself, but rather is a syndrome characterized by the composite of manifestations of acute lung injury that develops as a response to some pathologic event (Murray, Matthay, Luce, & Flick, 1988). Events that can lead to the development of ARDS in the postsurgical patient with previously healthy lungs include shock, sepsis, disseminated intravascular coagulation, cardiopulmonary bypass, oxygen toxicity, and trauma. Sepsis is one of the more frequently seen causes of ARDS in the critically ill patient. The incidence and mortality rate of septic ARDS is higher than for other causes of ARDS (Balk & Bone, 1983b; Kaplan, Sahn, & Petty, 1979; Pepe, Potkin, & Reus, 1982). The mortality rate for all cases of ARDS (all causes) is estimated to be between 50 and 60%, while the reported mortality rate associated with septic ARDS ranges between 80 and 90% (Kaplan et al., 1979; Jacobs & Bone, 1986; Murray et al., 1988). Secondary complications that may contribute to these figures include pulmonary emboli, pulmonary barotrauma secondary to treatment, cardiovascular problems, renal failure, gastrointestinal hemorrhage, nosocomial infection, and nutritional deficits that further compromise pulmonary function. Multiple-organ-failure syndrome is often associated with ARDS.

The major feature of ARDS is noncardiogenic pulmonary edema. Damage or injury to the alveolar–capillary membrane leads to increased membrane permeability to fluid and protein, which allows a protein-rich interstitial exudate to accumulate and eventually fill the alveoli, rendering them nonfunctional for gas exchange. The cause of the injury to the alveolar epithelium and the vascular endothelium is unclear at present. Elucidation of the parts played in the pathogenesis of ARDS by the inflammatory mediators, vasoactive substances, and perturbations of the coagulation and fibrinolytic systems seen in the syndrome is the subject of ongoing clinical investigation. Identification of pathogenetic mechanisms will allow medical treatments to become more precise and perhaps reduce the current controversy associated with the use of antiinflammatory drugs (including steroids). Studies have demonstrated that the efficacy of the steroidal agents varies depending on the underlying cause of ARDS (Bone, Fisher, Clemmer, Slotman, Metz, & Balk, 1987; Murray et al., 1988).

Surfactant defects also occur and lead to atelectasis, which in combination with the edema, cause decreases in both lung compliance and functional residual capacity. Intrapulmonary shunting occurs and hypoxemia subsequently develops (Bradley, 1987; Groer & Shekleton, 1989). The pulmonary capillary wedge pressure (PCWP) will remain below 18 cm H_2O (Bradley, 1987).

The clinical course of ARDS includes a latent period of apparent clinical stability that lasts for 6 to 48 hours after the injury. During the stable period hyperventilation and hypocapnia persist, with a mild increase in the work of breathing. Within 12 to 24 hours after injury, fine reticular infiltrates appear on the chest roentgenogram and indicate the development of perivascular fluid accumulation and interstitial edema formation. The next phase is that of respiratory insufficiency marked by tachypnea and dyspnea, the presence of crackles throughout the lung fields, decreased lung compliance (stiff lungs), and diffuse infiltrates on the chest roentgenogram. The final or terminal stage is characterized by severe hypoxemia that is refractory to oxygen administration and carbon dioxide retention, which leads to respiratory and metabolic acidosis (Balk & Bone, 1983b; Kirby & Taylor, 1986).

Intervention and Evaluation

The goal of therapy for impaired gas exchange is to improve ventilation and oxygenation. In order to accomplish this, perioperative factors causing impaired gas exchange must be minimized or eliminated. Supplemental oxygen therapy or assisted ventilation may be necessary in order to improve gas exchange. Expected outcomes of such therapy include adequate gas exchange as evidenced by arterial blood-gas values within the patient's normal range and absence of clinical manifestations of tissue hypoxia.

Oxygen Therapy

If the patient is hypoxemic on room air, supplemental oxygen must be administered. Fairley (1980) suggests that all postoperative patients receive oxygen until they are awake and stable. Patients who have preexisting cardiopulmonary disease, those who have had upper abdominal or thoracic surgery, and those who developed an oxygenation problem during the intraoperative period should receive oxygen until blood-gas values stabilize (Fairley, 1980). Selection of the amount and mode of delivery depend on the severity of hypoxemia and the presence of chronic hypercapnia (a history of obstructive lung disease). Patients with chronic obstructive pulmonary disease (COPD) should receive a low fraction of inspired oxygen (FiO_2) in order to maintain the hypoxic ventilatory drive. The venturi mask may be preferred for the patient with COPD, as low concentrations of oxygen (24 to 28%) can be delivered more precisely than with a nasal cannula. A higher concentration of oxygen can be delivered with a nonrebreathing (delivers an FiO_2 of up to 100%) or a rebreathing (delivers an FiO_2 of up to 60%) mask. Many patients find masks uncomfortable to use, however. Use of high concentrations of inspired oxygen over extended periods places the patient at risk for the development of oxygen toxicity. Therefore, use of this mode of treatment should be carefully monitored.

Assisted Ventilation

If alveolar ventilation at a level appropriate to meet metabolic needs and correct hypoxemia cannot be achieved or maintained through more conservative methods, then endotracheal intubation and mechanical ventilation must be initiated. Other indications for placement of an artificial airway and assisted mechanical ventilation include apnea or impending respiratory arrest, clinical presentation with severe hypoxemia, retention of carbon dioxide, acidosis, altered mental status such that the patient is unable to cooperate with the regimen, progressive exhaustion of the patient, and occasionally, the inability to remove airway secretions (Francis, 1983).

After the patient is placed on the ventilator and his or her condition is stabilized, the FiO_2 is set as low as possible to achieve a PaO_2 of 50 to 60 mm Hg (Bone & Stober, 1983). Prolonged administration of high concentrations of oxygen can lead to the development of oxygen toxicity (Bone, 1980). Deleterious effects of oxygen toxicity include suppression of the mucociliary and alveolar macrophage clearance systems and lung parenchymal damage. Early manifestations of toxicity include substernal chest pain, complaints of tickling in the throat, coughing, paresthesias, nausea, and vomiting.

If the patient is unable to attain a PaO_2 of 50 mm Hg or more on an FiO_2 of 50% or less, then positive end expiratory pressure (PEEP) therapy is usually indicated (Bone & Stober, 1983). PEEP improves oxygenation by reducing intrapulmonary shunting. Speculation about the mechanism through which this effect is accomplished include the recruitment of collapsed alveoli and the redistribution of edema fluid out of the alveolar space and into the extracellular space. It is known that PEEP increases the functional residual capacity and lung distensibility (Gray & Rogers, 1983).

The increased intrathoracic pressure induced by PEEP can lead to a reduction in venous return which, in turn, can cause a decreased cardiac output. The patient with underlying heart disease may have an increased PCWP in conjunction with a reduced cardiac output and may require inotropic therapy (Bone & Stober, 1983). PEEP also decreases mean arterial pressure and increases intracranial pressure, which can lead to cerebral hypoperfusion.

Continuous monitoring and meticulous care of the patient requiring mechanical ventilation are extremely important. Base-line measurements are taken to compare with subsequent changes in status. Chest roentgenography is performed after intubation to check the tube position. Chest auscultation is performed regularly in order to confirm tube placement and to check air distribution. Blood gases should be routinely monitored in order to assess the adequacy of the ventilation and exchange processes continually while on the ventilator. Ventilator settings, pressures, and flow rates should be checked at regular intervals. The ventilator tubing should be checked periodically for patency. Further impairment of gas exchange can be related to a worsening of the underlying condition, the onset of a new problem or complication of treatment, inappropriate ventilator settings, or malfunction or obstruction in the ventilator system (Glauser, Polatty, & Sessler, 1988).

Possible complications of mechanical ventilation include infection, decreased cardiac output, fluid volume excess, acid–base imbalance, oxygen toxicity, and tracheal laryngeal damage due to intubation. A current subject of speculation is whether prolonged ventilatory support results in disuse atrophy of the respiratory muscles. Another possible complication is barotrauma, which can present with subcutaneous emphysema, subpleural air cysts, pneumomediastinum, pneumoperitoneum, or pneumothorax (Dantzker, 1986; Marini, 1988). Tension pneumothorax is characterized by acute respiratory distress, rapid, thready pulse, JVD, and absent breath sounds over the involved area. This emergency situation requires immediate decompression. Barotrauma is most frequently seen in the presence of underlying lung disease and is most frequently associated with ARDS, aspiration-induced lung injury, and COPD (Dantzker, 1986). Nursing care of the mechanically ventilated patient is complicated by impaired verbal communication, which can be a significant additional stressor for the patient.

In order to avoid and/or minimize these potential problems, mechanical ventilation should be discontinued as soon as the patient's condition warrants. Weaning is the process of resuming spontaneous, independent ventilation after a period of dependence on mechanical ventilatory support. This is often a relatively quick and simple process, especially in surgical patients without cardiopulmonary impairment. In patients with an underlying cardiopulmonary problem or who have experienced respiratory failure, this process may be difficult and prolonged. Some patients may even become chronically dependent on the ventilator. Before weaning is started, the patient should be in the most stable and optimal metabolic, nutritional, and hemodynamic states possible. Variables that are routinely assessed to determine the patient's readiness to wean include the vital capacity, negative inspiratory force, minute ventilation, and maximal voluntary ventilation. The identification of more discriminating weaning parameters is the subject of much current research. Areas being researched include measurement of work of breathing, ventilatory pattern, and airway occlusion pressure (Marini et al., 1988).

Before weaning is initiated, the process should be explained to the patient. Since anxiety may be a factor in the ease with which the patient is able to be weaned, clear, concise information should be provided and the patient should be assured that all weaning attempts will be closely monitored.

Weaning is usually accomplished through the T-tube or T-piece intermittent spontaneous breathing method or the intermittent mandatory ventilation (IMV) mode. Another mode of weaning called pressure assist or pressure support ventilation (PSV) has recently been introduced. With the T-tube method, ventilatory support is periodically withdrawn and the patient is allowed to breathe spontaneously with supplemental, humidified oxygen. These spontaneous breathing periods are interspersed with periods of assisted mechanical ventilation and gradually increased in duration as the patient is able to sustain spontaneous ventilation. With the IMV method the patient is allowed to breathe spontaneously with periodic positive pressure breaths at a preset volume and rate. Weaning is achieved by gradually reducing the number of preset breaths the patient receives. The pressure support mode provides application of a low level of inspiratory pressure with every breath and the patient retains control of the cycle length and depth. This reduces the work of breathing for the patient to the extent that the air-flow resistance as a result of the endotracheal tube and ventilator circuitry is offset (Capps & Schade, 1988; Marini et al., 1988, Marini, 1988). The level of pressure support is gradually decreased until the patient is completely weaned from the ventilator. After discontinuation of assisted ventilation, the patient should be closely monitored for signs of respiratory deterioration.

ALTERED TISSUE PERFUSION

Altered tissue perfusion is defined as the state in which an individual experiences a decrease in nutrition and oxygenation at the cellular level due to a deficit in capillary blood supply. Alterations in tissue perfusion can occur within specific organ systems and, in the case of shock, throughout the general circulation. In the surgical patient a localized alteration in tissue perfusion occurs at the surgical site because of surgical disruption of the blood vessels, tissue edema, and swelling. Altered tissue perfusion due to pathology in the coronary and pulmonary circulations and shock are discussed in this section.

Altered Coronary Tissue Perfusion

Related Factors

Alterations in coronary perfusion can contribute to myocardial ischemia, which can lead to myocardial infarction, heart failure, shock, dysrhythmias, and possibly death. Coronary perfusion can be negatively affected by such factors as preexisting heart failure, thrombosis in the coronary vessels, intraoperative fluctuations in blood pressure, anesthesia-induced myocardial depression, and intraoperative hypoxemia. Some postoperative factors that increase myocardial oxygen demands and decrease the oxygen supply include shivering, blood loss and anemia, and infection. The sympathetic stimulation associated with pain, stress, and anxiety causes tachycardia, a rhythm that shortens diastole and, subsequently, coronary filling time. The physiologic stresses of surgery and healing increase tissue demands for oxygen. All of these factors can create an imbalance between oxygen supply and demand and ultimately cause myocardial ischemia. This is most likely to occur in the patient with preexisting heart disease.

Patients with a history of recent preoperative acute myocardial infarction (AMI) have a significantly increased risk of a postoperative infarct developing and reinfarction is associated with a mortality rate ranging between 50 and 70% (Tarhan, Moffitt, Taylor, & Giulioni, 1972; Mauney, Ebert, & Sabiston, 1970; Steen, Tinker & Tarhan, 1978). The risk of perioperative myocardial infarction has been found to be increased within the first 3 months after an AMI and to decrease progressively after that point declining significantly after 6 months (Tarhan et al., 1972). Reinfarction is also reported to occur more often in patients who are subjected to thoracic or abdominal procedures longer than 3 hours and in patients who experience preoperative hypertension or intraoperative hypotension (Mauney et al., 1970; Goldman et al., 1977; Steen et al., 1978; Goldman et al., 1978; Rao, Jacobs, & El-Etr, 1983).

Surgical risk in patients with accelerating or unstable angina may be analogous to that of patients with recent infarct (Goldman, 1983). Evidence of ventricular irritability or dysfunction associated with angina indicates an even greater operative risk. Severe ischemic heart disease usually requires corrective coronary artery bypass surgery in order to decrease the operative risk associated with any needed noncardiac surgery (Goldman et al., 1978; Tinker, Norback, Vliestra, & Frye, 1981; Goldman, 1983; Hermanovich, 1983).

In general, well-controlled essential hypertension is not considered a major risk factor for surgery, however, control of blood pressure during surgery is very important. Patients with hypertension are unable to tolerate hypotensive episodes caused by anesthesia or diuretic-induced hypovolemia. Rapid reduction of chronically elevated blood pressure to normotensive levels or below (mean pressure equal to or below 70 mm Hg) can impair cerebral perfusion. On the other hand, a profound increase in blood pressure as may occur during intubation or induction can produce myocardial ischemia. Intraoperative blood pressure must be closely monitored and maintained at or slightly below the preoperative level (Martin & Kammerer, 1983). Current practice is to continue antihypertensive therapy up to and including the day of surgery (Goldman, 1983). Sodium nitroprusside or nitroglycerin can be used to treat hypertensive episodes that may occur during or after surgery.

In addition to patients with preexisting cardiac disease, other high-risk patients include those who experience intraoperative hypotension and those who undergo emergency surgery. Postoperative myocardial infarction is four times more likely to develop in patients over 40 years old who have an emergency procedure (Goldman et al., 1977, 1978).

Assessment

Postoperative AMI usually occurs within the first week after surgery, with the incidence of AMI peaking within the first 3 to 5 days after surgery (Tarhan et al., 1972, Goldman et al., 1978; Steen et al., 1978; Goldman, 1983; Rao et al., 1983). This complication can be asymptomatic or "silent" in 20 to 60% of the surgical population, possibly because of residual anesthetic agents, analgesic medication, and incisional pain, all of which may mask ischemic coronary pain (Mauney et al., 1970; Tarhan et al., 1972; Goldman et al., 1977, 1978; Steen et al., 1978; Goldman, 1983). The acute development of hypotension, hypertension, dysrhythmias, or altered mental status in the surgical patient may herald the onset of a painless infarct. A possible lack of subjective information makes the monitoring and assessment of objective indicators of AMI, like ECG and enzyme changes, all the more important during the first week after surgery, especially in high-risk patients.

Positive isoenzyme studies combined with ECG changes and the patient's clinical picture are necessary to establish the diagnosis of acute myocardial infarction. Two enzymes released specifically from damaged myocardial tissue are creatine kinase (CK) and lactic dehydrogenase (LDH). Since total CK and LDH enzyme levels may be elevated after surgery, isoenzyme analysis allows differentiation between myocardial damage and surgical trauma. Isoenzymes are distinct molecular structures or fractions of the total enzyme that are separated during electrophoresis. The CK enzyme can be separated into three isoenzymes. The fraction of the total enzyme that is highly concentrated in cardiac muscle is the CK MB isoenzyme. In the presence of myocardial tissue necrosis, the level of CK MB in the serum will be elevated within 24 hours after the onset of symptoms. LDH has five isoenzymes and LDH_1 is specific for cardiac tissue damage. The serum level of LDH_1 will rise markedly within 48 hours after myocardial injury.

The ECG changes associated with transmural infarction reflect ischemia, injury, and necrosis. The first change, that of ischemia, is a tall and widened T wave that may exceed the height of the R wave. T-wave changes are often associated with ST-segment changes. Elevation of the ST segment above the isoelectric line is indicative of myocardial injury. The fully evolved stage of AMI is marked by ST-segment elevation, T-wave inversion, and the development of deep, wide Q waves and loss of R-wave voltage.

ECG evidence of subendocardial infarction differs from that of transmural infarction in that Q-wave development is absent in subendocardial infarction. Subendocardial infarction produces nonspecific ST- and T-wave changes. These ECG changes do not always absolutely correlate with the anatomic lesions, leading to the suggestion that the terms transmural and subendocardial should be replaced by Q-wave and non-Q-wave infarction (Phibbs, 1983; Alpert & Braunwald, 1984).

Intervention and Evaluation

The goals of treatment are to reduce myocardial ischemia and prevent further extension of the infarct. The expected outcomes include the absence of chest pain and the resolution of ECG and enzyme changes.

Therapy is directed toward reducing ischemia and restoring the balance between oxygen supply and demand. Ischemic chest pain is treated immediately with pharmacologic agents, which enhance coronary perfusion. Sublingual nitroglycerin may be given every 3 to 5 minutes up to three doses if the patient's systolic blood pressure does not drop. If pain continues to be unrelieved, then morphine sulfate can be given in small doses every 5 to 10 minutes until the pain subsides. Both of these medications can cause hypotension, which is treated by placing the patient in Trendelenburg's position and administering IV saline boluses should it occur.

The patient should be restarted on any antianginal medication taken prior to surgery. The patient without a history of chest pain can be started on longer-acting nitrate medication, calcium-channel blockers, or beta-adrenergic blockers in order to prevent any further chest pain. Early administration of beta-adrenergic blockers followed by oral therapy has been shown to limit infarct size (Hjalmarson et al., 1983), reduce myocardial oxygen demands, decrease heart rate and blood pressure (International Collaborative Study Group, 1984), reduce the severity of ischemia, prevent ventricular fibrillation (Norris et al., 1984), and decrease mortality after AMI (First International Study of Infarct Survival, 1986). These drugs should not be used in patients with heart failure, conduction defects, bradyarrhythmias, asthma, or hypotension (Sobel & Braunwald, 1984).

If chest pain persists, intravenous nitroglycerin can be administered in the normotensive patient and in the patient with chest pain associated with heart failure (Sobel & Braunwald, 1984). Once chest pain is relieved, the patient must be weaned from the medication and started on oral nitrate therapy.

The intraaortic balloon pump (IABP) is indicated for severe ischemic chest pain that is refractory to other treatment. The intraaortic balloon remains inflated during diastole and deflated during systole. It inflates just after the aortic valve closes and deflates just before the aortic valve opens. Timing with the ECG and arterial wave form is therefore crucial.

The physiologic effects of intraaortic balloon pumping reduce myocardial ischemia in several ways. Diastolic augmentation increases coronary and systemic perfusion. Deflation prior to the next systole reduces afterload and allows more complete emptying of the left ventricle with less stress. It also allows a reduction in left end diastolic pressure, a decrease in pulmonary congestion, and a reduction in cardiac output. Because the cardiac workload is reduced, myocardial oxygen consumption is decreased (Bolooki, 1977; Haak, 1983; Quaal, 1984). When the patient's condition has stabilized, the frequency of pumping is decreased and the patient is gradually weaned from the IABP.

The IABP is also used for the treatment of cardiogenic shock, acute mechanical defects associated with AMI and for perioperative support during surgery. Potential complications of the IABP include arterial thrombosis, infection and septicemia, bleeding, balloon rupture, arterial damage on insertion, limb ischemia, thrombocytopenia, and renal emboli (Quaal, 1984).

Intracoronary or intravenous thrombolytic therapy with streptokinase is currently being used during the early phase of AMI to dissolve intracoronary clots, restore coronary perfusion, and reduce the extent of injury after infarct. Intravenous tissue-type plasminogen activator, a newer agent that is more fibrin specific than streptokinase and produces fewer side effects, has also been used to restore perfusion in the coronary circulation (The TIMI Study Group, 1985). There are other thrombolytic agents that are currently in the investigational phase. Because these agents produce bleeding, their use is contraindicated after recent surgery (Brooks-Brunn, 1988; Gawlinski, 1987; Rethrop, 1985; Laffel & Braunwald, 1984). Further research is also needed on the use of coronary angioplasty after recent surgery, although this form of therapy may be useful for the stable patient who has undergone a relatively minor surgical procedure.

Interventions that promote rest and reduce anxiety are also essential to the care of the patient who has had an AMI. Physical and emotional rest reduces the incidence of factors that contribute to myocardial ischemia. Stress-management techniques such as relaxation and breathing exercises and guided imagery may need to be taught to the patient. The surrounding environment should be made as restful as possible. The presence of family and supportive others may also be a source of calm for the patient and visitation policies may need to be adjusted to accommodate such needs.

Altered Pulmonary Tissue Perfusion

Pulmonary embolism is the sometimes fatal consequence of venous thrombosis. Obstruction of the pulmonary arterial vasculature leads to wasted ventilation in the underperfused area (increased physiologic dead space), reduced functional lung volume, increased airway resistance, and increased intrapulmonary shunting. Hemodynamic abnormalities include increased right atrial and pulmonary artery pressures, which can result in pulmonary hypertension and right-sided heart failure.

Related Factors

Factors that increase the risk of thrombus formation and are induced by anesthesia, immobility, and the surgical procedure itself include hypercoagulability, increased stasis, and, in some cases, endothelial damage (see chapter 14). Clinical conditions associated with an increased risk of deep-vein thrombosis include orthopedic surgery (especially of the hip), prostate surgery, age over 40 years, chronic venous insufficiency, malignant neoplasm, use of oral contraceptives, obesity, and left heart failure (Rose, 1979). Fat embolism is a potential complication of trauma (see chapter 21).

Assessment

There does not appear to be a characteristic set of signs and symptoms of pulmonary embolism. Clinical manifestations vary and are nonspecific. The combined results of the Urokinase and Urokinase–Streptokinase Pulmonary Embolism Trials (1973, 1974) provided documentation of the frequency of signs and symptoms in 327 patients. Dyspnea occurred in the majority of patients. Chest pain was pleuritic in nature in submassive pulmonary embolism and ischemic in nature when the embolism was large. Apprehension and cough appeared in over half the patients and the incidence of hemoptysis and syncope was higher in submassive embolism. The most frequently documented signs included tachypnea, tachycardia, rales, increased pulmonic heart sound, and fever. Massive embolism was found to be associated with grossly elevated pressures in the right side of the heart and jugular venous distention.

Arterial blood-gas analysis often shows hypoxemia. A ventilation–perfusion scan may be done in an attempt to confirm the diagnosis.

Intervention and Evaluation

Treatment of pulmonary embolism includes administration of heparin or thrombolytic therapy (i.e., urokinase or streptokinase). Postoperative nursing care should be directed to the prevention of this disorder, and includes bed exercises, early mobilization, and use of antiembolism stockings. High-risk patients may be treated prophylactically with low-dose heparin (Rose, 1979; Kakkar, Lorrigan, & Fossard, 1975). Intermittent external pneumatic compression of the feet or calves by a cuff or boot that applies pressure and simulates muscular contraction has been shown to be effective in preventing thrombus formation (Rose, 1979).

General Circulatory Failure

Circulatory failure, or shock, is a pathophysiologic state in which tissue perfusion is totally inadequate to meet the metabolic requirements of the cells. Shock is a response to some assault or injury the body has experienced. Although the underlying cause may be different, common to all forms of shock is the insufficient flow of oxygenated blood and nutrients to the vital organs due to a reduction in cardiac output, a maldistribution of blood, or both (Sobel, 1984). Removal of the products of metabolism is also impaired, which will eventually lead to a state of acidosis.

Related Factors

Any condition that reduces the pumping ability of the heart or decreases venous return has the potential of causing the development of shock, the first stage of which is decreased cardiac output. Shock has been classified according to the precipitating cause.

Cardiogenic shock can be the result of extensive myocardial damage due to infarction or open heart surgery, as a sequela to heart failure, or as a result of prolonged arrhythmias. Cardiogenic shock is associated with a high mortality rate (75 to 90%) (Sobel, 1984; Resnekov, 1983). Other complications of acute myocardial infarction that can mechanically reduce cardiac output and predispose the patient to the development of shock include ventricular septal defect, papillary muscle rupture and cardiac tamponade.

Noncardiogenic causes of shock that may also be seen in the critically ill surgical patient include hypovolemia and sepsis. Hypovolemia is a decrease in the volume of the intravascular compartment and can be the result of actual loss of body fluids or sequestration of fluid outside the vascular compartment in a "third space" (see Chapter 9). Fluid may be lost through hemorrhage, excessive gastrointestinal or renal excretion, and through exudative lesions, draining wounds, or burns. Internal sequestration of fluid in a "third space" can occur in surgical wounds, skeletal muscle trauma, burns, ascites, intestinal obstruction, or paralytic ileus (Sobel, 1984). If the depletion in effective circulating blood volume that occurs as a result of these conditions is severe enough to reduce cardiac output and is not corrected quickly, hypovolemic shock can quickly develop. Hypovolemia is the most common cause of diminished systemic blood flow (Weil, vonPlanta, & Rackow, 1988) and hypovolemic shock is the form of shock most commonly seen (Billhardt & Rosenbush, 1986).

Septic shock is a response to infection. Approximately one third of the cases of septic shock are the result of infections caused by gram-positive organisms while the remaining two thirds are related to infections caused by gram-negative organisms. The majority of gram-negative infections leading to septic shock are due to the enteric coli. Septic shock is now considered to be a form of distributive shock in which vasomotor dysfunction alters the distribution of blood flow within the vascular compartment through either increased venous capacitance or shunting. The effective circulating volume is reduced without a decrease in the absolute amount of body fluid or impairment of cardiac function. Low arterial resistance and shunting are believed to characterize the hyperdynamic state of septic shock while increased arterial resistance and expanded venous capacity are believed to characterize hypodynamic septic shock due to gram-negative infection (Weil et al., 1988; Groer & Shekleton, 1989).

Assessment

Arterial pressure falls in response to decreased cardiac output. In response to hypotension, various compensatory mechanisms come into play. Sympathetic stimulation through baroreceptor reflexes causes an increase in heart rate and myocardial contractility, vasoconstriction, and redistribution of blood flow. Through these mechanisms cardiac output and arterial pressure are increased. For this reason, clinical detection of hypotension may occur in the later stages of shock, when compensation is no longer effective and therefore reliance on blood-pressure measurement alone may not be useful in the diagnosis of shock. Other clinical manifestations include rapid, thready pulse; cool, pale, and moist (clammy) skin; oliguria; and decreased pulse pressure. Respiratory activity will increase as chemoreceptors are activated in response to the development of acidosis. In contrast to other forms of shock, the hyperdynamic type of septic shock will be characterized in the early stage by high cardiac output, high central venous pressure, abnormal urine output, low peripheral resistance, and warm, dry extremities. The monitoring of great toe temperature has been advocated as an indicator of the adequacy of peripheral tissue perfusion while serum lactate levels can be used as an indicator of inadequate systemic perfusion.

If the underlying cause of shock remains uncorrected, continued sympathetic stimulation becomes detrimental. Mechanisms responsible for the progression of shock include altered hemodynamics in the capillary bed such that blood becomes trapped and stagnant in these beds and fluid moves into the interstitial space; the formation of microthrombi; the release of vasoactive substances such as histamine, bradykinin, and serotonin; and further depression of myocardial contractility. During this stage of progressive or decompensated shock the signs of extreme tissue hypoxia discussed earlier in this chapter will become apparent.

Intervention and Evaluation

The goal of treatment is restoration of adequate tissue perfusion and prevention of complications such as disseminated intravascular coagulation, gastric ulceration, acute renal tubular necrosis, and ARDS. Expected outcomes include the restoration of an adequate blood pressure and normal blood-gas values.

Treatment is directed at the underlying cause and includes intensive antibiotic therapy in septic shock, augmentation of cardiac performance in cardiogenic shock (see decreased cardiac output), and replacement of the effective circulating volume in hypovolemic shock. In hypovolemic shock, the basic defect is a loss in blood, fluid, or plasma volume. Thus the goal of therapy is to replace fluid losses. When hemorrhage has occurred, the circulating blood volume is replaced with blood products, but until the blood is available, volume can be expanded with crystalloid (normal saline or Ringer's lactate) or colloid solutions (Sobel, 1984). Fluid resuscitation in nonhemorrhagic shock is also accomplished with the latter solutions. In addition to correcting hypovolemia, it is important to identify the source of fluid loss, especially in nonhemorrhagic hypovolemia. Hemodynamic pressures are closely monitored during fluid replacement to avoid the complication of pulmonary edema. Pharmacologic agents such as isoproterenol and dopamine, which promote vasodilation, improve myocardial performance, and increase cerebral and renal perfusion, are also indicated.

DECREASED CARDIAC OUTPUT

Decreased cardiac output is defined as the state in which the amount of blood pumped by an individual's heart is decreased to the extent that the metabolic needs of the peripheral tissues are compromised. Cardiac output is the product of heart rate and stroke volume. Physiologic determinants of heart rate include the inherent automaticity of cardiac muscle as well as extrinsic neural and humoral factors. Physiologic determinants of stroke volume include the size of the left ventricle as well as the degree of myocardial fiber shortening. The extent of shortening is in turn determined by preload (ventricular end diastolic pressure or volume), the inotropic state of the cardiac muscle or contractility (the inherent force of ventricular contraction independent of load), and afterload (the ventricular wall tension developed during ejection) (Groer & Shekleton, 1989).

Related Factors

Decreased cardiac output is a response to pathologic conditions in which the physiologic determinants of cardiac output are disrupted such that heart rate and/or stroke volume decrease and compensatory mechanisms fail. Pathologic mechanisms that result in decreased cardiac output include damage to or loss or weakening of myocardial muscle tissue, aberrations in the rate and rhythm of the heart (dysrhythmias and conduction defects), abnormalities and incompetence of the cardiac valves, structural defects, increased vascular resistance, and constriction of the heart as occurs in cardiac tamponade or constrictive pericarditis.

Assessment

Early manifestations of decreased cardiac output reflect compensatory mechanisms of sympathetic stimulation and fluid retention. Reflex sympathetic activation causes an increase in cardiac rate and contractility as well as vasoconstriction and redistribution of blood flow to the heart and brain. Decreased renal perfusion results in activation of the renin–angiotensin system, which in turn causes aldosterone release. Stimulation of the volume receptors in the great vessels causes release of the antidiuretic hormone (ADH). Expansion of the extracellular fluid volume occurs as a result of the combination of depressed renal function and the actions of angiotensin II, aldosterone, and ADH on renal sodium and water reabsorption. This serves to augment the effective circulating blood volume and venous return to the heart, thus increasing ventricular end diastolic volume (preload), which helps to maintain cardiac output via the Frank–Starling mechanism (McCall & O'Rourke, 1985). This mechanism has physiologic limits, and the compensatory mechanisms described above increase systemic vascular resistance, afterload, and myocardial oxygen consumption, all of which can lead to further myocardial dysfunction. Clinical heart failure exists when these mechanisms are no longer able to maintain a cardiac output adequate for the metabolic needs of the body tissues.

Clinical manifestations of decreased cardiac output will reflect decreased systemic arterial pressure and tissue perfusion and increased venous and pulmonary vascular pressures as cardiac decompensation occurs. Hypotension, fatigue, weakness, pallor of the skin and mucous membranes, and restlessness occur as arterial pressure and tissue perfusion decrease. A profound decrease in cardiac output, such as that seen, for example, in cardiogenic shock, is associated with systolic blood pressure less than 80 mm Hg; cool, clammy (moist) skin; rapid, thready (weak) peripheral pulses; oliguria or anuria; cyanosis; confusion; and possibly chest pain (Sobel, 1984).

As the volume and pressure in the left atrium increase, a subsequent increase in the pulmonary vascular pressure will occur, leading to pulmonary congestion. Manifestations of pulmonary congestion include dyspnea, tachypnea, and bilateral rales (crackles) in the dependent lung fields. Cardiogenic pulmonary edema will be the result of a profound and rapid increase in pulmonary capillary hydrostatic pressure, which causes transudation of fluid from the capillaries into the interstitial space and alveoli. Clinical manifestations of pulmonary edema include extreme dyspnea, tachypnea, and use of the accessory muscles for breathing. The patient is anxious, often agitated, and frightened and feels as if he or she is suffocating. The sputum is frothy and pink tinged—a consequence of flooding the small and large airways with fluid. Cyanosis of the nailbeds, lips, and mucous membranes may be observed as the arterial PaO_2 decreases. Wheezes and fine, moist crepitant rales may be heard throughout the lung fields, making cardiac auscultation difficult. In addition to cardiac causes, hydrostatic pulmonary edema can occur after fluid overload.

Hemodynamic monitoring provides objective data regarding the extent of left ventricular dysfunction that may exist. In order to characterize the relation between clinical and hemodynamic states after myocardial damage due to AMI, Forrester et al. (1976, 1977) described four clinical subsets that correlate with cardiac index and pulmonary capillary wedge pressure (PCWP). These subsets can be used to assess short-term prognosis and to guide therapy after AMI (Table 7–5).

Hemodynamic monitoring is also helpful in differentiating between the causes of decreased cardiac output. For example, right ventricular infarction, which often occurs in the setting of inferior-wall infarction, reduces right ventricular function and cardiac output. The damage is clinically character-

Table 7–5 Clinical Subsets Correlated with Cardiac Index and Pulmonary Capillary Wedge Pressure

Clinical Subset*	Cardiac Index	Pulmonary Capillary Wedge Pressure	Mortality Rate (%)
I: No clinical signs of decreased cardiac output and heart failure	>2.2 liters/min/m²	<18 mm Hg	3
II: Isolated pulmonary congestion	>2.2 liters/min/m²	>18 mm Hg	9
III: Peripheral hypoperfusion. Hypovolemia may be related to right ventricular infarction	<2.2 liters/min/m²	<18 mm Hg	23
IV: Hypoperfusion and pulmonary congestion. Increased preload, increased afterload, and manifestations of cardiogenic shock. Poor prognosis.	Decrease < 2.2 liters/min/m²	Increase > 18 mm Hg	>51

*Hemodynamic monitoring is especially important for patients in the last two subsets.
Data from Forrester et. al. (1976) and Forrester, Diamond, and Swan (1977).

ized by jugular vein distention, clear lung sounds, and arterial hypotension. Right ventricular infarction can mimic cardiac tamponade and, to some extent, pulmonary embolism. Right ventricular infarction is characterized by an increase in mean right atrial and right ventricular end diastolic pressures, and a nearly normal or slightly elevated PCWP. Pulsus paradox (a 10 mm Hg inspiratory drop in systolic blood pressure) may be present in right ventricular dysfunction, a clinical feature often associated with cardiac tamponade. In cardiac tamponade, systolic right ventricular and pulmonary artery pressures are also normal and there is equalization of the right atrial, right ventricular diastolic, pulmonary artery diastolic, and pulmonary capillary pressures. This pattern may mimic right ventricular infarction except that the ECG does not reveal inferior-wall infarction in cardiac tamponade (Gore, Alpert, Benotti, Kotilainen, & Haffajee 1985). Also, the y descent of the right atrial tracing is preserved in right ventricular infarction whereas it may be smaller or even obliterated in cardiac tamponade (Resnekov, 1983). Pulmonary embolism produces an increase in right ventricular and pulmonary artery pressures, which distinguishes it from the other two conditions. Echocardiography and gated blood-pool scanning can further help to differentiate between these three abnormalities.

Ventricular septal defect and papillary muscle dysfunction or rupture can result in the development of an acute holosystolic murmur and manifestations of decreased cardiac output. Hemodynamic monitoring is also useful in distinguishing between these two conditions. Intraventricular septal perforation, which results from a massive transmural-wall infarction, can result in severe biventricular failure and a profound decrease in cardiac output. In this acute condition, oxygenated blood is shunted from the high-pressure left ventricle to the low-pressure right ventricle without going through the systemic circulation. Because oxygenated blood is leaking into the right ventricle, there is a "step-up" or an increase in the oxygen saturation of the blood from the right ventricle and pulmonary artery, which is a classic manifestation of this complication. There may also be a v wave in the PCWP, although it is not as prominent as that observed in mitral regurgitation (Gore et al., 1985). The other condition, papillary muscle dysfunction or rupture, which can also be a complication of AMI, causes tall v waves in the PCWP tracing, but there is no "step-up" in the oxygen saturation of the blood from the pulmonary artery and right ventricle. In both of these mechanical problems, left ventricular function can dramatically deteriorate if the defects are large. Hemodynamic monitoring facilitates early identification so that prompt management can be instituted. These complications do occur in a relatively small number of patients and, if severe enough, will require intraaortic balloon pump support, emergency catheterization, and emergency corrective surgery (Rackley, Russell, Mantle, Rogers, & Papapietro, 1981).

Intervention and Evaluation

Decreased cardiac output during the postoperative phase can be related to a number of factors. When this problem is associated with hypoxemia, acid–base disorders, sepsis, mechanical lesions, hypovolemia, or other problems previously mentioned, the goal of therapy is to correct the underlying disease process or abnormality. Decreased cardiac output related to left ventricular dysfunction that occurs in the setting of AMI or in the presence of preexisting heart disease necessitates interventions that increase contractility and reduce myocardial workload, preload, and afterload. Hopefully, successful management will result in the absence of clinical manifestations associated with decreased cardiac output.

Decreased cardiac output resulting from pump failure requires aggressive management to prevent further myocardial damage and hemodynamic deterioration. The hemodynamic subsets described by Forrester et al. (1976, 1977) are particularly useful in the care of these patients (see Table 7–5). No specific therapy is required for patients in Subset I, however these patients should be closely monitored for potential problems.

When the abnormality is primarily an increase in preload with pulmonary congestion (Subset II) diuretics are administered to the normotensive patient and vasodilators are used to reduce preload in the patient with an elevated blood pressure. With this therapy, the filling pressure is reduced to a range of 15 to 18 mm Hg.

Patients with peripheral hypoperfusion and decreased cardiac output without pulmonary congestion (Subset III) are considered to be hypovolemic. Hemodynamic monitoring is necessary to determine the cause of decreased cardiac output so that appropriate therapy can be instituted. The majority of these patients have decreased stroke volume and compensatory tachycardia, and thus fluid administration is used to increase the filling pressure and improve cardiac output. Hypoperfusion associated with hypotension and bradycardia, however, may be more responsive to atropine or temporary pacing.

Decreased cardiac output and pulmonary congestion (Subset IV) requires aggressive management with vasodilators to improve contractility. Vasodilators (nitroprusside or nitroglycerin) are used in the absence of hypotension when preload and afterload reduction is indicated. If use of a vasodilating agent results in a fall in blood pressure, dopamine is added to increase systemic pressure. The combination of these agents is often necessary in the treatment of severe heart failure. Dopamine, which exerts both alpha and beta effects, is useful in improving blood pressure and cardiac contractility at low to moderate doses. When the blood pressure is normal, dobutamine, which exerts primarily beta effects, is used to increase contractility and cardiac output.

The prognosis and clinical status are related to the cardiac output, and when it is within the range of 2.7 to 4.3 liters/min/m^2, the mortality rate is as low as 1%; however, when it falls below 1.8 liters/min/m^2, the patient is usually in cardiogenic shock (Alpert & Braunwald, 1984). Cardiogenic shock is an often fatal consequence of AMI, which occurs when there is massive left ventricular destruction. Aggressive therapy is aimed at increasing cardiac output, increasing contractility, reducing pulmonary congestion, reducing afterload and myocardial workload, and preventing further damage to the viable myocardial tissue. The combined use of dopamine and dobutamine (7.5 mg/kg/min each) has been shown to produce an improvement in hemodynamic status in patients with cardiogenic shock without the deleterious effects of administering each of these amines alone. This form of combination therapy is associated with an increase in cardiac output, blood pressure, and renal blood flow without an elevation of the PCWP. In cardiogenic shock, the PCWP is kept within the range of 18 to 24 mm Hg to maintain the cardiac index above 2 liters/min/m^2 (Rackley et al., 1981). If the filling pressure is elevated above 24 mm Hg, vasodilator as well as vasopressor therapy may be necessary (Rackley et al., 1981). If vasodilators are used, they are cautiously added and meticulously titrated, since further hypotension and ischemia can result with their use. For this reason, vasodilators may be reserved for the patient without hypotension. If the PCWP falls below 18 mm Hg, volume expansion is required to maximize preload and, subsequently, cardiac output. Continued hypotension with reduced cardiac output requires urgent insertion of the intraaortic balloon to prevent the vicious cycle of myocardial ischemia, necrosis, and further deterioration in left ventricular function (Resnekov, 1983). When arterial hypotension is life threatening, norepinephrine, a peripheral vasoconstrictor and positive inotropic agent, is used when other forms of therapy, including the IABP, fail to maintain diastolic pressure above 50 mm Hg in the previously normotensive patient (Sobel & Braunwald, 1984). Isoproterenol, another beta agonist, is associated with side effects such as tachyarrhythmias and increased myocardial oxygen consumption, thus this drug should not be used or, if it is used, it should be reserved for patients with extreme peripheral vasoconstriction and bradycardia.

Right ventricular infarction is associated with impaired right ventricular function, hypotension, and reduced cardiac output related to a reduction in left ventricular filling pressure. Therapy is usually directed toward improving the PCWP with fluid administration and enhancing contractility with inotropic agents such as dobutamine (Sobel & Braunwald, 1984).

Acute cardiogenic pulmonary edema is an emergency situation requiring prompt treatment. The dramatic increase in PCWP accompanied by pulmonary congestion can lead to death without immediate reduction in filling pressure. Interstitial and alveolar edema can produce severe hypoxemia in these patients, thus supplemental oxygen is administered by face mask and the patient is placed in the upright position to facilitate breathing. Mechanical ventilation and the use of PEEP therapy may be necessary to achieve a satisfactory PaO$_2$ at lower concentrations of inspired oxygen. Morphine sulfate is used in these patients to reduce anxiety and agitation; it also promotes some vasodilation and reduces venous return to the heart. Intravenous furosemide, a rapid-acting diuretic, is administered to promote diuresis and to reduce pulmonary congestion. Rotating tourniquets (inflated to a level 10 mm Hg below the diastolic pressure) may also be used to reduce venous return. Filling pressure may also be reduced by the use of vasodilators. Sodium nitroprusside is often preferred in this setting because it reduces preload and systemic vascular resistance (Ingram & Braunwald, 1984). Where there is associated bronchoconstriction, intravenous aminophylline is used and the heart rate is closely monitored, since this drug can cause serious tachyarrhythmias.

An accumulation of fluid within the pericardial space can cause acute cardiac tamponade. Since there is an obstruction to diastolic filling, left ventricular filling and cardiac output will be reduced and the patient will exhibit signs and symptoms of peripheral hypoperfusion. Cardiac tamponade results in an obstructive form of shock. Other manifestations include pulsus paradoxus, jugular venous distention, and muffled heart sounds. Treatment must be immediate and aggressive. It is essential that hemodynamic support is provided with intravenous fluids until aspiration of the fluid by pericardiocentesis can be accomplished. This procedure usually results in an improvement in the patient's clinical and hemodynamic status. After pericardiocentesis, the patient is closely monitored for recurrence of tamponade.

Disturbances in rhythm can potentially reduce cardiac output, especially in the patient with underlying heart disease. Thus, postoperative conditions that increase the frequency of arrhythmias should be immediately corrected. Life-threatening ventricular arrhythmias require antiarrhythmic therapy with intravenous lidocaine or procainamide. In the event that sustained ventricular tachycardia or ventricular fibrillation develop, direct-current (DC) cardioversion becomes necessary (Davis, 1983).

In the postinfarction setting, bradyarrhythmias are often associated with inferior–posterior and right ventricular infarction. Arrhythmias of this nature may be responsive to atropine administration. However, if the patient becomes hemodynamically compromised, a temporary transvenous pacemaker can be inserted. Atrial or atrioventricular sequential pacemakers may be required for patients with reduced left ventricular compliance who are dependent on the atrial systolic contribution (atrial kick) to diastolic filling (for example, patients with right ventricular infarction). Mobitz Type I second-degree AV block is usually transient and may require only observation. In contrast, Mobitz Type II second-degree AV block, which more often occurs in the setting of anterior-wall infarction, can progress to complete heart block, thus temporary pacing is necessary when this rhythm develops. Likewise, complete heart block, whether due to inferior- or anterior-wall infarction, requires pacemaker insertion. Prophylactic pacing is also required for left bundle-branch block or bilateral bundle-branch block (right bundle and either the left anterior or left posterior division) after AMI, since an increased risk for complete heart block is associated with these conduction defects (Sobel & Braunwald, 1984).

Vagal maneuvers (for example, carotid sinus massage) are used to reduce ventricular rate in supraventricular tachycardia (SVT); however, if this maneuver is unsuccessful, intravenous digitalis may be necessary. Other drugs used in the treatment of SVT include quinidine and procainamide. Parenteral verapamil (5 to 10 mg over 1 minute) may convert SVT, however, its use is contraindicated in patients with heart failure, cardiogenic shock, severe hypotension, second- or third-degree AV block, sick sinus syndrome, and in patients receiving parenteral beta-adrenergic drugs (Davis, 1983). In these patients, cardiac pacing techniques may be an option for terminating the arrhythmia. Emergency cardioversion may be necessary for patients in whom severe hypotension and hypoperfusion develop during an episode of SVT.

SUMMARY

Noncardiac surgery is associated with potentially life-threatening complications for the patient with underlying cardiopulmonary disease or who develops an alteration in oxygenation status because of surgery. Intraoperative and postoperative hypotension and hypoxemia can precipitate many complications that will further impair oxygenation status. The risk of elective surgery, however, can be reduced by control and stabilization of preoperative cardiopulmonary disease and early recognition of intraoperative and postoperative problems. Perioperative invasive monitoring of high-risk patients is extremely beneficial in reducing morbidity and mortality since this type of monitoring facilitates prompt identification and treatment of hemodynamic abnormalities. Improved outcome is also attributed to knowledgeable, well-planned nursing care. This care involves ongoing assessment, prevention of potentially life-threatening abnormalities, management of emotional and stress-provoking situations, and evaluation of the patient's response to therapy.

BIBLIOGRAPHY

Alpert, J. S., & Braunwald, E. (1984). Acute myocardial infarction: Pathological, pathophysiological, and clinical manifestations. In E. Braunwald (Ed.), *Heart disease: a textbook of cardiovascular medicine* (pp. 1262–1300). Philadelphia: W. B. Saunders.

Balk, R., & Bone, R. C. (1983b). The adult respiratory distress syndrome. *Medical Clinics of North America, 67,* 685.

Billhardt, R. A., & Rosenbush, S. W. (1986). Cardiogenic and hypovolemic shock. *Medical Clinics of North America, 70*(4), 853–876.

Bolooki, H. (1977). *Clinical applications of intra-aortic balloon pumping.* New York: Futura Publishing.

Bone, R. C. (1980). Treatment of severe hypoxemia due to the adult respiratory distress syndrome. *Archives of Internal Medicine, 140,* 85.

Bone, R. C., Fisher, C. J., Clemmer, T. P., Slotman, G. J., Metz, C. A., & Balk, R. A. (1987). A controlled clinical trial of high dose methylprednisolone in treatment of severe sepsis and septic shock. *New England Journal of Medicine, 317,* 653.

Bone, R. C., George, R. B., & Hudson, L. D. (1987). Acute respiratory failure. New York: Churchill-Livingstone.

Bone, R. C., & Stober, G. (1983). Mechanical ventilation in respiratory failure. *Medical Clinics of North America, 67,* 599.

Bradley, R. B. (1987). Adult respiratory distress syndrome. *Focus, 14*(5), 48–59.

Braunwald, E. (1984). The history. In E. Braunwald (Ed.), *Heart disease: a textbook of cardiovascular medicine* (pp. 3–13). Philadelphia: W. B. Saunders.

Brooks-Brunn, J. A. (Ed.) (1988). Symposium proceedings: Thrombolytic therapy for acute myocardial infarction: Critical care nursing update, 1988. *Heart and Lung, 17*(6), 741–792.

Buchbinder, N., & Ganz, W. (1976). Hemodynamic monitoring: Invasive techniques. *Anesthesiology, 45,* 146.

Burden, L. L. (1984). The person with angina pectoris. In C. E. Guzzetta & B. M. Dossey (Eds.). *Cardiovascular nursing, bodymind tapestry* (pp. 444–465). St. Louis: C. V. Mosby.

Capps, J. S., & Schade, K. (1988). Work of breathing: Clinical monitoring and consideration in the critical care setting. *Critical Care Nursing Quarterly, 11*(3), 1–11.

Carrieri, V., & Janson-Bjerklie, S. (1986). Dyspnea. In V. Carrieri, A. Lindsey, & C. West (Eds.), *Pathophysiological phenomena in nursing: human responses of illness* (pp. 191–218). Philadelphia: W. B. Saunders.

Cohen, C. A., Zagelbaum, G., Gross, D., Roussos, C., & Macklem, P. T. (1982). Clinical manifestations of inspiratory muscle fatigue. *American Journal of Medicine, 73,* 308–316.

Daily, E. K., & Schroeder, J. S. (1981). *Techniques in bedside hemodynamic monitoring.* St. Louis: C. V. Mosby.

Dantzker, D. (1986). *Cardiopulmonary critical care.* Orlando, FL: Grune & Stratton.

Davis, D. (1983). Diagnosis and management of cardiac arrhythmias in the postoperative period. *Surgical Clinics of North America, 63,* 1091.

Fairley, H. B. (1980). Oxygen therapy for surgical patients. *American Review of Respiratory Diseases, 122*(5), 37–44.

First International Study of Infarct Survival. (1986). Collaborative group: Randomized trial of intravenous atenolol among 16,027 cases of suspected acute myocardial infarction: ISIS-I. *Lancet, 2,* 57–66.

Forrester, J. S., Diamond, G. A., Chatterjee, K., & Swan, H. J. C. (1976). Medical therapy of acute myocardial infarction by application of hemodynamic subsets. *New England Journal of Medicine, 295,* 1356–1362, 1404–1413.

Forrester, J. S., Diamond, G. A., & Swan, H. J. C. (1977). Correlative classification of clinical and hemodynamic function after acute myocardial infarction. *American Journal of Cardiology, 39,* 137.

Francis, P. B. (1983). Acute respiratory failure in obstructive lung disease. *Medical Clinics of North America, 67,* 657.

Gawlinski, A. (Ed.) (1987). Symposium proceedings: Nursing interventions in limiting infarct size in the acute myocardial infarction patient: Nursing implications. *Heart and Lung, 16*(6), 739–800.

Glauser, F., Polatty, C., and Sessler, C. (1988). Worsening oxygenation in the mechanically ventilated patient. *American Review of Respiratory Diseases, 138,* 458–465.

Goldman, L. (1983). Cardiac risks and complications of noncardiac surgery: Review. *Annals of Internal Medicine, 98,* 504.

Goldman, L., Caldera, D. L., Nussbaum, S. R., Southwick, F. S., Krogstand, D., Murray, B., Burke, D. S., O'Malley, T. A., Ganroll, A. H., Caplan, C., Nolan, J., Carabello, B., & Slater, E. E. (1977). Multifactorial index of cardiac risk in noncardiac surgical procedures. *New England Journal of Medicine, 297,* 845.

Goldman, L., Caldera, D. L., Southwick, F. S., Nussbaum, S. R., Murray, B., O'Malley, T. A., Goroll, A. H., Caplan, C. H., Nolan, J., Burke, D. S., Krogstad, D.,

Carabello, B., & Slater, E. E. (1978). Cardiac risk factors and complications in noncardiac surgery. *Medicine, 57,* 357.

Goldman, L., Wolf, M., & Braunwald, E. (1988). General anesthesia and noncardiac surgery in patients with heart disease. In Braunwald, E. (Ed.), 1988. *Heart Disease and Disorders of Other Organ Systems,* (3rd ed.) (pp. 1693–1705). Philadelphia: W. B. Saunders.

Gore, J. A., Alpert, J. S., Benotti, J. R., Kotilainen, P. W., & Haffajee, C. I. (1985). *Handbook of hemodynamic monitoring.* Boston: Little, Brown.

Gray, B. A., & Rogers, R. M. (1983). Management of respiratory failure. In G. L. Baum, and E. Wolinsky (Eds.), *Textbook of pulmonary disease* (pp. 959–994). Boston: Little, Brown.

Groer, M. (1981). *Physiology and pathophysiology of the body fluids.* St. Louis: C. V. Mosby.

Groer, M., & Shekleton, M. (1989). *Basic pathophysiology: A holistic approach* (3rd ed.). St. Louis: C. V. Mosby.

Haak, S. W. (1983). Intra-aortic balloon pump techniques. *Dimensions in Critical Care, 2,* 196.

Hermanovich, J. (1983). The management of the cardiac patient requiring noncardiac surgery: Preoperative evaluation and management of the surgical patient with heart disease. *Surgical Clinics of North America, 63,* 985.

Hjalmarson, A., Herlitz, J., Holmberg, S., Ryden, L., Swedberg, K., Veden, A., & Wilhelmsson, C. (1983). The Gateberg metoprolol trial: Effects on mortality and morbidity in acute myocardial infarction. *Circulation, 67,* 26.

Ingram, R. H., & Braunwald, E. (1984). Pulmonary edema: Cardiogenic and noncardiogenic. In E. Braunwald (Ed.), *Heart disease: a textbook of cardiovascular medicine* (pp. 560–577). Philadelphia: W. B. Saunders.

International Collaborative Study Group (1984). Reduction in infarct size with early use of timolol after acute myocardial infarction. *New England Journal of Medicine, 310,* 9.

Jacobs, E., & Bone, R. (1986). Clinical indicators in sepsis and septic adult respiratory distress syndrome. *Medical Clinics of North America, 70*(4), 921–933.

Kakkar, V. V., Lorrigan, T. P., & Fossard, D. P. (1975). Prevention of postoperative embolism by low dose heparin: An international multicenter trial. *Lancet, 2,* 45.

Kaplan, R. L., Sahn, I. A., & Petty, T. L. (1979). Incidence and outcome of respiratory distress syndrome in gram negative sepsis. *Archives of Internal Medicine, 139,* 867.

Kirby, R., & Taylor, R. (1986). *Respiratory failure.* Chicago: Year Book Medical Publishers.

Laffel, G. L., & Braunwald, E. (1984). Thrombolytic therapy, a new strategy for the treatment of acute myocardial infarctions. *New England Journal of Medicine, 311,* 710–717, 770–776.

Larson, J., & Kim, M. (1987). Ineffective breathing pattern related to respiratory muscle fatigue. *Nursing Clinics of North America, 22*(1), 207–224.

Leasa, D., & Sibbald, W. (1988). Respiratory monitoring in a critical care unit. In D. H. Simmons (Ed.), *Current pulmonology,* (Vol. 9) (pp. 209–266). Chicago: Year Book Medical Publishers.

Macklem, P., & Roussos, C. S. (1977). Respiratory muscle fatigue: A cause of respiratory failure. *Clinical Science and Molecular Medicine, 53,* 419–422.

Marini, J. J. (1988). Mechanical ventilation. In D. H. Simmons, (Ed.), *Current pulmonology,* (Vol. 9) (pp. 164–208). Chicago: Year Book Medical Publishers.

Marini, J. J., Roussos, C. S., Tobin, M. J., MacIntyre, N. R., Belman, M. J., & Moxham, J. (1988). Weaning from mechanical ventilation. *American Review of Respiratory Diseases, 138*(4), 1043–1046.

Martin, D. E., & Kammerer, W. S. (1983). The hypertensive surgical patient: Controversies in management. *Surgical Clinics of North America, 63,* 1017.

Mauney, F. M., Ebert, P. A., & Sabiston, D. C. (1970). Postoperative myocardial infarction: A study of predisposing factors, diagnosis, and mortality in a high risk group of surgical patients. *American Surgeon, 172,* 497.

McCall, D., & O'Rourke, R. A. (1985). Congestive heart failure: Biochemistry, pathophysiology, and neuro-humoral mechanisms. *Modern Concepts in Cardiovascular Disease, 54,* 55.

Michaelson, C. (1983). *Congestive heart failure.* St. Louis: C. V. Mosby.

Murray, J. F., Matthay, M. A., Luce, J. M., & Flick, M. R. (1988). An expanded definition of the adult respiratory distress syndrome. *American Review of Respiratory Diseases, 138,* 720–723.

Norris, R. M., Barnaby, P. F., Brown, M. A., Geary, G. G., Clark, E., Logan, R. L., & Sharpe, D. N. (1984). Prevention of ventricular fibrillation during acute myocardial infarction by intravenous propranolol. *Lancet, 2,* 883.

Phibbs, B. (1983). "Transmural" versus "subendocardial" infarction: An electrocardiographic myth. *Journal of the American College of Cardiology, 1,* 561.

Quaal, S. J. (1984). *Comprehensive intra-aortic balloon pumping.* St. Louis: C. V. Mosby.

Rackley, C. E., Russel, R. O., Mantle, J. A., Rogers, W. J., & Papapietro, S. E. (1981). Modern approach to myocardial infarction: Determination of prognosis and therapy. *American Heart Journal, 101,* 75.

Rao, T., Jacobs, K. H., & El-Etr, A. A. (1983). Reinfarction following anesthesia in patients with myocardial infarction. *Anesthesiology, 59,* 499–505.

Resnekov, L. (1983). Cardiogenic shock. *Chest, 83,* 893.

Rethrop, K. P. (1985). Thrombolytic therapy in patients with acute myocardial infarction. *Circulation, 71,* 627.

Rose, S. D. (1979). Prophylaxis of thromboembolic disease. *Medical Clinics of North America, 63,* 1205.

Rose, S. D., Corman, L. S., & Mason, D. T. (1979). Cardiac risk factors in patients undergoing surgery. *Medical Clinics of North America, 63,* 1271.

Shekleton, M. (1987). Respiratory muscle fatigue. In D. Frownfelter (Ed.), *Chest physical therapy and pulmonary rehabilitation* (2nd ed.) (pp. 218–230). Chicago: Year Book Medical Publishers.

Shively, M. (1988). Effect of position change on mixed venous oxygen saturation in coronary artery bypass surgery patients. *Heart and Lung, 17*(1), 51–59.

Sobel, B. E. (1984). Cardiac and noncardiac forms of acute circulatory failure (shock). In E. Braunwald (Ed.), *Heart disease: a textbook of cardiovascular medicine* (pp. 578–604). Philadelphia: W. B. Saunders.

Sobel, B. E., & Braunwald, E. (1984). The management of acute myocardial infarction. In E. Braunwald (Ed.), *Heart disease: a textbook of cardiovascular medicine* (pp. 1301–1333). Philadelphia: W. B. Saunders.

Steen, P. A., Tinker, J. H., & Tarhan, S. (1978). Myocardial reinfarction after anesthesia and surgery. *Journal of the American Medical Association, 239,* 2566–2570.

Szaflarski, N. L., & Cohen, N. H. (1989). Use of pulse oximetry in critically ill adults. *Heart and Lung, 18*(5), 444–455.

Tarhan, S., Moffitt, E. A., Taylor, W. F., & Giulioni, E. R. (1972). Myocardial infarction after general anesthesia. *Journal of the American Medical Association, 220,* 1451.

The TIMI Study Group (1985). The thrombolysis in myocardial infarction trial: Phase I findings. *New England Journal of Medicine, 312,* 932.

Tinker, J. H., Norback, C. R., Vliestra, R. E., & Frye, R. L. (1981). Management of patients with heart disease for noncardiac surgery. *Journal of the American Medical Association, 246,* 348.

Tisi, G. M. (1979). Preoperative evaluation of pulmonary function: Validity, indications, benefits. *American Review of Respiratory Diseases, 119,* 293.

Urokinase pulmonary embolism trial: A national cooperative study. (1973). *Circulation, 47*(Suppl 2), 1.

Urokinase–streptokinase pulmonary embolism trial: Phase 2 results. (1974). *Journal of the American Medical Association, 229,* 1606.

Weil, M. H., vonPlanta, M., & Rackow, E. C. (1988). Acute circulatory failure (shock). In Braunwald, E. (Ed.), *Heart disease: A textbook of cardiovascular medicine* (3rd ed.). Philadelphia: W. B. Saunders.

Whitney, J. D. (1989). Physiologic effects of tissue oxygenation on wound healing. *Heart and Lung, 18*(5), 466–76.

Wolf, M. A., & Braunwald, E. B. (1984). General anesthesia and noncardiac surgery in patients with heart disease. In E. Braunwald (Ed.), *Heart disease: A textbook of cardiovascular medicine* (pp. 1815–1825). Philadelphia: W. B. Saunders.

ADDITIONAL READINGS

Anderson, F. D. (1988). Issues in the postresuscitation period. *Critical Care Nursing Quarterly, 10*(4), 51–61.

Andreoli, K. G., Zipes, D. P., Wallace, A. G., Kinney, M. R., & Fowkes, V. (Eds.) (1987). *Comprehensive cardiac care* (6th ed.). St. Louis: C. V. Mosby.

Awan, N. A., Amsterdam, E. A., & Mason, D. T. (1981). Vasodilator therapy in acute myocardial infarction: Enhancement of cardiac function and potential to limit infarct size. *American Heart Journal, 101,* 516.

Ayres, S. M. (1982). Mechanisms and consequences of pulmonary edema: Cardiac lung, shock lung, and principles of ventilatory therapy in adult respiratory distress syndrome. *American Heart Journal, 103,* 97.

Balk, R., & Bone, R. C. (1983a). Classification of acute respiratory failure. *Medical Clinics of North America, 67,* 551.

Bartlett, J. G., & Gorbach, S. L. (1975). The triple threat of aspiration pneumonia. *Chest, 68,* 560.

Brochard, L., Harf, A., Lorino, H., & Lemaire, F. (1989). Inspiratory pressure support prevents diaphragmatic fatigue during weaning from mechanical ventilation. *American Review of Respiratory Diseases, 139,* 513–521.

Burke, L. E., & Frein, J. (1983). Oxygen therapy in heart failure. In C. R. Michaelson (Ed.), *Congestive heart failure* (pp. 299–325). St. Louis: C. V. Mosby.

Bynam, L. J., & Pierce, A. K. (1976). Pulmonary aspiration of gastric contents. *American Review of Respiratory Diseases, 114,* 1129.

Cahill, J. M. (1968). Respiratory problems in surgical patients. *American Journal of Surgery, 116,* 362.

Campbell, P. B., & Waldhausen, J. (1983). Monitoring and perioperative interventions in the postoperative patient with heart disease. *Surgical Clinics of North America, 63,* 1057.

Criteria Committee of the New York Heart Association: Nomenclature and criteria for diagnosis of diseases of the heart and great vessels (1986). In M. Sokolous and M. B. Mellroy (Eds.), *Clinical cardiology* (p. 41), Los Altos, CA: Lange Medical Publishers.

Drew, B. J. (1989). Cardiac rhythm responses. 1. An important phenomenon for nursing practice, science and research. *Heart and Lung, 18*(1), 8–16.

Foex, P. (1981). Preoperative assessment of the patient with cardiovascular disease. *British Journal of Anaesthesia, 53,* 731.

Forgacs, P. (1979). Treatment of septic shock. *Medical Clinics of North America, 63,* 465.

Fromm, G. (1979). Using basic laboratory data to evaluate patients with acute respiratory failure. *Critical Care Quarterly, 1* (4), 43–51.

Goe, M., & Massey, T. (1988). Assessment of neurologic damage: Creatinine kinase BB assay after cardiac arrest. *Heart and Lung, 17*(3), 247–253.

Guyton, A. C. (1986). *Textbook of medical physiology.* (7th ed.). Philadelphia: W. B. Saunders.

Harmon, E., & Lillington, G. (1979). Pulmonary risk factors in surgery. *Medical Clinics of North America, 63,* 1289.

Heimer, D., & Scharf, S. M. (1983). History and physical examination. In G. L. Baum & E. Wolinsky (Eds.), *Textbook of pulmonary diseases* (pp. 223–234). Boston: Little, Brown.

Hill, N. S., Antman, E. M., Green, L. H., & Alpert, J. S. (1981). Intravenous nitroglycerin, a review of pharmacology, indications, therapeutic effects, and complications. *Chest, 79,* 69.

Huseby, J. S. (1982). Radiographic examination of the chest. In S. L. Underhill, S. L. Woods, E. S. Sivarajan, & C. J. Halpenny, (Eds.), *Cardiac nursing* (pp. 187–195). Philadelphia: J. B. Lippincott.

Isher, J. M., Cohen, S. R., Virmani, R., Lawrinson, W., & Roberts, W. C. (1980). Complications of the intra-aortic balloon counterpulsation device: Clinical and morphologic observations in 45 necropsy patients. *American Journal of Cardiology, 45,* 260.

Kigin, C. M. (1981). Chest physiotherapy for the postoperative or traumatic injured patient. *Physical Therapy, 61,* 1724.

King, T. K. C. (1983). Pulmonary gas exchange. In G. L. Baum & E. Wolinsky (Eds.), *Textbook of pulmonary disease* (pp. 99–116). Boston: Little, Brown.

Langlois, P., Gawryl, M., Zeller, J., & Lint, T. (1989). Accentuated complement activation in patient plasma during the adult respiratory distress syndrome: A potential mechanism for pulmonary inflammation. *Heart and Lung, 18*(1), 71–84.

Laszlo, G., Archer, G. G., Darrell, J. H., Dawson, J. M., & Fletcher, C. M. (1973). The diagnosis and prophylaxis of pulmonary complications of surgical operation. *British Journal of Surgery, 60,* 129.

Leaman, D. M., & Davis, D. (1983). Diagnosis and management of myocardial ischemia in the postoperative period. *Surgical Clinics of North America, 63,* 1081.

Marshall, B. E., & Wyche, M. Q. (1972). Hypoxemia during and after anesthesia. *Anesthesiology, 37,* 178.

Mecca, R. S. (1986). Respiratory failure in the postoperative period. In R. R. Kirby &

R. W. Taylor (Eds.), *Respiratory failure* (pp. 310–334). Chicago: Year Book Medical Publishers.

Morgan, T. E., & Edwards, L. H. (1967). Pulmonary artery occlusion. III: Biochemical alterations. *Journal of Applied Physiology, 22,* 1012.

Morrison, D. H., Dunn, G. L., Fargas, B. A. M., Moudil, G. C., Smedstad, K., & Woo, J. (1982). A double blind comparison of cimetidine and ranitidine as prophylaxis against gastric aspiration syndrome. *Anesthesia and Analgesia, 61,* 988.

Myers, D. L. (1986). Pharmacologic therapy of respiratory failure. In R. R. Kirby and R. W. Taylor (Eds.), *Respiratory failure* (pp. 478–496). Chicago: Year Book Medical Publishers.

Pennock, J. L. (1983). Perioperative management of drug therapy. *Surgical Clinics of North America, 63,* 1049.

Pepe, P. E., Potkin, R. T., & Reus, D. H. (1982). Clinical predictors of acute respiratory distress syndrome. *American Journal of Surgery, 144,* 120.

Rao, T. (1983). Cardiac monitoring for the noncardiac surgical patient. *Seminars in Anesthesia, 2,* 241.

Rice, V. (1987). Acid base derangements in the patient with cardiac arrest. *Focus, 14*(6), 53–61.

Rogers, R. M., & Gray, B. A. (1983). Recognition of acute and chronic respiratory failure and an algorithm for selecting therapy. In G. L. Baum & E. Wolinsky (Eds.), *Textbook of pulmonary diseases* (pp. 949–958). Boston: Little, Brown.

Shapiro, B. A., Harrison, R. A., & Kacmarek, R. M. (1985). *Clinical application of respiratory care.* Chicago: Year Book Medical Publishers.

Shoemaker, W. C., Appel, P., & Bland, R. (1983). Use of physiologic monitoring to predict outcome and to assist in clinical decisions in critically ill postoperative patients. *Amerian Journal of Surgery, 146,* 43–50.

Shoichet, S. H., DeBacker, N. A., & Webster, J. R. (1983). Contemporary management of the pulmonary patient: Preoperative, intraoperative, and postoperative evaluation and care. *Internal Medicine for the Specialist, 4,* 135.

Staub, N. C. (1978). Pulmonary edema due to increased microvascular permeability to fluid and protein. *Circulation Research, 43,* 143.

Stewardson, R. H., & Nyhus, L. M. (1977). Pulmonary aspiration. *Archives of Surgery, 112,* 1192.

Tantum, K. R. (1983). Respiratory care of the surgical patient with cardiac disease. *Surgical Clinics of North America, 63,* 1069.

Weigelt, J. A., Norcross, J. F., Borman, K. R., & Snyder, W. H. (1985). Early steroid therapy for respiratory failure. *Archives of Surgery, 120,* 536.

Wolfe, J. E., Bone, R. C., & Ruth, W. E. (1977). Effects of corticosteroids in the treatment of patients with gastric aspiration. *American Journal of Medicine, 63,* 719.

Wynne, J. W., & Modell, J. H. (1977). Respiratory aspiration of gastric contents. *Annals of Internal Medicine, 87,* 466.

Zeffren, S. E., & Hartford, C. E. (1972). Comparative mortality for various surgical operations in older versus younger age groups. *Journal of the American Geriatrics Society, 20,* 485.

8 Alterations in Nutrition

Joyce K. Keithley, D.N.Sc., R.N.

A key component in the care of critically ill surgical patients is the management of actual or potential nutrition problems. The nutrition-related nursing diagnosis most frequently made in critically ill surgical patients is "alteration in nutrition: potential for less than body requirements related to the effects of starvation and stress." Good nutritional status during the perioperative period ensures a smoother intraoperative course, better wound healing, fewer complications, shorter convalescence, and lower mortality rates (Askanazi, Starker, Olsson, Hensle, Lockhart, Kinney, & LaSala, 1986; Starker, LaSala, Askanazi, Todd, Hensle, & Kinney, 1986). This chapter focuses on the incidence and significance of malnutrition in surgical patients, metabolic factors involved in its onset, methods used to detect malnutrition, and nutritional support techniques to prevent or reverse malnutrition.

MALNUTRITION
Incidence and Significance

Based on reports in the literature, the incidence of malnutrition in surgical patients appears to range between 30 and 50%. Using anthropometric parameters, Bistrian, Blackburn, Hallowell, and Heddle (1974) reported the striking finding of 50% prevalence of protein-calorie malnutrition (PCM) among 131 surgical patients studied at an urban municipal hospital. Mullen, Gertner, Buzby, Goodhart, and Rosato (1979) studied the incidence of malnutrition in 161 elective surgical patients admitted to an urban Veterans Administration hospital. Ninety-seven percent of these patients had at least one abnormal measurement, and 35% demonstrated three or more abnormal nutritional and immunologic measurements. This study also demonstrated a significant correlation between malnutrition and postoperative morbidity and mortality.

In the past decade, selected nutritional assessment parameters have been tested to predict surgical outcome. Mullen et al. (1979) developed a linear predictive model, the Prognostic Nutritional Index (PNI), that related the risk of operative morbidity and mortality to base-line nutritional status. Of 16 nutritional and immunologic factors studied in developing the PNI, four parameters taken together (serum albumin, triceps skinfold, serum transferrin, and delayed cutaneous hypersensitivity) were significant in predicting postoperative morbidity and mortality. Buzby, Mullen, Matthews, Hobbs, and Rosato (1980) designed a prospective study to test the PNI on patients having abdominal surgery. Smale, Mullen, Buzby, and Rosato (1981) designed a similar study of cancer patients undergoing treatment. In both of these studies, patients with a PNI over 40% were at significantly greater risk for postoperative complications or death. The PNI is reviewed in greater detail later in this chapter.

Seltzer, Fletcher, Slocum, and Engler (1981) devised a method of instant nutritional assessment (INA) using only those data required by routine hospital admission laboratory tests. These investigators found that surgical intensive care unit patients with low serum albumin levels and low total lymphocyte counts had twice the complication rate and 4.5 times the death rate of those with both parameters in the normal range.

Rainey-Macdonald, Holliday, Wells, and Donner (1983) studied the relation of base-line nutritional tests to clinical outcome in 55 surgical and critically ill patients. Eight nutritional tests were evaluated on the basis of their ability to discriminate between patients who would have major septic complications and/or die and patients who would survive without major septic complications. Their results suggested that of the commonly employed nutritional tests serum albumin and serum transferrin were the most useful in identifying high-risk patients.

Roy, Edwards, and Barr (1985) proposed that weight loss alone might be used to assess rapidly and inexpensively nutritional status and to predict postoperative complications. Of 74 surgical patients assessed, there were no complications or deaths in patients with less than a 6% decrease from their usual body weights. Of the 27 patients having more than a 6% weight loss, 12 experienced postoperative complications; four of those patients died.

These and other studies continue to document the significance of malnutrition in hospitalized patients and to refine the specificity and sensitivity of various nutritional assessment factors in detecting malnutrition and predicting postoperative morbidity and mortality. With the assessment techniques and information now available, malnutrition can often be identified or prevented in critically ill surgical patients.

Pathogenesis of Malnutrition

Energy Reserves

In the normal adult, available stored energy amounts to about 250 g of glycogen, 6000 g of protein, and 15,000 g of fat. Carbohydrate stores (4 kcal/g), primarily in the form of liver and muscle glycogen, are relatively small, supply about 1,000 kcal, and meet basal energy needs for less than a day. (The term "calorie" is often used to mean either the calorie or the kilocalorie. The kilocalorie [kcal] is the unit of energy used in studying human nutrition and is the term that will be used in this chapter.)

Protein stores (4 kcal/g) account for approximately 24,000 kcal. Protein is stored in two forms—somatic and visceral. Somatic protein includes skeletal and smooth muscle stores; visceral protein stores include plasma protein, hemoglobin, several clotting components, hormones, and antibodies. Since all protein serves specific functions in the body, any protein loss or catabolism represents loss of essential function. For example, protein loss from the intercostal and diaphragmatic muscles may predispose the patient to inspiratory muscle weakness, hypoventilation, atelectasis, and subsequently, pneumonia; use of antibodies or other plasma proteins for energy may lead to sepsis as immunocompetence is compromised. Most significant to the surgical patient, loss of protein will impair the wound-healing process.

Fat (9 kcal/g) is the largest fuel reserve; approximately 135,000 kcal are stored as triglycerides in adipose tissue. Fat stores are excellent sources of energy because they can be used without sacrificing essential tissue or function.

Energy Requirements and Expenditure

Healthy adults require a protein intake of approximately 0.8 g/kg of body weight and a basal caloric intake of approximately 1,800 kcal per day. In contrast, critically ill surgical patients have a total calorie need of 32 − 40 kcal/kg per day and a total protein need of 1.5 − 2.0 g/kg per day. In addition to the total calorie and protein intake, the ratio of nonprotein calories to nitrogen is an important consideration. A ratio of 100:1 is necessary to achieve positive nitrogen balance in most critically ill patients. Also, the specific amino acid profile of the protein source is important. Several clinical studies comparing high branched chain amino acid formulas with standard amino acid formulas have demonstrated the benefit of the branched chain-enriched solutions in improving nitrogen retention, improving hepatic protein synthesis, and decreasing protein breakdown (Cerra, 1982; Cerra, 1987). The recommended percentage of calories from each nutrient source is: a.) protein: 20 − 25% of total calories, b.) carbohydrate: 40 − 50% of the total calories, and c.) fat: 30 − 40% of total calories (Cerra, 1987; Cerra, et al., 1990; Konstantinidis, et al., 1984; Negro & Cerra, 1988).

Several methods of estimating calorie requirements can be used. When available, indirect calorimetry is the preferred method of measuring energy needs. However, many clinical settings do not have the necessary equipment, or it cannot be used reliably. The classic equations of Harris and Benedict (1919) are therefore often used to estimate basal energy expenditure (BEE) based on weight, height, and age:

$$BEE_{men} = 66.47 + 13.75\,W + 5.0\,H - 6.74\,A$$
$$BEE_{women} = 655.10 + 9.56\,W + 1.85\,H - 4.68\,A$$

where W = weight in kilograms, H = height in centimeters, and A = age in years. Activity and injury factors (Table 8–1) are then added, in order to calculate resting energy expenditure (REE) precisely in critically ill surgical patients:

$$REE = BEE + \text{activity factor} + \text{injury factor}$$

After elective surgery, energy expenditure increases by as much as 20%. Major trauma or infection may increase this requirement to 50 to 80%; the presence of major thermal injuries may cause caloric requirements to double (Long, Schaffel, Geiger, Schiller, & Blakemore, 1979).

Effects of Starvation

When a person starves, glycogenolysis (glycogen breakdown) occurs to maintain blood glucose levels. Glycogen stores, which supply about 1,000 kcal, are usually exhausted within 15 to 20 hours. Next, protein is mobilized from skeletal muscle, converted to glucose in the liver, and released into the bloodstream to maintain blood glucose concentrations. This use of body proteins for fuel results in deterioration of body functions such as wound repair and immunocompetence, as mentioned earlier. The body, therefore, adapts by using fat, a more dispensable energy store; free fatty acids and ketones are the major fuels used by the brain and body. Another adaptation during starva-

Table 8–1 Activity and Injury Factors (Energy Expenditure)

Activity Factor	Injury Factor
Confined to bed = 1.2	Surgery = 1.1–1.2
Ambulatory = 1.3	Infection = 1.2–1.8
	Trauma = 1.3–1.6
	Burns = 1.5–2.0

Adapted with permission of Ross Laboratories, Columbus, OH. 43216, from *Critical Care Nursing Currents,* vol. 2, #2. Copyright 1984 by Ross Laboratories.

Table 8–2 Effects of Starvation

Body Store	Body Response
Glycogen (muscle, liver)—250 g (1,000 kcal)	Day 1—depletion of glycogen stores
Protein (somatic, visceral)—6,000 g (24,000 kcal)	Days 2–4—increase in catabolism of skeletal muscle to support gluconeogenesis
Fat—15,000 g (135,000 kcal)	Days 5–10—body fat becomes primary source of energy, and body adapts to conserve protein stores and energy expenditure
	Days 40+—remaining somatic and visceral proteins provide energy, resulting in edema, and eventually, death

tion includes a decline in metabolic rate. This, in conjunction with the predominant use of fat for energy, results in conservation of vital protein stores. In the final phase of starvation, fat stores are used up, and the entire energy requirement must be met by the remaining somatic and visceral protein stores. Depletion of these proteins is signaled by edema, and will ultimately result in death (Table 8–2).

Metabolic Response to Stress

The stress of major surgery, trauma, and sepsis triggers a series of complex metabolic changes that differ significantly from so-called simple starvation. In contrast to the starved patient, in whom adaptive mechanisms preserve protein stores and decrease metabolic rate, the stressed patient experiences accelerated protein breakdown and energy expenditure. Cuthbertson (1932) documented two distinct phases of metabolic response to stress or serious illness (Table 8–3). The first or "ebb" phase occurs immediately after the insult, lasts no more than 24 to 48 hours, and tends to preserve vital system function. In clinical practice, the ebb phase corresponds to the period of fluid resuscitation and restoration or maintenance of major system function. If the patient survives, the second or "flow" phase follows. The flow phase is subdivided into two subphases—acute and adaptive.

During the acute phase, stress hormones—catecholamines, growth hormone, glucocorticoids, and glucagon—stimulate accelerated breakdown of protein and fat stores. Proteolysis and lipolysis yield costly, but important, supplies of glucose for trauma patients. Proteolysis also provides glutamine,

Table 8–3   Metabolic Response to Stress

Ebb Phase
  Decreased circulatory volume, 24–48 hours' duration

Flow Phase
  Acute Phase
    Increased epinephrine, growth hormone, glucocorticoid, and glucagon release
    Increased protein and fat catabolism and gluconeogenesis
    Decreased insulin release
    Insensitivity to glucose and insulin, 3–5 days' duration
  Adaptive Phase
    Decreased or normal epinephrine, growth hormone, glucocorticoid, and glucagon secretion
    Decreased serum glucose levels
    Decreased protein catabolism
    Decreased insulin resistance

an amino acid that appears to be a specific fuel for the gut, and other amino acids that support protein synthesis at remote sites such as the wound and inflammatory foci. The acute phase is also characterized by decreased activity of insulin, the key anabolic hormone. In addition, high circulating levels of glucocorticoids reduce the sensitivity of tissues to insulin, while catecholamines inhibit its release (Porte & Bagdade, 1970). All of these factors interact to create a diabetes-like syndrome, marked by hyperglycemia and insensitivity to exogenously administered glucose and insulin. The administration of concentrated glucose solutions during the acute phase may exacerbate the hyperglycemia and lead to nonketotic hyperosmolar coma. The net effect of the acute phase is a highly catabolic hormonal environment that protects and defends the body at the expense of skeletal muscle.

Although the stress hormones have a major role in mediating the metabolic responses observed in critically ill surgical patients, they are not completely responsible for the catabolic changes that occur. With the recent aid of recombinant DNA technology, it is now known that at least two cytokines—tumor necrosis factor (TNF) and interleukin-2 (IL-2)—can initiate and perpetuate metabolic responses after injury and critical illness (Bessey, 1989). Endotoxin, a potent stimulus for TNF production, may gain access to the circulation in association with bacteremia or through the gut or wound. Transplant rejection, transfusion reaction and other strong antigen antibody reactions are associated with the elaboration of IL-2.

The gut has long been considered to be inactive or inert during critical illness, but actually may play a key part in the metabolic response to critical illness (Bessey, 1989; Wilmore, Smith, O'Dwyer, Jacobs, Ziegler & Wang, 1988). When the barrier function of the epithelium is impaired either by malnutrition or a massive direct insult such as major surgery, intraluminal bacteria can invade the host. This process, known as bacterial translocation, can promote a vicious cycle of repeated endotoxemia and systemic responses that leads to a prolonged hypercatabolic state. It is interesting to note that current parenteral nutrition solutions do not contain glutamine, an amino acid required for gastrointestinal epithelial cell proliferation and repair.

After 3 to 5 days, the acute phase gradually is replaced by the adaptive, or anabolic, phase. This phase is characterized by decreased levels of catabolic hormones, resolution of hyperglycemia and insulin resistance, and restoration of protein stores. Determining blood glucose level is an early and easy way to detect the transition from the acute to the adaptive phase. It is during the adaptive phase that nutritional support can be effectively used to reduce protein loss and promote protein synthesis.

Hypermetabolism, with or without organ failure, is the most common reason for admission to a surgical intensive care unit (SICU). It also accounts for over 85% of SICU deaths, and is the single greatest user of resources on a hospital surgical service (Madoff, Sharpe, Fath, Simmons, & Cerra, 1985). When hypermetabolism does not abate, complications are usually present, such as wound infection, anastomotic disruption, or intraabdominal abscesses. In some patients, the organ-failure process begins (Carrico, Meakins, Marshall, Fry, & Maier, 1986; Pine, Wertz, Lennard, Dellinger, Carrico, & Minshew, 1983). Predisposing factors to multiple-organ-failure syndrome include persistent, uncontrolled sources of infection; episodes of sepsis preceded by episodes of perfusion failure; severe episodes of perfusion failure alone; and persistent hypermetabolism, with or without uncontrolled septic sources. Once patients enter the organ-failure phase, the mortality rate begins to rise rapidly. Clinical malnutrition develops in a matter of days, and becomes a prominent feature in the disease process (Cerra, Siegel, Coleman, Border, & McMenamy, 1980; Long, Jeevanadam, Kim, & Kinney, 1977). Multiple-organ-failure syndrome is discussed in Chapter 1.

A number of current studies (Bessey, 1989; Lieberman, Shou, Torres, Weintraub, Goldfine, Sigal, & Daly, 1990; Reynolds, Daly, Zhang, Evantash, Shou, Sigal, & Zeigler, 1988) are examining strategies to manipulate the metabolic response to critical illness. These strategies include gut sterilization, new approaches to insulin administration and the use of growth hormones and immunomodulators, such as arginine, glutamine, and omega-3 fatty acids. In the future, it may be possible to attenuate the metabolic response, thereby preventing many of the metabolic alterations and complications that are now seen in critically ill surgical patients.

NUTRITIONAL ASSESSMENT

Nutritional assessment should be a routine part of the overall evaluation of critically ill surgical patients. The assessment process begins with a patient history and proceeds through physical examination, anthropometric measurements, and laboratory tests. From this data base, nurses can identify patients at nutritional risk, determine a plan of care to meet nutritional needs, and evaluate efficacy of the nutrition care plan through serial monitoring of nutritional status.

History

The history may be difficult to obtain in the critical care setting because of the patient's condition. If this is the case, family members may be asked if the patient has had any recent weight or appetite change, recurrent vomiting or diarrhea, recent surgery or trauma, any chronic illness, gastrointestinal disorder, or abnormal social or dietary habits that may lead to chronic debilitation, any allergies, or takes any medications (especially those that alter nutrient intake or metabolic processes, i.e., those that have the potential for drug–nutrient interaction). Patients who have received intravenous dextrose (5%) and water or saline solutions for more than 5 days are also at risk for malnutrition (Young, 1988).

Physical Examination

Clinical signs of nutrient deficits are a late manifestation of malnutrition, and as such, are usually not detected until the patient is grossly malnourished. A list of clinical signs indicative or suggestive of malnutrition appears in Table 8–4. Physical inspection may reveal the following: fat and muscle wasting; hair changes, such as sparseness, discoloration, or shedding; skin changes,

Table 8–4 Clinical Signs of Malnutrition

Area of Examination	Signs Associated with Malnutrition	Nutrient Deficiency
Hair	Dull, dry, sparse	Protein, zinc, linoleic acid
	Color changes	Copper
	Corkscrew hair	Vitamin C
Skin	Dry, flaking, scaly	Vitamin A, vitamin B-complex, linoleic acid
	Petechiae/ecchymoses	Vitamins C and K
	Follicular hyperkeratosis	Vitamin A, linoleic acid
	Cracks in skin, glove-and-stocking lesions, facial lesions, Casal's necklace	Niacin, tryptophan
	Nasolabial seborrhea	Riboflavin, vitamin B_6
	Acneiform forehead rash	Vitamin B_6
	Xanthomas	Excessive serum levels of low- or very-low-density lipoproteins

Table 8–4   *(Continued)*

Area of Examination	Signs Associated with Malnutrition	Nutrient Deficiency
Eyes	Cornea:	
	foamy plaques (Bitot's spots)	Vitamin A
	dryness (xerophthalmia)	Vitamin A
	softening (keratomalacia)	Vitamin A
	Pale conjunctivae	Iron
	Red conjunctivae	Riboflavin
	Blepharitis	B-complex vitamins, biotin
Lips	Swollen, red cracks at sides (cheilosis)	Riboflavin, niacin, vitamin B_6
	Angular stomatitis	Riboflavin, iron
Tongue	Glossitis	Vitamin B-complex
	Pale	Iron
	Papillary hypertrophy	Multiple nutrients
	Magenta tongue	Riboflavin
Gums	Bleeding	Vitamin C
Nails	Brittle, ridged, or spoon-shaped	Iron
	Splinter hemorrhages	Vitamin C
Musculo-skeletal	Pain in calves, thighs	Thiamine
	Osteomalacia	Vitamin D
	Rickets	Vitamin D
	Joint pain	Vitamin C
	Muscle wasting	Macronutrients
Neurologic	Peripheral neuropathy	Thiamine, vitamin B_6
	Hyporeflexia	Thiamine
	Disorientation or irritability	Vitamin B_{12}

such as dryness, flakiness, texture changes, or color loss; mucous-membrane changes, including swelling, redness, fissures, and bleeding; hepatomegaly; mental irritability; and apathy.

Anthropometric Measurements

Anthropometry indirectly measures body fat, lean body mass, and skeletal muscle—the body fuel stores used to provide energy during stress. These measurements are used to estimate changes in body fuel reserves and to predict morbidity and mortality related to malnutrition. Although a variety of standards are used to interpret anthropometric measurements, those developed by Frisancho (1984) are the most widely accepted for adults and the elderly. In critically ill patients, it is important to keep in mind that anthropometric measures may be significantly altered by the wide variations in fluid status that are so often seen in these patients. Therefore, pre-injury anthropometric measures, if available, provide the most accurate baseline for assessing trends and changes.

Body Weight

Weight and weight changes are the best general indicators of protein-calorie malnutrition. Rate of weight change is a prognostic indicator of the body's ability to survive the stress sustained from operative or skeletal trauma (Harvey, Moldawer, Bistrian, & Blackburn, 1981; Kinney, Duke, Long, & Gump, 1970; Seltzer et al., 1981; Studley, 1936). To ensure accuracy, weight measurements should be made on a platform balance scale. Patients who are confined to bed or unable to stand can be weighed accurately with a portable scale. If the physical condition permits, the patient should be weighed on admission to the critical care unit, and thereafter, at the same time each day, using the same scale. The presence of dressings, catheters, respiratory equipment, and casts or other items present at the initial weighing should be recorded on the flow chart or in the nurse's note. Changes during subsequent weighing and changes in weight due to amputation should also be noted. Weights are recorded to the nearest 0.2 kg or 0.5 lb.

Serial measurements of weight are important to establish whether the patient is responding to nutrition therapy or experiencing fluid shifts. This can be established by comparing the patient's weight change with the balance on the fluid intake and output record. Dehydration, overhydration, edema, and ascites may account for sudden changes in weight.

To determine the degree of weight change, compare the current weight and usual weight (based on patient or family recall), using the following formula:

$$\% \text{ weight change} = \frac{\text{usual weight} - \text{current weight}}{\text{usual weight}} \times 100$$

Evaluating the rate of weight change is difficult because weight normally fluctuates from day to day by 1.0 to 1.5 kg. Weight gain can be expected in postoperative or posttrauma patients who have undergone fluid resuscitation. Later weight loss in these patients may be attributed to diuresis. Moore (1959) noted that weight loss exceeding 500 g/day in postoperative patients is most likely the result of dehydration or diuresis. Guidelines, developed by Blackburn, Bistrian, Maini, Schlamm, & Smith (1977), for evaluating weight change are shown in Table 8–5.

Table 8–5   Evaluating Rate of Weight Change

Time	Significant Weight Loss (percent)	Severe Weight Loss (percent)
1 week	1–2	>2
1 month	5	>5
3 months	7.5	>7.5
6 months	10	>10

From "Nutritional and Metabolic Assessment of the Hospitalized Patient" by G. L. Blackburn, B. R. Bistrian, B. S. Maini, H. T. Schlamm, and M. F. Smith, 1977, *Journal of Parenteral and Enteral Nutrition, 1*(11). Copyright by the American Society for Parenteral and Enteral Nutrition. Reprinted with permission.

Height

Accurate determination of height is important in order to calculate body mass, creatinine-height index, and estimated basal energy expenditure using the Harris–Benedict equation. Height is measured without shoes, since standards used for interpretation of height data are based on height without shoes. The patient should stand upright, with heels together and back firmly against a measuring tape. Height is recorded to the nearest 0.5 cm. Such a measurement should be obtained on admission, before surgery. For critically ill patients who are unable to stand, information about height may be obtained from the patient or family or may be computed using measurement of the lower leg (knee height) using the following formulas:

$$\text{stature of men} = 64.19 - (0.04 \times \text{age}) + (2.02 \times \text{knee height})$$
$$\text{stature of women} = 84.88 - (0.24 \times \text{age}) + (1.83 \times \text{knee height})$$

Triceps Skinfold

Skinfold measurements provide an estimate of body fat reserves. Although many sites have been identified for measuring skinfold thickness, the triceps skinfold (TSF) is the most accessible. To measure the TSF, a fold of skin on the posterior aspect of the upper arm, midway between the shoulder and elbow, is grasped and gently pulled away from the underlying muscle. Calipers are applied to measure the skinfold. Ideally, three successive readings should be made, and the average recorded to the nearest 5 mm (0.5 cm). Conditions such as edema or subcutaneous emphysema may produce falsely high readings.

Skinfold measurements do not appear to be important predictors of outcome in stressed patients, relative to other parameters of nutrition assessment. This may be because little change occurs in the measurement during short stays in the intensive care or postoperative unit. Mullen, Buzby, Wald-

man, Gertner, Hobbs, & Rosato (1979) found that 33% of 64 patients undergoing elective surgery in a Veterans Administration hospital had TSFs less
than 90% of standard. In this group, TSFs were not useful in predicting morbidity or mortality, but were important, along with weight changes, in detecting protein-calorie malnutrition.

Mid-Upper Arm Circumference

The mid-upper arm circumference (MAC) is used to estimate skeletal muscle
mass and fat stores. MAC is determined by measuring the circumference of
the upper arm with a tape measure at a point midway between the shoulder
and elbow. MAC has little prognostic value in adults, but is usually measured
in order to calculate mid-upper arm muscle circumference and midarm muscle area.

Derived Anthropometric Measurements

Mid-upper arm muscle circumference (MAMC) is an indirect indicator of
muscle mass that is derived from the triceps skinfold and the mid-upper arm
circumference. It is calculated as follows:

$$\text{MAMC} = \text{MAC} - \frac{\pi \times \text{TSF}}{10}$$

where $\pi = 3.14$, MAC is measured in centimeters, TSF is measured in millimeters, and MAMC is measured in centimeters.

Midarm muscle area (MAMA) quantifies the surface area of muscle, medial neurovascular sheath, and bone at the cross section of the mid-upper
arm. When Heymsfield, McManus, Smith, Stevens, and Nixon (1982) corrected MAMA for bone area, they found an average discrepancy of 7.7% between calculated values and values measured by computerized tomography.
Bone-free MAMA (MAMA.BF) is considered to be a more sensitive measure of
longstanding malnutrition than MAMC. As with MAMC, however, daily or
weekly changes may be masked by fluid shifts, so a direct relation to protein
status is difficult to establish. The equations for MAMA and MAMA.BF are

$$\text{MAMA} = \text{MAC} - \frac{\text{MAMC}}{4\pi}$$
$$\text{MAMA.BF}_{males} = \text{MAMA} - 10$$
$$\text{MAMA.BF}_{females} = \text{MAMA} - 6.5$$

where MAMA and MAMA.BF are in square centimeters.

The body-mass index is an alternate way of describing degree of body
fatness. The assumption is that weight, when compared with height, is positively correlated with the degree of adiposity. Therefore, the higher the body-

mass index, the greater the relative amount of body fat. It is not a direct measure of body composition, since weight gain or loss can also occur because of changes in hydration or lean body mass. There are several body mass indexes, but the most frequently used is the Quetelet index:

$$\text{Quetelet index} = \frac{\text{weight}}{\text{height}^2} \times 100$$

where weight is measured in kilograms and height is measured in centimeters.

Laboratory Studies

Creatinine-Height Index

The creatinine-height index (CHI) is a method of estimating the amount of skeletal muscle mass. Creatinine is derived from the breakdown of creatine, an energy-containing complex found in muscle. Creatinine is excreted unchanged in the urine at a constant rate, in proportion to the amount of body muscle. The CHI is calculated by first measuring urinary creatinine using a carefully collected 24-hour urine specimen. This value is then compared with ideal urinary creatinine levels from a creatinine-for-height standard table, by means of the following equation:

$$\text{CHI} = \frac{\text{actual 24-hour urine creatinine}}{\text{ideal 24-hour urine creatinine for height}} \times 100$$

The patient's CHI is then compared with a CHI standard table to determine the degree of skeletal muscle depletion. Assuming an accurate 24-hour urine specimen has been collected, a CHI of 60 to 80% of standard indicates a moderate deficit in body muscle mass. A value of less than 60% for CHI indicates a severe deficit of body muscle mass (Blackburn, et al., 1977). Stress, fever, and trauma can increase urinary creatinine excretion. Increases in creatinine excretion from 20 to 100% have been found in seriously ill and injured patients (Schiller, Long, & Blakemore, 1979; Threlfall, Stoner, & Galasko, 1981).

Nitrogen Balance

Nitrogen balance is also used as an index of protein nutritional status. Nitrogen is released with the catabolism of amino acids and excreted in the urine as urea. As such, nitrogen balance indicates whether the patient is anabolic (positive nitrogen balance) or catabolic (negative nitrogen balance). Nitrogen balance is estimated by a formula based on urine urea nitrogen (UUN) excreted during the previous 24 hours:

$$\begin{aligned} \text{Nitrogen} \quad & \text{nitrogen} \quad \text{nitrogen} \\ \text{balance} = & \text{intake} \quad - \text{excretion} \end{aligned}$$

or

$$= \frac{\text{protein}\ \text{intake}}{6.25} - (24\text{-hour UUN} + 4)$$

where nitrogen balance is determined in grams, UUN = urinary urea nitrogen measured in grams, and 4 = nonurea nitrogen losses via feces, skin, sweat, and lungs measured in grams. In response to stress and increased protein demand, the body rapidly mobilizes its protein compartments, which results in increased production of urea and excretion of urea in the urine. With infection, an estimated loss of 9 to 11 g/day of UUN can be expected. In patients with major burns, 12 to 18 g/day of urea nitrogen may be expected in the urine (Blackburn et al., 1977). On the other hand, with adequate nutrition, one expects a positive nitrogen balance of 2 to 4 g/day.

The validities of the CHI and UUN are dependent on the accuracy of the 24-hour urine collection. Failure to obtain an accurate sample, abnormal renal function, and certain other conditions can result in underestimation of creatinine and nitrogen losses.

Visceral Proteins

Visceral protein status may be assessed by determining serum concentrations of albumin and transferrin. Serum albumin is the most frequently measured visceral protein. However, because of its relatively long half-life (17 to 20 days) and large body pool (4.0 to 5.0 g/kg), albumin levels cannot be used as an early indicator of protein malnutrition. Normal serum albumin concentrations range from 3.5 to 5.5 g/dl. In general, a serum albumin level of 2.8 to 3.5 g/dl represents moderate visceral protein depletion, and less than 2.8 g/dl denotes severe depletion (Bistrian, Blackburn, Vitale, Cochran, & Naylor, 1976).

Visceral proteins that respond more quickly to changes in nutritional status are retinol-binding protein, with a half-life of 12 hours, prealbumin, with a half-life of 48 hours, and transferrin, with a half-life of 8 to 10 days. Retinol-binding protein and prealbumin analysis are not yet available at many institutions; therefore determination of transferrin concentration is more widely used. Levels of serum transferrin, an iron-transport protein, can be measured directly or by an indirect measurement of total iron-binding capacity (TIBC). Blackburn et al. (1977) have developed the most widely used formula for computing serum transferrin:

$$\text{Serum transferrin} = (0.8 \times \text{TIBC}) - 43$$

where serum transferrin is calculated in milligrams per deciliter, and TIBC is measured in mg/dl. Normal values for serum transferrin are 170 to 250 mg/dl. Levels of 150 to 200 mg/dl are considered evidence of mild deficiency; 100 to 150 mg/dl, moderate deficiency; and levels less than 100 mg/dl are indicative of severe deficiency (Rudman, 1987). Because a variety of clinical conditions and incidents can alter serum albumin and transferrin levels, the patient's history must be considered in conjunction with these values for accurate interpretation.

Immune Function

Loss of immunocompetence is another indicator of visceral protein status, and is strongly correlated with malnutrition in stressed and starving patients. The most commonly used tests of immune function are total lymphocyte count (TLC) and skin testing, also called delayed cutaneous hypersensitivity testing.

The total lymphocyte count is derived from the white blood cell count (WBC) and the differential cell count:

$$TLC = WBC \times \frac{\text{the number of lymphocytes in differential}}{100 \text{ cells}}$$

where TLC is calculated in cells per cubic millimeter. As standards, Blackburn et al. (1977) recommend using 1,500 to 1,800 to represent mild depletion, 900 to 1,500 to represent moderate depletion, and less than 900 to represent severe depletion.

Adequate immunity can also be demonstrated by a positive reaction to multiple skin test antigens. In this test of immune function, antigens are injected intradermally in the forearm area and the response (redness and/or induration) is noted at 24 and 48 hours. A reaction area of 5 mm or greater response is generally considered positive. Commonly used antigens in current clinical use are candida, purified protein derivative (PPD), mumps, and tetanus. Lymphopenia and the lack of a positive response to skin test antigens place the patient at increased risk of infection, sepsis, shock, and other complications in the critical care unit. Both the total lymphocyte count and skin test results can be altered in patients who are receiving steroid or immune therapy or have conditions affecting immune function, such as sepsis.

New Indices

Recent adjuncts to the traditional method of assessing nutritional status are the Prognostic Nutritional Index and the Stress Index.

Prognostic Nutritional Index (PNI)

In 161 patients undergoing major elective surgery, Mullen et al. (1979) found that four nutrition assessment parameters, measured preoperatively, could assist in predicting major postoperative complications and survival. The PNI is calculated as follows:

$$PNI = 158 - 16.6(Alb) - 0.78(TSF) - 0.20(TFN) - 5.8(DH)$$

where PNI is a percentage, Alb = serum albumin in grams per deciliter, TSF = triceps skinfold thickness measured in millimeters, TFN = serum transferrin in mg/dl, and DH = delayed hypersensitivity (0 = nonreactive; 1 = <5 mm reactivity; 2 = ≥5 mm reactivity). A PNI of 40% indicates low risk, 40 to 49% indicates moderate risk, and 50% indicates high risk.

Stress Index (SI)

Bistrian (1979) devised a formula based on the premise that in mild to moderate stress about 50% of dietary protein is converted to urinary urea nitrogen, and 3 g of nitrogen loss is obligatory;

$$SI = 24\text{-hour UUN} - (1/2 \text{ dietary nitrogen intake} + 3)$$

where stress index values less than 0 indicate no significant stress, 1 to 5 mild stress, and more than 5 moderate to severe stress. Weekly determination of the stress index is a simple way to monitor response to treatment in critical illness.

Data Interpretation

Based on the findings of the nutritional assessment, the type and extent of malnutrition may be diagnosed (Table 8–6).

Table 8–6 Classification of Malnutrition

Protein Malnutrition (Kwashiorkor)	Protein-Calorie Malnutrition (Marasmus)	Combined Malnutrition (Mixed Marasmus–Kwashiorkor)
Decreased visceral proteins	Normal visceral proteins	Decreased visceral proteins
Anergy	±Anergy	Anergy
Decreased MAMC and CHI	Decreased MAMC and CHI	Decreased MAMC and CHI
Normal weight and TSF	Decreased weight and TSF	Decreased weight and TSF
Edema	Emaciated appearance	Wasted appearance with edema

Protein Malnutrition

In protein malnutrition (PM or kwashiorkor), the diet supplies calories chiefly in the form of carbohydrate (e.g., clear liquid, intravenous glucose), with little or no protein intake. Laboratory studies show a decline in visceral protein, but changes in anthropometric measurements are usually absent. Fat reserves and lean body mass tend to be normal, or loss is marked by edema. Thus, the patient appears deceptively well nourished.

Protein-Calorie Malnutrition

In protein-calorie malnutrition (PCM or marasmus) there is inadequate intake of both calories and protein (e.g., bowel obstruction, cancer cachexia). PCM, in contrast to PM, is characterized by a decrease in all anthropometric measurements, with obvious wasting of muscle and fat in the upper and lower extremities. However, visceral protein levels remain within normal ranges.

Combined Malnutrition

Combined malnutrition (mixed marasmus–kwashiorkor) is characterized by inadequate caloric and protein intakes, with a sudden increase in demand for protein intake. Typically, this results when a marasmic patient experiences a stress event. Laboratory values are similar to those found in PM, and anthropometric values are similar to those found in PCM. Without nutritional support, the patient follows a rapidly deteriorating clinical course.

Monitoring Profile

Adequacy of nutritional status and/or nutritional support techniques is monitored at regular intervals by serial measurements of nutritional assessment parameters. Fluid intake and output and daily weight measurements should be carefully recorded. It is recommended that nitrogen balance and changes in stress index be assessed once or twice weekly. Serum albumin, transferrin, and TLC should be evaluated weekly. Because measurements of triceps skinfold thickness, mid-upper arm circumference, arm muscle circumference, CHI, and skin-test reactivity change slowly, these measures may be obtained biweekly or monthly. The parameters given in Table 8–7 can be used as a general guide for determining when an alteration in nutritional status is present.

NUTRITIONAL INTERVENTION

Specific diagnoses related to the nutritional status of critically ill patients with the appropriate nursing interventions are highlighted in Table 8–8. Since critically ill patients often cannot eat and frequently have progressive weight

Table 8-7   Guidelines for Assessing an Alteration in Nutritional Status

Nutritional deficits	None	Mild	Moderate	Severe
% Ideal body weight	>90	80–90	70–79	<70
% Weight loss	0–5	5–15	15–25	>25
Serum albumin (g/dl)	>3.5	3–3.5	2.1–2.9	<2.1
TLC (thousands of cells/mm³)	>2.0	1.2–2.0	0.8–1.2	<0.8
Transferrin (mg/dl)	>200	150–200	100–150	<100
CHI % standard	>90	81–90	71–80	70–60
TSF % standard MAC	>90	51–90	31–50	<30
MAMC % standard	>90	51–90	31–50	<30

TLC = total lymphocyte count; CHI = creatinine-height index; TSF = triceps skinfold; MAC = midarm circumference; MAMC = midarm muscle circumference.

From "Malnutrition and Wound Healing" by M. E. Young, 1988, *Heart and Lung, 17*(1), pp. 60–69. Reprinted by permission.

loss, enteral or parenteral nutritional support may be necessary to maintain body weight and to diminish protein breakdown. Our understanding of the role of nutrition in critically ill surgical patients has increased dramatically in recent years. Traditionally, these patients were given large amounts of glucose and little or no protein and fat, which frequently led to complications such as respiratory failure due to excessive CO_2 production, hepatic steatosis, hyperglycemia, and excessive weight gain in the form of fat. Current nutritional support techniques and related nursing care practices are discussed in the following section.

Table 8-8   Selected Nutritional Nursing Diagnoses and Interventions for Critically Ill Surgical Patients

Nursing Diagnoses	Interventions	Expected Outcomes
Alteration in nutrition: less than body requirements related to accelerated rate of tissue breakdown due to hypermetabolic state	Assess and monitor laboratory and anthropometric parameters of nutritional status: Weigh patient daily Monitor variations in blood sugar, BUN, creatinine, electrolytes, fluid intake and output	Prevention of weight loss Maintenance of lean body mass
Alteration in nutrition: less than body requirements related to negative nitrogen balance due to hypermetabolism and immobility (see Chapter 14)	Establish minimal caloric and protein requirements per shift Obtain 24-hour urine collection for nitrogen and creatinine Reevaluate feeding intake based on nitrogen balance results Provide enteral/parenteral nutrition at prescribed rate Initiate passive and active range-of-motion exercises Keep strict calorie counts	Positive nitrogen balance

Table 8–8   *(Continued)*

Nursing Diagnoses	Interventions	Expected Outcomes
Potential for infection: sepsis related to enteral or parenteral nutrition support	Administer enteral feeding if gastrointestinal tract is functioning Reserve total parenteral nutrition for patients who cannot digest or absorb enteral feedings Avoid contamination of enteral or parenteral nutrition delivery systems Change central venous catheter dressing according to institution protocol Monitor temperature and other vital signs per intensive care routine Assess catheter insertion site for signs of inflammation or infection Change tubing/delivery systems every 24 hours or according to institution protocol Culture central venous catheter according to institution protocol Monitor catheter culture results and appropriate laboratory values If other catheters become infected (e.g., arterial line), central venous catheters should be changed prophylactically, and cultured according to institution protocol Administer antibiotics as prescribed	Free of sepsis; Afebrile Negative cultures Absence of redness, swelling, or drainage at catheter insertion site
Altered bowel elimination: diarrhea related to intolerance of tube feeding	Assess for tube-feeding-related causes of diarrhea: lactose intolerance, osmotic overload, bacterial contamination, rapid infusion, delivery of hot/cold formula, inappropriate composition Rule out non-tube-feeding-related causes of diarrhea: concurrent drug therapy, fecal impaction, low serum albumin, gastrointestinal dysfunction Start enteral feeding at prescribed rate and isotonic concentration Deliver feeding with an enteral pump Limit hang-time to a maximum of 4 to 8 hours, to avoid bacterial contamination.	Normal bowel function Normal bowel sounds Absence of diarrhea

Table 8–8   *(Continued)*

Nursing Diagnoses	Interventions	Expected Outcomes
	Provide adequate hydration Administer antidiarrheal medications as prescribed Monitor and record number and consistency of bowel movements Keep strict record of fluid intake and output Cleanse perianal area after each bowel movement and apply skin care products as indicated Apply fecal incontinence bag if indicated Monitor potassium levels	
Potential for aspiration of tube feeding	Confirm placement, patency, and security of tube before instituting tube feeding, and at 4 to 6-hour intervals thereafter Hold feeding and notify physician of questionable or improper placement, vomiting, difficulty breathing, abdominal distention Keep head of bed elevated to 30 degrees or higher at all times during infusion Add food coloring or methylene blue to enteral formula to prevent inadvertent IV administration Test pulmonary secretions with Labstix for glucose Assess for fever, changes in vital signs, pulmonary infiltration, purulent sputum	Prevention of aspiration Absence of respiratory dysfunction or distress No change in color or consistency of pulmonary secretions Pulmonary secretions negative for glucose
Alteration in fluid volume and composition related to glucose imbalance: hyperglycemia, hypoglycemia, or hyperosmolar, hyperglycemic, nonketotic dehydration	Administer enteral or parenteral feeding at constant rate Monitor serum and urine glucose every 6 hours, respiratory quotient, fluid intake and output Report serum glucose levels > 200 mg/dl to physician Observe for signs and symptoms of hyperglycemia (thirst, polyuria, confusion), hypoglycemia (sweating, hunger, weakness, tremors) Administer insulin as ordered Taper enteral or parenteral feedings gradually	Blood glucose level within normal limits

Enteral Nutrition

Enteral nutrition is the delivery of liquid nutritional products orally or through tubes introduced into one of several sites along the alimentary tract. If the gastrointestinal tract is functional, enteral nutrition is the preferred method of nutritional support in critically ill patients for several reasons (Hyman, Rodriguez, & Weissman, 1982; Orme & Clemmer, 1983). First, nutrient utilization is improved because the gut and portal system process nutrients in the normal fashion. Nutrients administered by the parenteral route (intravenously) bypass this mechanism and may have a role in altered nutrient oxidation and liver function (Starzl, Porter, & Putnam, 1975). Second, using the gut helps to maintain its normal mucosal structure and barrier function. Third, a gastrointestinal tract that is unused will have a start-up time of days to weeks once feeding is reinstituted (Pfeiffer, 1970). This phenomenon may explain why some critically ill patients demonstrate gastrointestinal (GI) dysfunction, such as diarrhea, when starting on clear liquids or tube feedings. Other reasons for providing nutrients by the enteral route include the fact that it is less costly than parenteral nutrition and is associated with fewer complications, especially since the introduction of small, soft feeding tubes that cause less discomfort, the recent availability of infusion pumps that prevent bolus infusion, and the availability of a large variety of commercially prepared enteral formulas.

Feeding Routes and Tubes

Routes for tube feeding include the traditional nasogastric, nasoduodenal, and nasojejunal feeding routes, and the surgically performed esophagostomy, gastrostomy, and jejunostomy methods of feeding. The percutaneous gastrostomy or PEG tube is increasingly popular since it is placed using an endoscopic approach rather than a surgical procedure (Eisenberg, 1989). Currently, the needle-catheter jejunostomy (NCJ) technique is gaining widespread acceptance as an effective means of providing nutritional support during the postoperative period (Bower, Talamini, Sax, Hamilton, & Fischer, 1986; Muggia-Sullam, Bower, Murphy, Joffe, & Fischer, 1985; Ryan & Page, 1984).

Dysfunction of the stomach and colon normally prevents oral or gastric feeding for 2 to 5 days postoperatively. However, the small bowel regains its motility and ability to absorb nutrients almost immediately, allowing infusion of the feeding into the small bowel distal to the site of operative procedures (Wells, Tinckler, Rawlinson, Jones, & Saunders, 1964). Enteral diets may be administered by NCJ immediately after surgery, although jejunal tolerance of a hyperosmolar feeding requires careful initiation and only gradual increase in concentration and rate (Hoover, Ryan, Anderson, & Fischer, 1980).

A number of feeding tubes that vary in length and diameter are now available. The large, red plastic "garden hose" variety tubes have been replaced by polyurethane and silicone tubes that are more pliable and less irritating to body tissues. Some of the commercially available feeding tubes include Flexiflo (Ross), Corpak (Corpak), Entriflex (Bismark), Keofeed (IVAC), and Dobbhoff (Biosearch). Feeding tube selection should be based on the formula required by the patient. Large-bore feeding tubes (10 to 14 French) are necessary when blended "house" formulas or viscous formulas are used. Commercially prepared formulas generally flow well through smaller bore (8 French or less) tubes.

Several of the tubes have radiopaque, mercury-weighted tips to facilitate insertion and to maintain proper position. Other types have tungsten or silicone tips. Silicone-weighted tips are very popular, but are lighter than tungsten or mercury tips, and dislodge more easily. The softness and pliability of the newer tubes necessitate the use of guide wires and stylettes for ease of insertion. Most of these guide wires are steel and come preassembled with the tube. Guide wires should be used only on initial insertion of the feeding tube. Reinsertion of the guide wire after a tube has been inserted may cause perforation of the feeding tube or slippage through an exit eyelet into the GI tract.

Formula Selection

The composition of enteral formulas varies greatly. Nutrient sources and osmolarity are major considerations in formula selection. In addition, caloric and lactose contents vary. A clinical dietitian can assist in choosing the formula that best meets each patient's requirements.

The digestive and absorptive capacities of the gastrointestinal tract should be considered when selecting nutrient sources. Nutrients may be present in their simplest forms—glucose, crystalline amino acids, medium-chain triglycerides—which require little or no digestion; or they may occur in more complex forms—polysaccharides, milk solids, corn oil—which must be digested. Critically ill patients with impaired digestive capabilities (e.g., pancreatitis, bile-duct obstruction) or altered absorptive capacity (e.g., short bowel syndrome) may require feedings containing simple nutrient sources. If the GI tract is fully functional, however, these formulas are not necessary, and a more complete formula, with intact protein, complex carbohydrate, and a higher percentage of fat is appropriate. In general, nutrients in simpler form are less palatable and should be administered through a straw or feeding tube.

Vitamin, mineral, and electrolyte contents also vary. Most commercial formulas are designed to meet the recommended dietary allowances (RDA) for vitamins in approximately 2 liters of formula. Care should be taken when choosing a formula for cardiac, renal, or hepatic patients requiring sodium and/or fluid restrictions. Critically ill patients with conditions characterized by excessive loss of electrolytes—GI fistulas, electrolyte-depleting nephropathies, or burns—may require electrolyte supplementation.

The osmolality of normal body fluids is about 300 mOsm/kg. Enteral products that are more concentrated than body fluids are hyperosmolar, cause water to be drawn into the gastrointestinal tract if given too rapidly, and may result in abdominal discomfort, diarrhea, and dumping syndrome. Most enteral products are hyperosmolar, although several products are isosmotic. In general, the closer an enteral feeding is to isosmotic, the lower the potential for hyperosmolar complications. Feedings delivered directly into the small intestine usually require the use of formulas as nearly isosmotic as possible.

Enteral products usually provide 1 kcal/ml at full strength. In other words, a volume of 1,000 ml is required to provide 1,000 kcal. Several newer formulas contain 1.5 or 2.0 kcal/ml and can be used when energy needs are high, such as for patients in hypermetabolic states or for patients who cannot tolerate large volumes of fluid. As a rule, the higher the caloric content of a formula, the higher the osmolarity. So the advantages of higher caloric content versus increased risk of hyperosmolar complications must be carefully weighed.

Lactose, the sugar normally found in milk, must be broken down into monosaccharides by the enzyme lactase in order to be absorbed. Certain disease states of the intestine, such as celiac sprue and regional enteritis can result in insufficient levels of lactase. Also, over half of all adults have a primary lactase deficiency, which results in lactose intolerance. Symptoms of lactose intolerance are bloating, gas, abdominal cramping, and diarrhea. Walike and Walike (1977) reported that in approximately 87% of patients given a large lactose load, such as that received in a typical blended formula, diarrhea developed. As a result of these findings, the lactose content of many new products has been minimized.

Classification of Formulas

Three general categories of enteral products are commercially available: nutritionally complete, specialized, and supplements. Some commonly used products and their compositions are listed in Table 8–9.

Nutritionally complete formulas supply protein, carbohydrate, fat, vitamins, and minerals in sufficient quantities to maintain the nutritional status of an individual receiving no other source of nourishment. The formulas in this category vary greatly in composition. Some formulas, such as the defined or elemental formulas, require minimal digestion and are clear liquid with minimal residue. Others, such as the meal replacement and blended feedings,

Table 8–9 Enteral Nutrition Products*

Product	Form	kcal/ml	N:kcal	Osmolality (mOsm)	Lactose
Nutritionally complete					
Ensure Plus	L, F	1.5	1:170	600	—
Isocal HCN	L, U	2.0	1:167	740	—
Osmolite HN	L, U	1.0	1:150	310	—
Sustacal	L, F	1.0	1:105	644	—
Enrich	L, F	1.0	1:178	400	—
Sustacal Pudding	Pd, F	1.6	1:220	NA	+
Vital	P, F	1.0	1:150	460	+
Pulmocare	L, U	1.5	1:125	409	—
Specialized					
Amin-Aid	P	2.0			—
Hepatic-Aid	P	1.6			—
Hepatic-Aid Pudding	P	1.6			—
Portagen	P	1.0			—
Supplements					
MCT Oil	L	7.7			—
Microlipids	P	4.5			—
Propac	P	2.0			—
Polycose Liquid	L	2.0			—

*Adapted from Enteral Nutrition Product Listings; Department of Pharmacy, Rush Presbyterian–St. Luke's Medical Center, Chicago.

L = liquid; F = flavored; U = unflavored; Pd = pudding; P = powder; NA = not available.

require full digestive and absorptive abilities and contain varying amounts of residue and lactose.

Specialized formulas have been formulated for use in patients with specific metabolic abnormalities. Formulas containing essential amino acids and histidine are available for use in patients with renal disease. Formulas with high branched-chain amino acid (leucine, isoleucine, valine) contents have been developed for patients with hepatic insufficiency who cannot use large quantities of non-branched-chain amino acids. Products that have a higher fat content have also been developed for pulmonary patients. Such formulations reduce carbohydrate load and minimize carbon dioxide production.

Supplements provide one single nutrient or combinations of only a few nutrients. Such formulas are nutritionally incomplete, however, and should be used only to supplement nutritional intake.

Methods of Administration

The preferred method of tube feeding administration is by continuous drip, usually over 8 to 24 hours. Continuous drip formulas can be administered by either gravity drip or infusion pump. Use of a pump is desirable for more accurate drip rates and to prevent accidental bolus delivery. Abdominal cramps, distention, nausea, and vomiting are usually avoided when feedings are administered by continuous drip.

Enteral feedings may also be administered by intermittent infusion. With this method, the prescribed volume of formula is administered over a 30 to 60 minute interval, with four to six feedings daily. Tolerance of intermittent feedings may be poor in patients who have inadequate absorptive capacity; such patients are better able to tolerate a consistent formula flow.

Bolus delivery, the least preferred technique, involves the rapid administration of a large volume of formula by syringe. Typically, the patient is fed a volume of 300 to 400 ml over a few minutes, four to six times daily. Feedings using this technique permit the rapid infusion of a large, hyperosmolar bolus of liquid, which may be poorly tolerated, and may result in diarrhea or other GI symptoms.

The following guidelines for tube feeding are generally recommended:

1. Start the feeding at isosmotic concentration and at a slow rate of flow, usually 50 ml/hr.
2. Observe the patient for glucosuria and/or diarrhea.
3. In the absence of glucosuria and diarrhea, gradually increase daily until the desired rate and strength are achieved. For intragastric feedings, the concentration is increased first, and then the rate of flow. With small bowel feedings, the rate is increased first, and then the concentration. Rate and concentration should not be altered simultaneously.
4. If the feeding is not tolerated, reduce the rate or concentration to levels tolerated by the patient.
5. Gradually advance again, giving the patient time to adjust to each increase.

Complications

Complications associated with enteral nutritional support are presented in Table 8–10. Interventions related to these complications are discussed in the following text.

Most mechanical and metabolic complications associated with enteral therapy in critically ill patients are preventable with proper tube placement, correct formula selection, and careful administration (Apelgren and Wilmore, 1983; Cataldi-Betcher, Seltzer, Slocum, & Jones, 1983). Problems with tube

Table 8–10   Complications associated with enteral nutritional support

Complication	Cause
Mechanical/anatomical	
Tube displacement	Tube inadequately secured
Mucous membrane irritation	Use of large-bore, inflexible feeding tubes
Localized infection at tube insertion site	Improper dressing care of gastrostomy and esophagostomy tubes; inadequate disinfection of insertion site
Feeding tube occlusion	Cessation of flow through tube
	Inadequate flushing of small-bore feeding tubes
Tracheoesophageal fistula	Prolonged oropharyngeal intubation with larger-bore feeding tube along with endotracheal or tracheal intubation
Metabolic	
Fluid imbalance	
Overhydration	Too rapid administration of feedings
Dehydration	Failure to meet fluid requirements
Tube-feeding syndrome (dehydration, prerenal azotemia, and hypernatremia)	Administration of highly concentrated formulas with inadequate attention to fluid needs
Electrolyte imbalance	
Excess	Failure to monitor electrolytes
	Improper selection of enteral product
	Inattention to electrolyte composition of feeding formulas
Deficit	Failure to monitor electrolytes
	Anabolism
	Inadequate delivery of required electrolytes
Glucose imbalance	
Hyperglycemia	Stress
	Sepsis
	Too rapid administration of carbohydrate formulas
	Diabetes mellitus
	Inadequate insulin coverage
Glucosuria	Excess glucose administration surpassing renal threshold
Hypoglycemia	Resolution of sepsis
	Insulin overdose
	Failure to withhold insulin when feeding discontinued
	Sudden inadvertent cessation of feeding after insulin administration
Hyperosmolar hyperglycemic nonketotic dehydration	Persistent prolonged glucosuria; glucose acts as osmotic diuretic

Table 8–10   *(Continued)*

Complication	Cause
Other	
Vitamin and trace mineral deficiencies	Inadequate administration of formula
	Prolonged infusion of diluted formulas
Protein and calorie deficiencies	Prolonged infusion of diluted formulas
	Scheduled feedings withheld
	Prolonged diarrhea (malabsorption)
Gastrointestinal/pulmonary	
Diarrhea	Hypoalbuminemia
	Too rapid administration of hypertonic solutions
	Lactose intolerance
	Bacterial contamination of formulas
	Medications
	Use of hot or cold formula
	Fat intolerance
Constipation	Prolonged use of antidiarrheal drugs
	Inadequate fluid intake
	Immobility
Nausea and vomiting	Too rapid administration of solution
	Formula intolerance
	Administration of refrigerated solutions
	Medications
	Paralytic ileus
	Gastric outlet obstruction
	Gastric atony
Gastric rupture	Gastric outlet obstruction (rare)
	Paralytic ileus
Aspiration	Regurgitation of formula
	Incompetent gastroesophageal junction leading to reflux
	Vomiting in moribund or comatose patient

From *Critical Care Nursing Quarterly* (formerly *Critical Care Quarterly*), 6(1), pp. 8–9. Copyright June 1983 by Aspen Publishers, Inc. Reprinted with permission.

insertion, such as misplacement in the trachea or perforation of the duodenum, can be lethal. Proper tube placement should always be confirmed by x-ray examination. The recent development of soft, pliable, small-bore tubes decreases the potential for lower esophageal sphincter incompetence, gastrointestinal irritation, and perforation.

Aspiration is one of the most dangerous complications of enteral feeding. Critically ill (weak, debilitated, intubated, and comatose) patients are especially vulnerable. The majority of the patients who were found to aspirate in the study conducted by Flynn, Norton, & Fisher (1987) had an artificial airway in place. Placement of the feeding tube in the small bowel significantly decreases the likelihood of aspiration in patients at risk because the tube is distal to the lower esophageal and pyloric sphincters. Use of metoclopramide before feeding tube placement has been found to enhance transpyloric intubation. This medication has also been found useful for patients exhibiting high gastric residuals with decreased emptying time (Perkel, Moore, Hersh, & Davidson, 1979; Whatley, Turner, Dey, Leonard, & Guthrie, 1984). Cuffed tracheal tubes also protect against large, life-threatening aspirations. Routinely checking for gastric distention and gastric residuals, and elevating the head of the bed at all times to an angle greater than 30 degrees are other techniques that may reduce the risk of aspiration.

Metabolic complications are frequently ascribed to parenteral therapy, but occur in enteral therapy as well. In a sample of 100 enterally fed patients, the following metabolic abnormalities were noted: hyperglycemia (29%), hypoglycemia (2%), hypernatremia (10%), hyponatremia (31%), hyperkalemia (40%), hypokalemia (8%), hyperphosphatemia (14%), hypophosphatemia (30%), hypomagnesemia (3%), hypozincemia (11%), and hypocupremia (3%) (Vanlandingham, Simpson, Daniel, & Newmark, 1981). These imbalances may be minimized by administering free water and by closely monitoring serum electrolytes, osmolality, blood urea nitrogen (BUN), fluid intake and output, and concurrent drug therapy.

Altered bowel elimination: diarrhea is the most commonly mentioned complication of tube feedings. Its frequency is reported at 10 to 20% (Heymsfield, Bethel, Ansley, Nixon, & Rudman, 1979). Flynn et al. (1987) report that diarrhea occurred in 60.3% of their sample. They also found that it occurred most often during the first 6 days of enteral feeding and that in 18.9% of the sample it was associated with a change in solution. Diarrhea can result when one or a combination of factors is present, including administration of hyperosmolar formulas, hot or cold formula, bacterial contamination of formulas or delivery sets, lactose intolerance, low serium albumin, low fiber content of formula, or concurrent drug therapy.

Administration of a hyperosmolar solution into the gut lumen often results in bloating, hypermotility, and osmotic diarrhea. Initial dilution of hyperosmolar solutions to a less hypertonic, isotonic, or even hypotonic concentration helps to eliminate this problem. In addition, delivery by continuous drip rather than bolus allows the gut to adapt to the constant osmotic load.

Kagawa-Busby, Heitkemper, Hansen, Hanson, and Vanderburg (1980) demonstrated that diets administered at room temperature or above seem to have no clinical effect on tube feeding tolerance. However, cold feedings caused cramping and diarrhea in two of six patients in their study group. Thus, cold feedings may increase the likelihood of gastrointestinal side effects in tube-fed patients.

Bacterial contamination of the feeding formula is preventable by adherence to strict, clean methods during preparation, storage, and administration of feeding solution. Schreiner et al. (1979) demonstrated a high rate (36%) of bacterial contamination of formulas in 115 neonates in an intensive care unit—probably introduced during the mixing and hanging of the formula by nursing personnel. Changing the feeding container and tubing every 8 to 24 hours also reduces the risk of excessive bacterial growth. Most critically ill patients are at increased risk for this complication because of compromised immune status.

Lactose intolerance may be caused by primary lactase deficiency or may be a consequence of malnutrition or disease. Undigested lactose creates a hyperosmolar load in the gut that precipitates dumping syndrome and osmotic diarrhea. Treatment requires the use of lactose-free feedings.

Serum albumin aids in maintaining colloidal osmotic pressure, which in turn increases the absorptive capacity of villous capillaries. Therefore, low serum albumin levels may result in decreased absorption by the villi, leading to malabsorption and diarrhea. Patients who require enteral nutrition frequently have lowered serum albumin levels as a result of chronic malnutrition or as a consequence of their primary disease.

Since most commercially available formulas are designed to be low in fiber, diarrhea may ensue. Thus, the addition of fiber to the feeding or the use of a fiber-enriched formula may be necessary.

Drug therapy may also be responsible for inducing diarrhea. Diarrhea is a common side effect of the penicillin-like antibiotics and magnesium-based antacids. If the medication cannot be discontinued, diarrhea can be expected to continue. Unless contraindicated, the use of antidiarrheals may be effective. These can often be administered through the feeding tube or directly into the formula.

Parenteral Nutrition

Parenteral nutrition is the intravenous administration of varying concentrations of glucose, amino acids, vitamins, electrolytes, trace elements, and sometimes fat. Parenteral nutrition is indicated in patients

1. with abnormalities of the GI tract that prevent adequate nutrient digestion and absorption (e.g., paralytic ileus, obstruction, fistulas, malabsorption syndrome, short bowel syndrome);
2. who require amounts of nutrients greater than can be delivered comfortably via the GI tract (e.g., burns or multiple trauma);
3. with severely restricted fluid intake, (e.g., renal and cardiac patients); and
4. with inadequate gag reflex, in whom bowel intubation is not possible.

Patients who have undergone major surgery may require a minimum of 3,000 kcal daily. Severely septic, traumatized, or burned patients may require

5,000 kcal/day or more to satisfy minimal energy requirements. Standard intravenous solutions of 5% glucose in water or saline contain only 170 kcal/ liter; therefore, patients would require the infusion of many liters of solution per day to meet minimal energy needs, which, of course, is not feasible.

Critical illness, such as sepsis, respiratory failure, trauma, acute renal failure, liver failure, and major surgery and its complications commonly require parenteral nutrition at some time during the course of the illness. For the surgical patient, the American College of Physicians (1987) has approved the following recommendations for the use of perioperative parenteral nutrition:

1. Perioperative use of parenteral nutritional support is recommended for *severely malnourished patients* having major surgery, such as intra-abdominal or noncardiac intrathoracic surgery.
2. Postoperative use of parenteral nutrition is recommended for selected groups of *moderately malnourished* and previously *well-nourished patients* having surgery that usually results in prolonged periods (10 days or more) of inadequate nutritional intake (pancreaticoduodenectomy, esophagogastrectomy involving total gastric resection). Some of these patients may receive nutrients through a feeding jejunostomy tube instead of total parenteral nutrition.
3. Postoperative use of parenteral nutrition is recommended for previously *well-nourished patients* who develop postoperative complications that are expected to result in prolonged periods (10 days or more) of inadequate intake (peritonitis associated with small bowel resection).

Several terms are used to describe the various types of parenteral nutrition; use of these terms is frequently confused in clinical practice. The most commonly employed definitions are given in Table 8–11.

Table 8–11   Common Definitions of Various Types of Parenteral Nutrition

---

Central venous nutrition (CVN)—parenteral nutrition solutions containing 10% or greater glucose concentrations, 4.25% or greater amino acid concentrations, plus electrolytes, vitamins, and trace elements, administered through a large central vein.

Peripheral venous nutrition (PVN)—solutions consisting of 5 to 10% glucose, 2.75% amino acids, plus electrolytes, vitamins, and trace minerals administered through a peripheral vein.

Total parenteral nutrition (TPN)—combines CVN or PVN with an intravenous fat emulsion.

Home parenteral nutrition (HPN)—parenteral nutrition provided in the home setting.

Central venous nutrition, with intravenous lipid, is usually the most effective form of support because of its ability to achieve a solution with high caloric density. Central venous solutions are hyperosmolar (1,700 mOsm/ liter) and contain approximately 1,000 kcal/liter. In patients with lower caloric needs, nutritional support through a peripheral vein, with an intravenous fat emulsion, is usually considered. The osmolarity of peripheral venous nutrition is about 700 mOsm/liter, with a total caloric content of less than 300 kcal/liter. Typical compositions of central, specialized, and peripheral venous nutrition solutions used at one tertiary care medical center are summarized in Table 8–12.

Table 8–12 Basic Parenteral Nutrition Formulas

Routine Central Venous Nutrition Solution		Peripheral Venous Nutrition Solution	
Each 1,000-ml bag provides:		Each 1,000-ml bag provides:	
Total calories = 1,010 kcal		Total calories = 285 kcal	
Crystalline		Crystalline	
amino acids	4.25%	amino acids	2.75%
Dextrose	25%	Dextrose	5%
Sodium	35 mEq	Sodium	35 mEq
Potassium	30 mEq	Potassium	30 mEq
Calcium	4.7 mEq	Calcium	4.7 mEq
Magnesium	5 mEq	Magnesium	5 mEq
Phosphorus	15 mM (30 mEq)	Phosphorus	15 mM (30 mEq)
Chloride	35 mEq	Chloride	35 mEq
Acetate	67.5 mEq	Acetate	50 mEq

1,850 mOsm/liter Total volume = 1,040 ml   710 mOsm/liter Total volume = 1,020 ml

Vitamins will be an automatic additive and will follow this protocol: A patient will receive 2 units of MVI-12 equivalent daily (20 ml). Trace elements will be an automatic daily additive for patients on CVN. The "trace element addition" provides the AMA recommendations for metabolically stable adult patients. Trace elements may be ordered for addition to PVN, and as single entities when needed.

Multiple Vitamin Addition:		**Trace Element Addition Provides:**	
2 units/day (20 ml) provides:		Zinc	3 mg
Ascorbic acid (vitamin C)	200 mg	Copper	1.2 mg
Vitamin A	6,600 IU	Manganese	0.3 mg
Vitamin D	400 IU	Chromium	12 μg
Thiamine hydrochloride	6.0 mg	Selenium	60 μg

Table 8–12 *(Continued)*

Multiple Vitamin Addition:		Trace Element Addition Provides:
Riboflavin	7.2 mg	Iodine 75 μg
Pyridoxine hydrochloride	8 mg	Additionally, molybdenum, 100 μg,
Niacinamide	80 mg	should be considered for
Dexpanthenol	30 mg	Home TPN or long-term TPN
Vitamin E	20 IU	patients
Biotin	120 μg	
B_{12} (cyanocobalamin)	10 μg	
Folic acid	800 μg	

Special Formulas

Renal Central Venous Nutrition Solution Formula revised: July 1986		Hepatic Central Venous Nutrition Solution	
Each 1,000-ml bag provides: Total calories: 1,340 kcal		Each 1,000 ml-bag provides: Total calories: 1,000 kcal	
Crystalline amino acids	2.75%	Crystalline amino acids	4% (BCAA*)
Dextrose	35% (350 g)	Dextrose	25%
Sodium	20 mEq	Sodium	35 mEq
Chloride	20 mEq	Potassium	30 mEq
Acetate	35 mEq	Calcium	5 mEq
Calcium	2.5 mEq	Magnesium	5 mEq
(Vitamins and trace elements)		Phosphorus	15 mM (30 mEq) aprox.
Electrolytes should be adjusted, based on patient requirements. Please note: There is no potassium in renal formula.		Chloride	30 mEQ
		Acetate	56 mEq

Total volume = 1,025 ml
Regular insulin may be added to
any of the solutions, if needed.
*BCAA = branched-chain amino acids

Adapted from Parenteral Nutrition Product Listings; Department of Pharmacy, Rush Presbyterian–St. Luke's Medical Center, Chicago. Revised 7/86

Advantages of peripheral venous nutrition include the absence of a central venous catheter and, therefore, a lower rate of sepsis. However, patients who need large amounts of protein and calories usually require central venous nutrition. The recent use of multi-lumen central catheters and venous access devices may minimize many of the complications associated with standard subclavian catheters.

Fat emulsions may be infused daily or twice weekly to prevent essential fatty acid deficiency and to boost caloric intake. These preparations are isosmotic and may be infused either peripherally or centrally. Lipid solutions have been used in the United States since 1977 and are now available in 10 or 20% concentrations. The 10% solutions provide 1.1 kcal/ml, and the 20% solutions, 2.2 kcal/ml.

Catheter Insertion

Parenteral nutrition solutions that have glucose as the major calorie source are generally hyperosmolar and tend to cause phlebitis or thrombosis if infused through peripheral veins. For this reason, intravenous access to a large central vein is imperative. Subclavian catheter insertion via infraclavicular venipuncture is the preferred method of central vein cannulation, primarily because it uses a flat, relatively immobile area on the chest, where it is usually somewhat easier to maintain a clean and intact dressing.

For long-term home parenteral nutrition, the catheters of choice are Hickman and Broviac-type catheters. These catheters are inserted in the operating room. The cephalic vein is generally used, and the tip of the catheter is placed just above or within the right atrium. The extravascular portion of the catheter is tunneled under the skin and is brought out at a point where the patient can easily see it and care for (Figure 8–1). The Dacron cuff around the extravascular portion of the catheter allows the growth of fibrous tissue, which anchors the catheter in place and acts as a barrier to bacteria. Most multi-lumen catheters have plastic caps that can be heparinized and sealed between nutrient infusions. Implantable venous access devices provide an alternative delivery system for patients unable to comply with the care requirements for permanent, indwelling, central catheters.

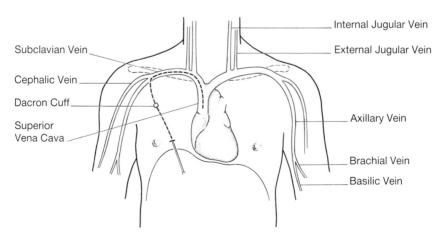

Figure 8–1. Catheter placement for long-term care.

Solution Delivery

The high flow rate of the superior vena cava allows hyperosmolar parenteral nutrient solutions to be diluted rapidly in the bloodstream, and to a large extent, eliminates the problems of phlebitis and thrombosis. These hyperosmolar glucose solutions must be given slowly at first. Usually, 1 liter is given in 24 hours, using a constant drip infusion maintained by an infusion pump. Depending on patient tolerance and blood glucose, urine glucose, and electrolyte levels, the rate is gradually increased, usually over 3 to 5 days, until the patient is receiving the prescribed amount.

Hyperosmolar parenteral solutions should be administered at a steady rate. If the administration rate drops, it should be corrected, rather than attempting to "catch up," since an excessive glucose load could result. When the central venous solution must be discontinued abruptly because of an emergency, $D_{10}W$ (10% dextrose in water) or $D_{20}W$ should be substituted and administered at the same rate, in order to maintain normoglycemia and to prevent hypoglycemia and insulin shock.

When hyperosmolar parenteral nutrition is no longer needed, it is important to decrease the amount infused gradually, to prevent rebound hypoglycemia. Typically, the infusion rate is decreased to one-half the usual rate for 12 hours. The solution is then switched to D_5W at 50 to 100 ml/hr for the next 12 hours, before complete cessation and removal of the subclavian catheter.

Hyperosmolar glucose solutions support the growth of organisms within 12 to 24 hours. Therefore, solutions should be changed every 12 hours or according to hospital policy and procedure. Filters, if used, and tubing are changed every day or with each bottle.

Fat Emulsions

The first dose of fat emulsion should be infused slowly to assess adverse reactions. Transient side effects from fat emulsion therapy include dyspnea, fever, chills, and pain in the chest and back due to embolism. Hepatomegaly, jaundice, and other delayed adverse reactions have been reported infrequently. The suggested starting rate is 1 ml/min for 15 to 30 minutes. If no adverse reactions are noted, the rate may be increased to a maximum of 125 ml/hr for the 10% fat emulsion or 60 ml/hr for the 20% fat emulsion. A single unit of lipid should not hang longer than 8 to 24 hours, intravenous tubing should be changed every 24 hours, and fat emulsions should not be administered through a filter.

Complications

Complications associated with parenteral nutritional support are presented in Table 8–13. Interventions related to these complications are discussed in the following text.

Table 8–13 Complications Associated with Parenteral Nutritional Support

Complication	Cause
Septic	
Catheter-related	Contamination of intravenous cannula during central vein catheterization
	Contamination via exit site
	Seeding of the catheter tip by blood-borne organisms
	Contaminated disinfectants
Bottle-related	Introduction of microorganisms into solution during preparation
	Additional medications added to TPN solution outside laminar air-flow hood
Staff-related	Poor hand washing techniques
	Inadequate use of disinfectant in administration techniques
Mechanical/anatomical	
Catheter insertion	
Pneumothorax	Unknown previous clavicular injuries making catheter insertion difficult
Hemothorax	
Hydrothorax	
Subclavian artery puncture	Improper patient positioning
Subclavian vein/artery laceration	Inadequate instructions given to patient, resulting in lack of cooperation
Brachial plexus injury	
Hematoma	
Catheter misplacement	Inexperience of physician inserting catheter
Air embolism	Possibly due to formation of fibrin sheath around catheter
Subclavian vein thrombosis	Hypercoagulability of individual patient
Air embolism	Failure to occlude catheter when changing tubings
Catheter occlusion	Inadequate rate of flow of solution through cannula
Metabolic	
Fluid imbalance	
Dehydration	Failure to meet fluid requirements
	Hyperglycemia; hypernatremia
Overhydration	Excess intake of solution above fluid requirements
Electrolyte imbalance	
Excess	Administration of excess amounts of both intracellular and extracellular ions
Deficit	
Intracellular (K^+, PO_4^-, Mg^{2+})	Inadequate administration of these electrolytes
	Anabolism

Table 8–13   *(Continued)*

Complication	Cause
Extracellular (Na$^+$, Cl$^-$, Ca^{2+})	Inadequate amounts of these electrolytes infused
Hyperchloremic acidosis	Administration of all electrolytes as chloride salts
	High gastrointestinal losses of base salts
Glucose imbalance	
Hyperglycemia	Metabolic response to injury
	Too rapid infusion of glucose solutions
	Sepsis
	Inadequate provision of insulin
Glucosuria	Renal threshold for glucose exceeded due to insulin resistance, too rapid administration of glucose solutions, or inadequate insulin coverage
Hypoglycemia	Sudden cessation of hypertonic glucose solutions
	Resolution of sepsis
	Insulin overdose
Hyperosmolar, hyperglycemic, nonketotic dehydration	Persistent prolonged glucosuria, causing osmotic diuresis
Other	
Essential fatty acid deficiency	Inadequate provision of fat emulsions in long-term TPN
Prerenal azotemia	Dehydration
	Improper calorie/nitrogen ratio
Trace mineral deficiencies	Long-term TPN with inadequate replacement of trace metals, especially, zinc, copper, chromium, and manganese
Vitamin deficiencies*	Inadequate maintenance therapy and failure to meet increased needs during stress
Vitamin excess	Fat soluble vitamins administered in excess of need not excreted via urine; stored in liver

*Usually water-soluble vitamins.

From *Critical Care Nursing Quarterly* (formerly *Critical Care Quarterly*), 6(1), pp. 8–9. Copyright June 1983 by Aspen Publishers, Inc. Reprinted with permission.

With proper patient monitoring and careful technique, most complications of parenteral nutrition can be prevented. When complications do occur, they may be classified into three categories: technical, metabolic, and septic.

Technical complications are the most common and are related to central catheter placement. Potential problems arising during central venous cannulation include pneumothorax, air embolus, catheter malposition, hemothorax, and hemopericardium. Technical complications associated with central venous catheterization can be minimized by thoroughly understanding the anatomy of the costoclavicular–subclavian area and strictly adhering to established cannulation techniques.

Metabolic complications include abnormalities of glucose, protein, and fat metabolism, as well as various mineral and electrolyte derangements. During the early years of TPN administration, many metabolic complications were related to improper administration technique and/or the infusion of inadequate or excessive amounts of substrates, vitamins, or minerals. With increased knowledge of substrate and micronutrient metabolism in various disease states, and improved patient monitoring, these complications are now reported with less frequency.

One metabolic complication that is particularly relevant to the critically ill surgical patient and which is receiving considerable attention in the literature is that of carbon dioxide retention. An excessive infusion of glucose can be detrimental to patients with compromised pulmonary status. Askanazi and his colleagues (1980, 1981, 1982) have confirmed the association of excessive glucose infusion rates with increased O_2 consumption, CO_2 production, alveolar ventilation, minute ventilation, and respiratory quotient in malnourished and hypermetabolic patients. For patients with inadequate pulmonary reserves, glucose-induced increases in carbon dioxide production may precipitate pulmonary failure. This may be particularly critical when weaning patients from ventilators. To avoid or treat CO_2 retention, Askanazi et al. (1982) propose substitution of 50% of the glucose calories with fat calories.

Septic complications may occur as a result of contaminated catheters, contaminated parenteral nutrition solutions, or both. Catheter sepsis may be minimized by strict adherence to aseptic catheter care. The catheter insertion site should be maintained with a dry, sterile, air-occlusive dressing that is changed according to protocol. Waterproof dressings should be applied to insertion sites located near a draining wound or tracheostomy. When the dressing is changed, the surrounding area should be inspected and cultures taken if there is any drainage from the area. Administration sets and tubing should be changed daily—usually with the first bag of the day—to minimize bacterial growth. Lipid emulsions, in particular, have been found to support bacterial growth (Moore, Guenter & Bender, 1986). Also, parenteral solutions should hang no longer than 8 to 12 hours.

Monitoring

As previously mentioned, mechanical, metabolic, and septic complications can be prevented with careful monitoring. Monitoring of patients on enteral or parenteral nutrition should include accurate measurement of temperature, pulse rate, respiratory rate, and blood pressure at least every 8 hours, urine sugar and acetone or blood glucose (Accu-check) levels every 6 hours, fluid intake and output every 8 hours, and daily body weights. Serum electrolytes, BUN, and glucose levels should be determined daily until serum levels stabilize, and every 2 to 3 days thereafter. Weekly measurements of serum calcium, phosphorus, magnesium, albumin, total and direct bilirubin, serum aspartate and alanine aminotransferases and alkaline phosphatase should be taken to ensure adequate mineral replacement and to determine liver function. Finally, periodic reassessment of nutritional status provides information about the overall adequacy of nutritional support techniques.

SUMMARY

Attention to the nutritional needs of the critically ill surgical patient is very important if the diagnosis "Potential for alteration in nutrition: less than body requirements" is to be prevented and/or treated. Critical care nurses must be prepared to assess nutritional status, request appropriate dietary consultation, administer nutritional support, and monitor the patient's ongoing status for any complications of treatment or further nutritional needs. The specialized nature of nutritional support requires that an interdisciplinary approach to the patient's needs be maintained. The critical care nurse at the patient's bedside must take responsibility for the coordination and continuity of care if nutritional needs are to be met.

BIBLIOGRAPHY

American College of Physicians, Health and Public Policy Committee. (1987). Perioperative parenteral nutrition. *Annals of Internal Medicine, 107,* 252–253.

Apelgren, K. N., & Wilmore, D. W. (1983). Nutritional care of the critically ill patient. *Surgical Clinics of North America, 63*(2), 497–507.

Askanazi, J., Nordenstrom, J., Rosenbaum, S. H., Elwyn, D. H., Hyman, A. I., Carpentier, Y. A., & Kinney, J. M. (1981). Nutrition for the patient with respiratory failure: Glucose vs. fat. *Anesthesiology, 54,* 373–377.

Askanazi, J., Rosenbaum, S. H., Hyman, A. I., Silverberg, P. A., Milic-Emili, J., & Kinney, J. M. (1980). Respiratory changes induced by the large glucose loads of total parenteral nutrition. *Journal of the American Medical Association, 243*(14), 1444–1447.

Askanazi, J., Starker, P. M., Olsson, C., Hensle, T. W., Lockhart, S. H., Kinney, J. M., & LaSala, P. A. (1986). Effect of immediate postoperative nutritional support on length of hospitalization. *Annals of Surgery, 203*(3), 236–239.

Askanazi, J., Weissman, C., Rosenbaum, S. H., Hyman, A. I., Milic-Emili, J., & Kinney, J. M. (1982). Nutrition and the respiratory system. *Critical Care Medicine, 10*(3), 163–172.

Bessey, P. Q. (1989). Metabolic response to critical illness. In D. W. Wilmore (Ed.) *Care of the surgical patient: A publication of the committee on pre and postoperative care.* New York: Scientific American Medicine.

Bistrian, B. R. (1979). A simple technique to estimate severity of stress. *Surgery, Gynecology, and Obstetrics, 148,* 675–678.

Bistrian, B. R., Blackburn, G. L., Hallowell, E. L., & Heddle, R. (1974). Protein status of general surgical patients. *Journal of the American Medical Association, 230*(6), 858–860.

Bistrian, B. R., Blackburn, G. L., Vitale, J., Cochran, D., & Naylor, J. (1976). Prevalence of malnutrition in general medical patients. *Journal of the American Medical Association, 235*(15), 1567–1570.

Blackburn, G. L., Bistrian, B. R., Maini, B. S., Schlamm, H. T., & Smith, M. F. (1977). Nutritional and metabolic assessment of the hospitalized patient. *Journal of Parenteral and Enteral Nutrition, 1*(1), 11–22.

Bower, R. H., Talamini, M. A., Sax, H. C., Hamilton, F., & Fischer, J. E. (1986). Postoperative enteral vs. parenteral nutrition. *Archives of Surgery, 121,* 1040–1045.

Buzby, G. P., Mullen, J. L., Matthews, D. C., Hobbs, C. L., & Rosato, E. F. (1980). Prognostic nutritional index in gastrointestinal surgery. *American Journal of Surgery, 139, 160–167.*

Carrico, C. J., Meakins, J. L., Marshall, J. C., Fry, D., & Maier, R. V. (1986). Multiple-organ-failure syndrome. *Archives of Surgery, 121,* 196–208.

Cataldi-Betcher, E. L., Seltzer, M. H., Slocum, B. A., & Jones, K. W. (1983). Complications occurring during enteral nutrition support: A prospective study. *Journal of Parenteral and Enteral Nutrition, 7*(6), 546–552.

Cerra, F. B. (1987). Hypermetabolism, organ failure, and metabolic support. *Surgery, 101*(2), 1–14.

Cerra, F. B., Lehman, S., Konstantinidis, N., Konstantinidis, F., Shronts, E. P., & Holman, R. (1990). Effect of enteral nutrient on in vitro tests of immune function in ICU patients: A preliminary report. *Nutrition, 6*(1), 84–87.

Cerra, F. B., Siegel, J. H., Coleman, B., Border, J. R., & McMenamy, R. R. (1980). Septic autocannibalism: A failure of exogenous nutritional support. *Annals of Surgery, 192,* 570–580.

Cerra, F. B., Upson, D., Angelico, R., Wiles, C., Lyons, J., Faulkenbach, L., & Paysinger, J. (1982). Branched chains support postoperative protein synthesis. *Surgery, 92,* 192–199.

Cuthbertson, D. P. (1932). Observations on the disturbance of metabolism produced by injury to the limbs. *Quarterly Journal of Medicine (New Series), 1,* 233–246.

Eisenberg, P. (1989). Enteral nutrition: Indications, formulas, and delivery techniques. *Nursing Clinics of North America, 28*(2), 315–338.

Flynn, K., Norton, L. C., & Fisher, R. (1987). Enteral tube feedings: Indications, practices & outcomes. *Image, 19*(1), 16–19.

Freund, H., Dienstag, J., Lehrich, J., Yoshimura, N., Bradford, R. R., Rosen, H., Atamian, S., Slemmer, E., Holroyde, J., & Fischer, J. E. (1982). Infusion of branched-chain enriched amino acid solution in patients with hepatic encephalopathy. *Annals of Surgery, 196,* 209–220.

Frisancho, A. R. (1984). New standards of weight and body composition by frame size and height for assessment of nutritional status of adults and the elderly. *American Journal of Clinical Nutrition, 40,* 808–819.

Harris, J. A. & Benedict, F. G. (1919). *A biometric study of basal metabolism in man.* Carnegie Institute, Washington, D.C., 189–193.

Harvey, K. B., Moldawer, L. L., Bistrian, B. R., & Blackburn, G. L. (1981). Biological measures for the formulation of a hospital prognostic index. *American Journal of Clinical Nutrition, 34,* 2013–2022.

Heymsfield, S. B., Bethel, R. A., Ansley, J. D., Nixon, D. W., & Rudman, D. (1979). Enteral hyperalimentation: An alternative to central venous hyperalimentation. *Annals of Internal Medicine, 90,* 63–71.

Heymsfield, S. B., McManus, C., Smith, J., Stevens, V., & Nixon, D. W. (1982). Anthropometric measurement of muscle mass: Revised equations for calculating bone-free arm muscle area. *American Journal of Clinical Nutrition, 36,* 680–690.

Hoover, H. C., Ryan, J. A., Anderson, E. J., & Fischer, J. E. (1980). Nutritional benefits of immediate postoperative jejunal feeding of an elemental diet. *American Journal of Surgery, 139,* 153–159.

Hyman, A. I., Rodriguez, J., & Weissman, C. (1982). Nutritional support of the critically ill patient. *Seminars in Anesthesia, 1*(4), 354–361.

Kagawa-Busby, K. S., Heitkemper, M. M., Hansen, B. C., Hanson, R. L., & Vanderburg, V. V. (1980). Effects of diet temperature on tolerance of enteral feedings. *Nursing Research, 29,* 276–280.

Kinney, J. M., Duke, J. H., Jr., Long, C. L., & Gump, F. E. (1970). Tissue fuel and weight loss after injury. *Journal of Clinical Pathology, 23* (Suppl. 4), 65–72.

Konstantinidis, N. N., Teasley, K., Lysne, J., Shronts, E., Olson, G., & Cerra, F. B. (1984). Nutritional requirements of the hypermetabolic patient. *Nutritional Support Services, 4*(2), 41–50.

Lieberman, M. D., Shou, J., Torres, A. S., Weintraub, F., Goldfine, J., Sigal, R., & Daly, J. M. (1990). Effects of nutrient substrates on immune function. *Nutrition, 6*(1), 88–91.

Long, C. L. (1984). Energy and protein requirements in stress and trauma. *Critical Care Nursing Currents, 2*(2), 7–12.

Long, C. L., Jeevanadam, M., Kim, B. M., & Kinney, J. M. (1977). Whole body protein synthesis and catabolism in septic man. *American Journal of Clinical Nutrition, 30,* 1340–1344.

Long, C. L., Schaffel, N., Geiger, J. W., Schiller, W. R., & Blakemore, W. S. (1979). Metabolic response to injury and illness: Estimation of energy and protein needs from indirect calorimetry and nitrogen balance. *Journal of Parenteral and Enteral Nutrition, 3*(6), 452–456.

Madoff, R. D., Sharpe, S. M., Fath, J. J., Simmons, R. L., & Cerra, F. B. (1985). Prolonged surgical intensive care: A useful allocation of medical resources. *Archives of Surgery, 120,* 698–702.

Moore, F. D. (1959). A general view of water, salt, and acid. In F. D. Moore, *Metabolic care of the surgical patient* (pp. 266–275). Philadelphia: W. B. Saunders.

Moore, M. C., Guenter, P. A., & Bender, J. H. (1986). Nutrition-related nursing research. *Image, 18*(1), 18–21.

Muggia-Sullam, M., Bower, R. H., Murphy, R. F., Joffe, S. N., & Fischer, J. E. (1985). Postoperative enteral versus parenteral nutritional support in gastrointestinal surgery: A matched prospective study. *American Journal of Surgery, 149,* 106–112.

Mullen, J. L., Buzby, G. P., Waldman, M. T., Gertner, M. H., Hobbs, C. L., & Rosato, E. F. (1979). Prediction of operative morbidity and mortality by preoperative nutritional assessment. *Surgical Forum, 30,* 80–82.

Mullen, J. L., Gertner, M. H., Buzby, G. P., Goodhart, G. L., & Rosato, E. F. (1979). Implications of malnutrition in the surgical patient. *Archives of Surgery, 114,* 121–125.

Negro, F., & Cerra, F. B. (1988). Nutritional monitoring in the ICU: Rational and practical application. *Critical Care Clinics, 4*(3), 559–572.

Orme, J. F., & Clemmer, T. P. (1983). Nutrition in the critical care unit. *Medical Clinics of North America, 67*(6), 1295–1304.

Perkel, M. S., Moore, C., Hersh, T., & Davidson, E. D. (1979). Metoclopramide therapy in patients with delayed gastric emptying: A randomized, double-blind study. *Digestive Diseases and Sciences, 24*(9), 662–666.

Pfeiffer, C. J. (1970). Gastrointestinal response to malnutrition and starvation. *Postgraduate Medicine, 47*(4), 110–115.

Pine, R. W., Wertz, M. J., Lennard, E. S., Dellinger, E. P., Carrico, C. J., & Minshew, B. H. (1983). Determinants of organ malfunction or death in patients with intra-abdominal sepsis: A discriminant analysis. *Archives of Surgery, 118,* 242–249.

Porte D., Jr., & Bagdade, J. D. (1970). Human insulin secretion: An integrated approach. *Annual Review of Medicine, 21,* 219–240.

Rainey-Macdonald, C. G., Holliday, R. L., Wells, G. A., & Donner, A. P. (1983). Validity of a two-variable nutritional index for use in selecting candidates for nutritional support. *Journal of Parenteral and Enteral Nutritional, 7*(1), 15–20.

Reynolds, J. V., Daly, J. M., Zhang, S., Evantash, E., Shou, J., Sigal, R., & Ziegler, M. M. (1988). Immunomodulatory mechanisms of arginine. *Surgery, 104*(2), 142–151.

Roy, L. B., Edwards, P. A., & Barr, L. H. (1985). The value of nutritional assessment in the surgical patient. *Journal of Parenteral and Enteral Nutrition, 9*(2), 170–172.

Rudman, D. (1987). Assessment of nutritional status. In E. Braunwald, K. J. Isselbacher, R. G. Petersdorf, J. D. Wilson, J. B. Martin, & A. S. Fauci (Eds.)., *Harrison's principles of internal medicine* (11th ed.) (pp. 390–393). New York: McGraw-Hill.

Ryan, J. A. Jr., & Page, C. P. (1984). Intrajejunal feeding: Development and current status. *Journal of Parenteral and Enteral Nutrition, 8*(2), 187–198.

Schiller, W. R., Long, C. L., & Blakemore, W. S. (1979). Creatinine and nitrogen excretion in seriously ill and injured patients. *Surgery, Gynecology, and Obstetrics, 149,* 561–566.

Schreiner, R. L., Eitzen, H., Gfell, M. A., Kress, S., Gresham, E. L., French, M., & Moye, L. (1979). Environmental contamination of continuous drip feedings. *Pediatrics, 63*(2), 232–237.

Seltzer, M. H., Fletcher, H. S., Slocum, B. A., & Engler, P. E. (1981). Instant nutritional assessment in the intensive care unit. *Journal of Parenteral and Enteral Nutrition, 5*(1), 70–72.

Smale, B. F., Mullen, J. L., Buzby, G. P., & Rosato, E. F. (1981). The efficacy of nutritional assessment and support in cancer surgery. *Cancer, 47,* 2375–2381.

Starker, P. M., LaSala, P. A., Askanazi, J., Todd, G., Hensle, T. W., & Kinney, J. M. (1986). The influence of preoperative total parenteral nutrition upon morbidity and mortality. *Surgery, Gynecology, and Obstetrics, 162,* 569–574.

Starzl, T. E., Porter, K. A., & Putnam, C. W. (1975). Intraportal insulin protects from the liver injury of portacaval shunt in dogs. *Lancet, 2,* 1241–1242.

Studley, H. O. (1936). Percentage of weight loss: A basic indicator of surgical risk in patients with chronic peptic ulcer. *Journal of the American Medical Association, 106*(6), 458–460.

Threlfall, C. J., Stoner, H. B., & Galasko, C. S. B. (1981). Patterns in the excretion of muscle markers after trauma and orthopedic surgery. *Journal of Trauma, 21*(2), 140–147.

Vanlandingham, S., Simpson, S., Daniel, P., & Newmark, S. R. (1981). Metabolic abnormalities in patients supported with enteral tube feeding. *Journal of Parenteral and Enteral Nutrition, 5*(4), 322–324.

Walike, B. C., & Walike, J. W. (1977). Relative lactose intolerance: A clinical study of tube-fed patients. *Journal of the American Medical Association, 238*(9), 948–951.

Wells, C., Tinckler, L., Rawlinson, K., Jones, H., & Saunders, J. (1964). Postoperative gastrointestinal motility. *Lancet, 1,* 4–10.

Whatley, K., Turner, W. W., Jr., Dey, M., Leonard, J., & Guthrie, M. (1984). When does metoclopramide facilitate transpyloric intubation? *Journal of Parenteral and Enteral Nutrition, 8*(6), 679–681.

Wilmore, D. W., Smith, R. J., O'Dwyer, S. T., Jacobs, D. O., Ziegler, T. R., & Wang, X. D. (1988). The gut: A central organ after surgical stress. *Surgery, 104*(5), 917–923.

Young, M. E. (1988). Malnutrition and wound healing. *Heart and Lung, 17*(1), 60–69.

ADDITIONAL READINGS

Anderson, C. F., Loosbrock, L. M., & Moxness, K. E. (1986). Nutrient intake in critically ill patients: Too many or too few calories? *Mayo Clinic Proceedings, 61,* 853–858.

Anderson, C. F., Moxness, K., & Meister, J. (1984). The sensitivity and specificity of nutrition-related variables in relationship to the duration of hospital stay and the rate of complications. *Mayo Clinic Proceedings, 59,* 477–483.

Apelgren, K. N., Rombeau, J. L., Twomey, P. L., & Miller, R. A. (1982). Comparison of nutritional indices and outcome in critically ill patients. *Critical Care Medicine, 10*(5), 305–307.

Baker, J. P., Detsky, A. S., Stewart, S., Whitwell, J., Marliss, E. B., & Jeejeebhoy, K. N. (1984). Randomized trial of total parenteral nutrition in critically ill patients: Metabolic effects of varying glucose-lipid ratios as the energy source. *Gastroenterology, 87,* 53–59.

Boles, J. M., Garre, M. A., & Youinou, P. Y. (1984). Simple assessment of the nutritional status in the critically ill patient. *Resuscitation, 11,* 233–241.

Boles, J. M., Garre, M. A., Youinou, P. Y., Mialon, P., Menez, J. F., Jouquan, J., Miossec, P. J., Pennec, Y., & LeMenn, G. (1983). Nutritional status in intensive care patients: Evaluation in 84 unselected patients. *Critical Care Medicine, 11*(2), 87–90.

Cerra, F. (1984). *Pocket manual of surgical nutrition.* St. Louis: C. V. Mosby.

Fischer, J. E. (Ed.). (1983). *Surgical nutrition.* Boston: Little, Brown.

Gilder, H. (1986). Parenteral nourishment of patients undergoing surgical or traumatic stress. *Journal of Parenteral and Enteral Nutrition, 10*(1), 88–99.

Goldstein, S. A. & Elwyn, D. H. (1989). The effects of injury and sepsis on fuel utilization. *Annual Review of Nutrition, 9,* 445–473.

Grant, J. P. (1986). Nutritional assessment in clinical practice. *Nutrition in Clinical Practice, 1*(1), 3–11.

Griggs, B. A., Ingalls, M., Ayers, N., & Champagne, C. (1984). *A Basic Nursing Guide to Providing T.P.N. for the Adult Patient.* Washington, D. C.: American Society for Parenteral and Enteral Nutrition.

Hoppe, M. C. (1983). Nutritional management of the trauma patient. *Critical Care Quarterly, 6*(1), 1–16.

Jones, K. W., Seltzer, M. H., Slocum, B. A., Cataldi-Betcher, E. L., Goldberger, D. J., &

Wright, F. R. (1984). Parenteral nutrition complications in a voluntary hospital. *Journal of Parenteral and Enteral Nutrition, 8*(4), 385–390.

Kaufman, C. S. (1981). Nutritional support of the trauma patient. *Nutritional Support Services, 1*(4), 11–13.

Keithley, J. K. (Symposium Guest Editor). (1989). Advances in nutritional support. *Nursing Clinics of North America, 24*(2). Philadelphia: W. B. Saunders.

Keithley, J. K. (1985). Nutritional assessment of the patient undergoing surgery. *Heart and Lung, 14*(5), 449–456.

Kohn, C. L. & Keithley, J. K. (1989). Enteral nutrition: Potential complications and patient monitoring. *Nursing Clinics of North America, 24*(2), 339–353.

Krey, S. H., & Murray, R. L. (Eds.). (1986). *Dynamics of nutrition support: Assessment, implementation, evaluation.* Norwalk, Conn.: Appleton-Century-Crofts.

Lakshman, K., & Blackburn, G. L. (1986). Monitoring nutritional status in the critically ill adult. *Journal of Clinical Monitoring, 2*(2), 114–120.

Lang, C. E. (1987). *Nutritional support in critical care.* Rockville, Md.: Aspen Publishers.

Lemoyne, M., & Jeejeebhoy, K. N. (1986). Total parenteral nutrition in the critically ill patient. *Chest, 89*(4), 568–575.

Lindholm, M., & Rossner, S. (1982). Rate of elimination of the intralipid fat emulsion from the circulation in ICU patients. *Critical Care Medicine, 10*(11), 740–745.

Long, C. L., Birkhahn, R. H., Geiger, J. W., & Blakemore, W. S. (1981). Contribution of skeletal muscle protein in elevated rates of whole body protein catabolism in trauma patients. *American Journal of Clinical Nutrition, 34,* 1087–1093.

McLaren, D. S., & Meguid, M. M. (1983). Nutritional assessment at the crossroads. *Journal of Parenteral and Enteral Nutrition, 7*(6), 575–579.

Mullen, J. L., Buzby, G. P., Matthews, D. C., Smale, B. F., & Rosato, E. F. (1980). Reduction of operative morbidity and mortality by combined preoperative and postoperative nutritional support. *Annals of Surgery, 192*(5), 604–613.

Pingleton, S. K., & Harmon, G. S. (1987). Nutritional management in acute respiratory failure. *Journal of the American Medical Association, 257*(22), 3094–3099.

Rombeau, J. L., & Caldwell, M. D. (Eds.) (1984). *Clinical nutrition: Vol. 1. Enteral and tube feeding.* Philadephia: W. B. Saunders.

Rombeau, J. L., & Caldwell, M. D. (Eds.) (1986). *Clinical nutrition: Vol. 2. Parenteral nutrition.* Philadelphia: W. B. Saunders.

Schlictig, R. J. & Ayres, S. M. (1988). *Nutritional Support of the Critically Ill.* Chicago: Year Book Medical Publishers.

Seltzer, M. H., Slocum, B. A., Cataldi-Betcher, E. L., Seltzer, D. L., & Goldberger, D. J. (1984). Specialized nutrition support: Patterns of care. *Journal of Parenteral and Enteral Nutrition, 8*(5), 506–510.

Williams, W. W. (1985). Infection control during parenteral nutrition therapy. *Journal of Parenteral and Enteral Nutrition, 9*(6), 735–745.

Alterations in Fluid Volume, Composition, Distribution and Acid–Base Balance

9

Jane Kray, M.S., R.N.

The dynamic nature of fluid balance in the body and the relationships relevant to electrolyte function are based on several physiologic principles governing these systems. A review of the basic physiology is included to familiarize the practitioner with terms and principles necessary for understanding fluid and electrolyte homeostasis.

BODY WATER

Water is the basic constituent of the human body. It normally comprises 45 to 60% of the total body weight of an adult. This figure is used as a guide to estimate an individual's body fluid content. There are several factors, such as distribution, sex, age, and obesity, that influence the body's water content and that must be taken into account when making fluid estimates (Table 9–1). When examining variations of body water content, the clinician is advised to identify groups at risk for body fluid imbalances. Of particular importance are the infant, the obese individual, and the elderly.

Distribution

In the body, fluids are distributed between two compartments and, normally, maintain a fairly constant relationship with respect to this distribution. The intracellular fluid compartment (ICF) contains the fluid inside all cells of the body and provides the aqueous medium for cellular metabolism. The extracellular fluid compartment (ECF) is comprised of the body fluid outside of cells that moves freely within the cardiovascular system, the organs, and the interstitial spaces. The extracellular fluid can be further subdivided into the plasma compartment and the interstitial fluid space, with approximately one

188

Table 9–1   Changes in Body Fluid with Age, Sex, and Weight

Age/sex/weight	Fluid proportion (%) of kilogram weight (approx.)
Premature infant	80
3 months	70
6 months	60
1–5 years	64
11–16 years	58
Adult male	55–60
Adult female	45–50
Obese adult	40–50
Emaciated adult	70–75
Over 65 years	40–50

From *Basic Pathophysiology: A Holistic Approach*, 3rd ed., by M. E. Groer and M. E. Shekleton, 1989, St. Louis: The C. V. Mosby Co. Reproduced with permission.

fifth of the ECF composed of plasma and four fifths occupying interstitial spaces. The ECF compartment also includes the transcellular or noncommunicating fluids such as intraocular fluid and cerebrospinal fluid (CSF). In humans, approximately two thirds of the total body fluid is contained in the intracellular and one third in the extracellular compartment.

Constituents

The water of the body performs many diverse physiologic functions. Of particular importance is the role of water as the primary solvent in which chemically active substances, gases, and nutrients are carried to the cells and waste products are removed from the tissues. The primary constituents of the aqueous portion of the body usually include electrolytes, proteins and nondisassociating compounds.

An electrolyte is a substance that disassociates in solution to form electrically charged particles called ions. Ionization produces positively charged particles called *cations* and negatively charged particles called *anions*. Body fluids contain both cations and anions, found both in the ECF and ICF.

Electrolytes help to maintain normal fluid distribution by contributing to osmolality, have a role in the regulation of the acid–base status, serve as mediators in chemical reactions, and contribute electrically to neuromuscular integrity. Often, the absolute amount of the particular substance does not signify its importance, but rather, its unique contribution to homeostasis depends on its specific function.

The sum of cations and anions in body fluids are equal. This means that the charges are exactly balanced in a normal state, with neither an excess nor a deficit of charge present. In effect, body fluids are electrically neutral solutions. This electrical neutrality must be maintained, and although the exact sum of cations and anions may be greater or less than 155, charges are always balanced. When electrolytes are lost or gained from the body, the physiologic mechanisms regulating cations and anions react to gain, or lose, sufficient quantities of like, or differing, charge to sustain electrical neutrality and thus homeostatic balance.

The concentrations of specific electrolytes differ markedly when comparing the ECF and the ICF. Summarized in Table 9–2 are the electrolytes of the body according to their normal concentrations and location within the body compartments.

Clinically important electrolytes include sodium, chloride, potassium, and calcium. Alterations in the concentrations of these ions can produce symptoms that, if untreated, threaten the life of the patient. The practitioner should possess a working knowledge of the normal values and functions of these electrolytes (Table 9–3).

Proteins are found in both the ICF and the ECF. The primary extracellular proteins are albumin, globulin, and fibrinogen. Intracellularly, proteinase is dominant. The proteins serve many functions, playing a part in the maintenance of intravascular volume as well as preserving the vascular buffering capacity.

The third category of body fluid constituents are the nondisassociating compounds, which include such substances as glucose, urea, and the respiratory gases. Glucose as the primary cellular energy source and the gases oxygen and carbon dioxide have important roles in maintaining the life of the organism and thus, are vital nonelectrolyte compounds.

Table 9–2   Electrolyte Concentrations in the Extracellular and Intracellular Fluid Compartments

	ECF (plasma) (mEq/liter)	ICF (muscle) (mEq/liter)
Sodium (Na^+)	140	12
Potassium (K^+)	4.5	160
Calcium (Ca^{++})	5.0	±2
Magnesium (Mg^{++})	1.5	34
Chloride (Cl^-)	104	2
Bicarbonate (HCO_3^-)	24	10
Sulfate (SO_4)	1	—
Phosphate (HPO_4)	2	140
Proteinates	15	54
Undetermined anions (usually organic acids)	5	Variable

Table 9–3   Normal Concentrations and Functions of the Major Body Electrolytes

Electrolyte	Serum concentration	Functions
Sodium (Na)	135–145 mEq/liter	Retention of fluid in body Generation and transmission of nerve impulses Maintenance of acid–base balance Replacement of potassium in cell Enzyme activities Regulation of osmolarity and electro-neutrality of cell
Potassium (K)	3.5–5.0 mEq/liter	Maintenance of regular cardiac rhythm Deposition of glycogen in liver cells Function of enzyme systems necessary for cell energy production Transmission and conduction of nerve impulses Regulation of osmolarity and electro-neutrality of cell
Calcium (Ca)	4.5–5.5 mEq/liter or 9–11 mg/dl	Formation of bone and teeth (calcium phosphate) Transmission of nerve impulse Muscular contraction Clotting of blood Maintenance of cell membrane permeability
Chloride (C)	97–104 mEq/liter	Transport of carbon dioxide (chloride shift) and maintenance of acid–base balance Formation of hydrochloric acid in stomach Retention of potassium Maintenance of osmolarity of cell

From *Basic Pathophysiology: A Holistic Approach,* 3rd ed., by M. E. Groer and M. E. Shekleton, 1989, St. Louis: The C. V. Mosby Co. Reproduced with permission.

TRANSPORT MECHANISMS

The fluid and electrolytes in the different compartments are not static entities but exist in a dynamic equilibrium across the membrane structures of the body. The concept of equilibrium implies exchange between the various compartments requiring mechanisms for transport of fluid and the constituents. There are two basic modes of transport operating across cell membranes: passive transport and mediated transport.

Passive transport is the movement of fluids and substance across body membranes by means of mechanisms that are governed by physical laws and do not require the expenditure of energy (Groer & Shekleton, 1989). There are three basic modes of passive transport in the body: diffusion, filtration, and osmosis.

Diffusion is the passive movement of solute particles across a membrane from an area of higher concentration to an area of lower concentration (down the concentration gradient). Particle size and electrical charge also influence diffusion. *Filtration* is the process by which water and diffusible substances move out of the solution with the greater hydrostatic pressure when a difference in hydrostatic pressure exists on two sides of a membrane. *Osmosis* is the diffusion of a solvent (water) across a selectively permeable membrane to an area where the concentration of solutes is relatively greater (Groer & Shekleton, 1989).

The various transport mechanisms are in operation in all body systems. Fluid exchanges involve both intercompartmental and intracompartmental components. Intercompartmental transport between the ECF and ICF usually involves mediated transport, or the passive modes of diffusion and osmosis. Intracompartmental exchange occurs in the ECF, usually between the plasma and interstitium and the primary operative mechanism is filtration.

Certain concepts need to be clear if transport mechanisms are to be understood. Concepts basic to the principles of water and solute transport include osmolality, tonicity, and permeability.

Osmolality, the number of particles present per kilogram weight of solvent, represents the governing force in water movement in the body. Taking into account all of the electrolytes and particulate constituents in body fluids, the normal "osmolality" of body systems is 290 to 305 mOsm/kg. A simple formula used to estimate osmolality in the clinical setting is

$$\text{Osmolality (mOsm/kg)} = 2\,[\text{Na}^+] + \frac{\text{BUN}}{2.8} + \frac{\text{glucose}}{18}$$

where BUN = blood urea nitrogen.

When the concentration of the extracellular compartment is altered, either by addition of solute or the loss of pure water, the osmolality is altered. Eventually, water movement takes place between the cells and the ECF to restore normal concentrations and, thus, normal osmolality relationships. The changes that take place because of water shifts into, or out of, the cells in response to osmolal changes constitute the basis of many fluid and electrolyte disorders.

The concept of tonicity is best exemplified by what happens to the cells when they are exposed to solutions of differing osmolalities. When the osmotic pressure is relatively equal on both sides of the membrane (concentrations of solutes are equal) the solutions are isomotic or isotonic to one another. They are also considered to be isosmotic if no volume change occurs between them. A solution that contains a lesser concentration of solutes than another solution is hypotonic in relation to the other. Water is hypotonic in relation to the body fluids. If a red blood cell is placed in a container of fresh water, water will move into the cell by the process of osmosis, causing the cell to swell and diluting the body fluid inside it. Eventually the cell will burst. A solution that has a higher concentration of solutes than another is hypertonic in relation to the other. A cell placed in a hypertonic solution would have the water drawn out of it by the process of osmosis, causing it to become crenated (wrinkled and shrunken) (Groer & Shekleton, 1989).

The concept of permeability is of prime importance in this discussion in that all biological membranes are semipermeable to some substances, but all are freely permeable to water. Permeating solutes can pass through the cell membrane and, thus, while initially added to the ECF, once diffusion takes place these substances also change the intracellular osmolality. Examples of permeating solutes are urea, methanol, and ethanol, and although the actual value of osmolality may be changed due to the addition of these substances, there will be no osmotic water shifts. Nonpermeating solutes, when added to the ECF, are unable to cross the cell membrane, usually because of electrical charge or particle size. They must remain in the extracellular compartment. Examples of nonpermeating solutes are glucose, mannitol, sodium, and chloride. Because of the relative isolation of these substances, above normal values will always change the osmolality of the ECF causing an osmotic water shift between the ECF & ICF compartment.

Passive diffusion across cell membranes of large polar molecules such as amino acids and sugars would occur slowly, if at all. Experimental evidence suggests that movement of such molecules must occur in some manner requiring special mechanisms built into the cell structure. It is thought that these molecules bind to specific sites on the cell membrane where their movement across the membrane is facilitated. This process, called *mediated transport,* can be further subdivided to include facilitated diffusion and active transport. Facilitated diffusion allows movement of substances down their concentration gradients much more quickly than could normally be expected. Active transport mechanisms can move substances against their concentration gradients at the expense of cellular energy. Carrier models have been proposed to explain both types of mediated transport, but as yet no carrier molecule has been identified. The mechanism by which energy is linked to active transport also remains a matter of speculation (Groer & Shekleton, 1989).

REGULATION

Water balance and extracellular fluid volume are primarily regulated by the influence of two hormones, ADH and aldosterone, and will be considered briefly in the context of control mechanisms.

Antidiuretic Hormone

Antidiuretic hormone (ADH) is produced in the hypothalamus, stored in the posterior pituitary gland, and responds primarily to changes in the osmolality of the ECF perfusing these cells. When released, ADH circulates to the kidney (where its site of action is the collecting ducts) and increases the permeability of these sites to water. When the level of ADH is increased, reabsorption of water will also increase, leading to decreased urine volume and increased urine osmolality. The overall effect of ADH is to influence renal water equilibrium to maintain osmolal balance between fluid compartments.

ADH release is stimulated in three ways:

- Hyperosmolality
- Neural input
- Decreased circulating blood volume, ultimately causing renal water retention.

The converse is also true, with ADH inhibition arising from hypo-osmolal states and situations in which blood volume is expanded.

Aldosterone

Aldosterone is a hormone secreted by the adrenal cortex that helps to regulate the sodium concentration of the ECF, thus influencing the extracellular volume. Because sodium is the major cation of the ECF, the volume of the ECF is maintained within fairly narrow ranges by retaining or excreting sodium. Aldosterone acts by altering the permeability of the distal tubules and collecting ducts of the kidney to sodium and potassium, which in turn causes changes in water reabsorption. In general, an increase in aldosterone secretion causes an increase in sodium resorption with concomitant water gain while promoting potassium excretion. When aldosterone is decreased, sodium excretion is augmented and potassium is retained by the kidney to cause an effective decrease in the volume of the extracellular fluid compartment. The role of aldosterone is intimately linked to renal physiology as its release is mediated by sensitive structures in the juxtaglomerular apparatus near the afferent arteriole of the kidney. This area, called the macula densa, releases the enzyme renin. Renin catalyzes the conversion of angiotensinogen manufactured in the liver, to angiotensin I, which is then converted by a series of reactions in the lungs to angiotensin II. Circulating angiotensin II stimulates the release of aldosterone from the adrenal cortex, which then acts on the distal tubules and collecting ducts of the kidney to increase sodium resorption, and potassium excretion with eventual water retention. These events expand the extracellular fluid volume.

Renin release is stimulated primarily by changes in the pressure-sensitive structures in the renal afferent arterioles. A decrease in perfusion pressure, caused by any factor that decreases the circulating blood volume delivered to the kidney, will cause renin release and aldosterone secretion. Examples include low cardiac output states, hemorrhage, shock, diuretics, or sodium depletion. The secretion of aldosterone attempts to increase renal perfusion by increasing the extracellular fluid volume. Once perfusion pressure is restored, negative feedback occurs to terminate renin release and aldosterone secretion.

In addition to renin, aldosterone secretion is influenced by plasma sodium levels, serum potassium levels, and adrenocorticotropic hormone (ACTH). These factors are summarized as follows: aldosterone is stimulated by hyponatremia, hyperkalemia, and *increased* ACTH; aldosterone is inhibited by hypernatremia, hypokalemia, and *decreased* ACTH.

Natriuretic Hormone

Natriuretic hormone is a third hormone that exerts some control over sodium content in the blood and thus affects the extracellular fluid volume. It is believed that this hormone originates from the right atrium of the heart in response to an elevated serum sodium level and promotes excretion of sodium in the proximal tubule of the kidney (Cosgrove, 1989).

DISTURBANCES OF FLUID AND ELECTROLYTE BALANCE

The care of patients experiencing disturbances of fluid and electrolyte balance often poses complex clinical problems for the critical care nurse. The nursing diagnostic categories include alterations in fluid volume, fluid distribution, and fluid composition. The categories will be discussed as separate entities in this textbook, although the practitioner is reminded that disturbances in the clinical setting may involve not one category but combinations of categories because of the complex nature of maintaining physiologic homeostasis.

Alterations in Fluid Volume

Alterations in fluid volume occur frequently in the clinical setting. In general, fluid volume disturbances can be viewed in relation to the site of the manifestation, that is, certain imbalances affect primarily the ECF or the ICF.

All fluids gained, or lost, from the body ultimately interface with the environment through the extracellular compartment. Ingested fluids pass into the ECF from the gastrointestinal (GI) tract and are eliminated by way of the kidney after renal perfusion by the plasma portion of the ECF. In addition to these "sensible" fluid gains and losses, "insensible" fluids are gained from the ingestion of foods and metabolic processes and lost from the pulmonary system, fecal wastes, and cutaneous sources. The normal fluid balance for a 24-hour period is summarized in Table 9–4.

Fluid balance can be estimated fairly accurately as apparent excesses or deficits are detected when alterations occur in the normal avenues for fluid

Table 9–4   24-Hour Water Balance

Intake	Excretion
Oral fluids, 1500 mg	Urine, 1500 ml
Solid food, 800 ml	Pulmonary vaporization, 400 ml
Metabolic sources, 300 ml	Cutaneous perspiration, 600 ml
(hydrogen oxidation:)	Fecal losses, 100 ml
Protein, 40 ml/100 g	
Fat, 100 ml/100 g	
Carbohydrate, 100 ml/100 g	
Total, 2600 ml	Total, 2600 ml

intake or elimination. However, if a therapeutic plan of intervention is to be designed, it must be remembered that any fluid change affects both the extracellular compartment and the intracellular compartment. Gains and losses generally occur from both compartments. Laboratory determinations reflect the state of the extracellular compartment, simply because the plasma is easily accessed by venipuncture. Excesses or deficits can be diagnosed initially by evaluating the ECF; however, fluid imbalances do eventually affect the ICF. The constitutional signs and symptoms exhibited by patients experiencing body fluid imbalances occur in relation to the magnitude of disruption in the ICF and/or the ECF. Fluid volume disturbances can thus be classified according to the major site of symptomatologic manifestation.

Osmolal Imbalances

Osmolal imbalances affect the normal distribution of water between the intracellular and extracellular fluid compartments and are synonomous with water imbalances or ECF imbalances. These imbalances occur because of a change in the amount of pure water in body fluids, as opposed to a change in water and solute. Osmolal disturbances may be considered concentration abnormalities, which can result in further volume imbalances.

Normal osmolality relationships between the ECF and ICF are maintained primarily by the extracellular cation sodium. The cell, impermeable to sodium and fully permeable to water, will experience volume changes in response to extracellular osmolality fluctuations. Thus, osmolal imbalances involve

1. a change in water relative to sodium, or
2. a change in sodium relative to water.

Regardless of the cause, an osmolal imbalance affects the concentration of intracellular solute with clinical signs and symptoms due to changes in cellular volume.

Hyperosmolal Imbalances

Hyperosmolal imbalances are fluid disturbances in which the osmolality of the ECF is increased above the normal 305 mOsm/kg. As a result of the increased ECF osmolality, water movement occurs from the ICF to the ECF, causing a deficit of the intracellular volume, i.e., cellular shrinking. The cellular volume deficit causes changes in cell morphology, as well as decreasing the amount of water available for cellular metabolism; the resulting symptomatology arises from these alterations.

Hyperosmolal imbalances can arise from two sources—a water deficit or a sodium/solute excess—both producing increased osmolality of the ECF and cellular crenation due to osmotic water loss from the cells. See Table 9–5 for possible causes for hyperosmolal imbalances.

Table 9–5   A Comparison of Hyperosmolality and Hypo-osmolality

Causes	Signs and Symptoms	Laboratory Findings
	HYPEROSMOLALITY	
Water deficit	Mild	Serum sodium
Decreased intake	Thirst	>150 mEq/liter
Dysphagia	Flushed skin	Hematocrit elevated
Decreased thirst	Dry mucous mem-	Elevated BUN, electrolytes
Coma, organic brain	branes	Osmolality >305 mOsm/
syndrome, stroke	Hyperthermia	kg
Water unavailable	2% body weight loss	Urine—low volume, high
NPO status	Moderate	specific gravity
Excessive loss	Oliguria	Decreased MCV
Diarrhea	Concentrated urine	Increased MCHC
Prolonged vomiting	Muscle weakness	
Fever/diaphoresis	Tremors	
Diabetes insipidus	Delirum	
Diabetes mellitus	2–6% body weight loss	
Mechanical ventila-	Severe	
tion	Anuria	
Hyperventilation	Hallucinations	
Polyuria	Tachycardia	
Diuretic therapy	Hyperpnea	
Burns	Respiratory arrest	
Sodium/solute excess	7% body weight loss	
Overt overingestion	Death	
Hypertonic IV solutions		
Protein tube feedings/		
high milk cream		
diets without ade-		
quate water intake		

Table 9–5   *(Continued)*

Causes	Signs and Symptoms	Laboratory Findings
	HYPO-OSMOLALITY	
Water excess	Mild	Serum sodium
Psychogenic polydipsia	Lack of thirst	<130 mEq/liter
Alcohol consumption	Moist skin	Decreased hematocrit
Renal disease/failure	Pitting edema	Hgb and MCHC de-
Inappropriate ADH se-	Rales	creased
cretion	Polyuria	Elevated MCV
Cirrhosis	Dilute urine	Urine volume increased
Congestive heart failure	Moderate	Decreased urine specific
Tap water enemas	Lethargy	gravity
IV infusions of D_5W	Confusion	Low electrolyte values
Sodium/solute deficit	Frank pulmonary	because of dilution
Poor dietary intake	edema	Osmolality <290 mOsm/
Diuretic therapy	Muscle weakness	kg
Renal disease	Twitching	
Aldosterone deficiency	Severe	
Vomiting	CHF	
Diarrhea	Convulsions	
Intestinal drainage/	Coma	
fistula	Death	
Cystic fibrosis		
Trauma		
Inflammation		
Nasogastric irrigation		
with water		
Ice chips		
D_5W IV fluids		

BUN = blood urea nitrogen; MCV = mean corpuscular volume; MCHC = mean corpuscular hemoglobin concentration; D_5W = 5% dextrose in water; CHF = congestive heart failure; Hgb = hemoglobin.

Assessment.   Symptoms of a hyperosmolal imbalance are related to the severity of the fluid alteration. Clinical findings are similar regardless of the cause of the hyperosmolality—either water deficit or solute excess. Common signs and symptoms and altered laboratory values that can be expected are summarized in Table 9–5.

Intervention.   The usual therapeutic regimen for hyperosmolal imbalance is aimed at correcting the underlying pathology and restoring the elevated osmolality of the ECF toward normal, thus preventing the loss of intracellular fluid due to osmotic fluid shifts. This is usually accomplished by administering water either orally, if the patient is able, or intravenously in the form of

5% dextrose in water (D_5W), if the patient is unable to drink or the condition is severe.

The volume of water replacement necessary can be calculated many ways. A simple method is as follows:

Mild: thirst is only symptom; 2% deficit/2% × 70 kg = 1400 ml
Moderate: thirst, dry mucous membranes, oliguria; 6% deficit/6% × 70 kg = 4200 ml
Severe: above plus mental signs; 7–14% = 5–10 liters

Regardless of the method of calculating fluid replacement, it is important to recognize that, in addition to the required replacement, the normal daily water needs must be met as well as treating the hyperosmolal state. The nursing interventions employed for a patient experiencing hyperosmolal imbalances require sensitive assessment skills and adequate communication with all members of the health care team.

Nursing responsibilities include

1. Accurate intake and output recordings, ensuring a net gain of water
2. Measurement of daily weight
3. Measurement of liquid stools/GI secretions
4. Accurate temperature assessment every 2 hours
5. Administration of fluids as ordered, encourage oral intake
6. Reporting a serum sodium above 145 mEq/liter
7. Monitoring for central nervous system symptoms
8. Frequent vital sign assessment
9. Osmolality estimations, if lab studies available

Expected Outcomes.   Provided that the initial etiologic factor has been corrected, expected outcomes of treatment of a patient with a hyperosmolal imbalance include an increased urine output, normal body temperature, weight gain, and the return of normal serum sodium values and normal central nervous system (CNS) function. These changes should be expected within 2 days of instituting a therapeutic treatment plan, although assessment must continue in order to ensure these outcomes.

Hypo-osmolal Imbalances

Hypo-osmolal imbalances are fluid disturbances in which the osmolality of the ECF is decreased below the normal 290 mOsm/kg. As a result of the decreased ECF osmolality, the intracellular concentration of solutes is greater than that of the ECF, causing a fluid shift into the ICF, producing cellular swelling. Intracellular volume expansion alters the morphology and chemical processes of the cell and produces signs and symptoms as a result of cellular swelling.

Hypo-osmolal imbalances arise from either a water excess or a sodium/ solute deficit, producing a decreased osmolality of the ECF and movement of water into the cells, with swelling due to this osmotic flux. See Table 9–5 for the general causes of hypo-osmolal imbalances.

Assessment.   The basis of the symptoms of a hypo-osmolal imbalance are related to the severity and time course of the disturbance. As the osmolality of the ECF decreases because of either water excess or sodium deficit, osmotic pressure differences cause a net movement of water into the cells, causing them to swell. The severity of symptoms is related to both the magnitude of the hypo-osmolality, as well as to the rapidity of the onset of the disorder. In general, gradual osmolality changes are tolerated better than those that occur rapidly. The time course of the disorder is probably more important than actual values for hypo-osmolal disorders. Common signs and symptoms and laboratory findings are included in Table 9–5.

Intervention.   The usual therapeutic regimen for hypo-osmolal imbalances is aimed at correcting the underlying pathology and restoring the osmolality of the ECF toward normal. In mild cases, simply withholding oral fluids and limiting IV intake is all that is necessary. In a 24-hour period, nearly 1000 ml of water can be eliminated by obligatory pulmonary, renal, and cutaneous losses. However, if severe neurological symptoms are present, it may be necessary to increase the ECF osmolality more rapidly by the administration of hypertonic sodium chloride solutions—either 3% or 5% concentrations. Administering 6 ml per kilogram of body weight of 5% hypertonic sodium chloride will increase serum sodium values approximately 10 mEq/liter and, given slowly, can produce clinical improvement and prevent death from CNS complications. Again, therapy depends on the severity of the symptoms.

Nursing interventions for a patient experiencing a hypo-osmolal imbalance are aimed both at prevention and assessment of clinical manifestations. These include

1. Accurate intake and output recordings
2. Measurement of daily weight
3. Frequent vital sign assessment
4. Assessment of subtle neurological changes
5. Fluid restriction, as ordered
6. Careful regulation of IV infusions
7. Reporting of serum sodium levels less than 130 mEq/liter
8. Prevention of hypo-osmolal imbalances by

   - limiting tap water enemas
   - irrigating nasogastric tubes with isosmotic solutions (normal saline) rather than pure water
   - replacing fluid losses with electrolyte solutions (isotonic ice chips, fruit juices)

9. Monitoring for signs of hyperosmolality in patients receiving hypertonic sodium chloride therapy

Expected Outcomes.   After correction of the underlying disorder, therapeutic outcome criteria for a patient experiencing hypo-osmolal imbalances include normalization of CNS changes, production of a lower volume of concentrated urine, normal serum sodium, electrolytes, and osmolality progressing toward a generalized state of well-being. These changes should be expected within 24 to 48 hours after treatment begins. It should be pointed out, however, that the nurse is uniquely qualified to assist in the prevention of this imbalance during routine care of many susceptible hospitalized patients.

Volume Imbalances

In contrast to osmolal imbalances, which are caused by concentration discrepancies between the ECF and ICF, the categories of volume imbalance include disorders that arise because of a loss of water and solute together from the extracellular compartment. Other terms for these disturbances include isotonic fluid imbalances or ECF alterations. Regardless of the terminology, these disorders involve either gains or losses of sodium and water together and, thus affect primarily the ECF without cellular or osmotic influences. Symptoms are thus exhibited as isotonic gains or losses from the extracellular compartments.

Extracellular Volume Excess

Volume excesses of the extracellular compartment are those in which the ECF is expanded, usually affecting both the plasma and interstitial components. Sodium and water are increased without osmotic cellular alterations.

The body's organ systems exhibit complex interrelationships in terms of fluid balance. In general, the factors that predispose an individual to an ECF excess relate either to an inability to excrete excess fluids, as in renal failure, or to an alteration in normal mechanisms to conserve fluids, as with cardiac insufficiency or hepatic disease, in which low renal perfusion as result of these illnesses "fool" the kidney into retaining fluid. Predisposing conditions for extracellular volume excess are listed in Table 9–6.

Assessment.   The basis of the symptomatology of the ECF excesses relates to an overloading of the ECF with sodium and water. Clinical findings are summarized in Table 9–6. Laboratory tests for ECF excess are not as easily defined as for other disorders but can include low hematocrit, low electrolyte values, low urine sodium, and normal osmolality.

Intervention.   A therapeutic treatment regimen for a patient with an ECF excess is aimed at correcting the underlying pathologic process and promot-

Table 9–6   A Comparison of Extracellular Fluid Excess and Deficit

Causes	Signs and Symptoms
EXTRACELLULAR FLUID EXCESS	

Overinfusion of IV saline
Renal failure/tubular disease
Cardiac insufficiency
Hepatic cirrhosis/ascites
Cerebral disease
Steroid therapy
Hypertonic fluid loads
	Mild
	    Puffy skin/eyelids
	    Weight gain (2.2 lb = 1 liter of
	        fluid)
	    Full veins
	Moderate
	    Dependent pitting edema
	    Elevated blood pressure
	    Jugular venous distention
	    Cough
	    Rales
	Severe
	    Frank congestive heart failure
	    Dyspnea
	    Tachypnea
	    Pulmonary edema
	    Frothy sputum
	    Elevated CVP/PAP

EXTRACELLULAR FLUID DEFICIT	

Gastrointestinal losses of sodium
    and water
  Vomiting (sodium 140/mEq/liter GI
    secretions)
  Diarrhea (sodium 60 mEq/liter fecal
    material)
  Fistula drainage
  Gastric or intestinal suction
Renal disease where sodium and water
    lost
Diuretics
Fever/sweating
Cutaneous burn loss
Hemorrhage
Third space/sequestration
Cutaneous burn loss
	Mild
	    Poor skin turgor
	    Dry mucous membranes
	    Dehydration
	    Weakness
	    Weight loss
	Moderate
	    Hypovolemia
	    Tachycardia
	    Orthostatic hypotension
	    Collapsed neck veins
	Severe
	    Vertigo
	    Syncope
	    Low CVP/PAP
	    Oliguria
	    Shock

CVP/PAP = central venous pressure/pulmonary arterial pressure.

ing the elimination of excess sodium and water. In general, sodium intake is restricted and diuretics are administered to promote water excretion. Drug therapy is tailored to individual patient requirements.

Nursing assessment is a valuable component in the care of patients with ECF excess. Nursing responsibilities include

1. Accurate intake and output recordings
2. Accurate measurement of daily weight
3. Monitoring for signs of edema, both pulmonary and dependent forms, and reporting findings to the physician
4. Performing careful skin care for edematous patients
5. Monitoring the cardiovascular system—check blood pressure and assess for jugular venous distention. Use central venous or pulmonary arterial pressures, if available.
6. Restricting fluids and sodium as directed by the physician. Certain medications such as carbenicillin, sodium bicarbonate, Metamucil, Alka-Seltzer, Bromo-Seltzer, and Fleets Enema contain moderate to large amounts of sodium; thus, use should be monitored and patient education should be attempted.
7. Regulating IV fluids carefully
8. Observing for side effects of diuretic therapy, particularly, potassium deficit and excessive fluid loss

Expected Outcomes.   In addition to correcting the underlying pathologic condition, successful treatment of an ECF excess generally produces the resolution of edema, restoration of normal cardiovascular and pulmonary function, increased urine output, and weight loss. Continued clinical treatment of the predisposing condition is necessary, with careful monitoring to prevent ECF excess, using assessment skills and patient education.

Extracellular Fluid Deficit

A volume imbalance in which the ECF shows a deficit involves the loss of sodium and water from the extracellular space. This is an isotonic volume deficit with symptoms related to losses solely from the ECF without cellular osmotic changes. Conditions that can result in ECF deficit are listed in Table 9–6.

Assessment.   The symptoms of an ECF deficit are related to an isotonic volume loss. Typical findings are summarized in Table 9–6. Laboratory tests that may confirm the diagnosis include an elevated hematocrit, concentrated electrolytes, low urine sodium, elevated serum proteins, low urine volume, and high urine specific gravity.

Intervention.   A therapeutic treatment plan for a patient experiencing ECF deficits is aimed at correcting the pathologic process, as well as replacing sodium and water loss. In general, the more rapid the ECF depletion the more serious the consequences, thus accurate assessment is of vital importance. Replacement fluids are given orally or intravenously in the form of sodium chloride until symptoms resolve.

Nursing interventions for the patient with an ECF deficit include

1. Accurate intake and output recordings
2. Frequent vital sign assessment
3. Observation of cardiovascular parameters:

   - orthostatic blood pressures
   - central venous or pulmonary arterial pressure determinations
   - venous collapse/tachycardia

4. Measurement of daily weight
5. Careful measurement of urine output and specific gravity
6. Replenish losses with isotonic fluid as directed by the physician

Expected Outcomes.   After successful resolution of the cause of the ECF deficit, patients with resolving ECF depletion should have improved skin turgor, elevated blood, central venous, and pulmonary arterial pressures, and increased urine output. Tachycardia should resolve, neck veins should fill, and orthostatic blood pressure changes should be eliminated. The patient's weight should return to normal and signs of shock (if present) should disappear. Laboratory values should normalize as plasma volume is restored.

Altered Distribution of Body Fluids

In the healthy individual, the normal distribution of body fluids is maintained by physiologic mechanisms to ensure adequate water content in the various fluid compartments. The formation of edema and "third space" sequestration are distribution imbalances that can be viewed as specialized forms of extracellular volume disturbances. Edema implies an interstitial fluid excess, while third space sequestration renders body fluid inaccessible, effectively causing an ECF deficit.

Edema

Edema can occur when oncotic pressure is low or venous hydrostatic pressure is high, preventing effective fluid reabsorption, as well as when elevated arterial hydrostatic pressure forces more fluid into the interstitium than can effectively be returned to the circulation by normal negative venous filtration forces. The fluid retained in the interstitial spaces as a result of these physiologic alterations is, in effect, an extracellular volume excess. The etiologic factors and the conditions commonly associated with edema formation are summarized in Table 9–7.

Table 9–7   Etiology of Edema

Etiologic factors	Associated conditions
Increased capillary permeability	Inflammatory reactions
	Burns
	Trauma
	Pulmonary Edema (noncardiogenic)
	Allergic reactions
Increased capillary hydrostatic pressure	
Na^+ retention and increased blood	Congestive heart failure
volume	Trauma and stress
	Renal failure
	Refeeding edema
	Adrenocortical hormone secretion
	Drugs; estrogen, phenylbutazone
Venous obstruction	Local obstruction
	Hepatic obstruction
	Pulmonary edema (cardiogenic)
Decreased plasma oncotic pressure	
Decreased synthesis of plasma proteins	Liver disease
	Malnutrition
Increased loss of plasma proteins	Nephrotic syndrome
	Burns
	Protein-losing enteropathy
Increased interstitial pressure	Lymphatic obstruction
(plasma protein lost to interstitium)	Increased capillary permeability

From *Basic Pathophysiology: A Holistic Approach,* 3rd ed., by M. E. Groer and M. E. Shekleton, 1989, St. Louis: The C. V. Mosby Co. Reproduced with permission.

Sequestration

The phenomenon of sequestration is associated with the accumulation in tissues or a body cavity fluids in excess of normal. In effect, that fluid is removed from the extracellular volume and rendered unavailable to the normal body fluid stores. Sequestration can occur as the result of the inflammatory process, mobilizing fluids to the site of tissue disruption, as well as from venous obstruction in various organ systems preventing fluid reabsorption. The conditions associated with fluid sequestration are summarized in Table 9–8.

Intervention.   In general, one can view edema as a form of ECF excess and sequestration as a type of ECF deficit, in terms of symptomatology, therapy, and nursing responsibilities when caring for patients experiencing these conditions. These disorders are generally indicative of serious underlying pathological processes, which may involve more than one fluid disturbance occurring simultaneously. The therapeutic treatment plan for patients experiencing

Table 9–8 Conditions Associated with Fluid Sequestration

Acute pancreatitis
Intestinal obstruction
Peritonitis
Postoperative inflammatory response
Intestinal fistula
Hepatic carcinoma
Cirrhosis

edema or sequestration should always include a thorough history and physical examination to correlate clinical findings with nursing diagnoses.

Alterations in the Composition of Body Fluid

Sodium

The minimum sodium requirement is approximately 5 g/day, which is easily met in a normal diet with added table salt. Once ingested, sodium is absorbed from the gastrointestinal tract. Excretion occurs by way of the urine, feces, and perspiration in approximately the same amount as that ingested.

Sodium balance in the body is regulated by hormonal influences, particularly by the mineralocorticoid aldosterone. Aldosterone increases the reabsorption of sodium and promotes the excretion of potassium in the renal tubules in response to renal perfusion changes and circulating sodium levels. Natriuretic hormone also promotes sodium excretion when serum values are elevated (Cosgrove, 1989).

Sodium is the major cation of the ECF, with normal serum concentrations of 135 to 145 mEq/liter. As the primary cation of the ECF, sodium's contribution to osmolality regulates the volume of the body fluid compartments.

$$\text{Osmolality} = 2 \times [\text{Na}] + \frac{[\text{BUN}]}{2.8} + \frac{[\text{glucose}]}{18}$$

Being relatively impermeable to the cell membrane, changes in the sodium content of the ECF alter the osmolal imbalance between the ICF and ECF causing osmotic fluid shifts between compartments.

Sodium helps to maintain neuromuscular integrity in body tissues. The active extrusion of sodium from the cells of excitable tissues (muscles, nerves) maintains an electrical potential across the cell membrane. When stimulated, an action potential is generated, sodium enters the cell, changing the electrical gradient, and is therefore responsible for depolarization. This phenomenon is particularly important in the sinoatrial node of the heart. Sodium also plays a part in chemical reactions with chloride and bicarbonate, thereby helping to regulate the acid–base balance of the body.

Pathologic states that alter the sodium balance tend to produce either an excess of sodium (hypernatremia) or a deficit (hyponatremia). Hypernatremia is defined by a serum sodium level greater than 145 mEq/liter. Hyponatremia is defined by a serum sodium value less than 135 mEq/liter. Because of sodium's intimate link with osmolality and water distribution, sodium imbalances usually occur as a result of a change in sodium relative to water producing hypernatremic or hyponatremic states. The common causes of sodium imbalance are summarized in Table 9–9.

Table 9–9   Causes of Sodium Imbalance

Hypernatremia (serum sodium greater than 145 mEq/liter)	*Hyponatremia* (serum sodium less than 135 mEq/liter)
SODIUM EXCESS	SODIUM DEFICIT
Overingestion	Poor intake
Excess IV infusions	Diuretic therapy
	Salt-wasting renal disease
	Aldosterone deficiency
	GI losses
	Cutaneous losses
	Replacement of sodium losses with pure water solutions
WATER DEFICIT	WATER EXCESS
Dysphagia	Psychogenic polydipsia
NPO status	Renal failure
Neurological alterations	Increased or inappropriate ADH secretion
Excessive GI losses	Low renal perfusion states
Diaphoresis	Rectal water absorption
Diabetes	Overinfusion of intravenous D_5W
Mechanical ventilation	
Hyperventilation	
Renal disease—polyuria	
Diuretic therapy	
Severe burns	

D_5W = 5% dextrose in water.

Assessment.   Hypernatremic states, by increasing the osmolality of the ECF, cause an osmotic gradient for water movement from the intracellular compartment to the extracellular compartment, producing signs and symptoms due to cellular crenation. The opposite is true of hyponatremic states; water movement occurs from the ECF to the ICF in response to the lowered osmolality of the ECF. Symptomatology related to hyponatremic states arises from cellular swelling as a result of osmotic fluid shifts. A summary of the symptoms associated with sodium imbalances is included in Table 9–10.

Intervention and Expected Outcomes.   Sodium disturbances are synonomous with osmolal fluid disturbances. The therapy and expected outcomes for hypernatremia are the same as those for hyperosmolal imbalances. Hyponatremia is treated the same way as hypo-osmolal fluid disturbances. This association obligates the clinical practitioner to evaluate any patient experiencing sodium alterations for related fluid disturbances, performing interventions for the appropriate osmolal imbalances.

Chloride

Chloride is the major anion of the ECF, with normal serum concentrations of 97 to 104 mEq/liter. Chloride concentrations are highest in the extracellular compartment, both in plasma and interstitial fluid. Intracellular chloride is minimal, on the order of 2 mEq/liter, found primarily in nerve tissue.

The minimal daily chloride requirement, although not exactly specified, tends to approximate that of sodium—approximately 5 g/day. Chloride requirements are met with a normal diet, and is contained in added table salt as NaCl. As with sodium, chloride is absorbed from the gastrointestinal tract. Excretion occurs in the kidneys, usually combined with phosphate and sulfate.

Chloride balance in the body is linked closely with sodium homeostasis. The hormone aldosterone, acting to promote increased sodium reabsorption in the renal tubule, causes chloride to be retained with the sodium in exchange for a potassium or hydrogen ion. Generally, disturbances in sodium levels also affect chloride in a proportional manner because of their common regulatory pathways.

Chloride functions in the body in tandem with sodium as the balancing anion in extracellular fluid. Thus, chloride content affects the osmolality of the ECF and helps to regulate fluid volume and distribution between compartments.

Chloride also plays a part in the acid–base balance of the body. Chloride and bicarbonate, as extracellular anions, compete for sodium binding in the maintenance of electrical neutrality. When chloride concentrations are low, the bicarbonate level is increased by renal reabsorption to maintain ionic balance, and blood pH becomes alkalotic. Excessive circulating chloride lev-

Table 9–10   Signs and Symptoms of Sodium Imbalance

Hypernatremia	Hyponatremia
CONSTITUTIONAL	
Dry mucous membranes	Moist mucous membrane
Flushed skin	Potential for
Hyperthermia	edematous tissue
Weight loss	Lack of thirst
Intense thirst	
CARDIOVASCULAR	
Tachycardia (if hyperthermic)	Potential pulmonary edema
Increased blood viscosity	
RENAL	
Oliguria	Polyuria
High specific gravity	Low specific gravity
Renal shutdown	
NEUROLOGICAL	
Muscle weakness	Lethargy
Tremors	Confusion
Delirium	*Convulsions*
Hallucinations	Coma
Coma	
RESPIRATORY	
(late)	
Hyperpnea	
Respiratory arrest	
LABORATORY FINDINGS	
Sodium above 145 mEq/liter	Sodium below 135 mEq/liter
Elevated hematocrit	Decreased hemtocrit
Concentrated electrolytes (increased BUN)	MCHC decreased
	MCV increased
Decreased MCV	Anion gap less than 8 mEq/liter
Increased MCHC	Osmolality less than 290 mOsm/kg
Anion gap above 16 mEq/liter	
Increased serum osmolality above 305 mOsm/kg	

BUN = blood urea nitrogen; MCV = mean corpuscular volume; MCHC = mean corpuscular hemoglobin concentration.

els promote renal excretion of bicarbonate and may alter the pH of the blood toward an acidotic state. In this manner, chloride becomes an integral component in maintaining normal acid–base equilibrium.

Pathologic states that alter the chloride content of the body can occur as a result of sodium disturbances, as well as independently of sodium imbalances. In general, chloride elevations, in combination with sodium elevations, are synonymous with hyperosmolal imbalances, and should be treated as such. Chloride deficits combined with sodium deficits are approached as hypo-osmolal imbalances in terms of recognition and therapeutic intervention. Less commonly, isolated chloride imbalances may occur in relation to acid–base disturbances. Potential causes of chloride imbalances are summarized in Table 9–11.

Assessment.   The signs and symptoms of chloride imbalance are summarized in Table 9–12.

Intervention.   Therapy for hyperchloremia consists, basically, of restricting the intake of chloride-rich substances and correcting metabolic acidosis if present. Hypochloremia is treated by replacing chloride losses and preventing complications associated with metabolic alkalosis.

Nursing responsibilities for chloride imbalances include

1. Monitoring intake and output carefully
2. Observing for respiratory variations associated with acid–base disturbances
3. Monitoring for signs of fluid disturbances
4. Administering medications as directed by the physician

Expected Outcomes.   Therapeutic outcomes for patients experiencing chloride imbalances depend greatly on the resolution of the underlying pathologic condition. Clinical improvement, generally, involves the correction of several disorders and, thus, assessment must continue throughout the course of the illness.

Table 9–11   Causes of Chloride Imbalance

Hyperchloremia (Cl⁻ greater than 104 mEq/liter)	Hypochloremia (Cl⁻ less than 97 mEq/liter)
Hyperosmolal states in combination with sodium	Hypo-osmolal states in combination with sodium
Excessive ingestion or over-infusion of IV solutions	Underingestion
	GI losses
	Renal disease

Table 9–12 Signs and Symptoms of Chloride Disturbances

Hyperchloremia	Hypochloremia
See Hyperosmolal imbalance if [Na$^+$] abnormal	See hypo-osmolal disturbances if [Na$^+$] abnormal
Renal bicarbonate loss	Renal bicarbonate gain
Metabolic acidosis	Metabolic alkalosis
Hyperventilation	Muscular hypertonicity
Delirium	Tetany
Weakness	Hypoventilation
Stupor	Seizures
Coma	

Potassium

The cation potassium exists in the body in amounts of approximately 50 mEq/kg. Of this total amount, 98% is located in the intracellular compartment, and 2 to 3% is found in the ECF. Normal serum values for potassium are 3.5 to 5.0 mEq/liter.

The normal potassium intake is approximately 100 mEq per 24-hour period, which is absorbed from the gastrointestinal tract after ingestion of potassium-rich foods such as bananas, green vegetables, citrus fruits, and potatoes. Potassium excretion occurs primarily through the kidneys. Fecal excretion accounts for a small amount, approximately 10 mEq/day.

Potassium is responsible for many vital functions in the body. By virtue of its largely intracellular distribution, potassium helps to regulate the osmolality of the body fluid compartments. Potassium is integral to normal neuromuscular function, influencing the conduction of impulses in nerves and muscles, including the heart. Potassium is also closely tied to the normal acid–base equilibrium. As a cation, potassium can exchange with hydrogen ions across the cell membrane, profoundly influencing pH changes in the ECF.

Potassium balance is regulated in the body based on the normal distribution pattern. While intracellular concentrations may fluctuate widely, the extracellular K$^+$ level is controlled within fairly narrow limits. Factors that affect extracellular potassium concentrations are discussed below.

Aldosterone influences serum potassium levels by augmenting sodium reabsorption. Sodium is retained by the renal tubule in response to aldosterone, and potassium is excreted in the urine in exchange for the sodium.

Potassium excretion also depends on renal sodium delivery and urine flow rates. As sodium delivery to the distal tubule increases, potassium excretion rises and vice versa. Increased urine flow augments potassium elimination.

Extracellular potassium distribution is affected by several factors. Systemic acid–base variations cause serum potassium fluctuations. Acidotic states tend to increase the amount of potassium in the ECF. Hydrogen ions move into the cell with acidemia, causing a potassium flux out of the cell, raising the K^+ concentration of the ECF. With alkalosis, hydrogen ions move into the ECF to buffer pH changes and potassium ions exchange for the hydrogen ions by moving into the cell. This preserves the electroneutrality of body fluids and decreases extracellular potassium concentrations.

The action of insulin also affects extracellular potassium levels. Potassium moves into the cells when glucose metabolism is augmented by insulin. When serum glucose levels are high, potassium levels are high. This situation can be remedied by insulin administration.

Extracellular potassium levels may be changed by factors that affect the integrity of the cell membrane. When cellular damage or death occur, potassium is liberated from the cell, increasing the potassium concentration of the ECF. The general causes of potassium imbalance are summarized in Table 9–13.

Hyperkalemia

Assessment.   Changes in the ECF serum potassium concentration can have profound effects in the body. The muscles are most affected by alterations in potassium balance because of the role of K^+ in depolarization of the muscle cell membrane. The muscle most seriously affected is the heart (Groer & Shekleton, 1989). Signs and symptoms of hyperkalemia are listed in Table 9–14.

Intervention.   The treatment for patients experiencing hyperkelemia is aimed at lowering serum potassium levels, especially if ECG changes are present. The therapy is tailored to the severity of the disorder.

Hyperkalemic states require that the nurse determine sources of potassium intake and eliminate any dietary or intravenous sources. Urinary output is critical for potassium elimination, and urine excretion should be promoted by administration of diuretics. Dialysis may be indicated if renal failure is present. The nurse should monitor and report serum potassium values greater than 5.0 mEq/liter to the physician. Blood transfusions, if required, should be administered, using fresh blood to eliminate the addition of excess potassium in stored blood. Cation exchange resins such as Kayexalate may be used to decrease GI absorption of potassium.

If cardiac symptoms are severe, drugs such as sodium bicarbonate or glucose and insulin may be administered to increase potassium movement into the intracellular compartment temporarily, reducing serum levels. Calcium (500 to 1000 mg) may also be administered to stabilize the cardiac action potential while measures are undertaken to lower serum potassium values definitively.

Table 9–13   Causes of Potassium Imbalance

Hyperkalemia (Serum K⁺ greater than 5 mEq/liter)	Hypokalemia (Serum K⁺ less than 3.5 mEq/liter)
INCREASED INTAKE	**DECREASED INTAKE**
Dietary excess	Dietary deficiency
Overinfusion of IV potassium	Alcoholism
Salt substitutes	Anorexia nervosa
Penicillin potassium	
CELLULAR REDISTRIBUTION	**CELLULAR REDISTRIBUTION**
Acidosis	Alkalosis
Hemolysis	Insulin shock
Rhabdomyolysis	Healing process
Crush injuries	
Serious burns	
Infection	
Hyperglycemia	
DECREASED EXCRETION	**INCREASED LOSS**
Acute renal failure	GI losses
Potassium-sparing diuretics	Prolonged vomiting
(spironolactone triamterene)	Laxatives/enemas
Mineralocorticoid deficiency	Diarrhea
(Addison's disease)	Gastric/intestinal
FACTITIOUS	suction
	Fistulas
Hemolysis of blood sample	Colostomies,
Tourniquet cell damage	ileostomies
	Renal losses
	Diuretics (Lasix,
	thiazides, mannitol)
	Mineralocorticoid
	excess (Cushing's
	syndrome)
	Interstitial
	nephritis
	Renal tubular
	acidosis

Hypokalemia

Assessment.   The clinical and laboratory indicators of hypokalemia are summarized in Table 9–14.

Intervention.   The primary therapeutic approach to hypokalemia involves prevention of excessive potassium losses. The development of hypokalemia

Table 9–14   A Comparison of Hyperkalemia and Hypokalemia

Signs and Symptoms	Laboratory Findings
HYPERKALEMIA	
Mild	$K^+ > 5.0$ mEq/liter
Twitching	Oliguria
Hyperreflexia	Hyperglycemia
Moderate	
Muscle weakness	
Paresthesias	
ECG—peaked T waves	
Intestinal colic	
Vomiting	
Severe	
Muscle paralysis	
Bradycardia ($K^+ = 7.0$)	
ECG—wide QRS/sine wave	
($K^+ = 9.0$)	
Death	
HYPOKALEMIA	
Mild	$K^+ < 3.5$ mEq/liter
Fatigue	Polyuria
Lethargy	
Decreased deep tendon reflexes	
Moderate	
Muscle weakness	
Abdominal distention	
Paralytic ileus	
Hypotension	
Ventricular arrythmias	
ECG—premature ventricular contractions,	
U waves	
Severe	
Paralysis of smooth and skeletal	
muscle	
ECG—ST depression	
Cardiac arrest	

may be prevented in part by the use of patient education by practitioners caring for patients at risk for potassium depletion. Dietary counseling and medication teaching may be important preventive measures.

If potassium loss is not preventable, then potassium supplementation, either orally or intravenously, must be undertaken to prevent the complications of potassium deficit. Dietary intake of foods rich in potassium may be augmented by the addition of 20 to 40 mEq of potassium per liter of IV fluid. Oral potassium supplements may also be administered to patients at risk for potassium depletion.

Intravenous potassium replacement requires dilution of potassium salts and slow administration to prevent phlebitis or possible cardiac arrest with too rapid an infusion. Guidelines for peripheral and central line infusions of potassium are provided by Lunger (1988). Adequate renal function must always be assessed prior to any potassium supplementation to avoid possible rebound hyperkalemia.

Hypokalemia potentiates digitalis preparations and patients receiving digitalis and diuretics may be at significant risk for digitalis toxicity regardless of the digitalis dosage. The care of patients with potassium imbalance requires thorough knowledge of the medication history, as well as appropriate planning prior to instituting any therapy aimed at restoring normal serum potassium concentrations.

The nursing care of patients at risk for potassium imbalances include interventions common to both disorders, as well as the specific recommendations discussed previously for each disturbance. General practices include

1. Frequent assessment of vital signs
2. Monitoring for pulse or ECG changes
3. Frequent serum potassium determinations (especially during replacement therapy)
4. Observation of neurological status for subtle or overt changes
5. Accurate intake and output determinations to assess renal function, as well as potential sources of potassium loss
6. Accurate medication history

Calcium

Calcium exists in the body primarily as the support matrix of the skeleton, as well as in the nails and teeth. The total body calcium content is approximately 20 g per kilogram of weight. Of this, 99% is bound to bony structures, with the remaining 1% circulating in the plasma portion of the ECF. Normal serum concentrations of calcium are expressed in either milligrams per deciliter or milliequivalents per liter. Serum calcium values of 9 to 11 mg/dl or 4.5 to 5.5 mEq/liter are considered to be within normal limits.

Calcium requirements vary with the age and sex of the individual. In general, children and the aged require larger amounts of daily calcium than the 0.8 g/day suggested for normal adults. Pregnancy and lactation also increase daily calcium requirements.

The usual source of calcium is dietary intake, primarily of milk and milk products. Once ingested, approximately 50% of the total intake is absorbed by the GI tract in the small intestine. Calcium excretion is both renal and fecal with potential losses through the skin when profuse perspiration occurs.

Normally 99% of the filtered calcium is reabsorbed in the kidney, with total excretion dependent on daily intake and effective absorption.

The function of calcium in the body relates to several physiologic processes. Calcium is important in the contractile function of skeletal and cardiac muscle, combining with ATP in the contraction sequence. Calcium tends to maintain or decrease neuromuscular irritability and decreases capillary permeability. In addition, normal conversion of prothrombin to thrombin in the coagulation mechanism depends on adequate calcium levels.

The regulation of calcium in the body depends on several factors. The hormone parathormone (PTH) is secreted by the parathyroid gland. PTH secretion is stimulated or inhibited in response to changes in the circulating serum calcium levels. Low serum calcium concentrations cause increased secretion of PTH. The release of PTH decreases renal excretion of calcium to restore serum levels near normal. The converse is also true. High calcium levels decrease PTH, promoting increased renal calcium excretion. PTH also affects the osteoclastic cells of the bone matrix. When serum calcium is low, osteoclastic cells release calcium from the bone to raise extracellular concentrations. The hormone calcitonin opposes osteoclastic activity, inhibiting calcium release from bone in response to elevated serum calcium levels.

Vitamin D and ultraviolet light also affect serum calcium levels. Sunlight is required by the body to synthesize vitamin D. Vitamin D allows increased absorption of calcium in the intestine and alters the response of bone calcium to PTH and calcitonin, thus affecting the ability of calcium to be released or retained in the skeletal matrix. Changes in these factors can easily alter the available circulating calcium level.

The relationship between calcium bound to bone and serum calcium is extremely important in that the skeleton provides a large reservoir of calcium from which the ECF levels can be maintained. Calcium is drawn from skeletal sources by osteoclastic activity when extracellular levels are low. Thus, alterations in serum calcium eventually have the potential to change skeletal structure, sometimes producing serious consequences.

Extracellular calcium exists, in the serum, partially bound to the plasma protein albumin and partially as free ionized particles. Plasma protein content will affect total calcium levels. Ionized calcium accounts for approximately one third of the total calcium concentration. Phosphorus levels also affect serum calcium levels in a reciprocal fashion. In effect, low calcium levels are associated with high phosphorus concentrations and vice versa. The causes of calcium imbalance are summarized in Table 9–15.

Hypercalcemia

Assessment.   The symptoms of hypercalcemia with associated laboratory findings are shown in Table 9–16.

Intervention.   The therapy for hypercalcemia is generally aimed at decreasing calcium intake and increasing calcium elimination. However, supportive

Table 9–15   Causes of Calcium Imbalance

Hypercalcemia (Serum Ca^+ greater than 11 mg/dl)	Hypocalcemia (Serum Ca^+ less than 9 mg/dl)
Excess intake	Inadequate intake
Milk products	Excess loss of GI secretions
Alkali medications	Intestinal drainage
(antacids)	Acute pancreatitis
Hyperparathyroidism	Diarrhea
Parathyroid tumors	Deficit of vitamin D
Excessive vitamin D intake	Hypoparathyroidism
Paget's disease	Parathyroidectomy
Neoplastic metastasis to bone	Immobilization bone
Prolonged immobilization	demineralization
Renal disease causing decreased	(decreases bony reservoir)
excretion	Excessive citrated blood
	transfusions (binds and
	inactivates calcium)

therapy is often necessary to correct serum values prior to definitive treatment. Often, isotonic sodium sulfate is administered (2 liters IV) to create a diuresis and improve excretion. Phosphate preparations may also be given orally or IV to improve renal calcium elimination. Steroids may be administered to inhibit calcium absorption. Definitive medical or surgical intervention for the underlying cause is often the sole recourse for the treatment of hypercalcemia.

Nursing interventions in the care of the hypercalcemic patient include

1. Accurate measurement of intake and output
2. Encouraging range-of-motion exercises and early ambulation for patients on bed rest
3. Monitoring of serum calcium levels
4. Assessment for neuromuscular changes
5. Restricting the intake of calcium rich foods/IV infusions
6. Straining urine for renal calculi.

Hypocalcemia

Assessment.   The clinical findings associated with hypocalcemia are listed in Table 9–16.

Intervention.   The therapeutic treatment regimen for hypocalcemia is aimed at correcting the underlying pathologic process, as well as at restoring normal calcium levels. Generally, mild hypocalcemia can be corrected by increasing

Table 9–16   A Comparison of Hypercalcemia and Hypocalcemia

Signs and Symptoms	Laboratory Findings
HYPERCALCEMIA	

Mild
  Anorexia
  Nausea
  Constipation
  Lethargy
 	
Moderate
  Skeletal muscle
    hypotonicity
  Bone pain
  Polyuria
  Renal calculi
 	
Severe
  Osteomalacia
  Pathologic fractures
  Cardiac arrhythmias
  Cardiac arrest
	$[Ca^+] > 11$ mg/dl or
	    5.5 mEq/liter
	$[PO_4] < 2.5$ mg/dl
	Positive Sulkowitch test (urine Ca^+)
	X-ray evidence of bone
	    demineralization and renal
	    calculi

HYPOCALCEMIA	

Mild
  Circumoral or digital
    paresthesias
  Muscle spasms
  Palpitations
 	
Moderate
  Hyperactive deep tendon reflexes
  Cardiac arrhythmias
 	
Severe
  Tetany
  (positive Chvostek's, Trousseau's
    signs)
  Laryngeal stridor
  Coagulopathy
  Seizures
	$[Ca^+] < 9$ mg/dl
	$[PO_4] > 4.5$ mg/dl
	Negative Sulkowitch test (urine)

dietary intake of calcium-rich foods along with the oral administration of calcium supplements such as calcium chloride, calcium lactate, and calcium gluconate. Vitamin D supplements are often prescribed in conjunction with calcium replacement. In general, 1.0 to 1.5 g/day of additional calcium will correct mild to moderate hypocalcemia.

If signs of tetany are present, calcium gluconate is the treatment of choice to restore serum levels rapidly and to ameliorate serious symptoms.

Doses of 200 to 300 mg are administered slowly, to a maximum of 1 g, until acute signs resolve. Calcium additives to IV fluids may then supplement oral therapy until normal serum values are restored.

Nursing interventions for the patient with hypocalcemia may include

1. Patient education related to dietary sources and supplemental medications
2. Monitoring for signs of tetany/impending seizures
3. Monitoring for signs of stridor/respiratory distress (have tracheostomy supplies nearby)
4. Administering IV calcium with care, as infiltration can cause tissue sloughing
5. Not mixing calcium solutions with phosphorus solutions, as precipitation may result
6. Administering calcium preparations with care to patients receiving digitalis, as potentiation may cause digitalis toxicity
7. Being aware that citrated blood products may potentiate hypocalcemia
8. Carefully recording intake and output, especially calcium-rich GI losses
9. Observing for calcium imbalances during replacement therapy. Thorough assessment and prompt treatment can help prevent dangerous consequences resulting from calcium imbalances.

ACID–BASE BALANCE

Basic Concepts

The acid–base parameter in the human body is one of the most complex physiologic systems in existence, designed solely to maintain the acidity of the body fluids within a range compatible for cellular function. Sophisticated control mechanisms provide protection against severe alterations in acid–base balance.

The pH is an expression of the relative acidity and alkalinity of the body fluid. More specifically, it is the negative logarithm of the hydrogen ion concentration per liter of solution. The pH value and the hydrogen ion concentration vary inversely, that is the higher the pH, the lower the hydrogen ion concentration and vice versa. The pH is determined using the Henderson–Hasselbalch equation:

$$pH = pK + \log \frac{base}{acid}$$

Because of the logarithmic relationship, a change in pH of 1 unit equates with a 10-fold change in hydrogen ion concentration.

There are two sources of hydrogen ions in human physiologic systems: volatile acids and nonvolatile or fixed acids. Volatile acids are those in which either the acid or its end product can be excreted from the body as a gas. The chemical reaction,

$$H^+ + HCO_3^- \rightleftharpoons H_2CO_3 \rightleftharpoons H_2O + CO_2,$$

describes the complete metabolism of carbohydrates and fats, producing water and carbon dioxide. The intermediate compound, carbonic acid, represents a volatile acid because the end product of its metabolism, CO_2, can be eliminated as a gas from the lungs. Normal metabolism results in the production of approximately 14,000 mEq of carbonic acid every 24 hours.

Nonvolatile, or fixed acids, include all other hydrogen-ion-donating substances in the body. These substances—lactic acid and pyruvic acid from incomplete fat and carbohydrate metabolism, as well as sulfuric acids and metabolic wastes from the oxidation of phosphoproteins—must either be metabolized or excreted in the urine to be eliminated from the body.

Acid–Base Regulation

To ensure the maintenance of normal serum pH values, three regulatory mechanisms exist to counteract severe alterations in hydrogen ion equilibrium. These mechanisms include chemical buffering, respiratory regulation, and renal compensation.

Chemical Buffering.   A buffer system consists of a combination of weak acid and its conjugate base that responds chemically in solution to accept or donate hydrogen ions in response to an acute change in pH. The ability to donate or accept hydrogen ions tends to minimize the effect of an excess acid or alkali load, thus lessening the magnitude of acid–base alteration that might occur had the buffer not been present. The extracellular fluid contains three chemical buffer systems:

1. The carbonic acid/bicarbonate pair
2. The phosphate buffer pair
3. The plasma proteins (buffering by configurational hydrogen changes)

Buffering is determined by the relationship between acid–base pairs as defined by the Henderson–Hasselbalch equation:

$$pH = pK + \log \frac{base}{acid}$$

This equation illustrates that pH cannot change unless the ratio of base to acid changes. Additionally, if it is accepted that if there are multiple buffer systems in a solution, all buffer ratios will change in relation to pH changes. This is exactly the case in the ECF; thus, sampling of one buffer system provides information related to the status of the others. In human plasma the carbonic acid–bicarbonate pair is used to make determinations of buffer status because it is the largest and most effective system and can also be regulated by the lungs and kidneys, thus providing information about those systems as well.

At normal pH, the Henderson–Hasselbalch equation dictates that the ratio of bicarbonate base to carbonic acid is approximately 20:1. The carbonic acid equation:

$$H^+ + HCO_3^- \rightleftharpoons H_2CO_3 \rightleftharpoons H_2O + CO_2$$

reveals that CO_2 is in direct equilibrium with the hydrogen ion concentration; thus without directly sampling the carbonic acid content, an inference to its value can be made from the arterial pCO_2.

Rearranging

$$pH = pK + \log \frac{[base]}{[acid]}$$

becomes

$$7.4 = 6.1 + \log \frac{[HCO_3^-]}{[pCO_2 x]}$$

The normal plasma bicarbonate level is near 24 mEq/liter. Normal pCO_2 is 40 torr. Normal pH depends on this ratio. If plasma bicarbonate is elevated, then CO_2 content must also be elevated to maintain the ratio. Conversely, alterations in the acid component, pCO_2, must obligate changes in the base HCO_3^- to sustain normal pH. These changes occur in the ECF to minimize pH variation.

An additional buffer system is contained in the red blood cells (RBCs) and operates through the chloride shift mechanism. Carbon dioxide in plasma is produced as a metabolic end product and is carried to the lungs for elimination in the RBCs as carbonic acid and carbamino complexes with hemoglobin. Carbonic acid dissociation occurs in the cell forming H^+ and HCO_3^- until the intracellular bicarbonate level exceeds that of plasma. As plasma becomes more acidic (low bicarbonate levels) a negatively charged chloride ion enters the RBC and a bicarbonate ion moves into the plasma to minimize pH changes. After pulmonary circulation, CO_2 levels are decreased, eliminating excess hydrogen ion, and the reaction reverses, sending chloride into the plasma in exchange for intracellular bicarbonate flux. This hemoglobin buffering is responsible for pH maintenance in the face of continuous CO_2 production.

Respiratory Regulation.   The respiratory system acts as a feedback system with the carbon dioxide concentration. Feedback control is possible because the CO_2 concentration is in equilibrium with the hydrogen ion concentration as demonstrated by the following equation:

$$H^+ + HCO_3^- \rightleftharpoons H_2CO_3 \rightleftharpoons H_2O + CO_2$$

Ventilation increases or decreases in response to the level of CO_2 in the plasma. When increased amounts of CO_2 are present, the respiratory system becomes more active and "blows off" the excess carbon dioxide, making less available to form carbonic acid. When the CO_2 level is decreased, the respiratory system becomes less active and retains carbon dioxide, making more available to form carbonic acid (Groer & Shekleton, 1989). Changes in the CO_2 concentration are sensed by central chemoreceptors, while peripheral chemoreceptors respond to pH, pCO_2, and pO_2 stimuli. The net effect after activation of the chemoreceptors provides either an increase or decrease in ventilation to restore normal pCO_2 and thus maintain normal pH values.

Renal Regulation.   The kidneys provide definitive resolution of acid–base disturbances through specialized mechanisms to maintain plasma bicarbonate levels and excrete excess hydrogen ions. Under normal circumstances, 99% of the filtered plasma bicarbonate is reabsorbed in the renal tubule in combination with the active secretion of hydrogen ions from the tubular cell into the urine. In effect, plasma bicarbonate is regenerated and hydrogen ions are eliminated in exchange for sodium, another positively charged ion, which is absorbed.

Two additional renal mechanisms exist for hydrogen ion elimination once all the filtered bicarbonate is reabsorbed: the phosphate buffers and ammonium formation. The phosphate buffer system forms complexes of excess hydrogen ions in the form of dihydrogen phosphate (H_2PO_4), which is excreted in the urine. Ammonia (NH_3), formed by amino acid metabolism, also retrieves hydrogen ions forming ammonium (NH_4^+) in the urine. Ammonium reacts with an anion such as chloride in the tubular fluid to form urinary salts, which are excreted. These two processes eliminate excess hydrogen ions, acidify the urine and generate new bicarbonate on the order of 50 to 60 mEq/24 hours in the process of maintaining the normal range of the systemic pH.

The regulatory systems differ with respect to reaction time, as well as to categories of acid capacity. In general, the first line of response to pH changes involves the chemical buffers followed closely by hemoglobin, which occurs almost instantaneously. Ventilatory responses occur within 10 to 30 minutes, and because they react only to carbonic acid disturbances, they regulate only volatile acid imbalances. Renal regulation can make permanent changes provided the kidneys are healthy. Renal responses are slow, requiring hours to days. However, under normal circumstances, the kidneys handle all fixed acids and thus regulate the rest of the daily acid–base load imposed on the body. The combination of chemical buffers, alveolar ventilation, and renal urine acidification provide strong regulation against systemic pH imbalances.

Alterations in Acid–Base Balance

Failure to maintain the hydrogen ion concentration of the body fluid within normal limits so that the pH is maintained at a value between 7.35 and 7.45 results in abnormal conditions known as alkalosis and acidosis. A change in pH indicates a disruption in the normal bicarbonate–carbonic acid ratio of 20:1 according to the Henderson–Hasselbalch equation. When the bicarbonate concentration of the blood rises or the carbonic acid concentration falls, the bicarbonate–carbonic acid ratio increases, and the pH becomes greater than 7.45, reflecting a decrease in the hydrogen ion concentration. This state is called alkalosis. When the bicarbonate concentration of the blood falls or carbonic acid concentration increases, the bicarbonate–carbonic acid ratio decreases, and the pH becomes less than 7.35, reflecting an increase in the hydrogen ion concentration. This is called acidosis. Cellular metabolism cannot proceed at excessively high or low pH levels. A pH less than 6.8 or greater than 7.8 is incompatible with survival, so that there is a very narrow range in which alterations in pH can be tolerated (Groer & Shekleton, 1989).

The diagnosis of an acid–base imbalance is based on several sources of information. Most important in the diagnostic process is the patient's medical history, including the course of the present illness. The clinician must elicit accurate details regarding symptomatology, as well as concomitant medical problems. Only then can laboratory determinations be used to classify acid–base imbalances.

Arterial blood-gas analysis is the primary diagnostic tool used to assess alterations in acid–base equilibrium. Common determinations on an arterial blood sample include the partial pressures of oxygen (pO_2) and carbon dioxide (pCO_2) as well as pH, bicarbonate concentration (HCO_3^-), and oxygen saturation. While pO_2 values give clues to the status of oxygenation, the remaining three parameters pH, pCO_2, and HCO_3^- directly aid in the diagnosis of acid–base imbalances. Normal values for these parameters are listed in Table 9–17.

A systematic approach to arterial blood-gas analysis is to examine the pH first. The pH value helps to determine the existence of an acid–base imbalance, however, it does not indicate the cause of the disturbance. After analyzing the pH to determine if an acid–base disturbance exists, one must examine the respiratory or carbonic acid component, the pCO_2, and the metabolic or

Table 9–17   Normal Arterial Blood-Gas Values

pH	7.35–7.45
pCO_2	35–45 torr
pO_2	80–100 torr
HCO_3^-	22–26 mEq/liter

noncarbonic acid component, the HCO_3^-, to elicit the cause of the acid–base imbalance. Depending on the cause, clinical conditions in which the hydrogen ion concentration is outside the normal range are classified as either metabolic or respiratory. The serum level of CO_2 is controlled by changes in alveolar ventilation and, thus, pH abnormalities produced by pCO_2 variations are termed "respiratory" or carbonic acid disturbances. Plasma bicarbonate levels are regulated by the renal system and pH changes associated with bicarbonate disturbances are called "metabolic" or noncarbonic acid imbalances. The four primary acid–base disorders include respiratory acidosis, respiratory alkalosis, metabolic acidosis, and metabolic alkalosis. In addition, mixed or combined acid–base disorders may also occur and are discussed later in the chapter.

Alterations in systemic pH are not well tolerated. In the event of a pH change, regulatory systems (buffers, respiratory, renal) react to attempts to return plasma pH to normal, restoring homeostatic balance. The attempt at normal pH restoration is termed *compensation* and occurs in a system not primarily responsible for the acid–base disturbance. Disturbances in the pCO_2 (respiratory parameter) stimulate renal compensation in the form of bicarbonate reclamation and hydrogen ion excretion. Metabolic imbalances primarily affecting the plasma HCO_3^- level produce changes in alveolar ventilation and pCO_2 to accomplish restoration of normal pH. In both instances, compensation tends to return the measured pH value in the arterial sample toward normal. By virtue of the Henderson–Hasselbalch equation, compensation occurs in the same direction as the primary disturbance. Elevations or deficits in the respiratory component obligate elevations or deficits in the renal component of the ratio and thus pH remains normal. The converse is also true.

The base excess is an additional value reported on arterial blood-gas analysis that can help in determining the degree of compensation present in an acid–base disturbance. The normal base excess ranges from $+2$ mEq/liter to -2 mEq/liter and is related to the base (HCO_3^-) content of the sample.

Bicarbonate levels are changed within the plasma primarily by renal mechanisms. However, hemoglobin buffering also alters bicarbonate levels in exchange for chloride in the chloride shift. Renal compensation alters the value of the base excess/deficit either positively or negatively by changing plasma bicarbonate reabsorption. The bicarbonate value can also indicate changes due to hemoglobin buffering. Alterations in the normal base deficit indicate that renal compensation is occurring; the value of HCO_3^- is also altered. If plasma HCO_3^- levels are abnormal, with a normal base excess value, the change in bicarbonate is due to hemoglobin buffering, thus, renal and additional buffering systems are not yet operative. The use of base excess/deficit values, coupled with additional clinical data, can give clues to the time course and source of compensatory mechanisms. The arterial blood-gas values for primary acid–base disturbances with compensatory changes are summarized in Table 9–18.

The etiologic factors, clinical manifestations, and compensatory mechanisms of the primary acid–base disorders are summarized in Table 9–19. Presented in Figure 9–1 is the Davenport diagram from which acid–base disorders can be identified. From this diagram it can be seen that respiratory acid–base disorders (Points II and III) cause shifts in pH that follow the buffer line while metabolic acid–base disorders (Points I and IV) cause shifts in pH that follow the pCO_2 isobar. Similarly, compensation involving respiratory

Table 9–18   Laboratory Characteristics of Primary Acid–Base Disturbances

State	Plasma pH	pCO_2(mm Hg)	HCO_3^- (mEq/liter)	Base Excess
Normal	7.35–7.45	35–45	22–26	+2.5 to −2.5
Acidosis				
Respiratory acidosis (uncompensated)	Low	High	Normal	Normal or negative
Respiratory acidosis (compensated)	Low normal	High	High	Positive value
Metabolic acidosis (uncompensated)	Low	Normal	Low	Negative value
Metabolic acidosis (compensated)	Low normal	Low	Low	Negative value
Alkalosis				
Respiratory alkalosis (uncompensated)	High	Low	Normal	Normal
Respiratory alkalosis (compensated)	High normal	Low	Low	Negative value
Metabolic alkalosis (uncompensated)	High	Normal	High	Positive value
Metabolic alkalosis (compensated)	High normal	High	High	Positive value

From *Moyer's Fluid Balance: A Clinical Manual,* 3rd ed. (p. 61) by J. Vanatta and M. Fogelman, 1982, Chicago: Year Book Medical Publishers. Copyright 1982 by Year Book Medical Publishers. Adapted by permission.

Table 9–19   Primary acid–base disorders

Condition	Other names	Signs and symptoms
Metabolic		

Primary base bicarbonate deficit
Ketones, chlorides, and/or organic acids replace HCO_3^- ions→deficit of base bicarbonate; ratio of 1 part H_2CO_3 to 20 parts HCO_3^- is decreased on HCO_3^- side
	Metabolic acidosis
	Primary alkali deficit
	Uncompensated alkali deficit
	Nonrespiratory acidosis
	Noncarbonic acid excess
		Deep, rapid breathing (Kussmaul)
		Shortness of breath on exertion
		Weakness
		Stupor
		Coma
		Laboratory findings
		  Plasma pH ↓7.35
		  Urine pH ↓6
		  Plasma HCO_3^- ↓ 25 mEq/liter in adults and ↓20 mEq/liter in children
		  Anion gap ≥ 16 mEq/liter

Primary base bicarbonate excess
Ratio of 1 part H_2CO_3 to 20 parts HCO_3^- is increased on HCO_3^- side, resulting in excess of base bicarbonate
	Metabolic alkalosis
	Primary alkali excess
	Uncompensated alkali excess
	Nonrespiratory alkalosis
	Noncarbonic acid deficit
		Depressed breathing (rate and depth)
		None are specific
		Hyperactive reflexes
		Muscle hypertonicity
		Paresthesias and cramping
		Tetany progressing to convulsions
		Mental confusion and obtundation
		Laboratory findings
		  Plasma pH ↑7.45
		  Urine pH ↑7.0
		  Plasma HCO_3^- ↑25 mEq/liter in adults and ↑20 mEq/liter in children
		  Plasma K ↓4 mEq/liter

Respiratory		

Carbonic acid deficit of extracellular fluid
CO_2 expelled due to hyperactive breathing; ratio of 1 part H_2CO_3 to 20 parts HCO_3^- decreased on H_2CO_3 side
	Respiratory alkalosis
	Hyperventilation
	Primary carbonic acid deficit
	Uncompensated carbonic acid deficit
	Hypocapnia
	Nonmetabolic alkalosis
		Vertigo/syncope
		Convulsions
		Paresthesias
		Tetany
		Unconsciousness
		Laboratory findings
		  Plasma pH ↑7.45
		  Urine pH ↑7.0
		  Plasma HCO_3^- ↓25 mEq/liter in adults and ↓20 mEq/liter in children
		  Plasma pCO_2 ↓

Etiologic factors	Compensatory mechanisms

Gain of strong acid by extracellular fluid
  Gain of exogenous acid
  Metabolic and organic acid overproduction and/or retention (underexcretion)
Loss of base from extracellular fluid
  Renal loss
  Intestinal loss
	Respiratory: $\downarrow$pH stimulates pulmonary ventilation; lungs blow off CO_2, and $\downarrow CO_2$ is available to form H_2CO_3; acid side is decreased
	Renal: kidneys retain base bicarbonate through preferential excretion of hydrogen ions→acid urine

Gain of HCO_3^- from extracellular fluid
  Gain of exogenous base
  Oxidation of salts of organic acids
Loss of acid from the extracellular fluid
  Gastrointestinal loss
  Renal loss
  Potassium depletion (may be renal or extrarenal)
  Chloride depletion
	Respiratory: lungs hold back CO_2 to build up H_2CO_3 side; breathing may be shallow and irregular; $\uparrow P{CO_2}$ of blood stimulates respiratory center
	Renal: kidneys excrete HCO_3^- ions and retain H^+ ions and nonbicarbonate anions to aid in restoring ratio and pH to normal range→alkaline urine (exception: Cl^- depletion; see text)

Anxiety, extreme emotion, hysteria, pain Intentional overbreathing Rapid breathing (hyperpnea) Mechanical overventilation CNS trauma/disease Thiamine deficiency Oxygen lack/deprivation High fever and other hypermetabolic states Encephalitis* Salicylate poisoning*	Renal: kidneys excrete HCO_3^- ions and retain H^+ ions and nonbicarbonate anions; by dropping bicarbonate level proper ratio is nearly restored→alkaline urine.

*Respiratory center directly affected.

Table 9–19   *(Continued)*

Condition	Other names	Signs and symptoms

Carbonic acid excess of extracellular fluid
Retention of CO_2 by the lungs causes an excess of carbonic acid; ratio of 1 part H_2CO_3 to 20 parts HCO_3^- increased on H_2CO_3 side
	Respiratory acidosis
	Primary CO_2 excess
	Uncompensated CO_2 excess
	Nonmetabolic acidosis
	Hypoventilation
	Hypercapnia
		Respiratory embarrassment/distress
		Headache
		Weakness
		Restlessness
		Lethargy/somnolence
		Disorientation
		Coma
		Laboratory findings
		  Plasma pH ↓7.35
		  Urine pH ↓6.0
		  Plasma HCO_3^- ↑29 mEq/liter in adults and ↑25 mEq/liter in children
		  Plasma pCO_2 ↑

mechanisms follows parallel buffer lines while renal mechanisms follow the pCO_2 isobars (Groer & Shekleton, 1989).

Respiratory Acid–Base Disorders

Primary respiratory acid–base disorders are those that occur in response to alterations in alveolar ventilation. Conditions that decrease ventilation cause an increase in the partial pressure of CO_2, which produces an acidosis due to carbonic acid excess. Conditions that increase ventilation lower the pCO_2, which produces an alkalosis caused by a primary carbonic acid deficit.

Respiratory Acidosis/Carbonic Acid Excess

Assessment.   Respiratory acidosis due to hypoventilation and CO_2 retention can produce symptoms in many physiologic systems. Patients with respiratory acidosis will exhibit signs of tissue hypoxia (restlessness, confusion, lethargy, somnolence, irritability, and CNS depression progressing to coma) and respiratory difficulty or distress depending on the precipitating cause. Tachycardia and arrhythmias may be present. The patient may be diaphoretic and restless, with cyanosis as a late sign.

Intervention.   The goals of therapeutic intervention for carbonic acid excess are aimed at alleviating the cause of the disorder and improving ventilation. Although mechanical ventilation may be necessary to sustain life, measures such as postural drainage, antibiotics, bronchodilators, and breathing exercises may also help to improve ventilatory function. Acidosis may be improved by the administration of exogenous buffer solutions. These include

Etiologic factors	Compensatory mechanisms
Any condition that causes hypoventilation and retention of carbon dioxide; Chronic pulmonary disease Neuromuscular disease CNS depression with respiratory center involvement Acute respiratory disease or failure Acute airway obstruction Obesity hypoventilation syndrome Pulmonary edema (cardiogenic and noncardiogenic) Trauma	Renal: kidneys conserve base bicarbonate while excreting hydrogen ions and nonbicarbonate anions→acid urine

From *Basic Pathophysiology: A Holistic Approach,* 3rd ed., by M. E. Groer and M. E. Shekleton, 1989, St. Louis: The C. V. Mosby Co. Reproduced with permission.

sodium bicarbonate, lactated Ringer's solution and Trishydroxy-aminomethane (THAM) solution. Bicarbonate therapy must be tailored specifically to the individual patient as overdosage can cause alkalemia.

In some instances, patients with chronic pulmonary disease experience ongoing carbonic acid excess and live in a constant state of compensated respiratory acidosis. Therapy is aimed at maximizing ventilatory function at a steady-state level and avoiding further insults to the pulmonary system. When these patients undergo surgery, careful attention must be paid to their respiratory status. The chronic condition makes the pulmonary patient a likely candidate for postoperative admission to the critical care unit for careful monitoring and, should complications arise, intensive treatment (see Chapter 7).

Nursing interventions for a patient experiencing carbonic acid excess include

1. Monitoring vital signs and respiratory rate, depth, and rhythm, noting synchrony of abdominal and chest-wall movement
2. Assisting in breathing treatments/postural drainage
3. Monitoring serum electrolyte values, especially potassium
4. Ensuring adequate hydration for secretion mobilization
5. Administering oxygen if necessary
6. Observing for signs of respiratory distress and instituting emergency measures as indicated
7. Maintaining mechanical ventilation at an appropriate level
8. Monitoring artcrial blood-gas values

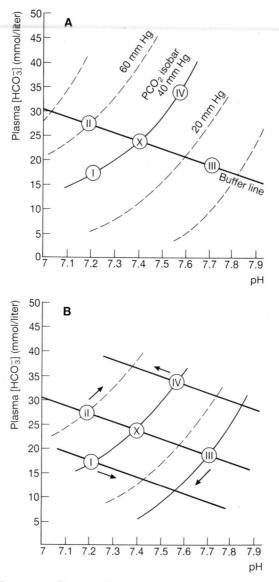

Figure 9–1. Davenport diagram: classical working diagram for studying acid–base imbalance. (A) Specific primary acid–base disorders are numbered as follows: I, metabolic acidosis; II, respiratory acidosis; III, respiratory alkalosis; IV, metabolic alkalosis. X refers to the normal state. The arrows in graph B indicate compensation for acidosis and alkalosis. Note that arrows point in direction of the normal pH. From *Basic Pathophysiology: A Holistic Approach,* 3rd ed., by M. E. Groer and M. E. Shekleton, 1989, St. Louis: The C. V. Mosby Co. Copyright 1989 by C. V. Mosby. Reprinted by permission.

Respiratory Alkalosis—Carbonic Acid Deficit

Assessment. Carbonic acid deficit is generally recognized by a rapid respiratory rate. Hyperventilation may cause paresthesias, headaches, vertigo, and eventually syncope in extreme conditions. Neuromuscular irritability may be present as evidenced by hyperreflexia with a potential for seizures. Respiratory alkalosis may also occur as a compensatory response to metabolic acidosis.

Intervention. Management of a carbonic acid deficit is aimed at eliminating the underlying cause of the disorder and normalizing ventilation. Hysterical reactions may require psychotherapy and CO_2 rebreathing with a paper bag. Mechanical ventilation should be adjusted to achieve arterial blood-gas values as close to normal as possible.

The nursing care of a patient with carbonic acid deficit may include some of the following:

1. Monitoring vital signs and respiratory rate, depth and rhythm, noting synchrony of abdominal and chest-wall movement
2. Administering sedatives and offering reassurance
3. Monitoring urine output and pH
4. Monitoring serum electrolyte values
5. Maintaining mechanical ventilation at an appropriate level
6. Monitoring arterial blood-gas values

Metabolic Acid–Base Disorders

Metabolic acid–base disorders arise from alterations in noncarbonic or "fixed" acid production or from disturbances in the plasma bicarbonate level. Most commonly, these disturbances are precipitated by medical illnesses that do not affect the respiratory system. An increase in the hydrogen ion concentration or a decrease in the base bicarbonate concentration produces a metabolic or noncarbonic acidosis. Conversely, bicarbonate excess or a decrease in the hydrogen ion concentration produces metabolic or noncarbonic alkalosis.

Metabolic Acidosis—Noncarbonic Acid Excess

Metabolic acidosis may develop as a result of excess acid being present or a loss of alkali from the body. An excessive amount of acid may result when exogenous acid is administered, when there is increased metabolic acid production (as in diabetic ketoacidosis), or when the kidneys are unable to excrete a normal endogenous acid load. When excess acid is present, a base bicarbonate deficit develops as bicarbonate reserves are depleted because of the buffering process. When 50% of the total buffer base is used, the acid will no longer be adequately buffered and the pH will drop.

A loss of alkali, or base, from the body may occur because the kidneys are unable to reabsorb HCO_3 or because alkali-rich body fluid is lost because of diarrhea or draining pancreatic or duodenal fistulas. Rapid dilution of the extracellular fluid with a base-free solution will also cause a primary base deficit (Groer & Shekleton, 1989).

Assessment.   Clinical manifestations of metabolic acidosis are variable and nonspecific and will coexist with those of the underlying condition (see Table 9–19). The patient experiencing noncarbonic acid excess may be disoriented and stuporous. CNS acidosis may produce twitching and convulsions leading to coma. Nausea and vomiting may occur. Respiratory compensation may result in a ventilatory pattern of increased rate and depth and, in fact, respiratory alkalosis may develop as a result.

The anion gap can be a useful diagnostic clue to the cause of metabolic acidosis. An elevated anion gap (AG greater than 16 mEq/liter) usually occurs when the concentration of non-chloride-containing acids increases. Conditions in which this occurs include methanol intoxication, salicylate poisoning, lactic acidosis, ketoacidosis, and ethylene glycol poisoning. The presence of unmeasured anions tends to displace the HCO_3^- in the serum, increasing the anion gap. The anion gap will be normal if acidotic states occur because of the addition of chloride-containing acids or defective renal bicarbonate reabsorption. Clinical significance of the anion gap is highly correlated to the patient's history. However, an elevated anion gap can alert the clinician to the presence of lactic acidosis if other sources of anion elevation have been ruled out.

Intervention.   The treatment of a noncarbonic acid excess is aimed at alleviation of the underlying cause of the disturbance. Supportive therapy tends toward increasing the bicarbonate concentration in the plasma to assist buffering and pH restoration. IV infusion of lactated Ringer's solution may be used conservatively. If the condition is severe, IV sodium bicarbonate may be used to augment plasma base stores partially. Insulin administration in diabetes mellitus promotes glucose utilization and a decrease in ketoacid production. Occasionally, dialysis may be necessary to remove severe excesses of fixed acids, especially if their concentration exceeds renal excretion capacity due to renal damage or failure.

The nursing care of the patient with metabolic acidosis may include the following interventions:

1. Monitoring intake and output with urine pH
2. Monitoring vital signs
3. Monitoring serum electrolyte values
4. Monitoring for neuromuscular changes and possibly instituting seizure precautions
5. Monitoring arterial blood-gas values

6. Monitoring respiratory rate, depth, and rhythm
7. Keeping emergency drugs and equipment available
8. Administering medications/fluid as ordered with observation for possible rebound alkalosis or hyperosmolal imbalances after the administration of sodium bicarbonate

Metabolic Alkalosis—Noncarbonic Acid Deficit

Metabolic alkalosis may develop as a result of either loss of acid from or the addition of excess bicarbonate to the body. The latter is usually the result of excessive exogenous alkali ingestion or administration (for example, milk-alkali syndrome). Excessive acid loss may occur as a result of vomiting or gastric suction. The sustained increase in the plasma HCO_3 level that occurs in response to this acid loss is stimulated by the loss of Cl^-. In fact, chloride depletion is the most common cause of metabolic alkalosis. Na^+ reabsorption is stimulated. The plasma HCO_3 is increased as Na^+, and HCO_3 (since Cl^- is not available) are reabsorbed by the kidney, and H^+ and K^+ are excreted because of their linkage with Na^+ reabsorption. This mechanism allows electrochemical balance to be achieved and the urine in this case will be acid. Chloride depletion may also be the result of chloride-rich diarrhea. Diuretic therapy involves the same basic mechanism. Since K^+ is also being lost, a hypochloremic–hypokalemic metabolic alkalosis can develop. Potassium depletion alone can cause metabolic alkalosis as well. Excess mineralocorticoid syndromes are characterized by metabolic alkalosis (Groer & Shekleton, 1989).

Assessment.   The symptoms of metabolic alkalosis or noncarbonic acid deficit are nonspecific since they will be related to both the underlying disorder, as well as to any electrolyte alterations that may be present. Neurological changes such as irritability and belligerence may be noted. Ionized calcium levels decrease with alkalosis, which may precipitate twitching, tetany, and convulsions. The respiratory pattern may be shallow, with periods of apnea as ventilatory compensation attempts to retain CO_2 for pH normalization (see Table 9–19).

Intervention.   As with all acid–base disturbances, therapy is directed toward eliminating the underlying pathology and attempting to restore pH to near normal. In general, prevention of excess bicarbonate ingestion can be accomplished through patient education. Electrolyte losses can be replaced orally or intravenously. IV infusions of chloride solutions such as Ringer's solution can replenish chloride deficits or KCl can be administered when K^+ loss has also occurred. The drug, Diamox (which is the carbonic anhydrase inhibitor, acetazolamide), is also useful in promoting renal bicarbonate excretion. In severe cases, administration of an acid such as ammonium chloride may be indicated. Ammonium chloride must be infused slowly with careful attention to arterial blood-gas parameters so as to prevent rebound acidosis.

Nursing care of the patient with noncarbonic acid deficit may include the following responsibilities:

1. Monitoring intake and output including GI losses and urine pH
2. Monitoring neurological and cardiovascular status
3. Monitoring vital signs
4. Monitoring respiratory, rate, depth, and rhythm
5. Monitoring arterial blood-gas values
6. Administering medications as ordered, with observation for side effects and rebound acidosis

Combined Acid–Base Disorders

In addition to the four primary acid–base disorders, critically ill patients may exhibit combined acid–base disorders. These complex imbalances often present a substantial challenge to the clinical practitioner. A mixed acid–base disorder is characterized by the concurrent existence of two or more of the primary acid–base disorders. The range of mixed disorders includes mixed metabolic and respiratory disorders, mixed metabolic disorders and triple disorders as presented below:

    I.   MIXED METABOLIC & RESPIRATORY
            Metabolic Acidosis & Respiratory Acidosis
            Metabolic Acidosis & Respiratory Alkalosis
            Metabolic Alkalosis & Respiratory Acidosis
            Metabolic Alkalosis & Respiratory Alkalosis
    II. MIXED METABOLIC
            Metabolic Acidosis & Metabolic Alkalosis
    III. TRIPLE DISORDERS
            Mixed Metabolic & Respiratory Acidosis
            Mixed Metabolic & Respiratory Alkalosis

In the first category, the combination of two similar states (metabolic acidosis and respiratory acidosis or metabolic alkalosis and respiratory alkalosis) represents failure of compensation, while the combination of opposite states (metabolic acidosis and respiratory alkalosis or metabolic alkalosis and respiratory acidosis) represents excessive compensation (Schrier, 1986).

A mixed acid–base disorder should be suspected if the pH is opposite that expected or there appears to be a lack of the anticipated response (Table 9–20). Diagnosis depends on a complete history and accurate laboratory data.

Treatment of one acid–base alteration in isolation has the potential for exacerbating the coexisting disorder in some instances. These combined acid–base alterations most often occur in critically ill patients, making diagnosis and restoration of normal acid–base balance extremely difficult. In this

Table 9–20   Mixed Acid–Base Disorders

Disorder	Compensation	pH
Type 1: Failure of compensation		
Metabolic acidosis and respiratory acidosis	PaCO$_2$ too high and [HCO$_3^-$] too low for simple disorders	↓ ↓
Metabolic alkalosis and respiraratory alkalosis	PaCO$_2$ too low and [HCO$_3^-$] too high for simple disorders	↑ ↑
Type 2: Excessive compensation		
Metabolic acidosis and respiratory alkalosis	PaCO$_2$ too low and [HCO$_3^-$] too low for simple disorders	Normal or slightly ↓ or ↑
Metabolic alkalosis and respiratory acidosis	PaCO$_2$ too high and [HCO$_3^-$] too high for simple disorders	Normal or slightly ↑ or ↓
Type 3: Triple disorders		
Metabolic alkalosis, respiratory acidosis or alkalosis, and metabolic acidosis	PaCO$_2$ and [HCO$_3^-$] not appropriate for simple disorders and anion gap >20 mEq/liter	Variable

From *Renal and Electrolyte Disorders* (p. 198), edited by R. Schrier, 1986, Boston: Little, Brown. Copyright 1986 by Little, Brown. Reprinted by permission.

population, these acid–base alterations will most probably be accompanied by some of the alterations in fluid volume, composition, and distribution that were discussed in preceding sections of this chapter. A representative sample of clinical situations in which a mixed alteration in acid–base balance can occur is presented in Table 9–21.

Metabolic Acidosis and Respiratory Acidosis

The combination of increased pCO$_2$ and an excess of fixed, noncarbonic acid are both contributing factors to a decreased pH in this combined disorder. Increased pCO$_2$ levels tend to increase renal bicarbonate reabsorption. However, excess fixed acid loads use up the additional bicarbonate, limiting the usual rise in plasma HCO$_3^-$. Combined acidosis can occur in patients who experience cardiopulmonary arrest. Elevated pCO$_2$ levels are common in conjunction with lactic acid production due to anaerobic glycolysis. pH values graphed against bicarbonate concentrations usually fall within Region 1 in Figure 9–2.

Table 9–21 Clinical situations in which mixed alterations in acid–base balance are likely to occur

Clinical Situation	Acid–base disturbance
Sepsis	Acute respiratory alkalosis
	Lactic acidosis
Salicylate overdose	Acute respiratory alkalosis
	Anion gap metabolic acidosis
Renal tubular acidosis or diarrhea with severe hypokalemia	Hyperchloremic metabolic acidosis
	Respiratory acidosis
Drug overdose (carbon monoxide, cyanide, ethylene glycol, methanol)	Metabolic acidosis
	Respiratory acidosis
Cardiopulmonary arrest/cardiogenic shock	Lactic acidosis
	Respiratory acidosis
Liver or cardiac failure plus diuretic therapy	Respiratory alkalosis
	Metabolic alkalosis
Mechanical overventilation plus nasogastric suction	Metabolic alkalosis
	Respiratory alkalosis
Chronic pulmonary disease plus diuretic therapy	Respiratory acidosis or alkalosis
	Metabolic alkalosis
Chronic renal failure plus vomiting	Metabolic acidosis
	Metabolic alkalosis
Surgical or ICU patients	Respiratory alkalosis or acidosis
	Metabolic alkalosis
	Metablolic acidosis

Adapted from "Disorders of Fluid and Electrolyte Balance" in *Diagnosis and Clinical Management* by J. Puschett, 1985, New York: Churchill Livingstone. Reproduced with permission.

Metabolic Alkalosis and Respiratory Alkalosis

The combination of hypocapnia and noncarbonic acid deficit contribute to the pH elevation associated with this mixed imbalance. Low pCO_2 values tend to promote renal bicarbonate excretion. However, plasma $[HCO_3^-]$ levels do not decrease but instead remain normal or slightly elevated because of metabolic derangements. Combined alkalosis can occur in mechanically overventilated patients losing hydrogen ions through gastric suction. pH values graphed against bicarbonate concentrations usually fall within Region 2 on Figure 9–2.

Metabolic Alkalosis and Respiratory Acidosis

Although the pH changes and compensatory mechanisms for these disorders appear to be offsetting, this combination occurs quite frequently in the clinical setting. Patients with chronically elevated pCO_2 values due to pulmonary conditions such as emphysema or neuromuscular disorders normally exist in a state of mild (compensated) respiratory acidosis. The onset of nausea and vomiting in the patient due to some other illness often precipitates a superimposed metabolic alkalosis. Blood-gas interpretation is often difficult because

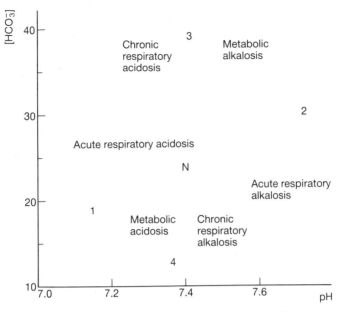

Figure 9–2.   Position of combined acid–base disorders on modified Davenport diagram. N = normal; 1 = metabolic acidosis and respiratory acidosis; 2 = metabolic alkalosis and respiratory alkalosis; 3 = metabolic alkalosis and respiratory acidosis; 4 = metabolic acidosis and respiratory alkalosis.

elevated bicarbonate levels are associated with compensated carbonic acid excess. Graphic representation is extremely helpful, with values for pH and HCO_3^- usually located in Region 3 of Figure 9–2.

Metabolic Acidosis and Respiratory Alkalosis

These disorders, while appearing to oppose each other in terms of pH disturbance, do occur in combination under several circumstances. An example of metabolic acidosis with respiratory alkalosis occurs as a result of salicylate poisoning. Respiratory stimulation occurs, lowering pCO_2, while salicylate metabolism increases the fixed acid content producing metabolic acidosis. Mechanically overventilated patients can also experience superimposed metabolic acidosis when lactic acid production increases as a result of widespread sepsis or tissue anoxia. pCO_2 values are generally low, coupled with decreased bicarbonate levels due to excess fixed acid buffering pH values graphed against bicarbonate concentration, and usually fall within Region 4 on Figure 9–2.

The diagnosis and treatment of mixed acid–base disturbances can prove exceedingly difficult. The critical care practitioner should rely heavily on information from the history of the illness and then correlate findings with arterial blood gases. Most often, treatment of mixed disorders proceeds in a slow and deliberate fashion, while monitoring clinical signs and serial blood-gas values. Substantial knowledge is required of practitioners instituting therapy for mixed disorders. Inadequate or infrequent assessment can lead to the correction of one disorder, while increasing the magnitude of the other. A rapid, dramatic change in pH following the correction of one component of a mixed disorder is generally not well tolerated by patients who are critically ill.

SUMMARY

Alterations in fluid volume, composition, distribution, or acid–base balance can make restoration of homeostasis in the critically ill surgical patient very difficult. These disorders can arise as a result of the primary, underlying disease process or as a result of surgical or medical treatment. The critical care nurse must monitor the patient closely in order to identify changes in the fluid, electrolyte, and acid–base status so that treatment can begin before these alterations become compounded or irreversible. Patience and prudence, coupled with constant vigilance, are the guiding principles to prevent unnecessary morbidity or mortality.

BIBLIOGRAPHY

Cosgrove, J. A. (1989). Atrial natriuretic peptide: A new cardiac hormone. *Heart and Lung, 18* (5), 461–465.
Groer, M. E., & Shekleton, M. E. (1989). *Basic pathophysiology: A holistic approach* (3rd ed.). St. Louis: C. V. Mosby.
Lunger, D. G. (1988). Potassium supplementation: How and why? *Focus on Critical Care, 15* (5), 56–60.
Vanatta, J., & Fogelman, M. (1982). *Moyer's fluid balance: A clinical manual.* Chicago: Year Book Medical Publishers.

ADDITIONAL READINGS

Arieff, A., & DeFronzo, R. (1985). *Fluid, electrolyte and acid–base disorders.* New York: Churchill-Livingstone.
Baltarowich, L. (1986). Chloride. *Emergency Medical Clinics of North America, 4*(1), 175–183.
Burgess, A. (1979). *Nurse's guide to fluid and electrolyte balance.* New York: McGraw-Hill.
Burke, S. (1980). *The composition and function of body fluids.* St. Louis: C. V. Mosby.
Cohen, J., & Kassiret, J. (1982). *Acid–base.* Boston: Little, Brown.
Davenport, H. (1974). *The ABC of acid–base chemistry.* Chicago: University of Chicago Press.

Doenges, M., Jeffries, M., & Moorehouse, M. (1984). *Nursing care plans: Nursing diagnosis in patient care.* Philadelphia: F. A. Davis.

Eastham, R. (1983). *A guide to water, electrolyte and acid–base metabolism.* Boston: Wright/PSG.

Goldberg, M. (1973). Computer-based instruction and diagnosis of acid-base disorders. *Journal of the American Medical Association, 223,* 269.

Goldberger, E. (1986). *A primer of water, electrolyte and acid–base syndromes.* Philadelphia: Lea & Febiger.

Groer, M. (1981). *Physiology and pathophysiology of the body fluids.* St. Louis: C. V. Mosby.

Jacobson, H., & Seldin, D. (1983). On the generation, maintenance, and correction of metabolic alkalosis. *American Journal of Physiology, 235*(4), 425–432.

Kaehny, W. (1983). Respiratory acid-base disorders. *Medical Clinics of North America, 67*(4), 915–928.

Keyes, J. (1985). *Fluid, electrolyte and acid–base regulation.* Monterey, CA: Wadsworth.

Laragh, J. (1985). Atrial natriuretic hormone, the renin–aldosterone axis, and blood pressure-electrolyte homeostasis. *New England Journal of Medicine, 313*(21), 1330–1340.

Littrell, K. (1983). Arterial blood gas analysis: The matching game. *Focus on Critical Care, 10,* 49–51.

Luckmann, J., & Sorenson, K. (1987). *Medical-surgical nursing: A psychophysiological approach* (3rd ed.) Philadelphia: W. B. Saunders.

Luke, R., & Galla, J. (1983). Chloride-depletion alkalosis with a normal extracellular fluid volume. *American Journal of Physiology, 245*(4), 419–424.

Maxwell, M. H., Kleeman, C. R., & Narins, R. G. (1987). *Clinical disorders of fluid and electrolyte metabolism.* (4th ed.) New York: McGraw-Hill.

McFadden, E., Zaloga, G., & Chernow, B. (1983). Hypocalcemia: A medical emergency. *American Journal of Nursing, 83,* 227–230.

Metheny, N., & Snively, W. (1983). *Nurse's handbook of fluid balance.* Philadelphia: J. B. Lippincott.

Nielsen, O., & Engell, H. (1986). The importance of plasma colloid osmotic pressure for interstitial fluid volume and fluid balance after elective abdominal vascular surgery. *Annals of Surgery, 203*(1), 25–29.

Puschett, J., & Greenberg, A. (1985). *Disorders of fluid and electrolyte balance: Diagnosis and management.* New York: Churchill-Livingstone.

Reid, I. (1985). The renin–angiotensin system and body function. *Archives of Internal Medicine, 145*(8), 1475–1479.

Rice, V. (1982). The role of potassium in health and disease. *Critical Care Nursing, 2,* 54–73.

Schrier, R. (Ed.) (1986). *Renal and electrolyte disorders.* Boston: Little, Brown.

Severinghaus, J., & Astrup, P. (1985). History of blood gas analysis. *Journal of Clinical Monitoring, 1*(4), 259–277.

Shapiro, B., Harrison, R., & Walton, J. (1982). *Clinical application of blood gases.* Chicago: Year Book Medical Publishers.

Siggard-Andersen, O. (1974). *The acid–base status of the blood.* Baltimore: Williams & Wilkins.

Ventrigeia, W. (1986). Arterial blood gases. *Emergency Medical Clinics of North America, 4*(2), 235–251.

10 Alterations in Rest and Sleep Patterns

Edward Goodemote, M.S., D.N.Sc., R.N.

Although the natural phenomenon of sleep consumes about one third of our lives, compared with other areas of science it has only recently received attention from the scientific community. A major breakthrough in the study of sleep occurred when Aserinsky and Kleitman (1953) discovered rapid-eye-movement sleep (REM) using an electrooculogram in the clinical laboratory. During the past 25 years, this major finding has opened new doors as researchers today study sleep not simply as a science, but as a clinical entity with aims focused on improved approaches for diagnosis and treatment of sleep disorders.

This chapter will bring together many of the most recent sleep research clinical findings and discuss how these findings can be used by nurses to improve the sleep of their critical care patients. Nurses in the ICU are in the unique position of being able to control many of the environmental factors that affect the sleep of their patients. Through better understanding of the signs and symptoms of sleep pattern disturbances, critical care nurses can recognize these problems and minimize their impact through early intervention.

BASIC SLEEP CYCLE

To understand the problem of sleep alterations/deprivation in the critical care setting, it is necessary first to review basic human sleep patterns and the neurological basis of sleep. There are two types of sleep: non-rapid-eye-movement sleep (NREM) and rapid-eye-movement sleep (REM). Within NREM sleep, there are four defined stages differentiated by specific alterations in the frequency and amplitude of polysomnography tracings recorded in the clinical laboratory setting. These stages are numbered 1, 2, 3, and 4, and are more specifically defined in Table 10–1. Since it is not necessary in most clinical applications to distinguish between Stages 3 and 4, sleep experts usually refer to these stages together as delta sleep. This name comes from the presence of prominent delta waves that appear on the human sleep electroencephalogram (EEG) recording during these stages.

Stage 1 sleep is referred to as a transitional period between wakefulness and the sleep state. During this period, which lasts up to about 7 minutes in young adults, mental processes change and thoughts begin to drift. Individuals are easily awakened and may subjectively report that they are still awake.

Stage 2 sleep is the first clearly defined stage of sleep. The duration of this stage in the first nighttime cycle is approximately 20 to 30 minutes in young adults. Stage 2 sleep is distinguished on EEG recordings by intermittent high-amplitude waves (K complexes) and sleep spindles (bursts of rapid electrical activity lasting 0.5 to 2.0 seconds).

Stages 3 and 4 (delta) follow Stage 2 and are identified on the electroencephalogram by slow, high-amplitude delta waves. It is difficult to awaken an individual from this stage of sleep, since it is the deepest sleep of the night. This stage is usually first entered 30 to 45 minutes after the initial onset of sleep. Although dream activity does occur in NREM sleep, it is generally recognized that these dreams are more thought-like and less animated than those occurring during REM sleep.

REM sleep periods in adults alternate with NREM sleep at about 70- to 90-minute intervals throughout the night. The first REM episode lasts approximately 5 minutes. Successive periods increase in duration ranging from 10 to 30 minutes.

Table 10–1   Basic Electroencepholographic (EEG) Characteristics of Sleep Stages

Stage	Characteristics
Wakefulness	Electroencephalogram exhibits alpha activity, and/or low voltage, mixed-frequency activity
Stage 1	Relatively low voltage, mixed-frequency EEG without rapid eye movements at 3 to 7 cycles per second (cps) — theta waves.
Stage 2	Sleep spindles (12–14 cps) and K complexes (well-delineated, slow, negative EEG deflections followed by a positive component) on relatively low voltage mixed-frequency EEG activity
Delta {Stage 3	Moderate amounts of high-amplitude, slow-wave activity (20–50% of 2 cps waves)
Stage 4	Large amounts of high-amplitude, slow-wave activity (over 50% are 2 cps or slower)
REM	A relatively low voltage, mixed-frequency EEG in conjunction with episodic rapid eye movements and low-amplitude electromyogram

Researchers further divide REM into two distinct types. The first, referred to as tonic REM, is characterized by near paralysis of the large postural and skeletal muscles. Phasic REM, in contrast, is characterized by increased cerebral metabolic activity, rapid eye movements, changes in respiratory and heart rates, and rapid changes in blood pressure. Systolic blood pressure readings may increase in bursts by as much as 40 mm Hg. These sympathetic central nervous system changes seem to occur in bursts closely associated with the rapid eye movements that define REM sleep.

Most dreaming occurs during the four to five REM periods of nighttime sleep. Since REM periods are typically of longer duration as the night progresses, it is not surprising that most dreaming is done during the second half of the night and that an individual awakens after the last dream period in the morning. Although the significance of dreams and the nature of their existence is not fully understood, it is theorized that these REM dreams may provide an opportunity for us to process many of the unresolved issues from our waking day.

SLEEP CYCLE AND AGE RELATIONSHIPS

Age is an important factor to consider when examining the sleep patterns of critical care patients. From birth through old age, a considerable amount of variability in both sleep amount and architecture occurs during the human life span.

The sleep cycle in the young adult (Figure 10–1A) begins as a relaxed wakefulness that progresses into Stage 1 sleep. After approximately 2 to 7 minutes, wave forms that identify Stage 2 patterns (sleep spindles and K complexes) begin to emerge. This stage lasts approximately 30 minutes, until the young adult enters a period of delta sleep.

After about 45 minutes of delta sleep, the young adult does not usually move directly into REM sleep. Instead, there is a brief retracing of steps back through Stage 2, and then to a first short REM period. As this first nighttime cycle is completed, another 70- to 90-minute cycle gradually begins.

Approximately five of these cycles occur in a normal night of sleep for a young adult. However, during the second half of the night, delta sleep almost completely disappears from the cycle, leaving individuals to move between Stages 1, 2, and REM. Often a spontaneous morning awakening occurs immediately after REM sleep. This explains why some individuals recall awakening at the end of a dream.

In contrast, infants sleep about 18 hours each day, with about 50% of their sleep time classified as REM. By about age 4, REM sleep accounts for only about 25% of the 10 to 12 hours per day that preschoolers sleep.

The sleep of preadolescents slowly decreases from 10 hours to about 7 to 8 hours, with 20% REM by the time adolescence is reached. From this age, sleep amount and architecture remain relatively stable until about age 40.

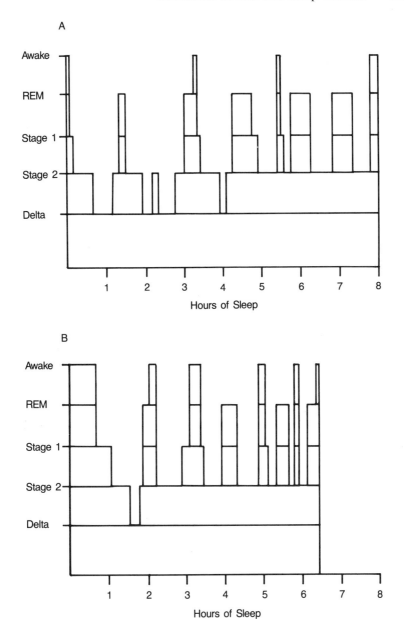

Figure 10–1. (A) Example of sleep cycle of the young adult. (B) Example of sleep cycle of the aged adult.

After age 40, a number of important changes occur in the sleep architecture and sleep amount of older adults (Figure 10–1B.) First, the amount of total sleep time gradually decreases to approximately 6.5 hours by age 60. Also, older adults often report more disruptions of sleep with frequent nighttime awakenings. This results in a lower sleep efficiency index (ratio of total sleep time to nocturnal time in bed). Researchers studying sleep in the elderly also report a reduction in the amount of time spent in Stage 4 sleep and an increase in the amount of transition or Stage 1 sleep. (Miles & Dement, 1980). In general, the amount of REM sleep decreases slightly and in parallel with the decrease in total sleep time (approximately 18% REM).

NEUROANATOMICAL BASIS OF SLEEP

A number of neurotransmitters may be responsible for initiating and maintaining both REM and NREM sleep. Serotonin (5- hydroxytriptamine), from the midbrain raphe and cortex has been implicated in the onset and maintenance of NREM sleep (McCarley & Hobson, 1975). Acetylcholine, in the gigantocellular tegmental field (FTG) seems to be closely associated with the onset of REM sleep, while norepinephrine, in the locus coeruleus, has been associated with the maintenance of wakefulness. In addition, other neurotransmitters, including dopamine, gamma-aminobutyric acid (GABA) and sleep-inducing peptides have been found to have a possible role in the neuroanatomical basis of sleep.

By manipulating areas of animal brain both pharmacologically and anatomically, researchers have begun to develop testable models to explain neuroanatomically how we move through the basic stages of sleep. In the McCarley and Hobson model (1975), the giant-cell field of the pontine tegmentum (FTG) (Figure 10–2) and the locus coeruleus areas of the brain are thought to interact, creating the REM–NREM cycle. The model proposes that the FTG activates the locus coeruleus with acetylcholine to stop the production of REM sleep. The locus coeruleus activation seems to be self-inhibitory, gradually allowing NREM sleep to appear. This process continues to repeat, therefore creating the REM–NREM cycle of sleep.

Mooncroft and Clothier (1986) proposed that wakefulness is maintained by the ascending reticular activating system via secretion of acetylcholine in combination with messages sent from the posterior hypothalamus to the cortex of the brain. At night, the basal forebrain causes synchronization of the brain waves, while the raphe system inhibits the ascending reticular activating system using serotonin. In this model, the NREM onset of sleep occurs as the FTG is inhibited by both the raphe system and the locus coerulus. As the input from these two areas decreases because of self-inhibition, the FTG becomes more active and begins producing REM sleep. Simultaneously, other cells of the FTG activate other brain areas with acetylcholine and produce eye movements in bursts, muscle twitches, and other characteristic

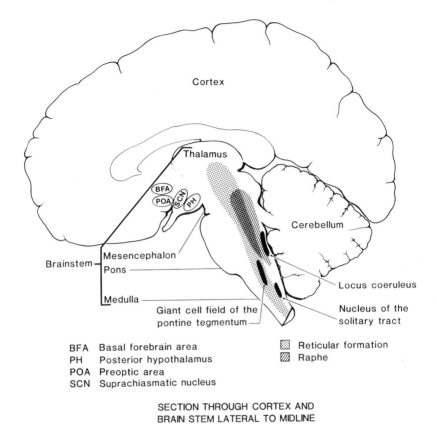

Figure 10–2. Section through cortex and brain stem lateral to midline. BFA = basal forebrain area; POA = preoptic area; SCN = suprachiasmatic nucleus; PH = posterior hypothalamus.

movements of REM sleep. In addition, this model postulates that FTG also activates the locus coeruleus, which slowly gains strength and then itself inhibits the FTG, causing the end of the REM period.

PHYSIOLOGIC CHANGES OF THE SLEEP STATE

Respiratory

It is universally accepted that respiratory changes occur during the sleep periods of normal healthy human beings. Of these changes, the most uniformly observed is the decrease in minute ventilation from the waking state that occurs in both REM and NREM sleep (Hudgel, Martin, Johnson, & Hill, 1984; Douglas, White, Pickett, Weil, & Zwillich, 1982; White, Weil and Zwillich, 1985). This decrease seems to be attributed to the lower tidal volume that has been reported to occur in Stages 2, 3/4 (delta), and REM (Douglas et al., 1982; White et al., 1985). With this decrease in minute volume, it seems then that hypoventilation is likely to occur during all stages of sleep.

Respiratory rate during NREM sleep seems to be regular and without much variability from the awakening state. During REM sleep however, the rhythmicity is often variable and may be associated with brief hypopneas and/or apneas.

In general, a critical care nurse should not attribute changes in respiratory rate of greater than five breaths per minute to normal respiratory sleep alterations. Certainly respiratory variations may occur during REM sleep, but these must be carefully distinguished from rate changes associated with clinical pathology.

Cardiovascular Changes

Sleep researchers acknowledge that there is an average reduction in the heart rate of individuals during the sleep state as compared with the resting state. However, men tend to have lower heart rates during sleep than women in the same age group (Brodsky, Delon, Denes, Kanakis, & Rosen, 1977; Sobotka, Mayer, Bauernfeind, Kanakis, & Rosen, 1981).

During NREM sleep, the heart rate seems generally to mimic the low steady metabolic rate of the total body, while during phasic REM sleep, periodic abrupt increases and decreases in the heart rate seem to occur. These changes are thought to be the result of alternating bursts of sympathetic and parasympathetic autonomic stimulation. In general, the reduced heart rate during sleep seems to be due to an increase in vagal tone. It has been reported that the incidence of ventricular arrhythmias may be more common in some individuals during sleep than during wakefulness (Guilleminault, Connolly, & Winkle, 1983).

Circadian Rhythms

Circadian rhythms are cyclical biological events that occur in patterns that require about 24 hours to complete. Common examples of physiologic processes associated with circadian cycles include body temperature variation, sleep–wake cycle, urinary excretion of electrolytes, and plasma cortisol and plasma growth hormone levels.

The average human circadian sleep–wake cycle is approximately 25 hours. Although many individuals have cycles as short as 22 hours or as long as 28 hours, most humans have a sleep–wake cycle longer than the sun-imposed 24-hour cycle on which daily activities are based. This means that individuals with 25-hour cycles will have to reset their daily biological clock by 1 hour each day to stay synchronized with the rest of the world.

To reset this clock, humans take advantage of time cues referred to by sleep researchers as *zeitgebers*. Common zeitgebers include alarm clocks, sunlight, work schedules, and meal times. These routines of daily life help to reset the clock to remain synchronized with the rest of the world.

Difficulties with circadian rhythms can occur when an individual's rest–activity schedule is no longer synchronized with his or her intrinsic biological circadian clock. For example, when sleep is attempted during hours customarily spent awake or when staying awake during hours usually spent asleep, the individual becomes desynchronized or phase-shifted within his or her circadian rhythm. Under such conditions, individuals often report poor-quality sleep with frequent arousals. During wakefulness, these same individuals describe feeling anxious, irritable, and restless, with difficulty concentrating and impairment of judgment. Quite often they also report gastric distress.

To stabilize this desynchronization in most adults takes 5 to 7 days and requires the engraining of new time cues (zeitgebers) into a person's sleep–activity schedule. As will be discussed later, the phase delay phenomenon is a common cause of sleep pattern disturbance in the critical patient.

SLEEP DEPRIVATION

A great deal of research has been reported on the behavioral and psychological effects of sleep deprivation on normal subjects. Although many of the reports are contradictory, Hartmann (1974) summarizes the data by stating that "most researchers report that sleep deprived subjects become increasingly angry, irritable, unfocused and antisocial" (p. 45).

When Stage 4 (delta) sleep was selectively disrupted in laboratory subjects, Agnew, Webb, and Williams (1967) noted that the subjects tended to be physically lethargic and depressed. In addition, studies by Moldofsky and Scarisbrick (1976) suggest that patients with delta depression may exhibit symptoms of increased sensitivity to pain and musculoskeletal tenderness.

During the early years of sleep research, reports of REM deprivation studies indicated that the probable effects included irritability, suspiciousness, and possible psychosis. Later works contradicted these results and found few if any harmful behavioral or psychological effects of REM deprivation. (Fishbein & Gutwein, 1977; Vogel, 1975; McGrath & Cohen, 1978) Later work by Vogel, Vogel, McAbee, and Thurmond (1980) suggests that REM deprivation increases motivational behavior and is even effective in treating some types of depression.

When humans are not allowed to progress into REM sleep, the body responds with a pressure to restore this type of sleep. Therefore, if a critical care patient is repeatedly awakened before his or her first REM period occurs, (normally 70 to 90 minutes after sleep onset) the next REM period will usually emerge before the expected cyclical time. A REM sleep period following REM deprivation is often more intense, with more eye movements and more vivid dreams. This phenomenon is referred to as "REM rebound," and may account for some of the bizarre dreams reported by critical care patients.

A number of clinical investigations of sleep disturbances and deprivation in the critical care setting are reported in the literature (Johnson, 1989; Fontaine, 1989; Richards & Bairnsfather, 1988; Rossi, Fitzmaurice, Glynn & Connors, 1987; Snyder-Halperin, 1985; Hilton, 1976; Hilton, 1985; Helton, Gordon, & Nunnery, 1980). These reports have documented that sleep disturbances in the ICU environment often occur, but they have been unable to conclude whether or not this problem is the cause of what is commonly termed "ICU syndrome."

In 1980, Helton et al. were able to demonstrate a moderate correlation between sleep deprivation and mental status changes. Unfortunately, the results in this study were limited, because of a lack of sensitivity in the mental status examination tool and difficulty making accurate sleep deprivation measurements.

Snyder-Halperin (1985) found that both physical and psychological changes can occur when noise interferes with sleep in the critical care setting. In addition, the researcher found that when critical care noise levels were introduced to sleeping volunteer subjects in a controlled sleep laboratory, mechanical noise was considered the most disturbing sound to subjects.

Richards and Bairnsfather (1988) reported significant differences between the sleep patterns of 10 critically ill subjects as compared with those of age- and sex-matched normal subjects. Sleep patterns were characterized using polysomnographic recordings. Critically ill subjects demonstrated significantly less total sleep time, a lower percentage of Stage 2 sleep and REM sleep, and a lower sleep efficiency index.

ASSESSMENT OF SLEEP PATTERNS

To understand the cause of current or potential sleep problems of a critical care patient, it is first necessary to elicit an admission sleep history. The history should be of appropriate depth and tailored to meet specific patient needs. It is often helpful to discuss the sleep history with family members and/or bed partners. Examples of suggested questions regarding the usual sleep pattern are listed in Table 10–2.

During hospitalization, a sleep assessment should become a standard activity of the daily nursing routine. Listed below are assessment questions that should be addressed on a daily basis:

1. Is the patient complaining of difficulty falling asleep or maintaining sleep?
2. What are the usual hospital bedtime and wake-up times?
3. Has the patient exhibited any of the following:
   Daytime sleepiness? Restless sleep? Frequent yawning? Listlessness? Frequent daytime napping? Ptosis (drooping eyelids)? Nystagmus (oscillatory movement of the eyeballs)? Conjunctival injection? Dark circles under the eyes?

4. Is the patient requesting sleeping medications?
5. Is the patient on any medications that might influence normal sleep patterns?
6. What routines/procedures are being performed during usual sleep hours? How often?

In the clinical sleep laboratory, sleep measurements are made with sophisticated equipment that monitors EEG (electroencephalogram), EOG (electrooculogram), and EMG (electromyogram) data. EEG tracings provide brain-wave information for determination of staging. EOG tracings detect and measure ocular movements characteristic of REM sleep, and submental EMG recordings provide muscle relaxation data. In combination, these parameters together provide the information necessary for staging of sleep.

In most critical care settings, the equipment necessary to make these sleep stage determinations is not available. The nurse must therefore rely on objective data obtained through observation to measure sleep amount and architecture. Fontaine (1989) found that observation of sleep using a structured observational tool was valid when compared with polysomnographic recordings.

Table 10–2   Prehospitalization Sleep History

1. Usual bedtime and usual wake-up time
2. Do you take daytime naps? If yes, at what time of the day? What is the normal duration of the naps?
3. Are you currently taking any medications for sleep or to stay awake? If yes, for how long? Does the medication help?
4. Do you have difficulty falling asleep? How long does it take to fall asleep? How often do you have difficulty falling asleep?
5. Do you wake up during the night? How often, and what is the duration of the wakeful period?
6. What helps you to fall asleep?
7. Have you ever had any of the following sleep-disturbing problems: Snoring? Sleep walking? Restless sleep? Nightmares? Nighttime awakenings to urinate (nocturnal enuresis)? Shortness of breath, coughing during the night? Palpitations? Nighttime indigestion and/or regurgitation? Tooth grinding (bruxism)?
8. What are your normal work hours and recreation/exercise schedule?
9. Do you smoke? How many packs per day? How many pack-years?
10. Do you use alcohol? How much, and how often?
11. What activities help you to sleep?
12. What is your preferred sleep environment? Number of pillows? Normal lighting? Room temperature?
13. What is your normal caffeine consumption?

In the most obvious sense, sleep as a level of consciousness can usually be distinguished from wakefulness by observation. However, in the critical care setting, the influence of narcotic analgesics, sedatives, anesthetic agents, or changes in level of consciousness make it difficult to distinguish sleep from wakefulness. In fact in many cases, without EEG monitoring, differentiation simply cannot be accomplished.

RELATED NURSING DIAGNOSES
Sleep Pattern Disturbance

The current NANDA (North American Nursing Diagnosis Association) nursing diagnosis, sleep pattern disturbance (Gordon, 1982, p. 150), is defined as a "disruption of sleep time causing discomfort or interference with the desired life activities." In this chapter, this diagnostic category is further subdivided according to specific causes or predisposing conditions that are applicable in the critical care setting (Table 10–3). Such specificity should allow the critical care nurse to better target possible treatments or interventions.

Signs and symptoms of sleep pattern disturbance are listed (Table 10–3) in two categories: (1) signs and symptoms that are less specific and occur regardless of cause and (2) signs and symptoms that are specific to sleep pattern disturbances due to particular causes. The list of signs and symptoms was based on defining characteristics identified through NANDA mechanisms (Johnson, 1989; Beyerman, 1987; Metzger & Hiltunen, 1987; Rossi, Fitzmaurice, Glynn, & Connors, 1987; Lo & Kim, 1986). Defining characteristics are separated according to the potential causes of sleep pattern disturbance in a critical care setting.

NURSING INTERVENTIONS

The first step toward ensuring that ICU patients receive the necessary amount of sleep should involve a daily sleep assessment. This assessment should address current concerns and may need to incorporate a sleep diary or log in which exact hours of observed sleep are charted. In addition, a detailed review of the prehospitalization sleep history (Table 10–2) may help to identify problem areas that may arise.

For example, patients who are accustomed to a 9 A.M. wake-up time will be in for a "rude awakening" when the noise of shift change and early morning vital signs disturbs their sleep at 6 or 7 A.M. This early awakening is not only uncomfortable for the patient, but also disrupts their ingrained circadian rhythm. Although it is unlikely that a nurse caring for the patient in this situation will be able to alter the ICU routine, he or she will be able to identify sleep pattern disturbance associated with circadian rhythm desynchronization as a potential problem.

Table 10–3   Defining Characteristics of Sleep Pattern Disturbance

Less-specific signs and symptoms

 Verbal complaints of difficulty falling asleep
 Verbal complaints of not feeling well rested
 Lethargy
 Listlessness
 Mild fleeting nystagmus
 Slight hand tremor
 Ptosis of the eyelids
 Dark circles under the eyes
 Frequent yawning

Cause-specific signs and symptoms

Sleep pattern disturbance associated with sensory/environmental conditions
 Early awakenings
 Interrupted sleep
 Increasing irritability
 Restlessness
 Disorientation
Sleep pattern disturbance associated with pain/physical discomfort
 Interrupted sleep
 Verbal complaints of pain (or signs and symptoms of pain)
 Increasing irritability
 Restlessness
 Frequent movements in sleep
Sleep pattern disturbance associated with circadian rhythm desynchronization
 Early morning awakenings
 Sleep pattern reversal
 Frequent daytime naps at irregular intervals
 Inability to fall asleep at conventional or desired bedtime
Sleep pattern disturbance associated with stress/anxiety
 Early awakenings with frequent movements during sleep
 Increased irritability
 Restlessness
 Disorientation
Sleep pattern disturbance associated with the use of CNS stimulants/depressants
 Frequent nighttime awakenings (lasting more than 5 minutes)
 Frequent sleep maintenance problems during the second half of the night
 As the period of drug ingestion lengthens, there is a progressive increase in
 sleep latency (time necessary to fall asleep)

Nursing interventions for sleep pattern disturbance in the critical care setting fall into two categories that are not mutually exclusive. First, there are interventions that can help to prevent sleep disturbances, and second, there are interventions for treatment of specific causes of sleep pattern disturbances.

Prevention Measures

Keep Nighttime Noise in the ICU Setting to a Minimum. The noise of paper wrapping on syringes and dressings can be especially irritating to patients who are trying to sleep. Whenever possible, prepare for treatments or procedures away from the bedside. Keep voices lowered during the nighttime, and if possible lower the volume of alarms and equipment. Whenever possible explain environmental sounds to lower patient anxiety.

Whenever Possible, Lighting Should Mimic Day/Night Schedules. Lighting has an important role in the synchronization of human circadian rhythms. If lighting can be diminished during the nighttime hours, patients will be less likely to dissociate from their sleep–wake cycle.

Nursing Assessment and Therapeutic Procedures Should Be Grouped Together Whenever Possible to Minimize the Interruptions of Sleep. As discussed earlier, the normal human needs a 70- to 90-minute uninterrupted period of time to complete one cycle of sleep. Nurses need to be aware of the amount of time their patients have been sleeping and whenever possible, patients should be allowed to complete one or two cycles before they are awakened.

Assist the Patient in Assuming a Comfortable Position for Sleep. Assumption of the usual and preferred position for sleep may help the patient to relax and achieve a restful sleep.

Be Aware That Sleeping Medications May Sometimes Be Disruptive to Sleep. When administering hypnotics, Hauri (1982) suggests that the following questions should be answered: How effective is the drug initially? How long is the drug effective? How are daytime performance and mood affected by treatment with the hypnotic drug? How does long-term use of the hypnotic affect sleep? What happens to sleep on cessation of hypnotic therapy?

  The most common hypnotics prescribed today include benzodiazepines, barbiturates, and a class of drugs referred to as nonbenzodiazepine–nonbarbiturates. (Examples of benzodiazepines are included in Table 10–4.) In general, hypnotics are effective only for short-term therapy, because they produce tolerance fairly quickly. In general, these agents have not been shown to be helpful for more than 28 consecutive nights. In most cases, they should be used intermittently, or for shorter periods of 1 to 2 weeks.

Treatment Interventions

Sleep pattern disturbance associated with sensory/environmental conditions

Treatment for this problem is most difficult because it is seldom possible to alter the ICU environment drastically or to relocate the patient to another less

Table 10–4 Common Hypnotic Drugs of the Benzodiazepine Class

Drug	Peak Concentration	Half-life Range of Active Metabolites	Sleep Effects	Other Notes
Flurazepam (Dalmane)	30–60 minutes after administration	74–160 hr	Decrease in stages 3 and 4, decrease in % of REM sleep, increase in Stage 2, reduces sleep onset time and the number of nighttime awakenings	Maintains effectiveness up to 4 weeks
Temazepam (Restoril)	2–3 hr after administration	8–38 hr	Decrease in amount of Stages 3 and 4 sleep, % of REM sleep remains unchanged, sleep onset time unchanged, sleep maintenance improved	Sleep may be disturbed after drug withdrawal
Triazolam (Halcion)	1.3 hr after administration	2–5 hr	Decreases sleep latency, increases total sleep time, reduces amount of stage 4 sleep, improves sleep maintenance	Sleep may be disturbed after drug withdrawal

acute setting. If sound is an issue, it may be possible to place cotton in a patient's ears or to mask the noise with a filtering device. Light can often be controlled by the use of curtains or screens. However, if these interventions, along with the preventive measures mentioned above, are ineffective, it is important to transfer the patient to a more appropriate environment as soon as possible.

Sleep pattern disturbance associated with pain/physical discomfort

Pain can be an important sleep-disturbing factor for patients in the ICU setting. Obviously, treatment with narcotic analgesics can help to relieve the pain and as a side effect can induce sleep through their hypnotic properties. It is important to be aware that the treatment in this instance can be a double-edged sword. Along with controlling the pain and inducing sleep, patterns of sleep can be disrupted by the frequent napping that occurs after administration of the medication. Also, many pain medications can block REM sleep, leading to REM rebound and a disruption of normal sleep architecture. Because of this possible side effect, which is discussed in greater detail later in this chapter, other techniques to minimize pain, such as relaxation, massage, and guided imagery, may be used by critical care nurses.

Sleep pattern disturbance associated with circadian rhythm desynchronization

In addition to control of lighting, it is important to monitor daytime naps carefully and even to discourage naps for patients who can remain alert and who are complaining of nighttime sleep difficulties. When naps are a necessity, as they often are in the ICU setting, they should be encouraged in the morning rather than in the afternoon. This is because afternoon naps consist mainly of delta sleep, which upon awakening can leave a patient feeling groggy and possibly disoriented.

As discussed earlier (see "Circadian Rhythms"), synchronization of an individual's rest–activity schedule is dependent on time cues known as zeitgebers. In addition to light, these include daily activities, clocks, and meals. To help ICU patients maintain their circadian rhythm, it is important to keep the patient awake for mealtime and to provide a clock for orientation.

Sleep pattern disturbance associated with stress/anxiety

In many cases, critical care patients are suffering from a life-threatening illness or recovering from a surgical procedure that can create a high level of anxiety for both the patients and their families. Stress itself leads to an increase in cortisol production that can block or shunt tryptophan, thereby causing insomnia. Restless sleep with frequent awakenings in this situation can best be treated by helping the patient to reduce his or her level of anxiety. Assess what your patient understands about his or her illness and help to allay any fears. For patients who are able to communicate, an explanation of a procedure or a clarification of a misconception may be the most important treatment for disrupted sleep.

Sleep pattern disturbance associated with the use of CNS stimulants or depressants

In the critical care setting these problems are most often associated with the use of pain or sleep medications. Over the short term, the difficulties most often encountered relate to desynchronization of the sleep–wake cycle related directly to medication-induced daytime naps. With prolonged use, however, these medications can cause REM deprivation and changes in normal sleep architecture. It is not always easy to balance the side effects and long-term effects of these medications on sleep, with the positive effects of pain control and short-term sedation. However, it is important to consider these potential negative effects when considering long-term therapy.

SUMMARY

Patients in the critical care setting often, by their own report, suffer from mild to severe sleep pattern disturbance. Unfortunately, the direct function of sleep and the consequences of this sleep disturbance or deprivation are unknown. To date, the sleep of critical care patients has received only moderate attention from the nursing research community.

As we move ahead in the field of sleep research, there are a number of critical research questions in this area that need to be addressed. For example:

1. How does sleep deprivation influence the rate of patient recovery?
2. What are the optimal environmental conditions that will facilitate sleep in the ICU setting?
3. How can ICU nurses more effectively assess the quality and quantity of their patients sleep?
4. Can nurses more efficiently monitor vital signs and other parameters to decrease sleep disturbance without jeopardizing patient care?

In conclusion, it is important to note that although there are many unanswered questions regarding sleep deprivation of critical care patients, we as nursing professionals cannot ignore the problem. With current knowledge, the best approach seems to be prevention. Through use of the preventative techniques described in this chapter and in other literature, it should be possible to increase the comfort level of ICU patients. Hopefully, nursing research will provide more insight and answers in the near future.

BIBLIOGRAPHY

Agnew, H., Webb, W., & Williams, R. (1967). Comparison of stage four and 1-REM sleep deprivation. *Perceptual Motor Skills, 24,* 851–858.

Aserinsky, E., & Kleitman, N. (1953). Regularly occurring periods of eye-mobility and concommital phenomena during sleep. *Science, 118,* 273–274.

Beyerman, K. (1987). Etiologies of sleep pattern disturbance in hospitalized patients. In A. M. McLane (Ed.), *Classification of nursing diagnoses: Proceedings of the seventh conference North American Nursing Diagnosis Association.* St. Louis: C. V. Mosby. pp. 193–198.

Brodsky, M., Delon, W., Denes, P., Kanakis, C., & Rosen, K. (1977). Arrhythmias documented by 24 hour continuous electrocardiographic monitoring in 50 male medical students without apparent heart disease. *American Journal of Cardiology, 39,* 390–395.

Douglas, N., White, D., Pickett, C., Weil, J., & Zwillich, C. (1982). Respiration during sleep in normal man. *Thorax, 37,* 840–844.

Fishbein, W., & Gutwein, B. (1977). Paradoxical sleep and memory storage processes. *Behavioral Biology, 19,* 425–464.

Fontaine, D. (1989). Measurement of nocturnal sleep patterns in trauma patients. *Heart and Lung, 18* (4), 402–410.

Gordon, M. (1982). *Manual of nursing diagnosis.* New York: McGraw-Hill.

Guilleminault, C., Connolly, S., & Winkle, R. (1983). Cardiac arrhythmia and conduction disturbances during sleep in 400 patients with sleep apnea syndrome. *American Journal of Cardiology, 52,* 490–494.

Hartmann, E. (1974). *The functions of sleep.* Chicago: University of Chicago Press.

Helton, M., Gordon, S., & Nunnery, S. (1980). The correlation between sleep deprivation and the intensive care unit syndrome. *Heart and Lung, 9,* 464–468.

Hilton, B. A. (1976). Quantity and quality of patients' sleep and sleep disturbing factors in a respiratory intensive care unit. *Journal of Advanced Nursing, 1,* 453–468.

Hilton, B. A. (1985). Noise in acute patient care areas. *Research in Nursing and Health, 8,* 283–291.

Hauri, P. (1982). *The sleep disorders: Current concepts.* Kalamazoo, MI: Upjohn.

Hudgel, D., Martin, R. Johnson, B., & Hill P. (1984). Mechanics of the respiratory system and breathing pattern during sleep in normal humans. *Journal of Applied Physiology, 56*(1), 133–137.

Johnson, S. E. (1989). Sleep pattern disturbance: Defining characteristics observable in practice. In R. M. Carroll-Johnson (Ed.). *Classification of nursing diagnoses: Proceedings of the eighth conference North American Nursing Diagnosis Association.* Philadelphia: J. B. Lippincott Co. pp. 368–370.

Lo, C., & Kim, M. (1986). Construct validity of sleep pattern disturbance: a methodological approach. In M. E. Hurley (Ed.), *Classification of nursing diagnoses: Proceedings of the sixth conference North American Nursing Diagnosis Association.* St. Louis: C. V. Mosby.

McCarley, R., & Hobson, J. (1975). Neuronal excitability modulation over the sleep cycle: a structural and mathematical model. *Science, 189,* 58–60.

McGrath, M., & Cohen, D. (1978). REM sleep facilitation of adaptive waking behavior: a review of the literature. *Psychological Bulletin, 85,* 24–57.

Metzger, K. & Hiltunen, E. (1987). Diagnostic content validation of ten frequently reported nursing diagnoses. In A. M. McLane (Ed.) *Classification of nursing diagnoses: Proceedings of the seventh conference North American Nursing Diagnosis Association.* St. Louis: C. V. Mosby. pp. 144–153.

Miles, L., & Dement, W. (1980). Sleep and aging. *Sleep, 3,* 119–220.

Moldofsky, H., & Scarisbrick, P. (1976). Induction of neurasthenic musculoskeletal pain syndrome by selective sleep stage deprivation. *Psychosomatic Medicine, 38,* 35–44.

Mooncroft, W., & Clothier, J. (1986). An overview of the body and the brain in sleep. In J. Gackenbach (Ed.), *Sleep and dreams.* New York: Garland Publishing.

Richards, K. C., & Bairnsfather, L. (1988). A description of night sleep patterns in the critical care unit. *Heart and Lung, 17*(1), 35–42.

Rossi, L., Fitzmaurice, J., Glynn, M., & Connors, K. (1987). Validation of the defining characteristics for sleep pattern disturbance. In A. M. McLane (Ed.) *Classification of nursing diagnoses: Proceedings of the seventh conference North American Nursing Diagnosis Association.* St. Louis: C. V. Mosby. p. 279 (abstract).

Sobotka, P., Mayer, J., Bauernfeind, R., Kanakis, C., & Rosen, K. (1981). Arrhythmias documented by 24-hour continuous ambulatory electrocardiographic monitoring in young women without apparent heart disease. *American Heart Journal, 101,* 753–759.

Snyder-Halperin, R. (1985). The effect of critical care unit noise on patient sleep cycles. *Critical Care Quarterly, 7,* 41–51.

Vogel, G. (1975). A review of REM sleep deprivation. *Archives of General Psychiatry, 32,* 749–761.

Vogel, G., Vogel, F., McAbee, R., & Thurmond, A. (1980). Improvement of depression by REM sleep deprivation. *Archives of General Psychiatry, 37,* 247–253.

White, D., Weil, J., & Zwillich, C. (1985). Metabolic rate and breathing during sleep. *Journal of Applied Physiology, 59*(2), 384–391.

11 Pain

Maureen E. Shekleton, D.N.Sc., R.N.

Pain is a complex subjective experience that involves physiologic, psychological, social, cultural, and for some, spiritual components. Pain is a phenomenon that is encountered frequently by the clinician, as it is a symptom of many pathophysiologic conditions and may be a response to treatment as well. Pain most often occurs as a response to some health problem; however, it becomes the disease in chronic pathologic pain syndromes. In many situations pain serves a protective function by alerting the individual to actual or potential tissue damage. It is considered a signal or warning sign in those situations and, as such, indicates the need for action. In other situations, such as incisional pain in the postoperative patient, pain serves no useful purpose. In fact, postoperative pain may impede recovery, prolong hospitalization, and even evolve into chronic pain (Smith & Covino, 1985).

Considered in this chapter are current definitions and theories of pain, the neurophysiologic basis for pain and the physiologic rationale for the treatment of pain as a response to a health problem. The nursing diagnosis, acute pain, is the major focus of this discussion of pain as a response to a health problem. Acute pain is defined as pain of relatively short duration for which there is a specific, identifiable cause. Postoperative pain is acute pain that results from planned, deliberate tissue injury and normally diminishes as healing proceeds. It has been identified as one of the "common problems in everyday hospital practice" (Leib & Hurtig, 1985, p. 164).

Aside from incisional pain there are other situations in which pain occurs as a response in the critically ill surgical patient. Invasive procedures and treatments such as the insertion of an indwelling venous catheter, debridement of burn wounds, and the maintenance of awkward positions during surgery and procedures can all cause additional pain with which the critically ill patient must cope (Bryan-Brown, 1986). Presented in Table 11–1 are different pathologic mechanisms that can cause pain, any of which may occur in the critically ill patient.

DEFINITIONS AND THEORIES

A variety of definitions of pain are found in the literature. There is probably no one definition of pain that completely describes the concept of pain as a human response to an actual or potential health problem. Pain has been defined as:

> "a subjective experience arising from activity within the brain in response to damage to body tissues, to changes in the function of the brain itself either as a result of damage due to injury or disease, or to changes of a more subtle nature perhaps depending upon biochemical changes which also appear to play a role in producing mental illness (Bond, 1984);
>
> "an unpleasant sensory and emotional experience associated with actual or potential tissue damage, or described in terms of such damage (International Association for the Study of Pain Subcommittee on Taxonomy, 1979);
>
> "an abstract concept which refers to (1) a personal, private sensation of hurt; (2) a harmful stimulus which signals current and impending tissue damage; (3); a pattern of responses which operate to protect the organism from harm (Sternbach, 1978);
>
> "whatever the experiencing person says it is, existing whenever he says it does (McCaffery, 1979).

While this list of definitions is not a comprehensive one, those presented do show the variety of types of definitions that have been proposed. Bond's definition is physiologic in nature while Sternbach's tends to be psychological. The Association's definition is a mix of the two approaches. McCaffery's definition falls outside of either approach. It is based on the fact that there is a cognitive component to the pain experience and thus it becomes a psychophysiologic phenomenon. Because of this cognitive component—which is determined by past experiences, anticipation, and sociocultural influences among other factors—the pain experience is unique to and, therefore, defined by each person. McCaffery's definition supports the clinical fact that the patient's subjective expression of pain is a more reliable indicator of the presence of pain than more objective indicators such as blood pressure and heart and respiratory rate changes.

Theories about the nature of pain have been developed over the years. The purpose of such theories is to explain the concept of pain in such a way that prediction and control of the phenomenon might be achieved in the clinical setting. The theories reviewed in the following text have been synthesized from a variety of sources and include the specificity, pattern, affect, and gate-control theories of pain (Ignelzi & Atkinson, 1980; Melzack & Wall, 1982; Meinhart & McCaffery, 1983a, 1983b).

Specificity Theory

The specificity theory is an extension of the work of Muller, who proposed that excitation of a particular receptor and sensory pathway elicited a particu-

Table 11-1   Major Causes of Pain

Abnormal Initiating Mechanism	Pathophysiology
I. Ischemia	Blood supply to involved area is reduced because of arteriosclerosis, external pressure on artery, vasospasm, or occlusion: when muscles do not receive an adequate supply of blood and oxygen for aerobic metabolism, anaerobic metabolism occurs, with accumulation of lactic acid and cellular breakdown with release of bradykinin and histamine, which stimulate the nerve endings
II. Increased arterial pulsation	The rhythmic stretch and relaxation of sensitive arterial walls with each systolic impulse stimulates pain receptors in response to the mechanical stretching
III. Pressure of mass on adjacent structure	Presence of a space-occupying mass exerts pressure on the nerves and displacement and traction on surrounding organs
IV. Spasm of a hollow viscus	Distention of an organ with air or fluid causes pain from overstretching of the tissues and the forcible peristaltic moving of the contents against resistance
V. Chemical irritation	Irritating chemical substances like hydrochloric acid, pancreatic enzymes, and bile come in contact with the naked nerve terminals in the peritoneum or pancreatic bed
VI. Inflammatory process	The elaboration of kinins, toxins, and other chemical substances in response to injury, invasion and multiplication of microorganisms, or other pathology lowers the threshold for pain; additionally the accompanying swelling from collection of exudate or edema puts pressure on nerves of adjacent organs
VII. Tissue injury A. External penetration	When tissue is damaged, the pain receptors in the free nerve endings in the

Clinical State	Character of Pain
Myocardial ischemia, myocardial infarction, angina pectoris, mesenteric infarct/ischemia, pulmonary infarction, chronic arterial occlusion, Raynaud's disease, compartment syndrome, sickle-cell crisis, cerebral thrombosis	Constricting, squeezing, burning, or heaviness, which may be provoked by exercise or stress
Malignant hypertension headache, migraine headache, arteritis, vascular headache	Throbbing and aching localized to involved area and sometimes accompanied by tenderness to pressure on area; pain increased by activity that increases systolic pressure such as exercise, bending over, fever, etc.
Intracranial mass, hemorrhage, neoplasm, hiatus hernia, urinary retention, torsion of ovarian cyst	Constant aching, most often severe, intensified by movement of involved area
Ileus, intestinal colic, intestinal obstruction, impacted stone in bile duct, gastroenteritis, labor, ureteral colic or spasm	Rhythmic cramping that increases to very severe and then subsides, with repetition every few minutes; in late obstructive disease pain becomes continuous as ischemia develops
Peptic ulcer disease, pancreatitis, heartburn, esophageal reflux, esophagitis	Steady burning or gnawing
Chest: pericarditis, pleuritis, pneumonia, myositis, acute tracheitis Abdomen: appendicitis, cholecystitis, peritonitis, diverticulitis, hepatitis, subphrenic abscess, pyelonephritis	Steady aching that frequently radiates and is accentuated with movement or increased abdominal pressure; when more severe, sharp and penetrating (knife-like)
Other: sinusitis, phlebitis, reaction to foreign body, prostatitis, acute pelvic inflammatory disease	Same as above
Surgical incision Wounds: Laceration, bruise, burn	Pricking, burning, aching in area affected

Table 11–1 *(Continued)*

Abnormal Initiating Mechanism	Pathophysiology
	skin and deeper structures are stimulated; the tissue reaction of swelling also stimulates the pain receptors responding to mechanical pressure
B. Internal disruption	Rupture or tear of a structure
VIII. Metabolic or toxic disorder	Metabolic abnormalities resulting in hypercalcemia, porphobilinogen, sodium and fluid depletion, and/or metabolic acidosis
	Pain from toxin ingestion or bite of black widow spider
IX. Osseous injury or lesion A. Skeletal bones	Disruption of continuity, tension on the periosteum, or alteration in the function of joints and overlying tissue (nerves, ligaments, tendons, or bursae) stimulate the pain receptors; if edema develops, pain is intensified from stimulation of pressure receptors
B. Vertebral column	Irritation of the fascia ligaments or tendons of the back, demineralization of the bones, or degenerative or traumatic changes in the disks with softening, loosening, and displacement of the nucleus pulposus, exerting pressure on (or stretching) adjacent ligaments and/or nerve roots
	Tumors extending from vertebral bodies or from extraspinal spaces through intervertebral foramens and other osseous lesions cause resorption of normal osseous tissue by production of sub-

Clinical State	Character of Pain
Dissecting aortic aneurysm, pneumothorax, mediastinal emphysema, rupture of esophagus, perforated duodenal ulcer, perforated viscus Ectopic pregnancy: tubal abortion, tubal rupture Rupture of uterus	Abrupt onset with quick progression to agonizing severity
Rupture of corpus luteum cyst, rupture of graafian follicle	Abrupt onset but pain of lesser severity than when larger organs are involved, and pain gradually subsides instead of becoming more severe
Hyperparathyroidism, acute intermittent porphyria, adrenal insufficiency, uremia, diabetic ketoacidosis	Abdominal pain of varying degrees of severity that may be continuous, colicky, or intermittent cramping
Heavy-metal poisoning, arachnidism, food poisoning	Severe cramping pain in abdomen
Fractures, sprains, ruptured tendons, scurvy, rickets, arthritis, bursitis, osteomyelitis, Paget's disease	Ache or deep pain in general area of lesion that is increased with movement and pressure on area
Sciatica, intervertebral disk disease, osteoarthritis of the spine, ankylosing spondylitis	Backache, which may be accompanied by abnormal posture, limitation of motion of the spine, and, if nerve root involved, radiation of pain, sensory alterations, and altered tendon reflexes; nerve root pain is exacerbated by sudden increases in intraspinal pressure as from coughing, sneezing, or straining
Primary extramedullary spinal cord tumors Secondary to: neoplastic diseases, lymphoma, tuberculosis	Same as above

Table 11–1   *(Continued)*

Abnormal Initiating Mechanism	Pathophysiology
	stances that lyse bone, resulting in bone deformity, pathologic fractures, and destruction and narrowing of the intervertebral disks
X. Muscular spasm or contraction	The contracting muscle compresses the intramuscular blood vessels with a reduction in flow of blood to the area but an increase in the metabolic rate of the muscle, resulting in relative muscle ischemia
XI. Nerve root, sensory ganglions, peripheral nerve disorders	Compression, stimulation, traction, or inflammation of nerve roots, sensory ganglions, or peripheral nerves results in pain
XII. Psychogenic, psychological needs, secondary gain	Various psychological factors are responsible for pain by precipitation of physiologic changes (vascular changes, muscle tenseness, hyposecretion and hypersecretion of glands), by conversion of an emotional conflict into a physical complaint, or by development of delusions

lar sensation. In the late 1800s a physician by the name of Max von Frey extended Muller's work and proposed a theory of the cutaneous senses in which specific pain receptors and nerve fibers for pain were postulated. The view of pain in the specificity theory is that of a specialized sense that is separate and distinct from all others. Receptors and tracts specific to the sensation of pain were thought to transmit stimuli to and evoke a response from pain centers located in the brain. Such an arrangement would dictate a fixed stimulus–response, relationship, which could be interrupted surgically. Phantom limb pain and the failure of surgical interruption of nerve tracts to cure pain are cited as clinical facts that do not support this theory.

Pattern Theory

In this theoretical approach pain was thought to be the result of the pattern of stimulation of nerves. Nerve endings and tracts were thought to be shared with other sensations, with pain being signaled by the spatiotemporal patterning of impulses. Physiologic research has not supported this approach, however, as specific tracts and nerve fibers have been shown to respond to painful stimuli.

Clinical State	Character of Pain
Tension headache, muscle cramp, muscle strain	Spasmodic muscular contraction, with knot in muscle sometimes palpable
Trigeminal neuralgia, glossopharyngeal neuralgia, herpes zoster, tabes dorsalis, entrapment neuropathies, neuritis (intercostal, peripheral, etc.)	Sharp, lancinating, or throbbing occurring in quick succession, and frequently triggered by end-organ stimulation
Hysterical pain, hypochondriacal pain, phantom pain (in some cases), spastic colon, delusional pain, conversion symptoms, psychosomatic pain, psychological augmentation of pain	Pain may be of any nature. Most frequently described as a sharp aching in the region of organ to which it is attributed

From *Decision Making for Patient Care* (pp. 266–269) by M. J. Aspinall, 1981, New York: Appleton-Century-Croft. Copyright 1981 by Appleton-Century-Croft. Reprinted by permission.

Subsumed under this heading are actually several theoretical orientations. Goldscheider first proposed that the critical variables in pain production were stimulus intensity and central summation. Weddell and Sinclair were adherents to the belief that excessive peripheral stimulation produces a pattern of impulse transmission that is interpreted centrally as pain. This approach is known as peripheral pattern theory. In contrast, Livingston emphasized central summation in an attempt to explain phantom limb pain and the pain of causalgia and the neuralgias. He postulated that abnormal spinal cord activity in the form of activation of closed, self-exciting loops (reverberating circuits) of neurons is responsible for these unremitting and untreatable pain syndromes. Another proponent of central summation theory was Gerard, who hypothesized that pools of synchronously firing spinal cord neurons develop in response to loss of sensory control of their firing and account for excessive and abnormally patterned discharges of impulses to the higher centers. Hebb suggested that pain is the result of such synchronized neural firing within the thalamocortical tract rather than the spinal cord. Related to central summation theory is sensory interaction theory, in which a specialized input-controlling system, which would prevent summation, was hypothesized. This approach served as a major foundation for future work. Noordenbos proposed that a change in the ratio of small fibers (which carry pain-producing nerve impulses) to large fibers (which inhibit that transmission) such that small fibers were favored would result in increased transmission, summation, and consequently, excessive pain.

Affect Theory

Basically, this theory states that pain has both sensory and affective aspects. Pain is seen not as a purely physical sensation but as one with overtones of feeling or affect as a response.

While each of the above theories addresses some aspect of pain, none accounts completely for the totality of the experience. None of the above theoretical approaches accounts for the motivational, cognitive, and cultural dimensions of pain and the interactions among them that make the experience unique for every individual. The notion of pain as a unidimensional experience was the theme of these approaches, rather than that of pain as a multidimensional experience associated with a variety of diverse mechanisms. In response to the deficiencies of these theories a more comprehensive theoretical framework was sought that would account for all of the following:

1. physiologic specificity of receptor-fiber units and central nervous system (CNS) pathways,
2. the role of spatiotemporal patterning in the transmission of impulses,
3. the influence of psychological variables on pain perception and response, and
4. clinical observations related to pain, such as the persistence, spread, and spatiotemporal summation of pain. (Melzack & Wall, 1982)

To this end, Melzack and Wall advanced a new theory.

Gate-Control Theory

First proposed in 1965, the gate-control theory postulates that a "gating" mechanism allows the modulation of pain impulses and, therefore, pain perception and response. Melzack and Wall (1982) have updated the original conceptual model to incorporate new facts and ideas while maintaining the validity of the conceptual model of "gating" and the propositions that underlie it. This theory is thought to be the most adequate explanation of the pain phenomenon currently available and, as such, has been very useful in stimulating discussion and research about the nature and treatment of pain (Bishop, 1980).

Propositions of this model include the existence of a spinal gating mechanism that is influenced by the relative activity of the large- and small-diame-
ter fibers and neural impulses descending from the brain, including some
activated by cognitive input. Pain is thought to occur when the output of the
spinal cord transmission (T) cells exceeds a critical level. The activity of the T
cells depends on the activity of the cells of the substantia gelatinosa (SG). The
gate is closed, that is T-cell transmission is inhibited, when the SG cells are
activated. The gate is opened, that is T-cell transmission is facilitated, when
the SG cells are inhibited. The SG-cell function is mediated by input from the
periphery as well as the CNS. Large-fiber input activates SG cells while small-
fiber input inhibits SG cells. A schematic diagram of the gate-control theory is
presented in Figure 11–1.

It is postulated that the spinal gating mechanism is most probably located in the substantia gelatinosa of the dorsal horn because the SG runs the
length of the spinal cord bilaterally, receives afferent input from both large
and small fibers, and influences cells that connect to the brain. The cells in
lamina V are most likely the spinal transmission (T) cells as they receive
afferent input from the small fibers of the skin, viscera, and muscles; are
influenced by fibers that descend from the brain; respond to a wide range of
stimulus intensities; increase their rate of firing in response to increased
intensities of stimulation; and their output is influenced by the relative activity
in the large and small fibers.

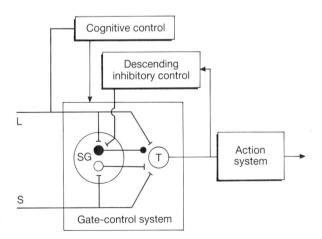

Figure 11–1. The gate-control theory: Mark II. The new model includes excitatory
(white circle) and inhibitory (black circle) links from the substantia gelatinosa (SG) to
the transmission (T) cells as well as descending inhibitory control from brain-stem
systems. The round knob at the end of the inhibitory link implies that its action may be
presynaptic, postsynaptic, or both. All connections are excitatory, except the inhibitory
link from SG to T cell. L = Large diameter fibers; S = Small diameter fibers. From *The
Challenge of Pain* by R. Melzack and P. D. Wall, 1982, New York: Raven Press. Copyright 1982 by Penguin Books Ltd. Reprinted by permission.

One of the more important points about the gate-control theory is that it allows for integration of all dimensions of the pain experience. The overt behavioral response that characterizes pain is determined by sensory, motivational, and cognitive processes that act on motor mechanisms of the central nervous system (Melzack & Wall, 1982). Integration of all these components is postulated to occur through parallel processing systems, which are schematically illustrated in Figure 11–2.

NEUROPHYSIOLOGY OF PAIN

It should be obvious from the preceding discussion that the pain-processing system is made up of large integrative neuronal networks. Inherent in this system are receptors, pathways, and neuroregulatory substances that allow the processing of nerve impulses between the peripheral and central nervous systems.

Physiologically, pain is viewed as a response to some stimulus. The usual painful stimuli may be placed into any one of three categories: thermal, mechanical, or chemical. In the case of acute postoperative pain, tissue injury is the initiating mechanism and the major stimulus for pain production is me-

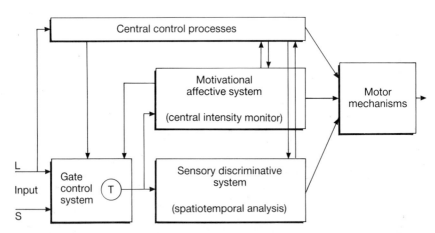

Figure 11–2. Conceptual model of the sensory, motivational and central control determinants of pain. The output of the T cells of the gate-control system projects to the sensory–discriminative system (via neospinothalamic fibers) and the motivational–affective system (via the paramedial ascending system). The central control trigger is represented by a line running from the large-fiber system to central control processes; these, in turn, project back to the gate-control system, and to the sensory–discriminative and motivational–affective systems. All three systems interact with one another and project to the motor system. L = Large diameter fibers; S = Small diameter fibers. From *The Challenge of Pain* by R. Melzack and P. D. Wall, 1982, New York: Raven Press. Copyright 1982 by Penguin Books Ltd. Reprinted by permission.

chanical, although with the use of electrocautery and antiseptic solutions, thermal and chemical stimulation may also occur. These noxious stimuli cause cell damage, which allows the release and activation of chemical substances with algetic (pain-producing) properties as part of the inflammatory response to injury.

The pain receptors are chemoceptive and can be stimulated by a variety of chemical substances that are released or activated in response to cell injury, including potassium and hydrogen ions, some amines, and peptides (Bond, 1984). Chemical substances that are most directly involved in the chemical interactions that mediate pain include histamine, serotonin, bradykinin, and prostaglandins (especially of the E series). These substances produce pain directly and increase the sensitivity of the receptors to noxious stimuli. They exert their effect individually and in combination with one another. Prostaglandins, which are generated from cell phospholipids via the arachidonic acid cascade, potentiate the effects of histamine and bradykinin. Bradykinin itself can stimulate the release of arachidonic acid and thus facilitates the synthesis of prostaglandins. Serotonin increases the vascular and noxious effects of both bradykinin and the prostaglandins and potentiates the action of histamine and bradykinin to decrease the sensory threshold of the nerves (Ignelzi & Atkinson, 1980; Zimmerman, 1981; Bond, 1984).

Receptors and Pathways

The nociceptors or pain receptors are undifferentiated free nerve endings that arise from unmyelinated or thinly myelinated axons. These receptors are polymodal, that is, they are able to respond to different types of noxious stimuli (heat, cold, chemical irritation, mechanical distortion) with different levels of sensitivity for each. For example, the most common receptor, a high-threshold receptor, responds readily to heat and irritant chemicals, while mechanical stimuli must be of moderate or greater intensity. Nociceptors demonstrate an augmented response to repetitive stimulation, in contrast to other somatic sensory organs, which show fatigue after repetitive stimulation (Ignelzi & Atkinson, 1980). This phenomenon, which is known as sensitization, is unique to the sensation of pain (Bishop, 1980).

The neuronal fiber types found to be associated with pain are the large, myelinated, fast-conducting sensory class A (alpha and delta) and the small, nonmyelinated, slow-conducting sensory class C fibers. The character of the fiber may be important in the differentiation of the type of pain experienced. There is some experimental evidence that stimulation of the A delta fibers results in clearly localized, pricking, or sharp "first" pain, while stimulation of the C fibers results in vague, dull, or aching "second" pain.

These fibers arise from bipolar neurons in the dorsal-root ganglion and the impulse passes from the periphery to the spinal cord through these cells. The afferent axon of these cells synapses in the dorsal horn gray matter, which has been subdivided into 10 concentric layers or laminae. Laminae II and III correspond to the substantia gelatinosa. At this level, synaptic connection can occur with either a spinal neuron, which is a link to motor and sympathetic reflexes, or with a second-order neuron within an ascending pathway, which allows passage of the impulse to higher levels of the central nervous system, including the somatosensory cortex, thalamus, reticular formation, and limbic forebrain. There are multiple ascending pathways organized with either long intersynaptic distances and few synapses (oligosynaptic) or short intersynaptic distances and many synapses (polysynaptic) (Smith & Covino, 1985). The oligosynaptic pathways allow rapid conduction of the impulse and localization of pain while conduction is relatively slower via the polysynaptic pathways and localization is not possible since there is no associated somatotropic organization.

The major ascending pathways for nociceptive afferents include the spinothalamic, spinoreticular, and spinocervical tracts. Anatomically, the spinothalamic tract is considered to have two parts: the neospinothalamic or lateral component and the paleospinothalamic or ventral component. The neospinothalamic tract projects to the posterior thalamic nuclei and is thought to be important in discrimination of spatial and temporal aspects of pain and touch. The paleospinothalamic tract projects to the medial and intralaminar thalamic nuclei and has many collaterals to the brain stem, which allows for interaction, and reflex activity. This branch is thought to participate in the less discriminative aspects of pain and aversive motivation. The spinoreticular tract projects to the brain stem and reticular formation. The spinocervical tract projects to the posterolateral ventral nucleus of the thalamus and may be involved in integration of the motor functions and behavioral responses to pain (Bishop, 1980; Ignelzi & Atkinson, 1980).

Ascending afferent information and spinal reflex activity is subject to selection, modulation, and control through the influence of descending inhibitory pathways (Bishop, 1980; Yaksh, Howe, & Harty, 1984.) Experimental evidence obtained using electrical stimulation and pharmacologic agents indicates that there are probably multiple pathways that exert inhibitory influences on nociceptive impulses (Terman, Lewis, James, & Liebeskind, 1984). Brain-stem structures are thought to be the site of origin of these pathways and the function of at least one is believed to include opiate mechanisms (Ignelzi & Atkinson, 1980; Zimmerman, 1981). Naloxone, a narcotic antagonist, only partially reverses stimulation-produced analgesia (SPA), providing evidence that a combination of opioid and nonopioid pathways exist (Meinhart & McCaffery, 1983a, 1983b). Pain and stress are known to activate these pathways, although the opioid and nonopioid pathways may respond to different types of stress (Terman et al., 1984; Phillips & Cousins, 1986).

Modulation of the afferent information can occur at any point in the path of transmission at which synapses occur. The first point at which modulation occurs, through the integration of ascending and descending input with additional local and peripheral nerve input, is in the substantia gelatinosa in the dorsal horn. Further integration occurs at the level of the brain stem, which contains many nuclei, and through which all information is transmitted via ascending and descending pathways in the reticular formation. Experimental evidence supports the nucleus raphe magnus in the medulla as the site of origin for at least one inhibitory pathway (Ignelzi & Atkinson, 1980; Phillips & Cousins, 1986). Ascending connections from the brain stem are with the thalamus, the third level of integration, where conscious perception of pain occurs. Thalamic nuclei serve as relays for thalamocortical projections. The final point of integration and perception is within the cortex (Ignelzi & Atkinson, 1980).

An example of how modulation works is seen in the inhibition of the response of the dorsal horn neurons to peripheral pain stimulation by electrical nerve stimulation. The inhibitory effect of nerve stimulation is thought to be the result of activation of both the inhibitory interneurons at the level of the spine and the descending inhibitory systems (Zimmerman, 1981). This is thought to be the mechanism of action of "counter-irritant" techniques for the relief of pain such as transcutaneous electrical nerve stimulation, massage, and acupuncture.

Neuroregulation

At each synapse there is the possibility of either facilitation or inhibition of the pain impulse (Dodson, 1985). Synaptic activity depends on the availability and function of various chemical neuroregulatory substances, which can be functionally subdivided into neurotransmitters and neuromodulators. Neurotransmitters or neurohormones are low-molecular-weight substances, with a short half-life, that act by binding to receptors of postsynaptic neurons. Neuromodulators are high-molecular-weight substances, with a relatively longer half-life, that may act by altering the synthesis, release, or activity of presynaptic neurotransmitters or by acting on postsynaptic receptor sites (Ignelzi & Atkinson, 1980).

In order to be accepted as a neurotransmitter, chemical substances must meet several criteria, including the presence of the substance and mechanisms for its synthesis and metabolism in neural tissue, its release with nerve stimulation, blocking or potentiation of its action by drugs with those actions, and the response to exogenous administration of the substance must be the same as that elicited by nerve stimulation (Smith, 1985). The two major transmitter systems include the monoamine and cholinergic systems (Ignelzi & Atkinson, 1980). Proven neurotransmitters include norepinephrine, epinephrine, dopamine, and acetylcholine. Other putative (or suspected) neurotransmitters involved in pain perception include substance P, serotonin (5 HT), somatostatin, gamma-aminobutyric acid (GABA), and histamine (Bishop, 1980; Meinhart & McCaffery, 1983a, 1983b; Phillips & Cousins, 1986).

Substance P is thought to be an excitatory transmitter released by the nociceptive afferents, but its activity appears to be dose related. At high doses it excites spinal cord and brain neurons, which are sensitive to nociceptive stimuli, and at low doses it causes the release of endorphins and inhibits nociception (Ignelzi & Atkinson, 1980). Substance P has also been found in a descending inhibitory system between the brain-stem raphe nucleus and the dorsal horn (Smith, 1985). Opioids inhibit the release and action of substance P (Bond, 1984). The ability of somatostatin to excite neurons in nociceptive pathways and its distribution within the CNS is similar to that of substance P (Ignelzi & Atkinson, 1980).

It appears that serotonin has a dual role as both an excitatory and inhibitory transmitter. Serotonin acts in the peripheral nervous system as an algesic substance that excites and sensitizes nociceptors. Acting on the dorsal horn neurons it appears to inhibit transmission of the pain impulse and is thought to be a transmitter involved in the descending inhibitory pathways. These paths are thought to be activated through the binding of the opiate receptors by either endogenous or exogenous opioids, and the subsequent stimulation of the descending neurons causes the release of serotonin at synapses within the spinal cord (Zimmerman, 1981; Phillips & Cousins, 1986). Depletion of serotonin has been found to decrease stimulation-produced analgesia (SPA) and injection of serotonin directly into the CNS or administration of its precursor, 5 hydroxytryptophan (5 HTP), has been found to restore analgesia (Gershon, 1986; Smith, 1985; Ignelzi & Atkinson, 1980). The availability of serotonin also affects the activity of morphine. The effects of morphine are enhanced with the injection of serotonin or with interference with its reuptake, and the effects of morphine are lessened with serotonin depletion or blocking with drugs (Dodson, 1985; Feinmann, 1985).

Norepinephrine acts in the opposite way. Depletion of norepinephrine has been found to enhance antinociception (Ignelzi & Atkinson, 1980). Increased norepinephrine levels can potentially lower the pain threshold and increase pain. Norepinephrine has been found to decrease the effectiveness of morphine (Gershon, 1986).

Dopamine also is thought to have some role in pain transmission and modulation. Administration of L-dopa (a dopamine precursor) increases the pain threshold and produces analgesia, presumably by increasing the dopamine level (Ignelzi & Atkinson, 1980).

Speculation about a mechanism that links depression and chronic pain has focused on abnormal levels of various neurotransmitters. Concentrations of serotonin and norepinephrine in the CNS indicate that overlap exists between affective and nociceptive paths. The results of clinical studies of the levels of these neurotransmitters in depressed individuals and the actions of antidepressant medications suggest that decreased concentrations of serotonin and norepinephrine may be a pathogenetic mechanism in depression. The evidence supports the existence of mutually interacting feedback loops between serotonin, norepinephrine, and enkephalin (Gershon, 1986).

Neuromodulators include the endogenous opioid peptides, which are morphine-like in their action. The identification and mapping of opiate receptor sites throughout the nervous system and in the gastrointestinal tract stimulated the search for endogenous substances capable of binding to these receptors. Although referred to generically as endorphins, three families or classes of these opioid peptides, based on their derivation from three distinct precursor molecules, have been recognized: 1) beta-lipotropin, which contains beta-endorphin; 2) enkephalin, which contains Met-enkephalin and Leu-enkephalin; and 3) dynorphin (Meinhart & McCaffery, 1983a, 1983b; Millan, 1986; Phillips & Cousins, 1986). The roles of these substances in the modulation and control of pain are very complex, with the effects depending on a number of interacting variables, including the particular substance; the receptor type being affected; whether action is occurring at the level of the brain, spinal cord, or periphery; the type and duration of the stimulus causing pain; the nature of the response; and the conditions of activity (Millan, 1986).

The actions of the endogenous opioids mimic the central and peripheral effects of morphine and other exogenous opioids. The enkephalins have a relatively short half-life in comparison to the endorphins, as the enkephalins are subject to rapid enzymatic degradation. The enkephalins are thought to inhibit the release of excitatory neurotransmitters and have been shown to inhibit the release of substance P and, subsequently, the transmission of noxious impulses when they bind to opiate receptors in the dorsal horn. In contrast, endorphin release can be stimulated by neurons in descending substance P pathways (Ignelzi & Atkinson, 1980). Beta-endorphin has an increased affinity for opiate receptors in the hypothalamus and pituitary gland. The enkephalins are considered weakly analgesic while the dynorphins are considered to have an analgesic potency 50 times greater than that of beta-endorphin (Meinhart & McCaffery, 1983a, 1983b).

The endogenous opioids are secreted in response to stress and pain (Meinhart & McCaffery, 1983a, 1983b; Millan, 1986). Elevated levels of these substances have been found after surgery (Cohen, Pickar, Dubois, Roth, Naber, & Bunney, 1981; Dodson, 1985). Other factors thought to stimulate endogenous opioids include fear, restraint, hypoglycemia, and elevated blood pressure (Puntillo, 1988). The effects of counter-irritant stimulation techniques such as acupuncture, transcutaneous electrical nerve stimulation, and massage, have been shown to be at least partially mediated through the mechanism of endorphin release (Lewith & Kenyon, 1984). There is some evidence that the placebo response may be mediated by endorphins as well (Levine, Gordon, & Fields, 1978).

At this time, information about the actions of the endogenous opioids is not complete and is the subject of much ongoing research. Elucidation of the mechanisms through which the endogenous opioids exert their effects may provide the means to control these systems in order to provide more complete pain relief in the clinical setting.

Effects and Manifestations of Pain

The observable behaviors associated with pain include vocalization, a startle response, a flexion reflex, and avoidance movements. Associated with these reflexive responses are the autonomic and learned responses that pain evokes (Abu-Saad & Tesler, 1986).

Learned responses can be highly individualized and often represent coping strategies that a person has used to deal with pain successfully in the past. Complex perceptual and cognitive processes at the higher levels of the CNS allow the integration of the nociceptive impulse with emotion, beliefs, expectations and the present situation. As a result of these processes, the meaning, quality, and intensity of the pain and the psychological and behavioral responses to it are determined in relation to the individual's personality, cultural background, learning history, and the present psychosocial context in which the pain is being experienced (Chapman, 1985).

The patient will voluntarily limit movement or activity that becomes associated with causing or increasing pain. Guarding (or splinting) is a protective rigidity that is adopted in order to limit pain caused by movement. Lack of or inadequate participation in the "stir-up" regimen (dangling, ambulation, bed exercises, coughing, and deep breathing) results in the following nursing diagnoses: potential for altered tissue perfusion related to thrombophlebitis or embolism, ineffective breathing pattern, and potential for ineffective airway clearance (See chapters 1 and 14).

The autonomic response includes input from both the sympathetic and parasympathetic systems. The initial response is that of activation, as in the reaction to any stressor the body encounters. The sympathetic system response is usually predominant at this point and blood will be shunted to the vital organs through peripheral vasoconstriction. The pulse and respiratory rates and blood pressure will be increased and the nurse may note pallor, perspiration, and dilated pupils. Sympathetic activation causes increased smooth muscle sphincter tone and decreased intestinal and renal motility. Intestinal secretions are also increased. The patient may experience nausea and vomiting. More serious results of sympathetic activity can include gastric stasis and dilation and urinary retention (Phillips & Cousins, 1986). This sympathoadrenal activation can have negative consequences in the critically ill patient, especially one with a compromised cardiovascular system, since myocardial ischemia, infarction, or failure may occur in response to the increased systemic resistance, decreased coronary filling time, increased cardiac workload, and increased myocardial oxygen consumption.

With severe acute pain, inhibition of the vasomotor center rather than sympathetic activation may occur. This causes peripheral pooling of blood, which is reflected by decreased blood pressure and, in turn, can result in decreased perfusion and tissue hypoxia. In the postoperative patient, pain should be prevented or treated as rapidly as possible in order to minimize these responses.

If pain persists, adaptation occurs, as the body cannot sustain prolonged sympathetic activation. The signs of sympathetic activation will no longer be present despite the continued presence of pain (Donovan, 1982). Adaptation may be due to parasympathetic system activity, inhibition of the sympathetic system or central inhibition at the level of the spinal cord (Abu-Saad & Tesler, 1986). Signs of parasympathetic stimulation may be seen in the patient with chronic pain in contrast to signs of sympathetic activity (Donovan, 1982).

Another consequence of pain are muscle spasms, which are part of the segmental and suprasegmental reflex responses to pain (Phillips & Cousins, 1986). Segmental reflex responses will be most intense in the areas of the body supplied by the same innervation as the operative site. Muscle spasms will produce pain directly and reduce gastric and renal motility. They also lead to both voluntary and involuntary immobility, the negative consequences of which are detailed in chapter 14. Both the reflex muscle spasms and reflex sympathetic activity elicited by pain have the potential to create a vicious cycle of pain as nociceptors can be further stimulated and sensitized by these reflexes (Zimmerman, 1981; Phillips & Cousins, 1986).

From the perspective of the whole person, pain will affect every aspect of the individual's ability to function and to interact with the environment. In response to pain, the appetite is depressed, the activity level and ability to concentrate are decreased, the normal sleep pattern is altered, social interaction is reduced, and attention may be focused exclusively on the pain (Wall, 1984). The presence of pain can make the patient more vulnerable to the effects of other stressors in the environment and lead to increased levels of anxiety and fear and sensory–perceptual alterations.

ASSESSMENT AND DIAGNOSIS

Concepts basic to assessment of the pain experience include threshold and tolerance. Threshold refers to a point at which some response to a painful stimulus occurs. There are two thresholds relevant to the evaluation of pain. The pain perception threshold is the point of initial response, or when pain is first perceived in response to a noxious stimulus. The severe pain threshold is the point at which pain becomes unbearable. Pain tolerance is measured by the interval between the two thresholds and represents the range of perception between these two points. While the lower threshold (perception) is relatively constant across individuals under laboratory conditions, the upper threshold depends on personal and social factors and, therefore, varies widely, accounting for individual differences in the level of pain tolerance (Bond, 1984).

Because pain is, by its very nature, a subjective, multidimensional experience, subjective indicators of its presence must be considered to be more reliable than objective indicators. Only the patient can indicate the location and radiation, intensity, character, and temporal pattern (duration and chronology) of the pain as well as the factors that precipitate, aggravate, and/or alleviate it. Harrison and Cotanch (1987) state that the following areas should also be included in assessment: the physical, psychological, and emotional causes of pain as well as the availability of support systems and the meaning of the pain to the patient. It is important to know whether the pain is perceived as a threat to life or continued quality and productivity of life by the patient. Additionally, the patient's usual coping style and past patterns of handling pain need to be assessed. This is information that only the patient and family can provide.

The source of the pain may be difficult to assess because of the phenomenon of referred pain. The actual pain sensation is perceived as being in a location different from the actual source of the pain and is a result of shared innervation, i.e., the location and the source of the pain are innervated by the same spinal segment. Examples include angina pectoris and the pain of a myocardial infarction being perceived in the jaw or arm, or an injury to the diaphragm or acute appendicitis or peritonitis presenting with shoulder pain. Headache is a commonly experienced result of the referred pain of temporomandibular joint syndrome (Meinhart & McCaffery, 1983a, 1983b).

Because of the nature of its innervation, visceral pain is diffuse and poorly localized and therefore also difficult to assess. While the organs are not supplied with nociceptors per se, they can respond to the mechanical pressure of distention or swelling. Examples include abdominal pain due to the accumulation of gas and/or fluid in the intestines, or flank pain due to bleeding in the kidney, which stretches the surrounding capsule.

Clinical assessment of pain needs to be regular, systematic, simple and quick, yet reliable, and should incorporate the multidimensional aspects of pain. The purpose of this assessment is to provide a basis for treatment by allowing selection of an appropriate intervention for managing the pain. Various instruments have been developed to make the assessment of this subjective phenomenon, pain, more objective and reliable. Donovan (1987) states that the ideal instrument for such assessment would have to be brief, easy to use, subjective, individualized and holistic.

Syrjala and Chapman (1984) report that there have been three major approaches to instrumentation for measuring pain: quantification of subjective reports, quantification of behaviors or activity that can be attributed to pain, and identification of physiologic correlates of pain. Instruments or tests may provide a measure of one (unidimensional perspective) or a combination of these areas (multidimensional perspective). Self-report scales are examples of simple, unidimensional tools by which the patient can rate the intensity of the pain being experienced. An example of a multidimensional measure of the total pain experience is the McGill Pain Questionnaire. The nurse must determine the best measure to use based on the patient's ability to comprehend and respond to the requirements of the instrument. McGuire (1984) provides a comparison of the properties of various instruments that have been designed to measure pain.

The self-report scales include verbal and nonverbal descriptor scales and visual analog scales. These may represent the most useful type of measure for critically ill patients who often have a decreased attention span and reduced ability to concentrate. They can be used and scored rapidly and easily and would provide a relatively objective means of evaluating the effectiveness of the pain treatment regimen.

The critically ill patient is not always able to communicate expressions of pain (Puntillo, 1988). A major challenge to the critical care nurse is assessment of the presence and amount of pain as well as the effectiveness of treatment for the pain. Since the subjective expression of pain by the critically ill patient is not always possible, the nurse must anticipate pain, interpret pain signals, and rely on less reliable objective indicators of pain. The nurse can use anticipatory information related to the type of surgery the patient has had. For example, pain should be expected in the patient who has had thoracic or abdominal surgery. In contrast, patients who have had intracranial surgery involving the skull and skin may have, at most, moderate pain, while those in whom neck muscles have been dissected (as for posterior fossa exploration) may have severe pain (Dodson, 1985). Severe muscle spasms may follow surgery or trauma to the bony skeleton (Phillips & Cousins, 1986). Often, in order to make the diagnosis of alteration in comfort, the critical care nurse must integrate observations of the patient's movements and facial expressions, blood pressure, and heart and respiratory rates with knowledge about the possible causes of pain in the individual patient (Harrison & Cotanch, 1987).

INTERVENTION AND EVALUATION

The expected outcome for a postoperative patient is complete relief of pain such that the patient indicates that he or she is comfortable. Such a goal is only infrequently attained, however. Donovan (1987) reports that inadequate relief of pain continues to be a major clinical problem. Pharmacologic undertreatment of pain can be partially attributed to clinicians' lack of understanding about tolerance and the differences between physical dependence, psychological dependence, and addiction (Coyle, 1987). The use of drugs with dependence potential in amounts necessary to attain adequate relief from postoperative pain is unlikely to result in addiction (Dodson, 1985; Bryan-Brown, 1986). Another reason for inadequate pain control in the critical care environment is that pain management may not be considered a top priority of care (Bryan-Brown, 1986; Puntillo, 1988). Another expected outcome is that pain relief is achieved without any adverse effects of treatment such as respiratory depression, hypotension, and decreased level of consciousness (Phillips & Cousins, 1986).

Two general categories of interventions for pain relief include pharmacologic and nonpharmacologic methods. Pharmacologic treatment is by far the most widely used approach in the surgical patient, although a combination of analgesic medication with a nonpharmacologic method may be needed by individual patients for the most effective pain relief. Nonpharmacologic methods are summarized in Table 11–2. With the exception of transcutaneous electrical nerve stimulation these methods do not require a physician's order and pose little, if any, risk to the patient (Donovan, 1982). Whipple (1987) includes stimulation-produced analgesia, stress-produced analgesia, acupuncture, and acupressure in a review of pain control interventions.

Table 11–2   Nonpharmacologic Methods for Controlling Pain

Technique	Physiologic Effect	Comments
Cutaneous stimulation Massage TENS* Heat Cold Vibration Mentholated rubs	Stimulates large fibers; modulates pain at SG–T gate in dorsal horn.	Most effective for local and superficial pain. Moderate stimulation is applied using a powder or lotion to minimize friction or a mentholated rub to increase stimulation. Sites of application include over the pain, around the pain, proximal to the pain, trigger points, acupuncture points, contralaterally. See McCaffery, M., & Chan P. (1975).
Auditory stimulation Comedy Music Distraction	Intense stimuli through thalamus, midbrain, and brain stem cause the production of modulating substances (i.e., endorphins and serotonin). Diversion of attention from the pain decreases the aversive nature of the stimulus. The resulting relaxation decreases muscle guarding at the site of the pain.	Most effective when used with headphones. Needs to match patient's taste. Effective for mild to moderate pain.
Breathing techniques	Same as auditory stimuli.	"He–who" breathing most broadly effective. Childbirth education classes are a readily available way to learn some of these techniques.
Relaxation and biofeedback	Increases blood flow and reduces muscle tension, which reduces the concentration of neurotransmitters at the site of pain. Also can be a type of auditory stimulus. May increase endorphins by way of corticol mechanisms.	For specifics, see Donovan, M. I. (1980, 1981).
Imagery and hypnosis	Alters perception of the noxious stimulus in the cerebral cortex. May produce relaxation. May increase endorphins through cortical mechanisms.	For specifics see Barber, J. (1978, 1980). See also Donovan, M. I. (1980, 1981).

*Transcutaneous electrical nerve stimulation.

From "Cancer Pain: You Can Help!" by M. Donovan, 1982, *Nursing Clinics of North America, 17,* p. 718. Copyright 1982 by W. B. Saunders. Reprinted by permission.

Analgesic medication can be classified according to the mode of action. Medications that act by inhibiting prostaglandin synthesis include the nonnarcotic analgesics and the nonsteroidal antiinflammatory drugs (NSAIDs). Aspirin and other NSAIDs inhibit the enzyme cyclooxygenase, which is necessary for the conversion of arachidonic acid in the prostaglandin cascade. This limits the amount of prostaglandin that can be generated. The opioid or narcotic analgesics alter pain perception by binding to the opiate receptors in the central and peripheral nervous system and activating descending inhibitory neurons that inhibit transmission of the impulse at the spinal cord level. The final class of medications, adjuvant analgesic drugs, does not produce analgesia directly but potentiates the effects of other drugs or counteracts their side effects (Coyle, 1987).

The choice of an analgesic most often depends on the intensity of the pain and the metabolic state of the patient. Conditions that can affect the pharmacodynamics and pharmacokinetics of a drug include renal failure, liver disorders, and preexisting drug or alcohol dependency. In the obese patient, absorption of oral medication can be reduced by decreased gastric emptying and absorption of injectable medication can be impaired by injection into fatty tissue. In the elderly patient a variety of conditions exist that can affect pharmacodynamics and pharmacokinetics: decreases in blood flow, protein binding, hepatic and renal function, and the general ability to adapt to physiologic and pathologic changes; increased sensitivity to CNS depressant drugs in target organs; and altered respiratory capacity (Dodson, 1985).

After the choice of the correct medication, decisions regarding the correct timing, dosage, and route of administration must also be made (Donovan, 1982). While many of these decisions are the responsibility of the physician, the effective use of analgesic medications is a responsibility of the nurse, who must exercise clinical judgment in administering the right amount at the right intervals for the most effective pain relief in each patient. The proper amount of medication will need to be assessed for each patient, as every individual will respond differently to analgesic drugs. There is no such thing as an "average" patient. Postoperative pain usually occurs with varying levels of intensity over time and certain activities will cause its exacerbation (Dodson, 1985). Analgesic medication should be administered before pain reaches its most intense level and before activities that will surely increase it. For severe pain, a routine schedule for administration rather than p.r.n. administration may help to control the pain by providing a more even and constant level of analgesia. The goal should be to prevent as well as treat pain (Bryan-Brown, 1986).

For patients experiencing moderate to severe postoperative pain, the most common method of administration of narcotic medication is by intramuscular or intravenous injection (Leib & Hurtig, 1985). The intramuscular method tends to produce a variable pattern rather than a constant level of analgesia. Respiratory depression may be more likely to occur with the high peak plasma levels of opioids caused by intramuscular or bolus IV administration (Dodson, 1985). Continuous intravenous infusion of small amounts of a narcotic allows a more constant serum level of the drug to be maintained, which in turn allows a more constant pattern of analgesia to be achieved. Furthermore, a more constant serum level of narcotic allows a lesser amount of drug to be used, decreasing the risk of development of tolerance and side effects (Harrison and Cotanch, 1987). This method obviously requires close nursing supervision and proper titration of the rate of administration of the drug to alleviate the patient's pain.

Patient-controlled analgesia (PCA) is another innovation, which allows patients to administer increments of medication to themselves. This method gives the patient more control and independence and allows the maintenance of a more constant level of pain control. Lange, Dahn, and Jacobs (1988) report that patients who received PCA used less medication overall and had fewer postoperative complications than a comparable group of thoracotomy patients who received intramuscular injections of analgesic medication. Medication is placed in an intravenous line connected to a button-switch–activated pump. The patient can activate the pump as often as is necessary until a predetermined dosage is reached. When the maximum dose is reached, the pump is deactivated until a preset minimal time period elapses (Paice, 1987). This method of analgesia administration may not be appropriate for many critically ill patients but it does represent a viable treatment option for those who are alert and oriented, such as burn and trauma patients, who often experience significant suffering due to pain (Harrison & Cotanch, 1987).

Another innovation is the direct administration of narcotic medication into the intrathecal and epidural spaces of the spinal cord. This method allows a maximum analgesic effect with minimal central depressant effects. Sensory and motor functions remain intact as well. This method may be the treatment of choice for patients at greatest risk for developing respiratory complications (see chapter 1) after surgery (Dodson, 1985). Contraindications to this method of narcotic administration include local or systemic infection, bleeding or clotting disorders, musculoskeletal or spinal abnormalities, certain preexisting neurological disorders, or inability to provide close, continual monitoring of patients (Leib & Hurtig, 1985). The catheter must be placed by an anesthesiologist.

Fear, anxiety, depression, stress, and fatigue are known to affect the perception of pain negatively. As discussed in section 2 of this book, these feelings can all be the result of or intensified by the critical care environment (Bryan-Brown, 1986; Harrison & Cotanch, 1987). The inability to rest and relax leads to feelings of fatigue and weakness. Cousins and Phillips (1986) propose that pain, anxiety, and sleep deprivation comprise a vicious cycle, which, if uninterrupted, can lead to anger and depression as the patient becomes demoralized and loses confidence in the ability of health care professionals to relieve the pain. These conditions may blunt the mental capacities needed to use such strategies as distraction or imagery to cope with pain.

The creation of an atmosphere conducive to pain relief is an intervention totally within the control of the nurse, but it may be very difficult in the critical care unit (Harrison & Cotanch, 1987). Nevertheless, if pain relief measures are to be maximally effective, critical care nurses must integrate measures for stress and anxiety reduction and promotion of sleep and rest into the plan of care. The design and decor of the critical care unit can be planned to be esthetically pleasing and peaceful as well as functional. Policies and procedures that allow maximum interaction with family, the presence of familiar objects in the environment, and distractions such as television and radio can be useful in promoting an atmosphere conducive to patient comfort.

Donovan (1982) states that the most effective intervention for the relief of pain is a positive approach by the nurse, which conveys to the patient an attitude that the presence of pain is acknowledged and will be treated. The author speculates that this type of approach may be effective because a placebo response is elicited. Studies have demonstrated greater pain relief in patients whose nurses attempted to communicate with them and apply individualized interventions (McMahon & Miller, 1978). A positive approach will also help to minimize anxiety, which may break a cycle of pain anxiety.

Providing information about and offering positive suggestions during treatments and invasive procedures can also be effective in helping the patient control the level of pain being experienced. Positive suggestions can help the patient focus on distractions or relaxation techniques during procedures. Providing information about how to move and how to splint the incision with a hand, pillow, or folded blanket can help patients ease their own pain. The work of Johnson and associates (Horsley, Crane, Reynolds, & Haller, 1981) indicates that patients use sensory and procedural information that is provided to them about a treatment to develop coping strategies for dealing with the event. Geach (1987) recommends viewing the patient as a partner in "pain work" as a means of increasing the patient's understanding of and participation in the treatment of pain.

Another part that the critical care nurse may play in the treatment of pain is that of coordinator of the different disciplines that may become involved in the patient's care. It is generally acknowledged that a multidisciplinary approach to the treatment of complex pain problems is necessary and beneficial. A clinical nurse specialist, clinical pharmacist, anesthesiologist, physical therapist, or clinical psychologist may contribute to the plan of care for a patient with a severe pain problem. The nurse at the bedside may be the only constant in this care and therefore carries the major responsibility for monitoring the patient's response and determining the effectiveness of treatment. The nurse can help to determine whether the currently prescribed analgesic regimen is the most appropriate one for that patient through a synthesis of information based on an understanding of the pharmacokinetics and pharmacodynamics of the drug and assessment of the type and amount of pain the patient is experiencing and the effect of the drug on that pain (Coyle, 1987).

Patients who have been relieved of their pain, even temporarily, will often need acknowledgment that their pain-related behavior was acceptable to others. The role of the nurse is one of support in this situation. At this stage the patient may also be very anxious about the reoccurrence of pain, and the nurse needs to review and reinforce with the patient those strategies that were most helpful in coping with the pain.

SUMMARY

The patient who is experiencing pain becomes vulnerable to the deleterious aspects of the critical care environment and, as a result, it may cease to be a positive force in the patient's recovery process. The critical care nurse has a responsibility to use every means at her or his disposal to alleviate suffering so that healing can proceed.

BIBLIOGRAPHY

Abu-Saad, H., & Tesler, M. (1986). Pain. In V. K. Carrieri, A. M. Lindsey, & C. M. West (Eds.), *Pathophysiological phenomena in nursing: Human responses of illness.* (pp. 235–269). Philadelphia: W. B. Saunders.

Barber, J. (1978). Hypnosis as a psychological technique in the management of cancer pain. *Cancer Nursing, 1,* 361–364.

Barber, J. (1980). Cancer pain: Psychological management using hypnosis. *CA: A Cancer Journal for Clinicians, 30,* 130–136.

Bishop, B. (1980). Pain: Its physiology and rationale for management. *Physical Therapy, 60*(1), 13–35.

Bond, J. J. (1984). *Pain: Its nature, analysis and treatment* (2nd ed.). New York: Churchill-Livingstone.

Bryan-Brown, C. W. (1986). Development of pain management in critical care. In M. Cousins & G. Phillips (Eds.), *Acute pain management* (pp. 1–19). New York: Churchill-Livingstone.

Chapman, R. (1985). Psychological factors in postoperative pain. In G. Smith & B. Covino (Eds.), *Acute pain* (pp. 22–41). London: Butterworth.

Cohen, M., Pickar, D., Dubois, M., Roth, Y., Naber, D., & Bunney, W. (1981). Surgical stress and endorphins. *Lancet, 1,* 213–214.

Coyle, N. (1987). Analgesics and pain. *Nursing Clinics of North America, 22,*(3), 727–741.

Dodson, M. E. (1985). *The management of postoperative pain.* London: Edward Arnold.

Donovan, M. I. (1980). Relaxation with guided imagery: A useful technique. *Cancer Nursing, 3,* 27–32.

Donovan, M. I. (1981). *Cancer care: A guide for patient education.* New York: Appleton-Century-Crofts.

Donovan, M. (1982). Cancer pain: You can help! *Nursing Clinics of North America, 17,* (4), 713–727.

Donovan, M. (1987). Preface to symposium on pain control. *Nursing Clinics of North America, 22*(3), 645–648.

Feinmann, C. (1985). Pain relief by antidepressants: Possible modes of action. *Pain, 23,* 1–8.

Geach, B. (1987). Pain and coping. *Image, 19*(1), 12–15.

Gershon, S. (1986). Chronic pain: Hypothesized mechanism and rationale for treatment., *Neuropsychobiology, 15,* Suppl. 1, 22–27.

Harrison, M., & Cotanch, P. H. (1987). Pain: Advances and issues in critical care. *Nursing Clinics of North America, 22*(3), 691–697.

Horsley, J., Crane, J., Reynolds, M., & Haller, K. (1981). *Preoperative sensory preparation to promote recovery.* New York: Grune & Stratton.

Ignelzi, R. J., & Atkinson, J. H. (1980). Pain and its modulation. *Neurosurgery, 6*(5), 577–590.

Lange, M. P. Dahn, M. S., & Jacobs, L. A. (1988). Patient controlled analgesia versus intermittent analgesia dosing. *Heart and Lung, 17*(5), 495–498.

Leib, R. A., & Hurtig, J. B. (1985). Epidural and intrathecal narcotics for pain management. *Heart and Lung, 14*(2), 164–174.

Levine, J., Gordon, N., & Fields, H. (1978). Evidence that the analgesic effect of placebo is mediated by endorphins. In *Pain abstract, 1.* Seattle: International Association for the Study of Pain.

Lewith, G. T., & Kenyon, J. N. (1984). Physiological and psychological explanations for the mechanism of acupuncture as a treatment for chronic pain. *Social Science and Medicine, 19*(12), 1367–1378.

McCaffery, M. (1979). *Nursing managment of the patient with pain.* (2nd ed.). Philadelphia: J. B. Lippincott.

McGuire, D. B. (1984). The measurement of clinical pain. *Nursing Research, 33*(3), 152–156.

McMahon, M. A., & Miller, Sr. P. (1978). Pain response: The influence of psycho-social-cultural factors. *Nursing Forum, 17*(1), 59–71.

Meinhart, N., & McCaffery, M. (1983a). Neurophysiological aspects. In N. Meinhart & M. McCaffery, *Pain: A nursing approach to assessment and analysis,* (pp. 27–89). Norwalk, CT: Appleton-Century-Crofts.

Meinhart, N., & McCaffery, M. (1983b). Pain syndromes. In N. Meinhart & M. McCaffery, *Pain: A nursing approach to assessment and analysis,* (pp. 213–241). Norwalk, CT: Appleton-Century-Crofts.

Melzack, R., & Wall, D. D. (1982). *The Challenge of pain.* New York: Penguin Books.

Millan, M. J. (1986). Multiple opioid systems and pain. *Pain, 27,* 303–347.

Paice, J. (1987). New delivery systems in pain management. *Nursing Clinics of North America, 22*(3), 715–726.

Phillips, G. D., & Cousins, M. J. (1986). Neurological mechanisms of pain and the relationship of pain, anxiety and sleep. In M. Cousins, & G. Phillips (Eds.), *Acute pain management,* (pp. 21–48). New York: Churchill-Livingstone.

Puntillo, K. A. (1988). The phenomenon of pain and critical care nursing. *Heart and Lung, 17*(3), 262–273.

Smith, G., & Covino, B. (Eds.) (1985). *Acute pain.* London: Butterworth.

Smith, T. W. (1985). The mechanisms of pain and opiod-induced analgesia. *Molecular Aspects of Medicine, 7,* 509–545.

Sternbach, R. A. (Ed.). (1978). *The psychology of pain.* New York: Raven Press.

Syrjala, K. L., & Chapman, C. R. (1984). Measurement of clinical pain: A review and integration of research findings. In C. Benedetti, C. R. Chapman, & G. Morricca, *Advances in pain research and therapy, 7* (pp. 71–101). New York: Raven Press.

Terman, G., Lewis, W., James, W., & Liebeskind, J. C. (1984). Endogenous pain inhibitory substrates and mechanisms. In C. Benedetti, C. R. Chapman, & G. Morricca, *Advances in pain research and therapy, 7* (pp. 43–56). New York: Raven Press.

Wall, P. D. (1984). Neurophysiology of acute and chronic pain. In C. Benedetti, C. R. Chapman, & G. Morricca, *Advances in pain research and therapy, 7* (pp. 13–25). New York: Raven Press.

Whipple, B. (1987). Methods of pain control: Review of research and literature. *Image, 19*(3), 142–146.

Yaksh, T. L., Howe, J. R., & Harty, G. J. (1984). Pharmacology of spinal pain modulatory systems. *Advances in Pain Research and Therapy, 7,* 57–70.

Zimmerman, M. (1981). Physiological mechanisms of pain and pain therapy, *Triangle, 20*(1/2), 7–18.

ADDITIONAL READINGS

Brown, R. M., & Pinkert, T. M. (1983). Mechanisms of pain and analgesia as revealed by opiate research: Summary and recommendations. *National Institute of Drug Abuse Research Monograph Series, 45,* 70–75.

Carron, H. (1981). Current concepts of pain mechanisms. *Urological Surveys, 31*(1), 1–2.

Dickenson, A. H. (1986). A new approach to pain relief? *Nature, 320,* 681–682.

Heft, M. W., & Parker, S. R. (1984). An experimental basis for revising the graphic rating scale for pain. *Pain, 19,* 153–161.

Jacox, A. (1977). *Pain: A source book for nurses and other health professionals.* Boston: Little, Brown.

McCaffery, M., & Chan P. (1975). *Finger acupressure.* Los Angeles: Price-Stern-Sloan.

Melzack, R. (1983). Concepts of pain measurement. In. R. Melzack (Ed.), *Pain measurement and assessment,* (pp. 1–5). New York: Raven Press.

Melzack, R., & Loeser, J. D. (1978). Phantom body pain in paraplegics: Evidence for a central "pattern generating mechanism." *Pain 4,* 195–210.

Radwin, L. (1989). Cues and strategies used in the diagnosis of pain conditions. In R. M. Carroll-Johnson (Ed). *Classification of nursing diagnosis: Proceedings of the eighth conference North American Nursing Diagnosis Association.* Philadelphia: J. B Lippincott Co. 381–387.

Ruch, T. C. (1979). Pathophysiology of pain. In T. Rush & H. Patton (Eds.), *Howell-Fulton-physiology and biophysics: The brain and neural function* (20th ed.), (pp. 272–324). Philadelphia: W. B Saunders.

Wall, P. D. (1978). The gate control theory of pain mechanisms: A reexamination and restatement. *Brain, 101,* 1–18.

Wall, P. D., & Melzack, R. (Eds.). (1984). *Textbook of pain.* New York: Churchill-Livingstone.

Alterations in Thermoregulation

12

Kim Litwack, Ph.D., R.N.
Lisa Mendelson, M.S., R.N.

Hyperthermia and hypothermia are common problems experienced by the hospitalized, critically ill, surgical patient. The increase or decrease in temperature is not the challenge facing either the patient or the nurse; it is the outcome of the alterations in temperature and the physiologic sequelae, including changes in metabolism, oxygenation, and cardiac and cerebral function. It is the purpose of this chapter to discuss alterations in thermoregulation, specifically focusing on hypothermia and hyperthermia, and to address nursing interventions specific to their management.

THERMOREGULATION

There are three basic components of the thermoregulatory system: the afferent system, the efferent system, and a neuronal control network. Each contributes to the maintenance of a normothermic state.

Afferent System

The afferent system is comprised of thermosensors, designed to sense increasing and decreasing temperature levels. Peripheral sensors, located in the cutaneous tissues of the fingertips and circumoral areas, and central sensors, located in the anterior hypothalamus, serve to activate the hypothalamic temperature-regulating centers.

Efferent System

The efferent components of thermoregulation serve as heat-generating and heat-dissipating mechanisms. Through reflex and semireflex thermoregulatory responses, including autonomic, somatic, endocrine, and behavioral changes, heat loss may be maximized or minimized, and heat production may be increased or decreased.

In response to cold temperatures, the body's response is to increase heat production and to minimize heat loss. Mechanisms designed to increase heat production include shivering (increasing metabolic activity), hunger (increasing intake of food energy sources), increase in voluntary activity (increasing muscle contraction), and increased secretion of catecholamines (increasing metabolism).

Heat, or chemical energy, is generated through a series of chemical reactions. This energy is the outcome of the metabolism of nutrients, specifically fats, proteins, and carbohydrates. Energy may be generated by means of glycolysis, the tricarboxylic acid cycle (TCA or Kreb's cycle), and gluconeogenesis. In addition to increasing heat production, the efferent system serves to decrease further heat loss via peripheral cutaneous vasoconstriction (shunting blood centrally), positioning (curling up), and horripilation ("goose bumps").

When faced with increased temperatures, the body responds by decreasing heat production and by increasing heat loss. Mechanisms designed to decrease heat production include anorexia (decreasing availability of food energy) and apathy and inertia (decreasing metabolic demand). In efforts to maximize heat loss, the body responds via peripheral cutaneous vasodilatation, sweating, and by increasing the respiratory rate (Flacke & Flacke, 1983).

Neuronal Control Network

In addition to afferent and efferent mechanisms for temperature regulation, there exists a neuronal control mechanism for integrating sensations of temperature changes; it is located in the hypothalamus, specifically, the preoptic anterior hypothalamus. Neurons located within the hypothalamus and spinal cord act as sensors to respond to internal and external environmental temperatures. When deviations from normal are sensed, the body responds by dissipating or by producing heat (Davis & Murphy, 1985). It is a negative-feedback system, as a rise in central temperature initiates mechanisms for losing heat while a fall in central temperature activates mechanisms for heat production and heat conservation.

Heat dissipation begins when the central temperature rises above 37.1°C (98.8°F), and increases sharply as central temperature increases. For every increase of 0.5°C in central temperature, heat loss is quadrupled, from about 20 to nearly 80 calories per second. Mechanisms of heat dissipation are initiated only with increases in central (core) temperature. Peripheral skin temperature has little influence.

Heat generation, in contrast, occurs with falling central temperatures and with falling skin temperatures. Unlike heat dissipation, skin temperature affects both the internal temperature at which heat generation begins and the magnitude of increase in heat generation per degree of fall of central temperature (Flacke & Flacke, 1983).

The goal of the hypothalamic regulatory center is to maintain a normothermic or euthermic state. Maintenance of a euthermic state optimizes energy consumption, metabolism, and assists in the maintenance of a normal acid–base balance.

Assessment

Temperature monitoring may reflect central (core) temperature or noncentral (peripheral) temperature. Central temperature reflects the temperature of blood flowing by the temperature-sensitive center of the hypothalamus. Currently, there are four sites used to reflect the central temperature: the tympanic membrane, the nasopharynx, the lower one third of the esophagus, and the pulmonary artery. The tympanic membrane and the nasopharynx reflect blood temperature of the internal carotid artery and its branches. The lower esophagus reflects blood temperature of the aorta. Pulmonary artery temperature monitoring is not the primary use of a Swan–Ganz catheter, but is useful in ongoing measurement of central temperature.

Noncentral temperature monitoring may be done rectally or via the axilla, skin, or oropharynx. Each has specific advantages and limitations that may apply in the critical care setting. Although noncentral temperature monitoring does not measure core temperature, it is useful to measure relative changes in body temperature. The advantages and disadvantages of various sites of temperature monitoring are identified in Table 12–1.

HYPOTHERMIA

Hypothermia is a condition marked by an abnormally low internal body temperature, typically below 96°F (35.5°C), that occurs when systemic heat loss exceeds heat production. Although patients may present to an emergency room in deep hypothermia (28°C), or may have deep hypothermia induced intentionally in an operating room setting (i.e., cardiac surgical procedures), it is likely that the nurse in a surgical critical care unit will face patients experiencing mild to moderate hypothermia (33 to 36°C). Results of a survey of 85 nurses conducted by Johnson (1989) indicate that nurses working in recovery room, intensive care and with neonates indicated that hypothermia is a relevant nursing diagnosis in their daily practice.

It is the patient's interaction with the environment that determines the degree of heat loss. The four main factors responsible for heat loss are radiation, convection, conduction, and evaporation.

Table 12–1   Comparison of Various Sites of Temperature Monitoring

Site	Advantages	Disadvantages
Rectal	Good with intubated patients Good with confused patients Good with all ages	Requires lubrication Risk of infection Varies with blood flow after peritoneal lavage, cystoscopy irrigation, after replacement of bowel into abdomen, and with hypoperfused bowel Cannot use with gastrointestinal bleeding, diarrhea, hemorrhoids, rectal surgery Risk of perforation
Skin	Noninvasive Good with children Disposable sensors Approximates core temperature, as forehead remains well perfused in hypothermic states	Varies with subcutaneous blood flow Sensors costly Difficult with diaphoretic patients
Axilla	Noninvasive Good with intubated patients Useful with all ages Good with agitated patients	Varies with blood flow/position, i.e., abduction and with cold peripheral IV fluids
Oropharynx	Accepted well by patients Convenient Requires no position changes Approximates core temperature when obtained in posterior sublinqual pocket	Reflects temperature of atmospheric gases Not good for agitated or obtunded patients Difficult after oral surgery or trauma Not used with infants

Radiation

Radiant heat loss is defined as the transfer of thermal or heat energy between objects in space through a process that depends only on the absolute temperature and nature of the radiating surfaces. Heat is transferred from a warm or hot surface, (i.e., the body) to a cooler one (the environment) through a vacuum, and does not require that the two surfaces be in contact with one another (Litwack, 1987). Radiant heat loss accounts for approximately 60% of heat lost to the environment, and is especially profound in neonates, the debilitated, and the elderly.

Convection

Most heat is lost from the surface of the body by convection, the transfer of heat to a fluid or gaseous medium. Heat loss by convection depends on the existence of a temperature gradient between the body surface and the ambient air (Petersdorf, 1974).

Convective heat transfer by the bloodstream to the skin is of vital physiologic importance and is under the control of the sympathetic nervous system. Convective heat transfer allows for dissipation of heat via vasodilatation and an increase in cutaneous blood flow. Convection may also prove protective, for with increasing hypothermia, cutaneous vasoconstriction prevents and diminishes further heat loss. Convective heat loss may occur in the operating room setting, particularly in laminar air-flow rooms, contributing to the hypothermia that may exist in the patient admitted to the critical care unit.

Conduction

Conduction refers to the transfer of heat by direct contact with a stable medium. Heat is conducted from deep body tissues to the skin surface, and from the skin to the air surrounding the body. The direction of heat flow is always toward the lower temperature.

Heat may be lost via conduction from a warm body to a cool operating room table, cool sheets, or drapes. Heating blankets may prevent or decrease conductive heat loss, but adds the responsibility of protecting the patient from thermal injury.

The resistance to conduction of heat from the internal organs to the skin is important physiologically. Fatty tissue acts as an insulator, preventing heat loss to the environment and, likewise, protecting the body from colder temperatures. Patients with minimal subcutaneous fat may be at greater risk for conductive heat loss.

Evaporation

Evaporation involves the transfer of heat that results when a liquid changes to a gas. Evaporation occurs when ambient temperature exceeds that of the body, and water is converted to water vapor. Evaporative heat loss may occur via perspiration (febrile or hypermetabolic states) or via respiration. Vaporization accounts for the loss of approximately 0.6 kcal of heat per gram of water.

Patient Characteristics

Although it is difficult to evaluate the true incidence of hypothermia, it is possible to identify patients at risk. The elderly patient in a poor state of nutrition and/or health is at risk for development of hypothermia on exposure. Elderly people may become hypothermic even with room temperatures set in the range of 60 to 70°F (Davis & Murphy, 1985). The intoxicated individual is at risk of accelerated heat loss that is associated with peripheral vasodilatation, depression of the heat-production center, and alteration of the temperature coefficient of the blood. The neonate is at risk because of an immature temperature-regulation center (Abels, 1986). Patients on medications, such as nonsteroidal antiinflammatory drugs and vasodilators, may also be at risk of hypothermia due to vasodilatation. General anesthetics do not induce hypothermia; they only depress the temperature regulatory system (Orkin & Cooperman, 1983). Accidental hypothermia has also been found in association with myxedema, pituitary insufficiency, Addison's disease, hypoglycemia, cerebrovascular disease, myocardial infarction, terminal cirrhosis, and pancreatitis (Petersdorf, 1974). Nurses surveyed by Johnson (1989) identified the most frequent causes of hypothermia as procedures that lead to exposed/uncovered body surfaces, changes in environmental temperature, circulatory and central nervous system pathology, and medications.

Assessment

Before hypothermia can be diagnosed the nurse must complete a patient assessment. The taking of a temperature provides a value, but it does not address the additional signs and symptoms that may be present and that may contribute to the morbidity of the hypothermic patient.

Prompt diagnosis of hypothermia is imperative to prevent the associated consequences of lowered body temperatures. Hypothermia results in decreased oxygen availability, by shifting the oxyhemoglobin dissociation curve to the left, therefore binding oxygen more tightly to hemoglobin. Shivering, associated with hypothermia, increases oxygen demand by 400 to 500% (Vaughn, 1984). Vasoconstricted tissues contribute to the development of metabolic acidosis. Many critically ill patients are already experiencing oxygen deficits and acid–base abnormalities due to cardiac and/or respiratory insufficiencies.

Hypothermia slows metabolically dependent processes, and may decrease drug biotransformation. Peripheral vasoconstriction makes subcutaneous and intramuscular medication administration unpredictable. Renal transport processes are also impaired, with a decrease in glomerular filtration rate. Gastrointestinal function is depressed and may result in the development of a paralytic ileus. Cardiac rate and rhythm disturbances may occur. Central nervous system depression may be profound, and may present as coma. Hyperglycemia is common because of the need for increased energy (Julien, 1986). Clinical signs and symptoms of hypothermia may be localized or generalized.

Localized Hypothermia

Localized hypothermia begins with a feeling of numbness and loss of sensation. The skin is initially white, then becomes erythematous and edematous. If exposure is not curtailed, frostbite will result, manifested by the formation of blisters and bullae, necrosis of tissue, and eventual gangrene (Davis & Murphy, 1985).

Localized hypothermia may be used clinically and intentionally. Two examples include selective destruction by freezing in cryosurgery and preservation of biological material. Cryogenic surgery has the advantages of safety and hemostasis. The preservation of red blood cells, spermatozoa, and other viable material by low temperature has become possible through the use of glycerol to protect cells from freezing. Hypothermia combined with hyperbaric oxygenation has been used to preserve organs, e.g., kidneys, for transplantation (Petersdorf, 1974).

Generalized Hypothermia

Generalized hypothermia results when core body temperature falls below 35°C (95°F). Patients will present with pallor and skin discoloration. Skin will be cool and dry to the touch. Patients may be shivering. It is not uncommon to find miotic pupils, slow, shallow respirations, and bradycardia. The most commonly identified defining characteristics identified by nurses surveyed by Johnson (1989) included cool skin, temperature less than 96°F, mottling, pallor, sluggish reflexes and decreased pulse. If severe, or allowed to continue, patients may become hypotensive and metabolic acidosis and ventricular dysrhythmias, most notably ventricular fibrillation, may develop. Unconsciousness and death may ensue.

As with intentional localized hypothermia, generalized hypothermia may be induced intraoperatively to permit surgical intervention to the heart and brain. Hypothermia may be induced via light anesthesia and surface cooling, or more effectively, via a pump oxygenator to provide extracorporeal circulation (Petersdorf, 1974).

Treatment of Hypothermia

Immediate care of the hypothermic patient is passive rewarming. The goal of passive rewarming is to maximize basal heat production (Abels, 1986). Wet, cold clothing and/or sheets should be removed. Warm, dry clothing and blankets should be wrapped around patients. If possible the ambient temperature should be increased. Most passive rewarming occurs outside of a medical setting or is used in conjunction with active rewarming.

Active rewarming may include external or internal techniques (Phillips & Skov, 1988). The use of active external rewarming, including the use of heated blankets, and immersion baths, is somewhat controversial. Peripheral vasodilatation occurs with external rewarming and may result in a paradoxical central cooling by shunting stagnant cold blood to the core. The myocardium becomes increasingly chilled, which may increase the likelihood of dysrhythmias (Abels, 1986). Peripheral vasodilatation may also precipitate hypovolemia as circulating blood volume pools peripherally.

Active core rewarming involves specific internal rewarming techniques and supportive therapy to keep the patient viable during rewarming. Core rewarming may include use of warmed intravenous fluids, warmed gastric lavage, inhalation of warmed, humidified oxygen, hemodialysis, peritoneal dialysis, and extracorporeal blood warming.

Supportive measures during rewarming include ongoing temperature monitoring, and intensive cardiorespiratory monitoring. ECG abnormalities are common, including atrial fibrillation and atrial flutter. If hypoxemia is present, ventricular dysrhythmias may occur. Oxygen therapy is mandated in the hypothermic patient, for shivering may increase myocardial oxygen demand by 400 to 500% (Vaughn, 1984).

Prevention of Hypothermia

Inherent in any discussion of hypothermia is the need to talk about prevention. The hazards of hypothermia can be prevented with attention and prophylactic intervention on the part of nurses. Obviously, ongoing temperature monitoring is imperative. In instances in which the probability of temperature loss is high, the ambient room temperature should be increased to prevent radiant and convective heat loss. The patient can be covered with warm blankets to reduce heat loss through exposure.

Cleansing solutions, intravenous fluids, irrigating solutions, and blood products may be warmed prior to use to prevent internal cooling. While a microwave oven is useful in warming fluids to 39°C (2 minutes on high power, 600 watts) microwave warming of blood products has been found to cause hemolysis and is therefore not recommended (Burchman, Datta, & Ostheimer, 1989).

Inspired oxygen and anesthetic gases can be warmed and humidified during use. Other techniques designed to prevent hypothermia include use of an esophageal thermal tube, heating mattress (Hoachimsson, Hedstrand, Tabow, & Hansson, 1987), and heated humidifier (Abels, 1986).

HYPERTHERMIA

Hyperthermia (fever) is defined as a state in which the core body temperature rises because of a storage of excessive heat (Groer & Shekleton, 1989). Increases in temperature may be attributed to a number of disease states and/or drugs. All infections, whether caused by bacteria, rickettsias, viruses, or parasites, cause fever. Mechanical trauma, e.g., a crush injury, frequently gives rise to fever. Infection is a common sequela of trauma. Many neoplastic diseases are associated with fever. Fever in these cases may be due to obstruction or infection produced by the tumor, or may be due to necrosis of tissue caused by chemotherapy. Tumors associated with fever include hypernephroma; carcinoma of the pancreas, lung, and bone; and hepatoma. Hematopoietic disorders, e.g., an acute hemolytic reaction, are characterized by fever. Ischemic injuries, e.g., myocardial, pulmonary, and cerebral infarctions, nearly always cause fever due to tissue necrosis. Acute metabolic disorders, such as thyroid crisis or addisonian crisis, are often associated with fever

(Petersdorf, 1974). There are a number of drugs, as well, that have been associated with fever.

The pathophysiologic mechanism for hyperthermia is unclear, but it is believed to be the result of an action on the temperature-regulating center in the hypothalamus (Abels, 1986). During hyperthermia, the body temperature increases and overrides the body's ability to lose heat. The increased heat is a response to a pyrogen, defined as a fever-producing substance. Foreign substances, such as viruses, bacteria, antigen–antibody complexes, and endotoxins, serve as sources of exogenous pyrogens. These agents or their by-products are pyrogenic in the body, and initiate a series of reactions that result in fever. First, phagocytic leukocytes are stimulated to produce endogenous pyrogens. This endogenous pyrogen circulates to the hypothalamus, stimulating the thermosensitive neurons to produce fever. The thermoregulatory center is then "reset," with the increased temperature being sensed as the new normal body temperature. Heat is then generated by shivering and peripheral vasoconstriction (Davis & Murphy, 1985).

The outcome of the increased temperature and heat generation have consequences that can negatively affect the critically ill patient, which include increased myocardial oxygen demand, increased work of breathing, increased cardiac workload, respiratory/metabolic acidosis, hypovolemia, and hypoglycemia. If not treated successfully, hyperthermia may result in death. Assessment must be thorough and intervention prompt.

Assessment

In addition to confirming the presence of an increased temperature, the hyperthermic patient will likely present with a number of additional clinical signs and symptoms, including weakness, hypotension, dizziness, tachycardia, headache, tachypnea, anorexia, and mydriasis. A patient presenting with these clinical signs should be further evaluated to locate the source of the elevated temperature. A fever workup should include physical examination; a medical history; laboratory tests, such as cultures of the blood, urine, and cerebrospinal fluid, determination of serum enzymes, particularly alkaline phosphatase and enzymes that measure hepatocellular function, blood smears, and bone marrow examination (when indicated); and chest roetgenograms.

When the source or site of infection cannot be located, additional tests may be employed, including radioactive scans, biopsies, exploratory laparotomy, and therapeutic antibiotic trials (Petersdorf, 1974). As infections and hemolytic and drug reactions are the most common causes of fever in the critically ill surgical patient, each will be discussed in greater detail.

Drug-Induced Hyperthermia

Drug-induced hyperthermia is responsible for approximately 10% of elevated temperatures in hospitalized patients (Cunha, 1986). Drug fever is an allergic or hypersensitive reaction to a medication. Drugs commonly implicated in producing fever are listed in Table 2–2.

The mechanism of drug-induced hyperthermia is not fully understood. The patient with a drug-induced fever will have a temperature of 102°F or above with bradycardia (Cunha, 1986). Once the drug causing the fever is discontinued, the temperature will return to normal within 72 hours. Acute temperature elevations and hypersensitivity reactions are managed with antipyretics and antihistamines.

Malignant Hyperthermia

Malignant hyperthermia is another pharmacogenic disorder. Triggering agents cause a release of intracellular calcium from the sarcoplasmic reticulum. This release of calcium is responsible for initiating a hypermetabolic state, characterized by tachycardia, hypoxemia, muscle rigidity, increased serum potassium, labile blood pressure, and dysrhythmias. Glucose and oxygen demands increase, promoting respiratory and metabolic acidosis. An unstable, hypoperfused myocardium can progress to circulatory collapse. The hypermetabolism causes elevations in temperature that may be as great as 1° every 5 minutes. Myoglobinuria is the outcome of prolonged muscular rigidity and may ultimately contribute to renal failure (Groer and Shekleton, 1989).

Malignant hyperthermia is considered to be an acute anesthetic event. It may be triggered by inhalation agents (fluothane, enflurane, or isoflurane),

Table 12–2   Medications Implicated in Drug Fever

Commonly	Frequently	Rarely, if ever
Antiarrhythmics	Allopurinol (Lopurin,	Antacids
Antibiotics*	Zyloprim)	Corticosteroids
Antihypertensives	Amphetamines	Digoxin (Lanoxin)
Antiseizure medications	Anticholinergics	Diphenhydramine
Barbiturates	Antiemetics	(Benadryl)
Diuretics	Antituberculosis drugs	Fibrinolytic agents
Narcotics	Antitumor drugs	Insulin
Sleep medications	Nonsteroidal antiinflam-	Oral contraceptives
Sulfonamide-containing	matory drugs	Salicylates†
laxatives	Thyroid medications	Vitamin preparations

*Except tetracyclines, erythromycin, clindamycin (Cleocin), aminoglycosides, chloramphenicol (Chloromycetin), vancomycin (Vancocin).
†May, in overdosage, induce very high fever.

From "Drug Fever" by B. Cunha, 1986, *Postgraduate Medicine, 80*(5), p. 124. Copyright 1986 by McGraw Hill, Salem, Massachusetts. Reprinted by permission.

succinylcholine, or ketamine—all anesthetic drugs. It is therefore imperative that anesthesiologists, and nurses responsible for the care of the postanesthetic patient, are able to recognize promptly and intervene immediately in cases of malignant hyperthermia.

Management includes discontinuation of all drugs, and hyperventilation with 100% oxygen. Metabolic acidosis is corrected with sodium bicarbonate. Tachycardia is treated with propranolol. Hypoglycemia and hyperkalemia are corrected with intravenous insulin and glucose, respectively. Myoglobinuria is managed with fluids and diuretics, administration of which is designed to "flush" the kidneys. Hyperthermia is treated with cooling through the use of antipyretic medications, lavage, and if severe, cardiopulmonary bypass. The interventions mentioned thus far are designed to treat symptoms of malignant hyperthermia. It is also important to treat the cause (calcium release). Dantrolene sodium (2.5 to 10 mg/kg) is given intravenously. Dantrolene sodium directly inhibits the release of intracellular calcium, halting the entire process.

Infection-Induced Hyperthermia

Bacterial

The leading cause of fevers of acute onset are bacterial infections. Bacteria cause fever because of the release of exotoxins by the microorganism. The exotoxins inhibit oxidative processes and protein synthesis within cells. Gram-negative bacteria can cause cell injury by the elaboration of endotoxins, the byproduct of bacterial cell death (Robbins, 1974). Identified in Table 12–3 are common bacteria that cause disease in humans.

Bacterial infections may present in the lungs, urinary tract, gastrointestinal tract, cerebrospinal fluid, bone, blood, skin, and heart. Sites of infections must be cultured, and antibiotic sensitivity determined. Treatment includes drug therapy and symptomatic care.

Table 12–3   Common Bacterial Infectious Agents

Gram-Positive	Gram-Negative
Staphylococcus aureus	Pseudomonas aeruginosa
Streptococci	Klebsiella enterobacter
Neisseria	Proteus
Clostridium	Escherichia coli
Mycobacterium	Salmonella
	Hemophilus
	Shigella

Viral

Viruses are difficult to culture and identify as sources of infection. Viruses act as exogenous pyrogens and may destroy cellular integrity in two ways. Viruses enter and survive in host cells by subverting the metabolism of the host for their own survival and growth requirements. Host cells are deprived of essential nutrients and are injured or die. Additionally, viruses within cells replicate rapidly within the cytoplasm of the cell, leaving only a destroyed carcass. The products of the dead cell constitute a source of injury to contiguous healthy cells. Viral ribonucleic acid (RNA) or deoxyribonucleic acid (DNA) may become incorporated into the genome of the host cell. The cellular transformation may result in cellular growth and viral replication or cell death (Robbins, 1974). Viral infections have been found in the gastrointestinal tract, respiratory tract, cerebrospinal fluid, blood, skin, and myocardium. Table 12–4 identifies commonly occurring viral infections. Viral infections are usually self-limiting, requiring only symptomatic management.

Fungal

While fungal infections have not been a major clinical problem in the United States, their incidence and accompanying morbidity and mortality have been steadily increasing. Fungal infections present as opportunistic infections in patients debilitated by malignancies, lymphomas, and leukemias. Additionally, patients treated with total body irradiation, immunosuppressive or cytotoxic drugs, and/or prolonged broad-spectrum antibiotic therapy as well as those suffering immune system dysfunction are at an increased risk for opportunistic infections.

Damage to cells is the result of an allergic necrosis caused by a progressive sensitization to fungal proteins. Febrile reactions are the outcome of the process of necrosis of tissue. Table 12–5 identifies common fungal infectious agents and their primary site(s) of infection.

Hemolytic-Induced Hyperthermia

A cardinal sign of an acute transfusion reaction is an elevation in body temperature. Transfusion reactions may present as allergic reactions, febrile reac-

Table 12–4 Common Viral Infectious Agents

Herpesviruses (including cytomegalovirus)

Adenoviruses

Papovavirus

Picornaviruses (including coxsackieviruses)

Myxoviruses (including influenza viruses)

Arbovirus

Hepatitis (including A, B, and C [non-A, non-B])

Table 12–5   Common Fungal Infectious Agents

Candida albicans (mucocutaneous/visceral)

Monosporium apiospermum (skin/subcutaneous tissue)

Sporotrichum schenckii (lymphatics)

Histoplasma capsulatum (respiratory)

Coccidioides immitis (respiratory)

Blastomyces dermatitidis (skin/viscera)

Aspergillus fumigatus (respiratory)

Cryptococcus neoformans (brain)

Actinomyces isrealii (mucocutaneous)

tions, or as acute hemolytic reactions. The increase in temperature may also be accompanied by urticaria, pruritus, chills, and tachycardia. Regardless of the type of reaction, the nursing orders are identical: STOP the transfusion; keep the IV open with 0.9% normal saline; and notify the physician and the blood bank (Litwack, 1987).

Treatment of Hyperthermia

Correction of hyperthermia requires treatment of both the cause (infection, atelectasis, hemolysis, etc.) and the symptom (increased temperature). Treatment of the causes of hyperthermia have been identified previously in this and other chapters. Treatment of the increased temperature includes cooling (light covering, sponge baths, ice packs to axillae and groin) and antipyretic therapy, including salicylates (ASA), acetaminophen (Tylenol) and nonsteroidal antiinflammatory agents (ibuprofen) (Davis & Murphy, 1985). The use of antipyretics as therapy is controversial, and many advocate their use only if clinically warranted, e.g., for symptomatic relief and comfort. Those against using antipyretics cite research that shows that bacterial growth is inhibited at higher temperatures. Additionally, antipyretics may mask the effects of antibiotic therapy and the course of the infection (Pierce, 1986).

SUMMARY

Hyperthermia and hypothermia will remain common problems of the hospitalized surgical patient, and therefore of the critical care nurse. Treatment of the patient experiencing alterations in thermoregulation includes prompt and ongoing assessment. It is not the change in temperature that presents the challenge but, rather, the physiologic sequelae that require prompt intervention. Changes in temperature affect metabolism and oxygenation, which may further complicate the condition(s) that caused the admission of the patient into the intensive care unit.

BIBLIOGRAPHY

Abels, L. (1986). *Critical care nursing.* St. Louis: C. V. Mosby.

Burchman, C., Datta, S. and Ostheimer, G. (1989). Delivery temperature of heated intravenous solutions during rapid infusion. *Journal of Clinical Anesthesia 1*(4), 259–261.

Cunha, B. (1986). Drug fever. *Postgraduate Medicine 80*(5), 124.

Davis, A., & Murphy, M. (1985). Alterations in body temperature. In M. Wiener and G. Pepper (Eds.). *Clinical pharmacology and therapeutics in nursing* (pp. 245–254). New York: McGraw-Hill.

Flacke, W., & Flacke, J. (1983). Alterations in temperature regulation. In F. Orkin and L. Cooperman (Eds.). *Complications in anesthesiology* (pp. 277–284). Philadelphia: J. B. Lippincott.

Groer, M., & Shekleton, M. (1989). *Basic pathophysiology: A holistic approach* (3rd ed.). St. Louis: C. V. Mosby.

Hoachimsson, P., Hedstrand, V., Tabow, F., & Hansson, B. (1987). Prevention of intra-operative hypothermia during abdominal surgery. *Acta Anaethesiologica Scandinavica, 31*(4), 339–7.

Johnson, S. E. (1989). Alteration in temperature regulation: Hypothermia. In R. M. Carroll-Johnson (Ed.). *Classification of nursing diagnoses: Proceedings of the eighth conference North American Nursing Diagnosis Association.* Philadelphia: J. B. Lippincott Co., pp. 378–380.

Julien, R. (1986). *Understanding anesthesia.* Menlo Park, CA: Addison-Wesley.

Litwack, K. (1987). Practical points in the management of hypothermia. *Journal of Post Anesthesia Nursing, 3*(5), 339–341.

Orkin, F., & Cooperman, L. (1983). *Complications in Anesthesiology.* Philadelphia: Lippincott.

Petersdorf, R. (1974). Chills and fever. In M. Wintrobe, G. Thorn, R. Adams, E. Braunwald, K. Isselbacher, & R. Petersdorf, *Harrison's principles of internal medicine* (7th ed.) (pp. 55–63). New York: McGraw-Hill.

Phillips, R., & Skov, P. (1988). Rewarming and cardiac surgery: A review. *Heart and Lung, 17*(5), 511–520.

Pierce, N. (1986). Undifferentiated acute febrile illness. In L. Barker, J. Burton, & P. Zieve, *Principles of ambulatory medicine* (2nd ed.) (pp. 311–316). Baltimore: Williams & Wilkins.

Robbins, S. (1974). *Pathologic basis of disease.* Philadelphia: W. B. Saunders.

Vaughn, M. (1984). Shivering in the recovery room. *Current Reviews for Recovery Room Nurses, 6*(1), 18–25.

ADDITIONAL READINGS

Biddle, C. (1985). Hypothermia: Implications for the critical care nurse. *Critical Care Nurse, 5*(2), 34–38.

Closs, S. J., Macdonald, I. A., & Hawthorn, P. J. (1986). Factors affecting perioperative body temperature. *Journal of Advanced Nursing, 11,* 739–744.

Cunha, B., & Tu, R. (1988). Fever in the neurosurgical patient. *Heart and Lung, 17*(6), 608–611.

Cunha, B., Digamon-Beltran, M., & Gobbo, P. (1984). Implications of fever in the critical care setting. *Heart and Lung, 13*(5), 460–465.

Enright, T., & Hill, M. (1989). Treatment of Fever. *Focus on Critical Care, 16*(2), 96–102.

Fallacaro, M., Fallacaro, N., & Radel, T. (1986). Inadvertent hypothermia: Etiology, effects, and prevention. *AORN 44*(1), 54–57, 60–61.

Faust, D. (1985). Malignant hyperthermia. *Alaska Medicine, 28*(1), 1–2.

Feldman, M. (1988). Inadvertant hypothermia: A threat in the postanesthetic patient. *Journal of Post Anesthesia Nursing, 3*(2), 82–87.

Frost, E., & Andrews, I. (1983). Recovery room care. *International Anesthesiology Clinics, 21*(1), 41.

Fruthaler, G. (1985). Fever in children: Phobia vs. facts. *Hospital Practice, 20*(11A), 49–53.

Greany, D., & Brown, M. (1986). Malignant hyperthermia: A concern for critical care nurses. *Focus on Critical Care, 13*(2), 52–57.

Grossman, M. (1986). Management of the febrile patient. *Pediatric Infectious Diseases, 5*(6), 730–734.

Hofland, S. (1985). Drug fever: Is your patient's fever drug-related? *Critical Care Nurse, 5*(4), 29–34.

Jordon, L. (1987). Malignant hyperthermia. *Today's OR Nurse, 9*(4), 12–18.

Kauffman, C., Jones, P., & Kluger, M. (1986). Fever and malnutrition: Endogenous pyrogen/interleukin-1 in malnourished patients. *American Journal of Clinical Nutrition, 44*(10), 449–452.

Rosenberg, H. (1985). Malignant hyperthermia. *Hospital Practice, 20*(3), 139–152.

Ryan, J. (1983). Unintentional hypothermia. In F. Orkin & L. Cooperman, *Complications in anesthesiology.* Philadelphia: J. B. Lippincott.

Simon, H. (1986). Extreme pyrexia. *Hospital Practice, 21*(5A), 123–124, 127–129.

Sissler, D. (1986). Malignant hyperthermia. *Journal of Pediatrics, 109*(1), 9–14.

Slotman, G., Jed, E., & Burchard, K. (1985). Adverse effects of hypothermia in postoperative patients. *American Journal of Surgery, 149*(4), 495–501.

Welch, T. (1986). Hypothermia: A nursing concern for surgical patients. *Today's OR Nurse, 8*(4), 20–22.

Wiener, M., & Pepper, G. (1985). *Clinical pharmacology and therapeutics in nursing* (2nd ed.). New York: McGraw-Hill.

Wyngaarden, J., & Smith, L. (1985). *Cecil textbook of medicine,* (17th ed.). Philadelphia: W. B. Saunders.

Young, M. (1987). Fever in the postoperative patient. *Focus on Critical Care, 14*(2), 13–18.

Altered Levels of Consciousness and Mentation

13

Janet M. Delgado, M.N., CNRN

The nervous system is very complex. It regulates or has influence on all other body systems. In addition, it receives information from and is influenced by other body systems. Because of the part that the nervous system plays in physiologic adaptation, nurses must be familiar with basic neurological function. In addition, because of its influence on other body systems, critical care nurses are bound to be faced with neurological disorders in patient populations whose primary problems are not neurological in origin. Neurological dysfunction can be the result of head or spinal cord injury, stroke, surgery, or neurological disease and can rapidly lead to life-threatening emergency situations. The critical care nurse must therefore be prepared to assess a patient's neurological status and to act rapidly. These dysfunctions are frequently predictable, occur in certain sequences or patterns, and can be managed successfully.

Neurological dysfunction is frequently characterized by changes or deterioration in an individual's level of consciousness and mentation. Therefore, the focus of this chapter will be on these two concepts. Also provided in this chapter is information about intracranial dynamics, neurological assessment and the nursing diagnoses, interventions, and evaluation required for a patient in the critical care setting with an altered level of consciousness and/or mentation.

CONSCIOUSNESS

Consciousness is composed of two physiologic components—arousal and content (Plum & Posner, 1982). It consists of the individual's awareness of self and his or her surroundings. Arousal is related to the appearance of being awake; and the content of consciousness is representative of an individual's cognitive and affective capabilities.

Consciousness is regulated by the reticular activating system (RAS), which is the physiologic basis for arousal and content of consciousness. The RAS originates in the brain-stem and radiates in an ascending manner to communicate with the cerebral cortex. The RAS is extensive and communicates diffusely with the cerebral cortex. For this reason an alteration in consciousness is often the first sign of neurological deterioration.

The brain-stem portion of the RAS is responsible for the arousal state. This inferior portion of the RAS allows periods of wakefulness and sleep. The state of arousal is determined neurochemically by neurotransmitters. If there is an alteration in the state of arousal, as in a coma state, it is likely that there is extensive bilateral cerebral involvement. The content of consciousness is regulated by the thalamocortical or superior portion of the RAS.

INTRACRANIAL DYNAMICS

In order to assist the reader to fully understand intracranial neuropathology, particularly intracranial hypertension, there are some fundamental physiologic concepts basic to intracranial dynamics that are presented in the following text. Understanding these concepts is vital if neurological dysfunctions and neurological emergencies are to be effectively managed. Recognizing an emergency situation and providing treatment for acute intracranial abnormalities is an integral part of critical care nursing.

Intracranial Components

The skull can be visualized as a semiclosed box consisting of brain tissue (approximately 85%), blood (approximately 6%), and cerebrospinal fluid (CSF) (approximately 9%). These three intracranial substances occupy a specific amount of volume. If there is an increase in the volume of any of these intracranial components, the other two volumes must decrease equally so that intracranial pressure (ICP) can remain at a stable level (Bruce, 1980). This relationship is summarized in the following equation, which reflects the modified Monro–Kellie hypothesis of intracranial volumes (V = volume):

$$V_{Blood} + V_{CSF} + V_{Brain} = V_{Cranial\ cavity}$$

Neurological lesions that occupy space and alter volume, such as tumors, abscesses, or fluid in the form of edema or hematomas can lead to an imbalance of this intracranial homeostasis, which results in neurological dysfunction. The individual components of the above equation and their interrelationships are discussed below.

Volume–Pressure Relationships

It is essential for nurses to understand volume–pressure relationships in order to prevent and treat neurological complications. When any of the intracranial contents increase in volume, the body's protective mechanisms must function in a dynamic fashion, maintaining a homeostatic equilibrium between brain mass, CSF, and cerebral blood volume. Fortunately, small increases in volume are initially compensated for by changes in the components of the cranial cavity. If cranial volume increases occur, the main compensatory mechanism is the displacement of cerebrospinal fluid into the spinal dural sac. When all compensatory mechanisms are exhausted and volume increases faster than it is displaced, ICP rises. At normal intracranial volumes, the ICP is low and remains low with even small increments in intracranial volume. As the intracranial volume increases, the brain loses the ability to compensate. It is at this time that even small additions of volume will result in a dramatic increase in ICP as illustrated in Figure 13–1. The rapid addition of a small volume, as in a vascular hemorrhage will cause more immediate and larger ICP increases and greater brain dysfunction than a much larger yet slowly growing mass. Therefore, the state of brain elastance must be considered as individuals who are experiencing a state of high elastance are at risk for considerable increases in ICP (Mauss & Mitchell, 1976).

Elastance is a property that reflects the stiffness or rigidity of the cranial contents. It reflects the relationship between changes in pressure and changes in volume (Miller, 1975). Elastance consists of a change in pressure with an accompanying change in volume (change in pressure/change in volume). Elastance is the inverse of a similar property in the lung, called compliance (change in volume/change in pressure). Therefore, a substantial in-

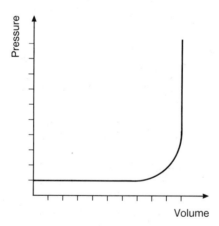

Figure 13–1.   Intracranial volume–pressure curve. Initial phase of compensation in compliant brain followed by marked increases in ICP with relatively small increases in volume as compensatory mechanisms are exhausted. From "Craniocerebral trauma" by S. L. Manifold, 1986, *Focus on Critical Care, 13*(2). Reprinted by permission.

crease in ICP with a small increase in intracranial volume would demonstrate a state of high elastance.

In summary, increases in volume in the three basic components of the cranium can alter intracranial dynamics. In addition, there are other factors such as hemodynamics, CSF, and ventilatory status that influence intracranial dynamics.

Intracranial Hemodynamics

The blood supply to the brain is carried by two vertebral and two carotid arteries. Blood from the cranium leaves primarily via the two internal jugular veins. In the noncompromised brain, cerebral blood flow (CBF) should remain fairly constant, at about 15% of the cardiac output, resulting in a constant cerebral blood volume (CBV). Either a markedly increased or markedly decreased CBV can have damaging consequences. Two factors that may alter CBF and CBV are the loss of autoregulation and decreased venous outflow.

Autoregulation is the ability of the brain's blood vessels to maintain a stable cerebral perfusion pressure by automatic alterations in the diameter of resistance vessels. The body attempts to maintain a constant CBF by vasodilation and vasoconstriction. Vessel walls constrict or dilate according to the ICP and the arterial pressure in the periphery. Autoregulation often fails when ICP is increased above 30 mm Hg. If autoregulation is not intact, as the systemic blood pressure increases, CBF increases and thus the volume of blood in the brain increases. Again if autoregulation fails, as systemic blood pressure decreases markedly, the CBF passively decreases, resulting in cerebral ischemia.

Venous outflow from the head and neck circulates through the external jugular veins and the vertebral veins; however, the principal drainage is via the internal jugular veins. In close proximity to the internal jugular veins are muscles that enable the neck to flex and rotate. The contraction of area muscles could partially occlude or reduce blood flow out of the brain. Such a partial occlusion in a compromised brain could restrict blood flow out of the brain. Increased intrathoracic and intraabdomical pressures may also decrease venous outflow. Decreased venous outflow has the effect of increasing cerebral blood volume.

Cerebrospinal Fluid

Cerebrospinal fluid is continually being produced in the ventricular system and reabsorbed back into the circulatory system. CSF is a clear watery fluid that cushions and protects the brain and spinal cord from injury. It is formed in the choroid plexus in the lateral, third, and fourth ventricles. CSF circulates through the ventricular system and is reabsorbed into the venous sinuses by granulations or villi in the subarachnoid space.

The total volume of CSF in the brain can be increased by an increase in the production of CSF, decreased reabsorption of CSF, or blockage of the CSF circulation. The production of CSF is fairly constant; therefore, an increased amount of CSF itself is rarely a cause of increased intracranial volume. There are rare cases of increased CSF production, resulting in an increase in intracranial volume. This occurs with rare tumors of the choroid plexus usually found in infants. Intracranial hypertension will result if CSF cannot travel via its usual pathways in the ventricular system or if it cannot be reabsorbed into the bloodstream by the arachnoid villi. Noncommunicating hydrocephalus is a condition in which the flow of CSF is blocked. The flow of CSF can be blocked by intracranial hemorrhage, tumors, or herniation of brain tissue. With noncommunicating hydrocephalus, the CSF cannot reach the subarachnoid space, and therefore cannot be reabsorbed into the circulation via the arachnoid villi. Communicating hydrocephalus is a condition in which there is less reabsorption of CSF. In this situation, the path of CSF is not blocked, but something prevents the reabsorption of CSF. Reabsorption of CSF by the arachnoid villi can be altered by meningeal tumors or inflammation or by a subarachnoid hemorrhage that can alter CSF access to the villi.

However, given the time, as with slow-growing tumors, the CSF system can use three compensatory mechanisms to decrease the volume of CSF in the brain and therefore decrease intracranial pressure. The system will attempt to displace CSF from the cranium to the spinal sac. In addition to this displacement, the CSF makes further attempts to reach homeostasis by increasing the absorption rate of CSF into the venous system (Shapiro, 1975). Also, the CSF system will attempt to compensate by forming less CSF. However, if the pathways are blocked or reabsorption is altered, these protective mechanisms cannot function.

Ventilatory Factors

Ventilatory factors influence ICP by affecting the hemodynamics of the cerebral blood vessels. Cerebrovascular dilation can be augmented by hypercapnia, hypoxemia, and certain volatile agents. CBV is directly affected by the partial pressure of arterial carbon dioxide ($PaCO_2$). Individuals in a state of high elastance who also have chronic obstructive pulmonary disease, increased tracheal secretions, and chronically increased ICP will be greatly affected by increased levels of $PaCO_2$, since carbon dioxide is a potent cerebral vasodilator. The elimination of excess CO_2 by hyperventilation is effective in decreasing ICP. Yet caution should be taken with prolonged excessive hyperventilation, since a $PaCO_2$ of less than 23 mm Hg can cause such excessive vasoconstriction that cerebral hypoxia and ischemia may result (Nikas & Konkoly, 1975). Within the normal range, the partial pressure of arterial oxygen (PaO_2) has essentially no effect on CBF. However, if PaO_2 is less than 50 mm Hg, CBF will increase.

In addition, the normal physiologic changes that occur during the rapid-eye-movement (REM) stage of sleep may have cumulative effects on the compromised brain (Hulmes & Cooper, 1968). This may be a result of the increased CBF that occurs because of the increased metabolic activity and increased CO_2 production that occurs during the REM phase of sleep. Shallow breathing, hypoventilatory cycles, or sleep apnea can lead to increases in CBF due to the dilating effects of CO_2 on cerebral vessels. These facts are interesting to compare with the clinical observation that neurological deterioration of patients usually occurs at night.

NEUROLOGICAL ASSESSMENT

The neurological examination is multifaceted, and serves a twofold purpose: to localize neurological lesions and to assess an individual's functional status.

Physiologic Integrity

In a critical care setting, clinicians need a quick method to screen an individual for physiologic integrity of the central nervous system. This method is commonly known as the "neuro-check." This technique is by no means comprehensive nor is it a substitute for a complete neurological examination. It is, however, a screening tool that can be used in an emergency or as a guide toward a more comprehensive examination. Nurses can use information from the neuro-check to be alerted to impending changes in neurological status, to plan nursing interventions, and to evaluate treatment strategies.

The four components of the neuro-check include level of consciousness, motor and sensory signs, eye signs, and changes in vital signs. The specific components of the "neuro-check" and the anatomic areas of control and assessment information are identified in Tables 13–1, 13–2 and Figure 13–2.

Functional Status

Assessment of functional status provides nurses with information about the effects of neurological dysfunctions on activities of daily living and self-care to which patients will need to adapt. The assessment model presented in Table 13–3 is based on categories of human functioning that include consciousness, mentation, movement, sensation, integrated regulation and coping with disability (Mitchell, Cammermeyer, Ozuna, & Woods, 1984).

The focus is to guide the nurse in examining functional ability related to the activities covered in each category. The nurse evaluates functional ability by interviewing, observing, and examining the patient and family. Data must be reviewed and areas of dysfunction noted considering the impact of the dysfunction on the individual's and family's life. Use of an assessment model will assist the nurse in the identification of nursing diagnoses in the planning and evaluation of care of patients with neurological dysfunction.

Mental Status

Commonly seen in the practice of critical care nursing are neurobehavioral disorders such as dysphasia, dementia, and confusion. The critical care nurse

Table 13–1   Components of the Neuro-Check

Assessment Area	Regulated By	Assessment Information
Consciousness	Reticular activating system (RAS)	Awareness of self and surroundings
Content	Thalamocortical or superior portion of RAS	Reflects cognitive and affective abilities, including orientation to self, place, time
Arousal	Neurotransmitters Brain-stem portion of RAS	Requires determining degree of stimulation necessary to arouse the patient
Motor strength and sensation		Must assess in combination with appropriateness of response
Strength	Nerve tracts Sensory fibers Motor fibers Sensory receptors	Assess bilateral hand grasps and upper/lower extremity strength (see Table 13–2) and assess for presense of posturing (see Figure 13–2)
Sensation		Response to light touch and pain (sharp or dull)
Eye signs		
Pupillary size	Cranial nerve III	Compare bilaterally
Reaction to light	Cranial nerve II/III	Examine in semidarkened room and observe for unilateral/direct/consensual pupillary constriction
Symmetry of movements	Cranial nerve III/IV/VI	Observe consensual movement inferiorly, superiorly, laterally, medially
Vital signs		
Pulse pressure	Brain-stem	If widening—irreversible brain damage
Heart rate		If bradycardic—irreversible brain-stem damage
Respirations		If aberrant—brain-stem damage

Table 13–2 Muscle Strength Rating Scale

5 Full muscle strength; offers maximal resistance to examiner, against gravity

4 Offers some resistance to examiner, against gravity

3 Able to raise limb against gravity; offers no resistance to examiner

2 Joint motion present, moves limb across surfaces; unable to raise limb against gravity

1 Palpable muscle twitch

0 No movement

F Abnormal flexion (decorticate posturing) (see Figure 13–2)

E Abnormal extension (decerebrate posturing) (see Figure 13–2)

Note: A score of 1–5 represents an appropriate motor response, but may reflect a dysfunctional motor system. A score of 0, F, or E represents an inappropriate response.

needs to be familiar with the basic elements in assessing mental status. Some patients may need serial exams with a simple bedside screening tool. Patients who have brain tumors or who have experienced trauma or a stroke should have a comprehensive mental status examination to document any cognitive or emotional changes. The critical care nurse can use the findings of the mental status evaluation to evaluate how neurobehavioral changes have affected the patient's ability to function and to assist the patient in adapting to his or her illness.

Comprehensive Mental Status Examination

There are eight basic components to the comprehensive mental status examination: assessment of the level of consciousness, attention, behavioral observations, language, memory, constructional ability, higher cognitive functions, and related cognitive functions (Strub & Black, 1977). A brief description of these components is given in Table 13–4.

Clinical Mental Status Tools

There are a multitude of instruments available to provide clinicians with a quick screening method to assess mental status at the bedside. Some of these tools are more appropriate in the evaluation of mental status than others. Before a mental status screening instrument is used in practice, the clinician needs to explore the origins of the development of the instrument, the reliability of the instrument, the applicability to the population being assessed, and whether the instrument actually evaluates mental status (validity). Mental status questionnaires that are commonly used in the clinical setting include the Short Portable Mental Status Questionnaire (SPMSQ) (Pfeiffer, 1975), the Cognitive Capacity Screening Examination (CCSE) (Jacobs, Bernhard, Delgado, & Strain, 1977), and the Mini-Mental State Examination (MMSE) (Folstein, Folstein, & McHugh, 1975).

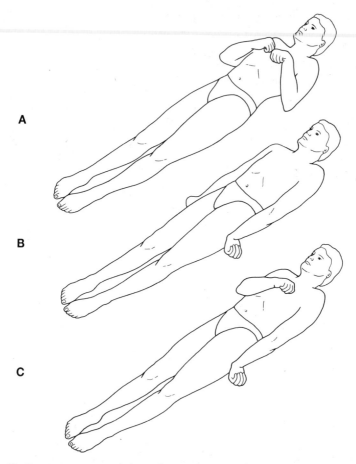

Figure 13–2. Decorticate and decerebrate responses. A: Decorticate response. Flexion of arms, wrists, and fingers with adduction in upper extremities. Extension, internal rotation, and plantar flexion in lower extremities. B: Decerebrate response. All four extremities in rigid extension with hyperpronation of forearms and plantar extension of feet. C: Decorticate response on right side of body and decerebrate response on left side of body. From *Mosby's Comprehensive Review of Critical Care* by D. Zschoche, 1986, St. Louis: The C. V. Mosby Co. Reprinted by permission of the author.

NURSING DIAGNOSES RELATED TO ALTERED LEVELS OF CONSCIOUSNESS AND MENTATION
Altered Cerebral Tissue Perfusion

The cells of the central nervous system are very sensitive to an alteration in tissue perfusion that results in hypoxia, as the brain's major source of energy is the metabolism of simple sugars. Oxygen is used rapidly by cerebral tissue, and oxygen consumption by the brain accounts for 20% of total basal oxygen

Table 13–3 Functional Assessment Categories

Category	Function
Consciousness	Arousal Self-awareness
Mentation	Thinking Remembering Perceiving Language Problem solving
Movement	Expressing (facial) Speaking Walking Transferring Eating (chewing, swallowing) Blinking ⎱ combined movement Seeing ⎰ and sensation
Sensation	Smelling Hearing Feeling (touch, temperature, pain, pressure, position, form, shape, etc.)
Integrated regulatory function	Eating (ingesting, digesting) Eliminating Breathing Circulation Temperature control Sexual response Emotion
Coping with disability	Self-care competence Role competence Coping (adapting, coping, supporting, growing)

From *Neurological Assessment for Nursing Practice* (p. 7) by P. Mitchell, M. Cammermeyer, J. Ozuna, and N. F. Woods, 1984, Reston, VA: Reston Publishing Co. Copyright 1984 by Reston Publishing Co. Reprinted by permission.

consumption, although the brain accounts for only 2% of the total body weight. Disruption of central nervous system function by hypoxia results in a wide range of clinical manifestations, which reflect physiologic dysfunction, such as restlessness, uncooperativeness, inability to concentrate, or any change in the level of consciousness from lethargy to unconsciousness, to name a few (Groer & Shekleton, 1989). These signs and symptoms will accompany those of the underlying cause of the altered tissue perfusion. If cerebral hypoxia persists, ischemia and cell death will occur, possibly leading to permanent brain damage or death.

Cerebral blood flow is determined by the diameter of the cerebrovascular bed as well as by the cerebral perfusion pressure (Nikas, 1987). Factors

Table 13-4   Components of a Comprehensive Mental Status Examination

Component	Description
Consciousness	Range of alertness to comatose. As definitions differ, it is important to *describe* behavioral responses.
Attention	Attention to a *specific* stimulus for a minimum of 30 seconds.
Behavioral observations	Attention to appearance, response to examiner, emotional status, hygiene.
Language	Attention to communication and understanding of words, speed, tone, and volume of speech. Reflects left cerebral hemisphere functioning.
Memory	Differentiating between instant recall, recent memory, and remote memory.
Constructional ability	Identifies person's ability to draw two- or three-dimensional figures or shapes. Reflects occipital, parietal, and frontal lobe coordination and functioning.
Higher cognitive functions	Evaluates knowledge, problem-solving, judgment, and analytical skills. Requires concentration, language, and memory skills.
Related cognitive functions	Evaluates ability to carry out high-level sensory and motor perceptual acts. May present as inability to perform a task or inability to recognize familiar objects.

affecting the diameter of the cerebrovascular bed, such as the property of autoregulation and the concentrations of carbon dioxide and oxygen, were discussed in the first section of this chapter. Cerebral perfusion pressure (CPP) is the difference between the mean arterial pressure (MAP) and intracranial pressure (ICP) (CPP = MAP − ICP). Normal CPP is approximately 80 mm Hg. Cerebral blood flow will be impaired if the CPP is 50 mm Hg or less. In the compromised brain, even a CPP at the lower limits of normal may be inadequate for meeting metabolic demands (Waltz & Sundt, 1968; Bruce, 1980). Any factor that affects either the arterial or intracranial pressure has the potential to alter cerebral perfusion pressure and, therefore, cerebral blood flow.

Autoregulation of the diameter of the arterioles is most effective when MAP is in the range of 50 to 150 mm Hg. Mean arterial pressure can be calculated (if it is not being directly monitored) by the following formula: MAP = diastolic BP + 1/3 pulse pressure. Cerebral blood flow will decrease when the MAP falls below 50 mm Hg and will increase when MAP rises above 150 mm Hg. The danger with arterial hypertension is the potential for breakdown of the blood–brain barrier and development of cerebral edema (Nikas, 1987). Arterial hypotension is more likely to be a problem in the critically ill surgical patient and can be the result of any number of conditions, including bleeding, anesthesia, trauma, or fluid volume depletion due to loss or inadequate replacement.

Normal intracranial pressure is a measure of the force being exerted by the volume of the intracranial contents against the walls of a closed, nonexpandable cavity—the cranial vault of the skull. Intracranial pressure will rise in response to an increase in any of the three components of intracranial volume without a proportionate, reciprocal decrease in the others. Clinical manifestations of intracranial hypertension, or an ICP greater than 25 mm Hg, occur when compensatory mechanisms fail to match the increase in volume and the total intracranial volume increases (Table 13–5). As explained earlier in this chapter, the extent of the increase in ICP depends on several factors,

Table 13–5 Physiologic and Clinical Correlates of Increased Intracranial Pressure

Stage	Intracranial Pressure	Effects
Stage 1	No rise in intracranial pressure is associated with an expanding mass.	Compensation phase; no change in vital signs
Stage 2	Slight increase in the mass of the brain results in great elevations of intracranial pressure.	End stage of compensation; changes in vital signs are slight to moderate
Stage 3	Intracranial pressure can approach arterial blood pressure.	Beginning of decompensation, also called the preterminal stage; signs and symptoms that may be observed in the patient include deterioration in the level of consciousness, abnormalities in the respiratory pattern, rise in the systolic blood pressure, a widening of the pulse pressure, bradycardia, and cardiac arrhythmias
Stage 4	The autoregulatory mechanism that normally responds to increased levels of carbon dioxide by dilating cerebral arteries to supply nutrients and oxygen to the brain is nonfunctional. If the condition is not improved, arterial and intracranial pressure will become equal, resulting in cessation of blood flow and death.	Decompensation phase; symptoms as noted in Stage 3 continue; death results if there is not immediate reversal of the condition

including elastance, the rate and amount of the increase in volume, and the total volume of the intracranial cavity.

Patients with space-occupying lesions (hematomas, hemorrhages, abscesses, or tumors), head trauma (accidental or surgical), edema, or hydrocephalus are at risk for development of intracranial hypertension. If generalized edema occurs, the resulting distended brain may actually mechanically obstruct the subarachnoid villi, where CSF is reabsorbed into the circulatory system. Intracerebral bleeding or hematomas cause a rapid increase in volume, which can displace and compress brain tissue and lead to rapid increases in ICP, obstruction of CSF or venous outflow, herniation syndromes, and even death (Langfitt, 1975; Shapiro, 1975). With slowly expanding lesions such as tumors, the brain compensates for the increase in volume by displacing and shifting its contents. Sometimes this shifting is very gradual and symptoms are not apparent until there is a great deal of intracranial involvement; it is at this point that a state of high elastance is achieved. The patient with a large tumor that is in a state of high elastance will exhibit signs of neurological deterioration.

Pathologic increases in intracranial pressure can be compounded by the compensatory responses to hypoxia as cerebral blood flow is compromised. When the oxygen supply is diminished because of decreased CBF, the blood in the brain will become acidotic as glycolysis shifts from the aerobic to the anaerobic pathway and cerebral vasodilation will occur, resulting in increased CBF. Increased permeability of the cerebral capillaries occurs as a response to hypoxia and contributes to the formation of cerebral edema (Groer & Shekleton, 1989). All of these compensatory responses contribute to the vicious cyclic progression of intracranial hypertension (Figure 13–3). Nursing care activities have also been found to increase ICP (Walleck, 1987).

Herniation Syndromes

One of the consequences of intracranial hypertension is herniation of the brain. When the contents of the cranium can no longer compensate for an increase in one of the components (brain tissue, blood, or cerebrospinal fluid), the brain tissue begins to shift and displace itself through the openings or linings of the cranial cavity. This displacement of tissue is called herniation. When herniation occurs, the patient will exhibit severe neurological deficits as the brain tissue becomes damaged and necrotic.

Critical care nurses need to be able to recognize rapidly the occurrence of herniation, establish the baseline level of brain function remaining, and plan treatment strategies to protect the patient from further harm (Mitchell, 1981). It is important for critical care nurses to be skilled in the assessment of patients with altered cerebral tissue perfusion and the potential for herniation of the brain.

The cranial vault is divided into anterior and posterior cavities or fossa. The tentorium cerebelli, an inflexible portion of the dura, creates these two cavi-

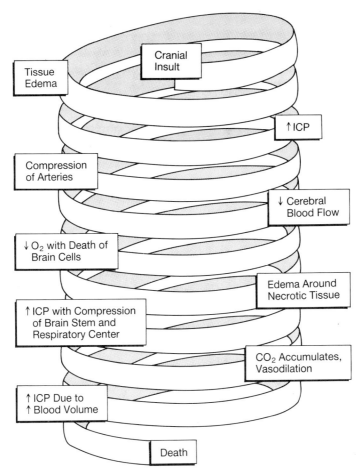

Figure 13–3. Cyclic progression of increased ICP. From *Neurologic Problems: A Critical Care Nursing Focus* (p. 52) by M. Snyder and M. Jackle, 1981, Bowie, MD: R. J. Brady. Copyright 1981 by R. J. Brady Co. Reprinted by permission.

ties. The tips of the temporal lobes, called the uncus, and the third cranial nerve are supratentorial structures and rest near the edge of the tentorium. If herniation occurs, these areas can become severely damaged by the tentorium, and cause the patient to exhibit life-threatening symptoms. There is also another fibrous meningeal tissue, the falx cerebri, which separates portions of the right and left hemispheres. Brain tissue can also herniate laterally through this lining. If there is a space-occupying lesion or generalized swelling in the posterior fossa, the cerebellum and midbrain will begin to herniate upward through the tentorium. In addition to tentorial herniation, the foramen magnum at the base of the skull is another potential site for intracranial herniation. In this case, the areas of the brain that are displaced downward are the cerebellar tonsils.

Brain herniation syndromes are identified mostly by clinical signs including pathologic eye signs, unresponsiveness, and aberrant ventilatory patterns, which are late indicators of increased intracranial pressure (Hickey, 1986). The treatment of progressive brain herniation is managed jointly by physicians and nurses and is discussed in chapter 19. The ideal situation is to identify the potential for herniation and prevent its occurrence or progression. Invasive ICP monitoring allows for ongoing monitoring of rising intracranial pressure and response to treatment. ICP monitoring is discussed in greater detail in chapter 19.

The occurrence of head trauma, Reye's syndrome, intracranial hemorrhage, hydrocephalus, massive strokes, rapidly growing tumors, or persistent cerebral edema that occurs after cardiac arrest are all conditions in which intracranial monitoring and ongoing evaluation may be required. In addition to expecting the occurrence of intracranial hypertension with various conditions, researchers have found the use of a particular assessment tool to be very helpful in making the decision to use ICP monitoring. The Glasgow Coma Scale (GCS) (see Table 21–2) allows assessment of the symptoms one would expect with progressive herniation syndromes. Scores of 7 or below on the GCS have been associated with high intracranial pressures (Bruce, Berman, & Schut, 1977; Ropper, Kennedy, & Zervas, 1983). In addition to monitoring individuals with pathologic states, ICP monitoring may be used in the immediate postoperative period to evaluate individuals who have had cranial surgery. The potential for infection is increased when ICP monitoring is used because it is an invasive procedure and of concern when meningeal layers are penetrated since immunologic factors are not present in the CSF (Nikas, 1987).

Altered Thought Processes

In practice, critical care nurses will encounter many individuals who have alterations in complex thought processes, including disorientation, difficulty with abstract thinking, decreased attention span, impaired memory, difficulty with problem solving, difficulty with decision making, altered or inappropriate behavior, and hallucinations. An individual who has an altered level of consciousness is unable to function effectively or safely in his or her environment.

Sensory–Perceptual Alterations

Individuals can experience sensory–perceptual difficulties because of the changes that occur with neuropathology. This is a condition in which individuals experience a change in the quantity, quality, and/or understanding of stimuli from within their person and from the environment. Most sensory–perceptual problems that appear in the patient population with neurological dysfunction have a significant impact on an individual's higher cortical functioning and the ability to integrate information accurately. Stroke, trauma, and tumors, particularly pituitary tumors, are all conditions that may cause sensory–perceptual difficulties. Examples of sensory perceptual alterations are presented in Table 13–6.

Potential for Injury

Individuals with neurological dysfunction are frequently at risk for injury because of neuropathology, perceptual deficits, alteration in thought processes, or motor–sensory limitations. Seizures, confusion, decreased sensation and dysphagia are all conditions that may predispose the patient to injury. Risk factors pertinent to the neurologic population include history of injuries, altered mobility, altered sensation (pain, temperature, vision, hearing), confusion, and poor judgment. Potential causes of injury in patients with neurological dysfunction are identified in Table 13–7.

Table 13–6 Sensory–Perceptual Alterations

Alteration	Possible Defect	Presenting Definition
Visual-field deficits	Lesion in visual pathways	Defects in field of vision
Agnosia		
Visual	Lesion in occipital cortex	Inability to recognize familiar sights
Auditory	Cortical lesion of temporal lobe	Inability to recognize familiar sounds
Tactile	Cortical lesion of parietal lobe	Inability to recognize familiar objects by touch
	(Note: requires intact neuronal pathways for sight, hearing, and touch)	
Anosmia	Disruption of olfactory pathway	Absence of sense of smell
Unilateral Neglect	Problems with integration and interpretation of sensory information	Disregard for one side of body or one half of space in environment
Anosognosia	Problems with integration and interpretation of sensory information	Unawareness or denial of presence of hemiplegia. May cause major safety hazards

Table 13–7   Potential Causes of Injury in Neurologically Impaired Patients

Neurological Disorder	Potential Deficits
Seizures	May compromise respiration and ventilation
	May result in loss of consciousness
	May cause bradycardia
	May result in aspiration
	May result in drowsiness and/or confusion
	Resultant anoxia may cause cognitive deficits, mental retardation, or death
	Loss of motor control
Confusion	May not recognize dangerous situations
	May not be able to communicate discomfort or pain
	May not recognize boundaries or restrictions (side rails, IV tubing)
Sensation deficit	↓ tactile sensation, ↓ response to pain, and/or temperature
	↓ visual sensation, ↓ awareness of environmental hazards
	↓ auditory sensation, ↓ awareness of environmental warning signals
Dysphagia	Inability/difficulty in swallowing may ↑ potential for aspiration

Self-Care Deficits

The cognitive, motor, sensory, and perceptual alterations that occur with neurological disease can have a great impact on a person's ability to care for himself or herself. A diagnosis of self-care deficit is confirmed when an individual is unable to feed, bathe, dress, or toilet himself or herself. The degree of self-care deficit that an individual exhibits depends upon the neurological signs and symptoms present. The self-care deficit may be partial, such that a patient with fine-coordination problems may need assistance opening milk cartons. The self-care deficit may be total, as in a comatose patient. However, because of the multisystem patient problems seen in the critical care setting, it is more likely that a critically ill patient would need assistance with most, if not all, self-care activities.

Impaired Verbal Communication

Patients with neuromuscular problems and those with cortical disorders may have difficulty with verbal communication. Impaired verbal communication describes a condition in which a person may have difficulty in speaking appropriately or have difficulty in using language. It is important to note that there is a difference between a person's ability to articulate or speak and his or her ability to use language. Stroke, tumors, head injury, Parkinson's disease, multiple sclerosis, and myasthenia gravis are all pathologic conditions that can impair verbal communication. Some of the characteristics of the diagnosis that are common to the neurological population include slurred speech (dysarthria), nasal speech, difficulty following commands, difficulty in expressing self with appropriate language (dysphasia), fluent, yet incomprehensible speech, and total lack of ability to use language (aphasia). The most commonly occurring language problems are related to the reception and expression of words and are summarized in Table 13–8.

Impaired Physical Mobility

The motor deficits associated with many neurologic disorders can limit an individual's ability to move. Independent movement is a body function that is highly valued in our society, and the loss or impairment of movement has devastating effects on the patient and family. Impaired physical mobility can occur suddenly, such as after a head injury, stroke, peripheral nerve damage, or an amputation. The loss of physical mobility can also happen gradually over a period of months or even years as occurs with degenerative or demyelinating diseases. The diagnostic characteristics of impaired physical mobility that are most relevant to the neurological population include inability to move voluntarily, decreased or absent muscle strength, impaired coordination, and impaired position sense.

Table 13–8 Disorders of Language

Type of Dysphasia	Lesion Site	Impact on Patient
Expressive	Frontal lobe (Broca's area)	Unable to express self using language. Patterns of speech are not fluent. Comprehends written and verbal language. Demonstrates understanding by following simple commands.
Receptive	Temporal lobe (Wernicke's area)	Unable to interpret language. Patterns of speech are fluent, and exhibits frequent spontaneous unintelligible speech. Writing is either absent or unintelligible. Does not comprehend written or verbal speech.
Mixed	Temporal or frontal lobes or connecting fibers between speech centers	Mixed disorder—unable to express self or interpret language. No spontaneous speech or attempts at verbal or written language made. Does not comprehend written or verbal communication.

Two nerve tracts are involved in executing a voluntary motor act, the pyramidal and extrapyramidal systems. The pyramidal system transmits the impulses that allow skilled voluntary movement to occur. The extrapyramidal system contributes both excitatory and inhibitory influences on voluntary motor activity. These influences aid posture, muscular tone, the initiation of movement, equilibrium, and postural reflexes (Delgado & Billo, 1988). The pyramidal and extrapyramidal deficits that may be present in the neurologic population are identified in Table 13–9.

Motility Deficits Related to Cognition

The inability to perform previously learned voluntary movements when requested to do so is termed apraxia. The person with apraxia does not have a paralysis or sensory loss and has no difficulty in understanding instructions; he or she is unable to integrate motor function cognitively, and is therefore unable to carry out the motor act. Apraxias are associated with focal lesions on the cerebral cortex and with diffuse brain disorders (Chusid, 1982). The three types of apraxia are motor, ideational, and ideomotor, which are summarized in Table 13–10.

A person who is experiencing impaired physical mobility is at risk for all the effects of immobility discussed in detail in chapter 14. The nursing diagnostic category "potential for disuse syndrome" can be used in care planning to identify all the potential problems for which an immobile person is at risk.

Impaired Tissue Integrity

Individuals with neurologic dysfunction have a particularly high risk of development of impairment of the skin and underlying tissue. Immobility and sensory and vasomotor deficits are the most direct causes of skin breakdown; however, even a decreased level of consciousness predisposes a patient to

Table 13–9 Pyramidal and Extrapyramidal Mobility Deficits

Pyramidal deficits	
Paresis	Decline in muscular strength and force Seen in central and peripheral nervous system disorders May be seen in patients after a stroke
Paralysis	Total absence of muscular strength Seen in central and peripheral nervous system disorders May be seen in patients after spinal cord injury
Extrapyramidal deficits	
Movement disorders	Tremors, rigidity, bradykinesia, postural instability Seen in imbalance of acetylcholine and dopamine Seen in patients with Parkinson's disease

Table 13–10 Types of Apraxia

Type	Lesion Site	Deficit	Assessment
Motor	Precentral gyrus	Inability to manage movement of extremities; thought to be due to altered memory patterns related to movement.	Request patient to select an object, raise hand, or pick up a piece of paper.
Ideomotor	Supramarginal gyrus	Inability to carry out motor acts upon request, although patient may be able to carry out the same act spontaneously when not consciously aware of his or her motor acts.	Request patient to open a bottle, to imitate the clinician performing an act, such as folding a piece of paper, and asking the patient to perform a habitual act such as handing the patient a toothbrush and telling him or her to show you how to use it.
Ideational	Diffuse	Inability to carry out complex acts that are purposeful. Patient may be able to perform parts of act correctly, but not the act as a whole.	Ask the patient to perform a complex act such as combing hair. He or she must be able to pick up the comb, hold it with the teeth of the comb facing hair, and be able to pull the comb through hair.

problems with skin integrity. Problems with skin and tissue integrity can have an impact on an individual's general health, mobility, self-esteem, and rehabilitation potential. The most common risk factors for impaired skin and tissue integrity in the neurological population include impaired physical mobility, decreased sensation, weakness and paralysis, and reports of pain or numbness.

An area of skin, typically over a bony prominence, under mechanical pressure can develop tissue hypoxia, which leads to the development of a decubitus or pressure ulcer. With excessive or prolonged mechanical pressure, the pressure on the skin exceeds capillary pressure, which causes loss of local circulation and cellular death. Prolonged tissue pressure leads to the additional destruction of the cutaneous and underlying tissues. Impairment of skin and tissue integrity as a result of impaired physical mobility is discussed in detail in chapter 14.

All individuals with motor, sensory, and vasomotor losses are at risk for development of skin impairment. Critical care nurses can have a great impact on the health of a patient's skin. If the patient is totally immobile, it is vital to establish a turning schedule of every 1 to 2 hours. The standard protocol of turning a patient every 2 hours is probably not frequent enough in a patient with decreased vasomotor tone. In order to establish an individualized turning schedule, after each position change the nurse must thoroughly assess the previously dependent areas of the patient's skin. It is normal to see a pink area immediately after the patient is repositioned. However, the patient's skin should not be reddened after approximately 10 minutes. Unfortunately, routine position changes do not provide the best opportunity to assess the condition of the skin thoroughly; the ideal opportunity to complete a methodical skin assessment is while bathing the patient.

Altered Nutrition: Less Than Body Requirements

Many individuals with neurological dysfunction are at risk of losing weight because they have an inadequate intake of nutrients. Individuals in a high stress state such as a neurological disorder or critical illness have increased nutritional needs, which are discussed in chapter 8. The primary reason why individuals with neurological dysfunction are at risk for losing weight is because of paresis or paralysis of muscles. This paresis or paralysis interferes with either their ability to procure food or their ability to chew and swallow. Most of these individuals do not have a problem with the digestion of their nutrients. Strokes, neuromuscular diseases, and cranial nerve disorders are all pathologic conditions that can impair nutritional status in this manner.

The critical care nurse may note that cold thin liquids are more difficult for the weak patient to swallow. Liquids may pool in the mouth, placing the patient at risk for pulmonary aspiration or they may drool out so that the patient never receives the nutrients. Early recognition of these signs will allow clinicians to plan alternative methods of feeding the patient with muscular weakness.

Alternative methods of feeding can span a wide range of techniques. The critical care nurse may find that certain foods such as warm, thicker fluids are easier for the patient to manipulate and swallow. On the other hand, the nurse may find that the muscular weakness interferes so much with the act of chewing and swallowing that the patient may need enteral feedings. The principles of nutrition and enteral feedings are presented in detail in chapter 8.

Ineffective Coping

Patients and families face great challenges in their ability to cope with neurological dysfunctions. The critical care nurse has the capacity to identify potential and actual problems associated with coping. The general concepts associated with coping are presented in chapter 4.

The principal cause of ineffective coping patterns in the patient population with neurological dysfunction is the recognition of a disability. The unique elements of neurological disabilities is that they can either be sudden or insidious, that they can be progressive in nature, and that they are frequently permanent. The attributes of the disability may be physical or behavioral such as sensory–perceptual deficits, motor deficits, or cognitive deficits. In addition, these same physical and behavioral deficits can have devastating effects on an individual's life, having an impact on job, social activities, hobbies, and on the roles of parent, spouse, and member of a community. Any neuropathologic state that results in a loss, change in daily activities, or lifestyle predisposes patients and families to ineffective coping. The diagnostic characteristics related to ineffective coping that are common to the patient population with neurological dysfunction include verbalization of inability to cope, inability to make decisions, destructive behavior, and inability to express concerns.

Patients or their families may find that they are dealing with problems in an effectual or ineffectual manner. The critical care nurse must assist the patient and the family in identifying short-term coping strategies, and thus promote optimal physical and psychological health. Coping strategies that are effective in the critical care setting may not be effective for long-term adaptation to neurological dysfunction. The critical care nurse must identify and then inform and collaborate with other members of the health care team as to what coping strategies the patient has used successfully in the past.

The critical care nurse can provide patients and families with information about the disease process so that they can begin to plan to adapt to anticipated changes in their lifestyles. Further assessment and specific interventions will be planned once the patient is transferred out of the critical care unit; however, the initial information provided by the critical care nurse can provide a strong framework upon which others can build during the rehabilitation process.

NURSING INTERVENTIONS
Maintaining Cerebrovascular Perfusion

Maintaining adequate cerebrovascular perfusion is of utmost importance in a patient with intracranial hypertension. Unless ICP monitoring is being used, it is not possible to know a patient's intracranial status at a given point in time. If ICP monitoring is not available, the nurse has only the patient's clinical status and responses to activity by which to formulate an evaluation. Many patient care activities have been noted to have an influence on intracranial pressure, some of those include: suctioning, turning the patient, touch, pain, and emotional and environmental stimuli (Mitchell & Mauss, 1978; Mitchell, Mauss, Lipe, & Ozuna, 1982; Shalit & Umansky, 1977; Boortz-Marx, 1985; Mitchell, Habermann-Little, Johnson, VanInwegen-Scott, & Tyler; 1985). The critical

care nurse should attempt to minimize the harmful effects of these procedures and situations. Relevant nursing interventions are summarized in Table
13–11.

Maintaining an Optimal Physiologic Environment

A seriously compromised nervous system can lead to a life-threatening emergency, especially if the ventilatory and cardiovascular systems are affected.
Ineffective breathing pattern and ineffective airway clearance can lead to impaired gas exchange and/or pneumonia. Individuals with spinal cord injuries
and demyelinating and degenerative diseases that affect the ventilatory and
cardiovascular systems are particularly at risk. Promotion of an effective
breathing pattern and maintaining a clear airway must be a priority of care.

In many neuropathologic states, particularly if there is an alteration in
the patient's consciousness, urinary and fecal incontinence is a problem. The

Table 13–11   Relationships Between Patient Activities and Increased Intracranial
Pressure (ICP)

Mechanism	Activity or Condition	Nursing Intervention
Increase in cerebral blood volume secondary to:		
1. Rise in blood pressure		
a. Isometric muscle contractions	Turning, moving up and down in bed, pushing self in bed	Turn sheet, encourage patient to allow passive movement
	Decerebrate/decorticate posturing	Avoid stimuli that cause posturing, if possible; phenothiazines, pancuronium (Pavulon) may help
b. Rebound phase of Valsalva maneuver	Straining at stool	Prevent constipation; use stool softeners, suppositories as dictated by state of consciousness
	Pushing self, moving in bed	Encourage patient to exhale while turning, pushing
c. Emotional stimuli	Family visits, conversation about fears, concerns	Weigh risk versus benefit for each person; avoid conversations held "over" patient about condition
2. Decreased venous outflow		
a. Transient mechanical obstruction to jugular, vertebral, and intrathoracic venous systems	Head and body position that obstructs flow: rotated head; flexed, extended neck; extreme hip flexion	Keep head in neutral position when possible, avoid neck flexion and extension both in resting posture and during procedures Slight head-up position promotes venous drainage

Table 13–11 *(Continued)*

Mechanism	Activity or Condition	Nursing Intervention
b. Increased intrathoracic and intraabdominal pressure	Any activity that causes a Valsalva maneuver	See previous intervention re: Valsalva
	Body positions that increase pressure: prone, extreme hip flexion	Avoid such positions
	Positive end-expiratory pressure ventilation (PEEP) in some patients	Head up position may help some; avoid multiple activities in patients who increase ICP with PEEP
3. Cerebral vasodilatation secondary to hypercapnia or marked hypoxia ($Pa_{O_2} < 50\text{-}60$ mm Hg)	Occluded airway	Keep airway patent; if suctioning necessary, use intermittent, brief (15 seconds or less) periods; may help to preoxygenate patient
Increase in cerebrospinal fluid (CSF) volume: Transient increase in intracranial CSF due to obstruction of basal cisterns	Head position that temporarily occludes CSF outflow to spinal sac: head rotation, neck extension	Avoid head rotation whenever possible; side-lying position may be helpful to patients with decreased CSF absorption (such as postsubarachnoid hemorrhage)

From *AACN's Clinical Reference for Critical Care Nursing* by Kinney, M. R., et al. (Eds.), 1981, New York: McGraw-Hill Book Co. Reproduced by permission of the C. V. Mosby, Co., St. Louis.

patient may not be aware of or be able to communicate the need to evacuate the bladder or bowel. While physiologically unstable, patients frequently have an indwelling catheter. Since the presence of a long-term indwelling urinary drainage catheter places the patient at risk for urinary tract infections, it is most desirable to remove indwelling catheters as soon as the patient is stable. Urinary incontinence may occur after the removal of an indwelling catheter and urine can be a very potent skin irritant. Frequent inspections for soiled bed linens are important. The nurse may be able to identify or predict a pattern of incontinence based on observation of the patient and knowledge of types and amounts of enteral and parenteral intake the patient receives. A regular toileting schedule can be established based on this pattern.

The alert patient, with decreased or no sensation to parts of his or her body can be taught to be relatively independent in maintaining the integrity of the skin. Patients can be trained to examine bony prominences and dependent areas such as the back and buttocks. This visual examination can be performed by paraplegics by using hand-held mirrors with long handles. If the patient does not have sufficient mobility of his or her arms to use a mirror, a family member can be taught the appropriate techniques.

The paralyzed patient and family need to be taught that it is important to stimulate circulation to dependent areas of the body. The critical care nurse can demonstrate this principle each time the patient is turned or repositioned. Once the patient is stable enough to sit up in a chair, this basic premise must not be neglected. While up in a chair, the patient must be repositioned every 15 to 30 minutes. The importance and value of repositioning *must* be conveyed to the patient and family.

Maintaining a Safe Environment

Patients with neurological dysfunction need to be protected from harm. Individuals with alterations in their thought processes are particularly at risk for unintentionally hurting themselves or entering unsafe situations.

The nurse needs to provide the patient with the adaptive devices that may be needed, such as eyeglasses, hearing aids, or dentures. Being able to see and hear clearly will enhance the patient's ability to perceive and interpret stimuli appropriately. Having dentures will improve the patient's self-esteem, allow communication, and facilitate the ability to chew food thoroughly and decrease the potential for aspiration.

The nurse must frequently attempt to reorient the patient to time, person, and place and to activities and procedures that will be experienced (Kroner, 1979). This process of reality orientation may need to occur often if the patient is confused or has an impaired memory. Verbal reorientation may not be enough and the patient may benefit from cues in the environment such as large calendars, clocks, or other mechanisms that would prompt and help orient a patient. Particularly in a critical care setting, with the constant overwhelming stimuli, nurses must be cognizant of controlling the lighting in the patient's room to mimic day and night cycles. However, bright lights may be contraindicated in certain neurological conditions such as migraine, meningitis, or aneurysms.

Since memory is often impaired, the patient may forget daily care routines and the nurse may need to reiterate the routines to the patient constantly. In addition, the nurse needs to maintain as standardized a routine as possible in order to decrease anxiety and frustration in a patient with memory impairment. Frequent family visits or the presence of personal belongings help establish reality orientation. When giving instructions or information, the nurse may need to separate the data into small steps that the patient can follow. If the patient is easily confused or distracted, it is best if one person interacts with him or her at a time.

Providing Initial Rehabilitation

The critical care nurse can have a dramatic impact on a patient's future functional ability and quality of life. This impact depends on the participation of the critical care nurse in the patient's initial rehabilitation. Rehabilitation is an intense process by which an impaired person is assisted and supported in acquiring and maintaining an optimal health status. Such an optimal health status is related to an individual's ability to maintain physiologic, psychological, functional, and social well-being independently. O'Brien and Pallet (1978) note that, in order for rehabilitation to be effective, a rehabilitation program must commence early in the course of the illness and must continue to be integrated into the total care of the patient at all levels of health care.

In physical rehabilitation, the critical care nurse's primary objective is to foster the patient's optimal functioning, prevent unnecessary deterioration, and decrease the occurrence of complications such as joint contractures and muscle atrophy. The nurse can use information derived from assessment and from the physical and occupational therapists and rehabilitation clinical nurse specialist involved in the patient's care to evaluate the patient's overall level of function. Passive range-of-motion exercises should be performed on all joints at least every 4 hours and in repositioned joints after position changes. If the patient is at risk for intracranial hypertension, vigorous active range-of-motion exercises are contraindicated, particularly movements of extreme flexion or those that would prompt a Valsalva maneuver. The patient should be encouraged to move paretic extremities and to guard the extremities against injury if sensory–perceptual alterations are present.

Patients with autonomic dysfunction or those who have been on prolonged bed rest may experience postural instability when a standing posture is assumed. These patients may be safely transferred using a gait belt, a wide rigid belt used by therapists for balance and mobility training. In a patient with a stabilized spinal cord injury, it is most advantageous if balance training and sitting programs are introduced in the critical care unit. Balance training is reviewed in chapter 19. When instituting such a program, the nurse will need to evaluate the patient's physiologic responses critically. At the onset of a balance training program in an individual with decreased postural tone, symptoms of orthostatic hypotension are common and may recur if the program progresses too rapidly.

Many neurological conditions result in bowel and bladder dysfunctions. If not addressed at the onset of the illness these dysfunctions could predispose the patient to complications such as urinary tract infections, renal reflux, and decubiti, which are detrimental to recovery and overall health. In addition, if bowel and bladder training programs are started early, the patient is more likely to adapt successfully. The basic principles of bowel and bladder training programs are presented in chapter 19. However, it is important to note that bowel and bladder dysfunctions are as complicated as the neuropathology that causes them; therefore it would be most beneficial if the critical care nurse consulted with a neuroscience or rehabilitation clinical nurse specialist in order to develop an individualized program.

Promoting Effective Communication

Patients who cannot speak are often seen in the critical care unit. Barriers such as wired jaws, tracheostomies, or endotracheal tubes (to name a few) can interfere with a patient's ability to speak. If the patient is alert, alternative methods of communication can be devised between the nurse and patient, such as tapping, pointing, writing, or even eye signals. Similar methods can be devised for patients who have a problem with either interpreting language or expressing themselves using language due to neurologic dysfunction. A comprehensive program should be planned with the assistance of a speech pathologist; however, some basic techniques will be presented in this section.

A person with receptive dysphasia may hear gibberish or even groups of meaningless words. Since the immediate goal is communication, not speech therapy, the nurse must find ways to communicate events and procedures to the patient and ways to identify the patient's needs. Since the problem in this case is with the interpretation of language, an effective strategy would be to minimize the use of spoken language. A strong emphasis on nonverbal communication is important. Lengthy verbal explanations can be confusing to the patient, and should be avoided. Pointing to objects or using a communication board with pictures of objects can be very effective. The nurse can point to a chair and say "sit chair" if the patient is to sit in a chair. On the same note, if the patient appears to want to communicate, the nurse should encourage pointing or use of the communication board.

A person with expressive dsyphasia is frequently frustrated because he or she can understand others, but cannot express his or her own thoughts. The nurse should encourage the patient to speak, instructing him or her to concentrate on using verbs and nouns. The nurse can explain procedures verbally and ask for indications that the patient comprehends. The patient's attempts at speech may be frustrating and the nurse should encourage slow, clear speech patterns. If the patient is difficult to understand, the nurse should encourage repetition or the use of another communication method. It is important to acknowledge the patient's efforts at speech and the associated frustration.

A patient with global dysphasia is much more difficult to treat. In this case, the nurse needs to identify the primary deficit and make attempts at communicating, using methods for both receptive and expressive dysphasia.

Providing Family Support

Interacting with distraught families is a familiar occurrence in the critical care setting. The family's responses and functioning can have a great impact on the patient's outcome. The critical care nurse must ensure that the patient and family have been provided with the necessary support to promote optimal functioning.

Upon the patient's admission to the critical care unit, the immediate objective of the health care team is to stabilize physiologic function. It is at this time that the critical care nurse will first encounter the patient's family. During the initial admission phase, the nurse will be able to begin to assess the family's response to the illness and the supportive resources available to the patient and family. The nurse should also relay information about the patient's status and what the family can expect while the patient is in the critical care unit. The nurse must use this opportunity to identify the family's priority questions and address or refer these questions as appropriate.

On the family's first visit, the nurse should accompany the family to the patient's bedside and again be available for questions. The family should be encouraged to touch and speak with the patient. Once the family has become familiar with the critical care unit, the nurse must assess their readiness to become involved in the patient's care. If the patient has a permanent injury or a long-term deficit, family participation in care will eventually be a necessity; however, early involvement in the patient's physical care gives many family members a feeling of comfort.

First-Level Discharge Planning

Discharge planning must be initiated as soon as the patient enters the health care system. Discharge planning is an organized and systematic approach to making decisions about a patients' progression through the health care system. This involves transitions from one health care phase to another until the patient is able to return to home and the community. In order for the process of discharge planning to be successful, the patient, the family, and a multidisciplinary health care team must all become actively involved.

The critical care nurse must execute the initial steps in planning for the patient's discharge. The critical care nurse will compensate for the patient's lost functional ability while initiating a teaching plan for any knowledge deficits that present.

Rarely will a patient be discharged to the community directly from the critical care unit; however, if such an exceptional situation happens, it poses a real challenge to all involved. I have noted this situation to occur with ventilator-dependent quadriplegic patients who are not going to enter a rehabilitation setting. In such circumstances, the critical care nurse and other members of the health care team would need to teach at least one member of the family the skills needed to care for the patient at home.

Since direct discharge from the critical care unit is a rare occurrence the critical care nurse's role in discharge planning usually involves promoting a smooth transition for the patient to the acute or general care unit. The critical care nurse can facilitate the continuity of care by informing the acute care nurse of the assessments and plans that have been made in the critical care unit. Furnishing such information provides the acute care nurse with a strong framework upon which care planning can proceed and progress and the discharge-planning process can continue.

EVALUATION OF NURSING CARE

In the critical care setting, the evaluation of nursing care is typically based on the patient's responses to life-threatening situations. Critical care nurses are concerned with maintaining if not improving the patient's physiologic status.

In a patient with severe intracranial hypertension, using techniques to minimize increases in cerebral pressure and preventing complications may be the extent of critical care nursing interventions. Providing support for the family of a dying patient may be the most effective intervention that the critical care nurse can provide. If the patient survives the initial stage of neurological insult, evaluation focuses on the degree of adaptation and level of independence achieved.

The deficits that most neuropathologic states produce have an impact on the patient's ability to perform activities of daily living and function independently. These deficits may be transient or permanent in nature. The critical care nurse is able to influence the patient's ability to either overcome or adapt to neurological deficits.

A temporary deficit, such as the slight paresis of an arm, can cause extreme apprehension in a patient. Interventions to maximize early mobility of that arm can be a very effective intervention for a patient to overcome such a transient deficit, and may shorten the patient's recovery and rehabilitation time. A permanent deficit such as permanent paralysis, sensory–perceptual loss, or loss of bowel and bladder function pose a different challenge for the critical care nurse and should, therefore, be evaluated differently. The patient and family will have more opportunities to become active in goal setting, particularly with short-term goals. Sometimes evaluating the adaptation to a permanent deficit is more psychologic in nature. In order to survive psychologically, patients with severe losses may have difficulty accepting these losses and may even need to deny losses or deficits for a time. The critical care nurse needs to allow the time the patient may need, but also needs to be articulate about the permanence of a condition. Clearly addressing the presence of a permanent deficit should not be done in a negative manner, as the patient's hope could be lessened. Rather, the positive aspects and achievable goals should be discussed.

SUMMARY

An alteration in the level of consciousness is an early, reliable and sensitive sign of neurological deterioration (Hickey, 1986). Although an alteration of consciousness is an early indicator of neurological deterioration, it is not a precise indicator of the degree of pathologic involvement. Once alterations in consciousness are noted, the nurse needs to look for further deterioration in physiologic integrity.

BIBLIOGRAPHY

Boortz-Marx, R. (1985). Factors affecting intracranial pressure: A descriptive study . . . Nursing care activities, patients' body positions, and environmental stimuli. *Journal of Neuroscience Nursing, 17,* 89–94.

Bruce, D. (1980). Cerebrospinal dynamics and brain metabolism. In J. H. Wood (Ed.) *Neurobiology of cerebrospinal fluid I*. New York: Plenum.

Bruce, D., Berman, W., & Schut, L. (1977). Cerebrospinal fluid pressure monitoring in children: Physiology, pathology, and clinical usefulness. *Advances in Pediatrics, 24*, 233–290.

Chusid, J. G. (1982). *Correlative neuroanatomy and functional neurology*. Los Altos, CA: Lange Medical Publications.

Delgado, J. M., & Billo, J. M. (1988). Care of the patient with Parkinson's disease: Surgical and nursing implications. *Journal of Neuro-Science Nursing, 20*, 142–150.

Folstein, M. F., Folstein, S. E., & McHugh, P. R. (1975). Mini-mental state: A practical method for grading the cognitive state of patients for the clinician. *Journal of Psychiatric Research, 12*, 189–198.

Groer, M. E. & Shekleton, M. E. (1989). *Basic pathophysiology: A holistic approach* (3rd Ed.). St Louis: C. V. Mosby.

Hickey J. V. (1986). *The clinical practice of neurological and neurosurgical nursing* (2nd ed.). Philadelphia: J. B. Lippincott.

Hulmes. A., & Cooper, R. (1968). Cerebral blood flow during sleep in patients with increased pressure. *Progress in Brain Research, 30*, 77–81.

Jacobs, J. W., Bernhard, M. R., Delgado, A., & Strain, J. J. (1977). Screening for organic mental syndromes in the medically ill. *Annals of Internal Medicine, 86*, 40–46.

Kinney, M. R., Dear, C. B., Packa, D. R., & Voorman, D. M. N. (Eds.) (1981). *AACN's Clinical reference for critical care nursing*. New York: McGraw-Hill.

Kroner, K. (1979). Dealing with the confused patient. *Nursing, 11*, 72–77.

Langfitt, T. W. (1975). Pathophysiology of increased intracranial pressure. In M. Brock & H. Dietz (Eds.). *Intracranial pressure I*. New York: Springer-Verlag.

Mauss, N. K., & Mitchell, P. H. (1976). Increased intracranial pressure: An update. *Heart and Lung, 5*, 919–926.

Miller, J. (1975). Volume and pressure in the craniospinal axis. *Clinical Neurosurgery, 22*, 76–105.

Mitchell, P. H. (1981). Neurological disorders. In M. R. Kinney, C. B. Dean, D. R. Packa, & D. M. Voorman (Eds.). *AACN's clinical reference for critical care nursing*. New York: McGraw-Hill.

Mitchell, P. H., Cammermeyer, M., Ozuna, J., & Woods, N. (1984). *Neurological assessment for nursing practice*. Reston, VA: Reston Publishing.

Mitchell, P. H., Habermann-Little, B., Johnson, F., VanInwegen-Scott, D., & Tyler, D. (1985). Critically ill children: The importance of touch in a high-technology environment. *Nursing Administration Quarterly, 9*, 38–46.

Mitchell, P. H., & Mauss, N. K. (1978). Relationship of patient-nurse activity to intracranial pressure variations: A pilot study. *Nursing Research, 27*, 4–10.

Mitchell, P. H., Mauss, N. K., Lipe, H., & Ozuna, J. (1982). Effects of patient–nurse activity on ICP. In K. Shulman (Ed.). *Intracranial pressure IV*. Berlin: Springer-Verlag.

Nikas, D. L. (1987). Critical aspects of head trauma. *Critical Care Nursing Quarterly, 10*(1), 19–44.

Nikas, D., & Konkoly, R. (1975). Nursing responsibilities in arterial and intracranial pressure monitoring. *Journal of Neurosurgical Nursing, 7*, 116–122.

O'Brien, M. T., & Pallet, P. J. (1978). *Total care of the stroke patient*. Boston: Little, Brown.

Pfeiffer, E. (1975). A short portable mental status questionnaire for the assessment of organic brain deficit in elderly patients. *Journal of the American Geriatrics Society, 23,* 433–441.

Plum, F., & Posner, J. (1982). *The diagnosis of stupor and coma* (3rd ed.). Philadelphia: F. A. Davis.

Ropper, A., Kennedy, S., & Zervas, N. (1983). *Neurological and neurosurgical intensive care.* Baltimore: University Park Press.

Shalit, M. N., & Umansky, R. (1977). Effect of bedside procedures on intracranial pressure. *Israeli Journal of Medical Sciences, 13,* 881–886.

Shapiro, H. (1975). Intracranial hypertension: Therapeutic and anesthetic considerations. *Anesthesiology, 43,* 445–469.

Strub, R., & Black, F. W. (1977). *The mental status examination in neurology.* Philadelphia: F. A. Davis.

Walleck, C. A. (1987). Intracranial hypertension: Interventions and outcomes. *Critical Care Nursing Quarterly, 10*(1), 45–57.

Waltz, A., & Sundt, T. (1968). Influence of systemic blood pressure on blood flow and microcirculation of ischemic cerebral cortex: A failure of autoregulation. *Progress in Brain Research, 30,* 107–112.

ADDITIONAL READINGS

Booth, K. (1982). The neglect syndrome. *Journal of Neurosurgical Nursing, 14,* 38–43.

Conway-Rutkowski, B. L. (1982). *Carini and Owens' neurological and neurosurgical nursing.* St. Louis: C. V. Mosby.

Delgado, J. M. (1983). *The effect on intracranial pressure of turning children to the lateral position.* Unpublished master's thesis, University of Washington, Seattle.

Gastaut, H. (1970). Clinical and electroencephalographical classification of epileptic seizures. *Epilepsia, 11,* 102–113.

Harper, J. (1988). Use of steroids in cerebral edema: Therapeutic implications. *Heart and Lung, 17*(1), 70–75.

Kahn, R. L., Goldfarb, A. L., & Pollack, M. (1960). Brief objective measures for the determination of mental status in the aged. *American Journal of Psychiatry, 117,* 326.

Kaufman, D. M., Weinberger, M., Strain, J., & Jacobs, J. (1979). Detection of cognitive deficits by a brief mental status examination. *General Hospital Psychiatry, 1,* 247–255.

Mattis, S. (1976). Mental status examination for organic mental syndrome in the elderly patient. In L. Bellak & T. Karasu (Eds.). *Geriatric psychiatry: A handbook for psychiatrists and primary care physicians.* New York: Grune & Stratton.

Snyder, M. (1983) *A guide to neurological and neurosurgical nursing.* New York: John Wiley.

Snyder, M., & Jackle, M. (1981). *Neurologic problems: A critical care nursing focus.* Bowie, MD: Robert Brady.

14 Impaired Physical Mobility

Maureen E. Shekleton, D.N.Sc., R.N.

Movement is essential for the maintenance of both physiologic and psychological well-being in humans. Movement provides the means for nonverbal communication and the expression of emotion, for self-defense, and for satisfaction of basic and secondary needs. The ability to adapt to ever-changing conditions depends to a great extent on the individual's level of mobility.

In order for the level of physical mobility to be within normal limits, the nervous and musculoskeletal systems and the proprioceptive sense must be intact and functioning. Trauma (surgical or accidental), disease, or altered levels of consciousness can impair the function of these organ systems with the result of altering the normal level of physical mobility. Restriction of movement may also be voluntary or prescribed. It is interesting to note that prior to World War II, immobilization in the form of imposed bed rest was the treatment of choice for most medical and surgical conditions and after child birth. Pathologic complications that occurred were considered to be the inevitable result of the primary disease process. It was an observation that the incidence of complications appeared to be less in injured soldiers who were rapidly mobilized because of conditions imposed by the war that led to questions about the true benefits of bed rest as a therapeutic measure. These questions, which arose from clinical observations, led to research studies in which the negative consequences of immobility on normal body function were documented; these are discussed later in this chapter.

Whenever an individual experiences a departure from the normal level of physical mobility, impaired physical mobility becomes the focus of treatment. Impaired physical mobility is defined as a state in which the individual experiences or is at risk of experiencing limitation of physical movement (North American Nursing Diagnosis Association definition).

The critically ill surgical or trauma patient will almost certainly experience some degree of impairment of physical mobility. The ability to move will be diminished or restricted for a variety of reasons related to both illness and treatment. The etiology of impaired physical mobility may vary depending on the underlying pathology. For example, Keenan (1989) compared the etiology of impaired physical mobility in neurotrauma and multitrauma patients. The etiologies of intolerance to activity, decreased strength and endurance and neuromuscular impairment were present in both types of patients, but musculoskeletal impairment and pain and discomfort were etiologies present in only the multitrauma patients.

Aside from generalized weakness, the presence of pain, an altered level of consciousness, or any of the other direct effects of illness, the critical care environment and postsurgical treatment can also cause severe restriction of the patient's ability to move or be moved. The presence of drainage devices, bulky dressings, casts, splints or traction, intravenous and arterial lines, and attachment to a ventilator and/or various monitoring devices make even limited movement difficult. Instability of the patient's condition may even be a contraindication to movement. The actions of medication may also adversely affect the patient's ability to move. The effects of immobility may even be already present in the postoperative patient who is brought to the unit after an extended period spent in surgery in one position.

ASSESSMENT OF IMPAIRED PHYSICAL MOBILITY

The degree to which physical mobility is impaired can be assessed using four qualitative measures described by Spencer, Valbona, & Carter (1965). A judgment can be made based on how many of the following conditions are actually present.

1. Physical inactivity, which is manifested by a reduction in body movement;
2. Physical restriction or limitation of movement, which is manifested by an imposed reduction of movement;
3. Constancy of body posture in relation to gravity, which results in a loss of the body's ability to respond and adapt to changes in position and posture; and
4. Sensory deprivation, which causes a reduction in the stimuli to move and which results in even more physical inactivity.

The more of these conditions are present, the greater will be the degree of impairment of physical mobility being experienced by the patient. For example, in a comatose patient all four conditions are present and the degree of impairment of physical mobility is total. In contrast to this is a fully alert, recovering trauma patient whose leg remains in a cast and traction and in whom the degree of impairment of physical mobility is moderate to severe, with all conditions present except sensory deprivation. In further contrast is the patient who is ambulatory but has a cast in place for treatment of a fractured arm. The degree of impairment is minimal since only the condition of an imposed reduction of movement is present.

EFFECTS OF IMPAIRED PHYSICAL MOBILITY

The effects of impaired physical mobility reflect a lack of use and are both functional and metabolic in nature. No body system is immune to the consequences of impaired physical mobility (Groer & Shekleton, 1989). A classic study, conducted in the middle to late 1940s, documented the effects of prolonged immobility in four young, healthy, normal, male volunteers (Deitrick, Whedon, & Schorr, 1948). Physiologic parameters such as heart rate, muscle size and strength, metabolic rate, response to position change, and levels of excreted metabolic products were measured during three separate 6-week periods—before, during, and after immobilization. The data from each period were analyzed to determine changes that had occurred and the length of time necessary for recovery from these changes. The results of this study have been replicated consistently in other studies of the response of normal subjects to immobility. Interestingly, the effects of immobility seen in normal subjects correspond to the experience of astronauts on prolonged space missions, in whom weightlessness simulates immobility. In fact, studies conducted by the Air Force and the National Aeronautics and Space Administration are among those that have increased the body of knowledge about the consequences and treatment of prolonged immobility (Fisher & Fisher, 1980; Goode, 1981; Lynch et al., 1967; Mack & LaChance, 1967; Ryback, Lewis, & Lessard, 1971).

The effects of immobility seen in healthy subjects are a result of deconditioning. Deconditioning was defined by Spencer et al. (1965) as loss of functional capacity secondary to lack of use. These effects include the following:

- Decreased basal metabolic rate,
- Decreased blood volume and red cell mass,
- Increased urinary excretion of calcium, phosphorus, and nitrogen waste products,
- Decreased muscle mass,
- Decreased endurance for physical activity,
- Increased pulse rate, and
- Inability to tolerate position change.

Some of the effects of impaired mobility observed in ill persons have not been observed in healthy subjects participating in immobility studies. In clinical situations the effects of impaired mobility listed above occur concomitantly with pathologic processes that, in the critically ill patient, may be quite severe. The effects of impaired physical mobility in an ill individual can eventually lead to the following problems (Groer & Shekleton, 1989):

- Loss of endurance for physical activity,
- Decreased physical stability,
- Impaired oxygenation processes,
- Chemical disequilibrium,
- Altered patterns of elimination, and
- Impaired tissue integrity.

These problem areas are preventable but have the potential to develop if treatment to minimize the duration and degree of impaired mobility is inadequate. It cannot be emphasized enough that prevention of the complications of immobility is primarily the responsibility of the nurse. This is one area where the outcomes depend totally on independent nursing judgment and action.

Loss of Endurance

The problem of loss of endurance for physical activity, or activity intolerance, can be attributed to both diminished functional capacity of the muscles and an increased cardiac workload. It is related primarily to the loss of functional capacity of the muscles that accompanies lack of use (deconditioning). Functional capacity is determined by frequency, duration, and intensity of use. Loss of functional capacity occurs when these variables are less than optimal, as in the ill patient whose activity level is reduced. Loss of functional capacity is characterized by loss of muscle mass, tone, strength, and endurance.

The loss of muscle mass is related to the principle that metabolic processes tend to balance one another: a reduction in catabolic processes leads to a reduction in anabolic processes and, subsequently, to a reduction in available cellular energy and in cell size. The reduction in cell size that occurs as a result of impaired physical mobility is referred to as *disuse atrophy*.

The loss of muscle mass and strength resulting from disuse is observable and measurable. An example is the observable difference in the size of two limbs seen after removal of a cast from one of them. Deitrick et al. (1948) found a 4 to 10% loss of mass in the thighs and a 10 to 12.5% loss of mass in the calves. Loss of muscle strength in the immobilized legs measured between 13 and 20%. Deitrick et al. (1948) concluded that recovery of preimmobility muscle mass and strength in these normal subjects took between 4 and 6 weeks. One can expect that the effects will be intensified in ill individuals in whom metabolic processes are already altered by the disease process.

The muscles most affected by immobility are the antigravity muscles of the lower limbs. This fact lends support to the theory that the normal stresses of gravity are important in maintaining function and development. This is also true of muscle tone, a state of constant, partial contraction of the muscles. Maintaining an upright position requires a greater degree of muscle tone than lying in bed, and muscle tone will diminish during an extended period spent lying in a recumbent position. The loss of muscle tone further contributes to the loss of mass and strength because it represents a further reduction in the use of the muscles.

As stated previously, the problem of loss of endurance for physical activity (or activity intolerance) can also be attributed in part to an increased cardiac workload. Cardiac workload is increased because of the increased venous return of blood from the lower extremities that is passively mobilized upon assumption of a recumbent position. Stroke volume will be increased to accommodate the increased venous return.

Inactive or immobilized individuals also have a relative tachycardia as compared with active or athletic individuals of the same age and with the same physical characteristics. A progressive increase in the resting pulse rate was documented by both Deitrick et al. (1948) and Taylor, Henschel, Brozek, & Keys (1949). This increase in pulse rate was found to be greater in magnitude during exercise and required twice as long to return to preexercise levels in the immobilized as compared with the normal subjects. Results of these studies also demonstrated that the pulse rate did not return to normal (preimmobility) levels for at least 6 to 8 weeks after resumption of regular activity.

Tachycardia in the inactive individual is thought to be the result of dominance of sympathetic effects in contrast with the active individual in whom vagal or parasympathetic effects predominate. Tachycardia contributes to an increase in cardiac workload by increasing the amount of work performed per unit of time. Because the diastolic period of the cardiac cycle is shortened, ventricular and coronary filling time is also shortened. An increased demand for energy therefore occurs concurrently with a decreased ability to meet that demand.

Clinical manifestations of loss of endurance for physical activity include weakness, easy fatigability, and an increased pulse rate, especially during activity or exercise. Loss of endurance will lead to a further reduction in physical activity since an individual will match the level of actual activity to the physical capacity or tolerance for such activity. Closely related problems are those of impaired oxygenation processes and chemical disequilibrium, since decreased levels of available oxygen and disruption of normal metabolic processes will affect the amount of energy available for activity. Loss of endurance is, therefore, a central feature in the vicious cycle created by impaired physical mobility.

Decreased Physical Stability

After a period of impaired physical mobility, an individual's physical stability, or the ability to maintain steady movement in or to change position to the upright position without losing balance, will also be impaired. This individual will have difficulty in maintaining equilibrium while in motion in an upright, weight-bearing position because of the generalized body weakness, loss of joint mobility, osteoporosis, and postural hypotension that occur as sequelae of the immobility being experienced (Groer & Shekleton, 1989).

Weakness is the result of muscle atrophy and the slowing of metabolic processes that occurs as a result of decreased activity. When a muscle atrophies it can no longer generate the same amount of force, i.e., the strength of the muscle is decreased. The general slowing of metabolic processes means that less energy for activity is available. Stability is affected because it becomes extremely difficult to perform activities that require the use of energy, such as attaining and maintaining the upright posture.

Loss of joint mobility is the result of the pathologic changes that occur in the muscle and connective tissue surrounding the joints in response to decreased joint movement. The muscles, because of decreased use and loss of tone become either stretched from being held in a lengthened position or contracted from being held in a shortened position. Fibrosis of the surrounding connective tissue will fix the muscles in these positions. Fibrosis occurs because the normally areolar nature of the connective tissue is maintained by stretching through repeated movement. If movement of the joint is limited or absent, this tissue becomes denser, fixed, or less resilient, i.e., fibrosed. Stiffness of the joints may be the first sign of loss of joint mobility. Because of these changes, the joint becomes progressively more resistant to movement and eventually may become fixed in one position, a condition referred to as a *contracture*. Once contractures have begun to form, a greater than normal energy expenditure is required to overcome the added resistance in the joint.

Assumption of the bed-lying position for any period makes an individual susceptible to the development of several different contracture deformities. The critical care nurse needs to pay particular attention to how a patient is positioned in the bed-lying position as well the frequency of position changes, since the critically ill surgical patient may be unable to leave the bed for several days after surgery. Contractures can form vary rapidly and, once formed, often require months of therapy to reverse, with the possibility that functional mobility may not be restored completely. Flexion deformities, especially of the back, hips, and knees, and footdrop may develop as a result of the alignment of the body in the recumbent position. Functional alignment of the bones and muscles for the weight-bearing position is not supported in this position, as is illustrated in Figure 14–1.

Another factor that works to reduce physical stability as a result of immobility is a reduction in bone mass, or osteoporosis. The processes of bone formation and resorption, under normal conditions, are in balance with one another. Activity and movement with the resultant mechanical stress on the bones is thought to stimulate bone growth through a piezoelectric effect. When that stress is removed (as when impaired physical mobility occurs), the process of bone resorption is favored. It is a known fact that the bones of athletic individuals are heavier than those of sedentary individuals. As the matrix is broken down, the mineral constituents of the bone are released into the general circulation and the excesses will be excreted in the urine. The urinary loss of calcium leads to other problems, which are discussed later in

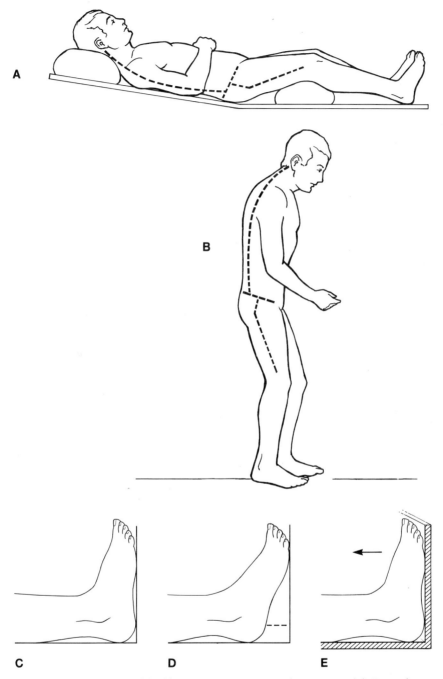

Figure 14–1. Effects of bed-lying position on upright posture. (A) Recumbent. (B) Upright. (C) Normal position of the foot. (D) Usual position of foot with individual in supine position. It is this position that promotes the development of a footdrop contracture deformity. (E) Corrected position. A support should be used to maintain the normal anatomic position of the foot. From *Basic Pathophysiology: A Holistic Approach,* 3rd ed., by M. E. Groer and M. E. Shekleton, 1989, St. Louis: The C. V. Mosby Co. Reproduced with permission.

this chapter. Deitrick et al. (1948) found that the level of urinary calcium in immobilized subjects rose on the second to third day after immobility began, indicating that bone resorption begins soon after the usual level of mobility is reduced.

Individuals who are at greatest risk for the development of osteoporosis are postmenopausal females and patients in whom a pathologic process or treatment (e.g., steroid therapy), which also affects the processes of bone formation and resorption, exists concurrently with the impaired physical mobility. If osteoporosis is severe enough, pathologic fractures of the bones may occur. The neck of the femur, the ribs, and the lower end of the radius are most susceptible. Vertebral compression can also occur, resulting in back pain, which is a common complaint after long periods of immobility and which can become chronic. Weight bearing under these conditions can become very difficult and, again, an effect of immobility is seen to contribute to further impaired physical mobility.

Postural or orthostatic hypotension has been observed consistently in all of the studies of immobilized individuals cited thus far. These studies have also demonstrated that it occurs despite intact sympathetic nervous system responses and that it occurs more frequently when subjects are raised passively to the upright position. Normally, as an individual assumes the upright position from a sitting or lying position, baroreceptor reflexes elicit an immediate sympathetic response to any reduction in arterial pressure. This response causes constriction of the splanchnic and peripheral blood vessels, which prevents pooling of the blood in the lower extremities. Failure of these vessels to constrict, as seen in immobilized persons, results in rapid pooling of blood in the lower extremities. Subsequently, decreased venous return, decreased cardiac output, and reduced arterial pressure result in a feeling of dizziness or faintness, or possibly even loss of consciousness upon arising (Thomas, Schirger, Fealey, & Sheps, 1981; Levy & Talbot, 1983). It is thought that postural hypotension due to immobility is the result of changes in the reactivity of the vessels themselves rather than to any aberrance in sympathetic function. This change in reactivity is thought to be the result of disuse similar to the loss of tone seen in unused muscles (Groer & Shekleton, 1989). Another possible contributory factor is the loss of the pumping action of the muscles on the blood vessels of the lower extremities. During periods of immobility the muscle tone will be diminished and the number of contractions of the muscles of the lower extremities will be reduced, thus minimizing any effect the muscles have on preventing venous pooling. Deitrick and coworkers (1948) were able to diminish the fainting response by wrapping the subjects' legs with elastic bandages.

Impaired Oxygenation Processes

Several of the effects of immobility compound one another to disrupt normal oxygenation processes in the immobilized individual. Among these responses to impaired physical mobility are a reduction in blood volume and red-cell mass, decreased cardiac output, ineffective breathing pattern and airway clearance, and potential for altered tissue perfusion related to thrombus and embolus formation. The disruption of oxygenation processes may be an especially significant problem in the critically ill patient.

A reduction in blood volume and red-cell mass adversely affects the oxygen-carrying capacity of the blood. The decrease in cardiac output that is secondary to venous stasis will adversely affect the transport process by which oxygen is delivered to the body tissues and carbon dioxide is removed. The combination of these two conditions results in a reduction in oxygen-delivery capability, which has implications for periods during which the body's oxygen requirements might increase. There will be a decreased ability to supply oxygen in the face of an increased demand, which may precipitate a crisis in the already precarious hemodynamic status of the critically ill patient.

Ventilatory ability is also affected by immobility. Ventilation is the mechanical act of drawing oxygen from the atmosphere into the alveoli of the lungs and expelling carbon dioxide from the alveoli into the atmosphere. An ineffective breathing pattern characterized by reduced chest and lung expansion is the result of the pressure created in the supine position by the abdominal organs and the bed against the diaphragm and thoracic cage. This will be compounded by the pattern of breathing caused by anesthesia and surgery (see chapter 1) as well as by poor posture in bed and the use of constrictive bandages, binders, or clothing.

Ineffective airway clearance related to stasis of secretions has not been observed in healthy subjects participating in immobility studies. Persons at greatest risk for ineffective airway clearance during a period of immobility are those who are totally unable to move or in whom ventilatory function is already impaired, mucus secretion is excessive or thicker than usual, or the cough reflex is suppressed. The critically ill surgical patient will most likely fit this description. Impaired physical mobility further complicates this situation because of position, reduced efficiency of the normal mucociliary clearance mechanism, and the ineffective breathing pattern described in the preceding paragraph. When an individual is in the upright position, the bronchioles are in a vertical plane and mucus will be distributed in a fairly uniform manner. In the supine position the bronchioles will be oriented along a horizontal plane and mucus will pool on the lower side. The cilia on the upper sides of the bronchioles may become dried, which can damage the cilia. The cilia on the lower side of the bronchioles may not be able to move the volume of pooled mucus effectively. Additionally, the diameter of the lumen of the bronchioles is decreased in the supine position, and this effect will be intensified by the pooled secretions. These changes are illustrated in Figure 14–2.

These conditions predispose the patient to the development of hypostatic pneumonia or a mucus plug. Pneumonia is an inflammatory process characterized by consolidation due to exudate filling the alveolar spaces. This inflammation can be the result of an infectious process or the aspiration of

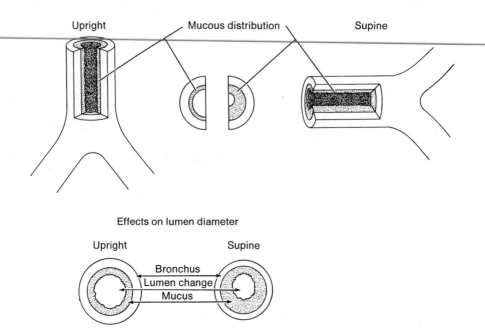

Figure 14–2. Effect of recumbent position and gravity on distribution of respiratory tract secretions and diameter of bronchiolar lumen. From *Basic Pathophysiology: A Holistic Approach,* 3rd ed., by M. E. Groer and M. E. Shekleton, 1989, St. Louis: The C. V. Mosby Co. Reproduced with permission.

food, vomitus, or chemical agents into the respiratory tract. The immobilized patient is at risk for development of pneumonia for two reasons. First, accumulated secretions can act as a medium for the growth of microorganisms and thereby lead to infection. Secondly, the supine position predisposes an individual to aspiration. The signs and symptoms of pneumonia include fever, dyspnea, cough, pallor, malaise, and cyanosis if hypoxemia due to the shunting of blood around nonfunctional alveoli is severe. Consolidation will appear as radiopaque or as a hazy area on the chest roentgenogram in the dependent areas of the lung fields (Sanchez, 1986). Breath sounds over the affected lung tissue will be absent or bronchial in nature.

Venous thrombosis is another condition that may develop as a result of impaired physical mobility and that can contribute to the disruption of normal oxygenation processes (Moser & Fedullo, 1983). Most commonly, thrombi develop in the deep veins of the legs and can spread the entire length of a vein. Blood does not clot within the blood vessels under normal conditions, so obviously some abnormal condition(s) must be present for this to occur. Conditions that enhance the formation of intravascular thrombi include endothelial damage or changes in the vessel, venous stasis, and increased blood viscosity or coagulability (Groer & Shekleton, 1989).

Venous stasis is the only one of these conditions that is directly affected by immobility. Immobility contributes to venous stasis through loss of the pumping action of the muscles and because of the structure of the veins themselves. During inactivity, the pooling of blood in dependent areas of the body is enhanced because the pumping action created by muscular contraction and that promotes venous return is greatly diminished. Veins are affected because of the relatively slow flow of venous blood and because the many bifurcations and valve pockets within the veins contribute to localized areas of stasis during periods of immobility.

It is believed that stasis may create a local environment in which thrombin is concentrated and sequestered from inactivation by the liver. Venous stasis alone does not cause thrombus formation. Other factors must also be present, and surgical patients are predisposed to development of factors that can enhance thrombus formation. Hypercoagulability associated with an increase in the number and the adhesiveness of the platelets and a rise in the prothrombin time has been observed after both surgical and accidental trauma. These changes have been found to be greatest on the 10th day after the injury, which coincides with the time most thromboembolic episodes occur. There is also some evidence that fibrinolysis is inadequate, which may be the result of impaired plasminogen activation. The intimal endothelium of a thrombosed vessel is usually found to be normal, but sites where invasive treatment measures such as placement of intravascular cannula have been used may serve as focal points for a thrombotic process to begin. In the surgical population, the greatest risk of thromboembolism exists in patients who have experienced injury or surgery of the pelvis and/or lower extremities or prolonged general anesthesia. In the critically ill patient population, a history of venous thrombosis with residual venous obstruction or right ventricular failure as well as immobility serve as predisposing factors for thrombus formation.

Clinical manifestations of venous thrombosis depend on whether a superficial or deep vein has been affected. There will be visible redness along the affected vein as well as tenderness and hardness on palpation if a superficial vein is affected. Deep-vein thrombosis following immobilization after surgery or during bed rest and illness usually occurs in the soleal veins of the calf. Local pain on compression of the calf may be the only sign. If venous return is blocked, swelling of the leg will occur. If the thrombus is less extensive, a measurable increase in calf circumference may occur, with redness, warmth, and tenderness in the affected area. Movement will aggravate the pain and Homan's sign (calf and popliteal pain upon dorsiflexion of the foot) is often present. Systemic signs of an inflammatory process (fever, leukocytosis, an increased erythrocyte sedimentation rate, and an increased pulse rate) will also be present.

Thrombosis is a serious complication of immobility because of the potential it poses for embolism. The site of embolism secondary to thrombosis of the systemic veins is most frequently the pulmonary vasculature. Most clinically significant pulmonary emboli have been found to be the result of thrombosis in the lower-extremity veins. It is estimated that at least 10% of all episodes of deep-vein thrombosis lead to pulmonary embolism, which subsequently results in a mortality rate of 10%.

Signs and symptoms of a pulmonary embolism depend on the size of the embolus and the portion of the pulmonary circulation in which it lodges. A large embolus from the femoral or iliac trunk that occludes the pulmonary artery will cause sudden death, preceded by a period of intense dyspnea accompanied by cyanosis and gross neck-vein distention. Smaller emboli can pass through the right side of the heart and pulmonary artery to become lodged in smaller branches of the pulmonary circulation. Clinical manifestations can include dyspnea of sudden onset and chest pain. Other signs and symptoms will be those of right-sided heart failure due to increased pulmonary vascular pressure and resistance. If cardiac output drops to the point at which tissue perfusion is jeopardized, signs of cerebral hypoxia such as restlessness, confusion, or diminished consciousness may also appear.

Chemical Disequilibrium

Normal chemical equilibrium of the body is disrupted by impaired physical mobility through the following pathophysiologic mechanisms: a negative calcium balance, a negative nitrogen balance, and an alteration in fluid distribution in the dependent parts of the body. Calcium is excreted in the urine as bone resorption occurs in response to immobility. Deitrick et al. (1948) demonstrated that urinary excretion of calcium began within the first week of immobility and reached a peak during the fourth to sixth week of immobility. Dietary absorption of calcium is also impaired during periods of immobility, leading to increased fecal excretion. Not only can these conditions cause a negative calcium balance, but the increase in urinary calcium can negatively affect normal elimination processes as well.

The nitrogen balance provides a gross measure of protein utilization by the body. A negative nitrogen balance occurs when the loss of nitrogen due to the breakdown of protein exceeds the replacement of nitrogen. The urinary excretion of nitrogen, which occurs in healthy immobilized individuals on the fifth or sixth day after immobilization, is thought to reflect the depletion of muscle tissue as atrophy occurs. This is supported by the fact that the urinary sulfur–nitrogen ratio remains stable during periods of impaired physical mobility, indicating that sulfur-rich tissue such as that found in skeletal muscle is being catabolized. Factors that may exacerbate the loss of nitrogen and that are especially relevant to the critically ill surgical patient are poor nutritional status and pathologic states, such as stress and trauma (accidental and surgical), in which protein is being catabolized rapidly. The consequence of a negative nitrogen balance is lack of adequate nitrogen for protein synthesis, which will impair tissue repair and healing. With severe protein depletion the plasma protein concentration will eventually decrease as well.

Fluid will shift from the intravascular to the interstitial compartments in the dependent areas of the body as a result of the increased hydrostatic pressure secondary to venous stasis. Blood pools in the dependent areas of the body due to the cumulative effects of gravity, the nature of the veins as capacitance vessels, and the loss of the pumping action of the muscles. The hydrostatic pressure of the blood at the venous end of the capillary bed will increase proportionately as the volume of pooled blood increases. When the hydrostatic pressure gradient becomes higher than the osmotic pressure gradient, the Starling forces will be disrupted such that the movement of fluid out to the intravascular compartment is favored. If the plasma protein concentration is less than normal, the Starling forces will be disrupted more readily. The result is dependent edema. Edematous tissue can be uncomfortable and is more easily injured than normal tissue. Edema of the lower extremities can make walking and standing difficult, impairing physical mobility even further.

Altered Patterns of Elimination

The effects of impaired physical mobility can disrupt normal elimination patterns of both the bladder and bowel. Constipation does not result directly from decreased mobility but occurs as a result of weakness of the abdominal and perineal muscles and decreased gastric motility, which are direct consequences of immobility. Decreased gastric motility may contribute to the feelings of bloating and anorexia that many immobilized individuals experience. Other factors, such as dietary changes, stress, lack of privacy, difficulty using a bedpan, and inhibition of the urge to defecate in the supine position may also contribute to constipation.

Normal patterns of urinary elimination can be disrupted by renal calculi, retention of urine, and urinary tract infection. Like constipation, stone formation and infection are not direct results of immobility per se but can occur because of alterations in the composition and acidity of the urine and urinary stasis, which are direct effects of immobility. Urinary calcium remains in solution through the action of citric acid and the acidic condition of the urine. During periods of immobility, the calcium concentration increases at the same time that fewer acid products of metabolism are being formed and the pH of the urine is rising. The alkalinity of the urine and the altered ratio between citric acid and calcium concentrations favoring the calcium concentration will enhance the precipitation of calcium salts from the urine, thereby promoting the formation of renal calculi.

Stasis also favors precipitation of calcium salts out of solution in the urine. Because of the effects of gravity, the recumbent position causes pooling of the urine in the dependent part of the bladder, and complete emptying of the bladder may be very difficult. Urine will also pool in the dependent calyces of the kidney as illustrated in Figure 14–3. This effect will be intensified if the patient has difficulty voiding in the sitting or lying position. The presence of stagnant urine in the kidneys and bladder increases the chances that an infectious process might develop. Retention of urine can cause distention of the bladder to such a degree that small tears develop in the bladder mucosa, providing a site for infection to develop. Development of an infection will even further enhance the conditions that promote renal calculi formation: urine alkalinity will continue to increase and cellular debris from the inflammatory process can serve as nuclei for stone formation.

Clinical manifestations of renal calculi include hematuria, colicky flank pain, backache, and nausea and vomiting. Constipation, bloating, urinary retention or infection, and renal calculi create discomfort for the patient, which may lead to further impairment of physical mobility.

Impaired Tissue Integrity

The potential for impaired tissue integrity exists in all ill and/or debilitated patients with impaired physical mobility. The potential for this serious and devastating problem will be compounded by the presence of a negative nitrogen balance, since tissue repair and synthesis will be retarded. Prevention of impaired tissue integrity should be a major focus of the nursing care of the immobilized patient.

Various terms are used to describe impaired tissue integrity related to impaired physical mobility, including pressure sore, pressure ulcer, decubitus ulcer, and bedsore. All these terms refer to a lesion that is the result of

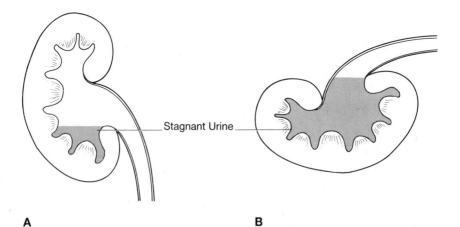

A   **B**

Figure 14–3.   Effect of position and gravity on distribution of urine in calyces of kidneys. (A) Upright position. (B) Recumbent (supine) position promotes stasis of urine in dependent calyces and inhibits complete emptying of urine. From *Basic Pathophysiology: A Holistic Approach,* 3rd ed., by M. E. Groer and M. E. Shekleton, 1989, St. Louis: The C. V. Mosby Co. Reproduced with permission.

ischemic injury to the skin and subcutaneous tissues due to prolonged pressure, shearing forces, and/or friction. The term pressure sore or ulcer is most descriptive of what is believed to be the primary cause.

The consequences of development of a pressure sore to the individual are pain, discouragement and depression, increased susceptibility to infection, loss of body fluid, and further impairment of physical mobility. Development of a pressure sore may prolong hospitalization, delay rehabilitation, and impose economic hardship as well (Parish, Witkowski, & Crissey, 1983). The consequences to the health care system include higher morbidity and mortality rates and increased health care costs related to an increased need for institutionalization and nursing care. In a review of the literature on pressure ulcers, Maklebust (1987) reports the following statistics: approximately 60,000 persons die from pressure-sore-related complications each year; the cost estimates to heal each pressure ulcer range between $5000 and $40,000; and presence of a pressure ulcer can cause as much as a 50% increase in nursing care costs. It is obvious, then, that prevention of the development of pressure ulcers could result in great cost savings to the health care system and prevent much suffering in already ill and debilitated patients.

Any patient experiencing impaired physical mobility is at risk for the development of a pressure sore, although the potential is greater in certain groups of patients. A patient with impaired sensory input or motor function is at greater risk than a patient with intact sensory and motor function who is on bed rest. It is estimated that the incidence of pressure sores is as high as 85% in the patient population with injured spinal cords, and is the cause of up to 8% of the deaths in that population (Reuler & Cooney, 1981).

Other factors that place a patient at greater risk for the formation and nonhealing of a pressure sore are malnutrition (protein deficiency and negative nitrogen balance and lack of adequate amounts of vitamin C), anemia, dehydration, hyperglycemia, maceration (moistness and softening of the skin), heat, circulatory impairment, and corticosteroid therapy (catabolism is increased) (Schappler, 1989). Recent weight loss and low hemoglobin levels have been associated with the development of pressure ulcers (Iverson-Carpenter, 1989). These conditions may reflect an alteration in nutritional status, which predisposes the patient to tissue breakdown. Edematous tissue is more prone to pressure damage, as the blood supply is already impaired and waste products remain because of the existing disruption of the Starling forces in the capillary bed. Excessive moisture on the skin can be the result of wound drainage, perspiration, condensation from humidified oxygen-delivery systems, and fecal and urinary incontinence. Reuler and Cooney (1981) state that the presence of moisture increases the risk of pressure-sore formation fivefold. Heat increases tissue metabolism and the need for oxygen, making already hypoxic tissue even more susceptible to ischemic injury. Age must also be considered in the pathogenesis of a pressure sore, as the incidence increases in the elderly (Groer & Shekleton, 1989). Of significance to the critically ill population, Stotts (1987) found, in a sample of 67 patients admitted to the cardiovascular or neurosurgical services of a tertiary care hospital, that length of hospitalization and severity of illness were even more important determinants of pressure-ulcer development than age-specific characteristics. Stotts (1988) also found that pressure ulcers developed more frequently in patients undergoing cardiovascular surgery as compared with those undergoing neurosurgery, and speculated that this is related to preexisting impairment in tissue perfusion. Sites of the most severe ulcers seen in this sample were the knee and lateral malleoulus. There were indications from the data obtained in this study that the early postoperative period may be an important time for the prediction of pressure-ulcer development in patients who have undergone cardiovascular or neurological surgery.

Obesity can either decrease or increase susceptibility to pressure-sore development. Adipose tissue, in small quantities, can serve a protective function by cushioning the bony prominences against the effects of pressure. This function is thought to be most applicable to persons older than 75 years of age. On the other hand, adipose tissue is not as well vascularized or as resilient as other types of body tissue so it is more vulnerable when subjected to sustained pressure and shearing forces (Natow, 1983).

As stated previously, pressure is the essential element in the formation of a pressure sore. In fact, development of a pressure sore is a function of a time–pressure relationship (Stotts, 1988). Obviously, the skin and subcutaneous tissue can tolerate some pressure, or sitting and lying would be impossible. Externally applied pressure that exceeds that of the capillary bed obstructs blood flow, resulting in tissue hypoxia. Ischemic injury occurs if the hypoxic condition is allowed to persist beyond a critical time threshold. If a tissue pressure greater than 32 mm Hg remains unrelieved beyond this point the vessels will collapse and thrombose (Maklebust, 1987). If the pressure is relieved prior to this point, circulation is restored through the physiologic mechanism of reactive hyperemia. The local histologic changes, documented through both light and electron microscopy, seen in response to pressure are as follows: gross changes, pallor (early), edema and reactive hyperemia (later); with moderate pressure (100 mm Hg for 2 hours), patchy congestion of the skin vessels, subcutaneous edema and moderate inflammatory infiltrate; and with sustained pressure (100 mm Hg for 6 hours), intense inflammatory infiltrate, degenerating muscle fibers, loss of cross striations, and swelling of myofibrils (Constantian, 1980, p. 20).

Other factors important to note in the pathogenesis of a pressure sore are the varying degrees of pressure tolerance exhibited by different body tissues and the gradient and distribution of the pressure. Fat and muscle are more susceptible to ischemic injury than the skin (Cherry & Ryan, 1983). Rather than being distributed and dissipated over large areas of the body surface, pressure is concentrated over bony prominences close to the body surface that have less subcutaneous fat and muscle padding. These are the sites at which pressure ulcers are most likely to develop (Figure 14–4). Localized pressure areas can also be created by external devices such as casts and

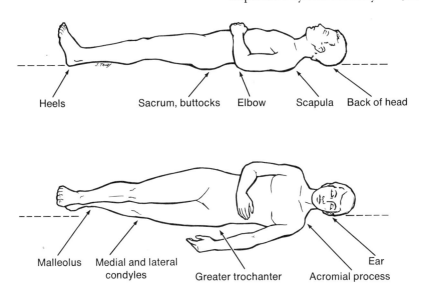

Heels   Sacrum, buttocks   Elbow   Scapula   Back of head

Malleolus   Medial and lateral   Ear
            condyles   Greater trochanter   Acromial process

Toes   Knees   Iliac crest   Ear unless the
                                                head is supported

Figure 14–4. Pressure points in various body positions. (A) Supine. (B) Side. (C) Prone. These are the sites at which pressure sores are most likely to form. From *Basic Pathophysiology: A Holistic Approach,* 3rd ed., by M. E. Groer and M. E. Shekleton, 1989, St. Louis: The C. V. Mosby Co. Reproduced with permission.

traction apparatus, catheters, tubing, or loose foreign objects in the bed that exert a constant pressure.

Subcutaneous tissue damage may be quite extensive, with the greatest damage occurring at the bony interface because of the way in which pressure is dissipated across the subcutaneous soft tissues to the bone. Pressure is transmitted between the surface and the bone in a cone-shaped pattern with its base at the bone surface. A wider area of subcutaneous damage may therefore exist than that which is apparent on the skin's surface.

Another type of mechanical stress that can contribute to the formation of a pressure sore is *shearing force*. This occurs when adjacent, parallel surfaces of tissues move in such a way that the end result is relative displacement of these tissues with respect to one another. When a patient is moved or repositioned in bed without being lifted or is allowed to slide down in the bed the skin surface may adhere to the bed while the bone slides in the direction of movement. The deeper tissue will slide with the bone while subcutaneous tissue attached to the dermis remains in position with the skin. The result is stretching of the tissues and kinking and damage of the blood vessels. Subcutaneous fat is particularly vulnerable to damage because of its lack of tensile strength (Reuler & Cooney, 1981). Shearing force is thought to be particularly relevant to the development of sacral pressure sores (Maklebust, 1987). Deep massage over bony prominences may inadvertently cause shear and, therefore, should be done with care.

Friction is the force resulting from two surfaces that come into contact with one another while moving in opposite directions. The effect of the friction generated when skin is dragged across sheets can be abrasion or removal of the outermost layer of skin. This effect is exaggerated by moisture. Removal of the outermost layer of skin enhances the potential for infection as well as making the skin more susceptible to pressure damage.

The clinical manifestations of the effects of pressure present on a continuum. Intervention will depend on the stage of pressure-induced damage that is present. The initial change is that of *blanchable erythema*. This appears as a red spot that turns white when compressed and immediately recolors when the compression is relieved. This area may appear slightly elevated and feel warm to the touch. If sensation to the area is intact, the patient may complain of pain or tenderness. With removal and avoidance of repeated pressure, the skin will return to normal within 24 hours, as permanent damage has not occurred. If pressure is unrelieved, the second stage in the formation of a pressure sore will present as *nonblanchable erythema*. The area will be more sharply defined, the color will be more intense (a dark red to cyanotic) and will not fade when the area is compressed. The affected area may feel cool and soft to the touch. If sensation is intact, there will be pain and tenderness. With prompt relief of pressure, the damage is reversible but may take 1 to 3 weeks to return to normal. Treatment of both blanchable and nonblanchable erythema includes avoidance of pressure on the affected area and keeping the area cool and dry until the tissue returns to normal.

If pressure is unrelieved, damage will progress to the third stage, *decubitus or pressure dermatitis*. This stage is characterized by disruption of the epidermis. Vesicles, bullae, scaling, and crusting (serous and hemorrhagic) appear. If sensation is intact, there will be pain and tenderness. Pressure must be relieved immediately and unruptured vesicles and bullae should remain intact to prevent contamination. Cool compresses can be used, but in order to avoid maceration the site should not be covered with material that holds moisture, such as plastic. Heat, which increases the metabolic demands of the tissues, must be avoided; the use of warm compresses, heat lamps, or heating pads is therefore contraindicated (Tepperman & Devlin, 1983). Topical agents that reduce the effects of inflammation can be applied. Healing is possible but will require 2 to 4 weeks. Treatment must be prompt and aggressive if progression to the next stage is to be prevented.

The fourth stage is the development of a true *pressure ulcer*. The early ulcer appears as a superficial erosion of the epidermis with indistinct borders, an irregular shape, and a glistening erythematous base surrounded by an area of decubitus dermatitis or nonblanchable erythema. A chronic or true pressure ulcer will develop if pressure persists. The base of the chronic ulcer appears flat and dusky red in color. The tissue does not bleed easily and various tissues (muscle, tendon, bone, etc.) may be exposed, depending on the depth of the ulcer. Because of the pressure-gradient phenomenon a relatively small surface opening may expose a much larger necrotic cavity beneath the skin, with wide undermining and extensive fat necrosis. The skin surrounding the chronic ulcer is warm, indurated, and erythematous and blanches very little with pressure (Parish et al., 1983).

A pressure sore can form rapidly and once formed will continue to deteriorate unless treatment is very aggressive. Illustrated in Figure 14–5 is the sequence of events in the formation and perpetuation of a pressure sore. Pressure ulcers present with varying degrees of tissue damage, and choice of an appropriate treatment will depend on the extent of that damage. Pressure ulcers are categorized according to the following grading system (Enis & Sarmiento, 1973; Shea, 1975). Grade I ulcers are partial-thickness skin alterations confined to the epidermis and dermis. Grade II ulcers are full-thickness tissue alterations that extend through the subcutaneous tissue. These low-grade pressure ulcers are the most common (Reuler & Cooney, 1981) and treatment is amenable to nonsurgical interventions, which are most often determined through independent nursing judgment and decision making. In contrast, Grade III ulcers, which involve the deep fascia, and Grade IV ulcers, which involve bone, require surgical repair, including debridement and closure with skin and tissue flaps in addition to aggressive systemic treatment to correct any underlying medical conditions such as infection, malnutrition, and anemia that can perpetuate the tissue damage. Nonsurgical interventions are geared toward prevention of further tissue damage and promotion of wound healing. Further tissue damage is prevented through relief of additional pressure and avoidance of infection. Wound healing is promoted through local wound care and attention to nutritional needs.

Pressure can be relieved and avoided through frequent repositioning or through the use of a variety of devices that can be used to support specific pressure areas (e.g., gel flotation pads, sheepskin, foam boots), aid in turning or moving a patient (e.g., Stryker frame, CircOLectric bed), or support the entire body surface to change, minimize, or equalize pressure distribution across the body surface (e.g., air mattress, water bed, air-fluidized bed, foam eggcrate mattress).

Infection causes further tissue destruction and retards healing. More importantly, infection and sepsis are potentially life-threatening complications of a pressure ulcer (Reuler & Cooney, 1981). The organisms most frequently involved in infection of a pressure ulcer include the normal microbes found on skin. Organisms from the gastrointestinal tract most often infect

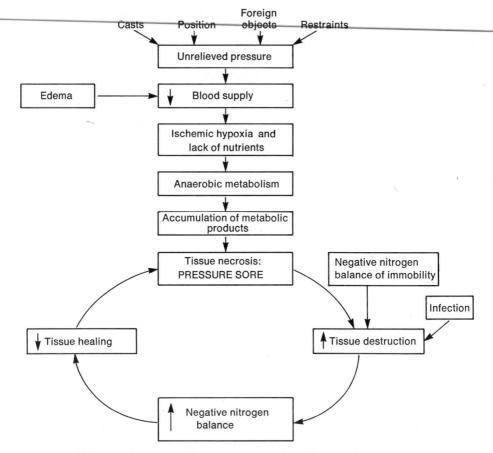

Figure 14–5. Pathogenesis of pressure sore and resulting cycle once pressure has developed. From *Basic Pathophysiology: A Holistic Approach,* 3rd ed., by M. E. Groer and M. E. Shekleton, 1989, St. Louis: The C. V. Mosby Co. Reproduced with permission.

pressure ulcers below the waist (Gurevich, 1983). Necrotic tissue must be debrided, as it provides a potential site for infection.

The ulcerated area must be kept clean, and agents that stimulate granulation tissue formation can be applied. Because of the nature of the injury, healing occurs through second-intention connective-tissue repair. Basically, the site is filled with highly vascular granulation tissue over a matrix of fibrin. Eventually, collagen fibrils are deposited, which serve as the basis for scar formation. Fowler (1987) provides a review of local wound care, which consists of cleansing, possibly debriding, and using an appropriate material to dress the wound.

Poor healing may be the result of many factors (which were reviewed earlier in this chapter) that may be present because of the immobility and the critical nature of illness being experienced. Nutrition is especially critical, as second-intention healing requires more tissue synthesis than primary-intention healing. In contrast to normal repair of healthy tissue, in which an 80% growth rate is seen by the third day, less than a 70% growth rate at 14 days has been observed in biopsied pressure-ulcer tissue (Sieggreen, 1987). Natow (1983) recommends a diet high in protein and carbohydrates and a moderate amount of fat. Vitamin C and zinc supplements are suggested for patients who have or are at risk for development of a pressure sore.

TREATMENT OF IMPAIRED PHYSICAL MOBILITY

No body system escapes the consequences of impaired physical mobility, and each of the resulting problems just discussed has the potential to reduce the level of physical mobility even more. The problems are related and compound one another (Groer & Shekleton, 1989). The severity of the effects of impaired physical mobility is directly proportional to the duration and the degree of the impairment being experienced by the patient. These effects will progressively worsen, and some changes may become irreversible if effective treatment is not begun immediately.

The goal of treatment of impaired physical mobility is prevention of all of the pathologic effects of immobility discussed above. The nursing diagnostic category, potential for disuse syndrome, has been approved for clinical use and testing through the 1987–1988 diagnosis review cycle of the North American Nursing Diagnosis Association (NANDA). This category has been defined by NANDA as "the state in which an individual is at risk for deterioration of body systems as a result of prescribed or unavoidable musculoskeletal inactivity" (Carroll-Johnson, 1989, p. 530; Esposito, Tracey & McCourt, 1989 pp. 464–468.) Risk factors include all of the conditions that lead to impaired physical mobility discussed earlier in this chapter. Interventions to prevent all of the potential effects of impaired physical mobility are incorporated within this one category, which is recommended for use in planning the care of an at-risk patient (Shekleton, 1989). If any of the pathologic sequelae of impaired physical mobility should occur, the revised care plan would incorporate the appropriate nursing diagnosis, for example, impaired tissue integrity or altered tissue perfusion.

Lack of endurance and decreased physical stability can be prevented or minimized by range-of-motion exercises for all the joints while on bed rest, early ambulation, and positional changes and isometric and isotonic exercises (if not contraindicated) (Lentz, 1981). Weight-bearing activities will promote bone deposition and thus help decrease the amount of calcium being lost. Structural and functional integrity of the muscles, connective tissue, and joints can be maintained through anatomic positioning of the limbs and joints. Early initiation of such nursing measures in the critically ill patient may have a significant impact on successful rehabilitation and long-term outcomes. The use of elastic or anti-embolism stockings to prevent venous pooling in the extremities will help prevent postural hypotension as well as thromboembolic phenomena.

Coughing and deep-breathing exercises and change of position will prevent ineffective airway clearance and promote a more effective breathing pattern through excursion of the respiratory muscles. Frequent position changes will also prevent stasis of urine in the kidneys and bladder and relieve pressure on the different body parts. When movement is not possible or is extremely restricted, as may be the case with the critically ill surgical patient, there are a variety of mechanical aids that can be used to relieve pressure and prevent contracture development. It is important to remember that, once a pressure sore has formed, it is extremely difficult to treat. Prevention is the best treatment. Successful prevention begins with an assessment of the potential for impaired tissue integrity based on identification of the risk factors for each patient with impaired physical mobility. Gosnell (1987) provides a review of the various assessment instruments available for use (Williams, 1972; Gosnell, 1973; Gruis & Innes, 1976; Norton, McLaren, & Exton-Smith, 1981; Abruzzese, 1985; Bergstrom, Braden, Laquzza, & Holman, 1985; Stotts, 1985; Waterlow, 1985; Pritchard, 1986; Bergstrom, Demuth & Braden, 1987). Parish et al. (1983) outline five strategies essential to a successful pressure-sore prevention program:

1. Remove pressure at all body support–surface interfaces;
2. Minimize shearing forces;
3. Maintain a clean and dry skin surface;
4. Implement supportive therapy when needed;
5. Treat concurrent disease. (p. 119)

Use of a commode rather than a bedpan and adequate amounts of fluid and roughage in the diet will promote normal elimination processes. The diet should also include high-protein acid–ash foods to improve the nitrogen balance and maintain the acidity of the urine. Methods of promoting adequate enteral and parenteral nutrition are discussed in detail in chapter 8.

SUMMARY

Impaired physical mobility will occur to some degree in every critically ill surgical patient. Impaired mobility can lead to the development of other problems that will complicate recovery should they occur. Each patient will respond to impaired physical mobility in an individual and unique way. For this reason, the critical care nurse must be knowledgeable about the potential consequences of immobility and constantly be alert for their development. Should they occur, treatment must be immediate and aggressive in order to halt their progression and promote recovery.

The preventive measures that constitute the treatment of impaired physical mobility are all within the realm of independent nursing judgment and action. The critical care nurse must make treatment of impaired physical mobility a priority if the patient is to attain optimal health status.

BIBLIOGRAPHY

Abruzzese, R. S. (1985). Early assessment and prevention of pressure sores. In B. Y. Lee (Ed.), *Chronic ulcers of the skin* (pp. 1–19). New York: McGraw-Hill.

Bergstrom, N., Braden, B., Laquzza, A, & Holman, V. (1985). The Braden scale for predicting pressure sore risk: Reliability studies. *Nursing Research, 34*(6), 383.

Bergstrom, N., Demuth, P., & Braden, B. (1987). A clinical trial of the Braden scale for predicting pressure sore risk. *Nursing Clinics of North America, 22*(2), 417–428.

Carroll-Johnson, R. M. (1989) (Ed.). *Classification of nursing diagnoses: Proceedings of the eighth conference North American Nursing Diagnosis Association.* Philadelphia: J. B. Lippincott Co.

Cherry, G. W., & Ryan, T. J. (1983). Pathophysiology. In L. C. Parish, J. A. Witkowski, & J. T. Crissey, *The decubitus ulcer* (pp. 11–20). New York: Masson.

Constantian, M. (Ed.) (1980). *Pressure ulcers: Principles and technique of management.* Boston: Little, Brown.

Deitrick, J., Whedon, G., & Schorr, G. (1948). Effects of immobilization upon various metabolic and physiologic functions of normal men. *American Journal of Medicine, 4,* 3–36.

Enis, J., & Sarmiento, A. (1973). The pathophysiology and management of pressure sores. *Orthopedics Review, 2,* 25–34.

Esposito, M., Tracey, C. & McCourt, A. (1989). Nursing diagnosis: Potential for disuse syndrome. In R. M. Caroll-Johnson (Ed.). *Classification of nursing diagnoses: Proceedings of the eighth conference North American Nursing Diagnosis Association* (pp. 464–468). Philadelphia: J. B. Lippincott Co.

Fisher, W., & Fisher, A. (October 1980). Medical implications of space. *Topics in Emergency Medicine, 2,* 137–149.

Fowler, E. M. (1987). Equipment and products used in the management and treatment of pressure ulcers. *Nursing Clinics of North America, 22,*(2), 449–461.

Goode, A. (1981). Microgravity research: A new dimension in medical science. *Lancet,* 767–769.

Gosnell, D. (1973). An assessment tool to identify pressure sores. *Nursing Research, 22,* 55–59.

Gosnell, D. (1987). Assessment and evaluation of pressure sores. *Nursing Clinics of North America, 22,* 399–417.

Groer, M. E. & Shekleton, M. E. (1989). *Basic pathophysiology: A holistic approach* (3rd ed.). St. Louis: C. V. Mosby.

Gruis, M., & Innes, B. (1976). Assessment: Essential to prevent pressure sores. *American Journal of Nursing, 76*(11), 1762–1764.

Gurevich, I. (1983). Infected decubiti: The problem of patient placement and care. *Topics in Clinical Nursing, 5*(2), 55–63.

Iverson-Carpenter, M. (1989). A descriptive study of the etiologies and defining characteristics of pressure sores. In R. M. Carroll-Johnson (Ed.). *Classification of nursing diagnoses: Proceedings of the eighth conference North American Nursing Diagnosis Association* (pp. 275–280). Philadelphia: J. B. Lippincott Co.

Keenan, K. (1989). Clinical validation of the etiologies and defining characteristics of the nursing diagnosis impaired mobility. In R. M. Carroll-Johnson (Ed.). *Classification of nursing diagnoses: Proceedings of the eighth conference North American Nursing Diagnosis Association* (pp. 291–295). Philadelphia: J. B. Lippincott Co.

Lentz, M. (1981). Selected aspects of deconditioning secondary to immobilization. *Nursing Clinics of North America, 16*(4), 729–737.

Levy, T., & Talbot, J. (1983). *Research opportunities in cardiovascular deconditioning* (Contract No. NASW-3616). Washington, D.C.: National Aeronautic and Space Administration.

Mack, P., & LaChance, P. (1967). Effects of recumbency and space flight on the bone density. *American Journal of Clinical Nutrition, 20,* 1194–1205.

Maklebust, J. (1987). Pressure ulcers: Etiology and prevention. *Nursing Clinics of North America, 22*(2), 359–377.

Moser, K., & Fedullo, P. (1983). Venous thromboembolism. *Chest, 83,* 117–121.

Natow, A. B. (1983). Nutrition in prevention and treatment of decubitus ulcers. *Topics in Clinical Nursing 5*(2), 39–44.

Norton, D., McLaren, R., & Exton-Smith, A. (1981). Pressure sores. In J. A. Horsley, *Preventing decubitus ulcers: CURN project.* (pp. 104–149). New York: Grune & Stratton.

Parish, L. C., Witkowski, J. A., & Crissey, J. T. (1983). *The decubitus ulcer.* New York: Masson.

Pritchard, V. (1986). Pressure sores: Calculating the risk. *Nursing Times, 82*(8), 59–61.

Reuler, J. B., & Cooney, T. G. (1981). The pressure sore: Pathophysiology and principles of management. *Annals of Internal Medicine, 94*(5), 661–666.

Ryback, R., Lewis, O., & Lessard, C. (1971). Psychobiologic effects of prolonged bed rest (weightless) in young, healthy volunteers (study II). *Aerospace Medicine, 42,* 529–535.

Sanchez, F. (1986). Fundamentals of chest x-ray interpretation. *Critical Care Nurse, 6*(5), 41–61.

Schappler, N. (1989). Impaired skin integrity: Actual and potential in orthopedic patients. In R. M. Carroll-Johnson (Ed.). *Classification of nursing diagnoses: Proceedings of the eighth conference North American Nursing Diagnosis Association* (pp. 345–348). Philadelphia: J. B. Lippincott Co.

Shea, J. D. (1975). Pressure sores: Classification and management. *Clinical Orthopaedics and Related Research,* October (112), 89–100.

Shekleton, M. (1989). Potential for disuse syndrome care plan. In M. J. Kim, G. D. McFarland, & A. M. McLane. (Eds.). *Pocket guide to nursing diagnoses.* St. Louis: C. V. Mosby.

Sieggreen, M. Y. (1987). Healing of physical wounds. *Nursing Clinics of North America, 22,*(2), 439–447.

Spencer, W., Valbona C., & Carter, R., Jr. (1965). Physiologic concepts of immobilization. *Journal of Physical and Medical Rehabilitation, 46,* 89–100.

Stotts, N. (1985). Nutritional parameters as predictors of pressure sores in surgical patients. *Nursing Research, 34*(6), 383.

Stotts, N. A. (1987). Age specific characteristics of patients who develop pressure ulcers in the tertiary-care setting. *Nursing Clinics of North America, 22*(2), 391–398.

Stotts, N. A. (1988). Predicting pressure ulcer development in surgical patients. *Heart and Lung, 17*(6), 641–647.

Taylor, H., Henschel, A., Brozek, J., & Keys, A. (1949). Affects of bed rest on cardiovascular function and work performance. *Journal of Applied Physiology, 11,* 223–239.

Tepperman, P., & Devlin, M. (1983). Therapeutic heat and cold. *Postgraduate Medicine, 73*(1), 69–76.

Thomas, J., Schirger, A., Fealey, R., & Sheps, S. (1981). Orthostatic hypotension. *Mayo Clinic Proceedings, 56,* 117–125.

Waterlow, I. (1985). A risk assessment card. *Nursing Times,* November, 49, 51, 55.

Williams, A. (1972). A study of factors contributing to skin breakdown. *Nursing Research, 21*(3), 238–243.

ADDITIONAL READINGS

Barbenel, J. C., Ferguson-Pell, M. W., & Beale A. Q. (1985). Monitoring the mobility of patients in bed. *Medical and Biological Engineering and Computing, 23*(5), 466.

Birkhead, H., Haupt. G., & Mayers, R. (1963). Circulatory and metabolic effects of prolonged bed rest in healthy subjects. *Federation Proceedings, 22,* 520.

Browse, N. (1965). *The physiology and pathology of bedrest.* Springfield, IL: Charles C Thomas.

Carnevali, D., & Brueckner, S. (1970). Immobilization reassessment of a concept. *American Journal of Nursing, 70,* 1502–1507.

Downs, F. (1974). Bed rest and sensory disturbances. *American Journal of Nursing, 74*(3), 434–438.

Horsley, J. A. (1981). *Preventing decubitus ulcers: CURN project.* New York: Grune & Stratton.

Kottke, F. J. (1966). The effects of limitation of activity upon the human body. *Journal of the American Medical Association, 196,* 117–122.

Lee, B. Y. (Ed.) (1985). *Chronic ulcers of the skin.* New York: McGraw-Hill.

Lerman, S., Canterbury, J., & Reiss, E. (1977). Parathyroid hormone and the hypercalcemia of immobilization. *Journal of Clinical Endocrinology and Metabolism, 45*(3), 425–428.

Lynch, T. N., Jensen, R. L., Stevens, P. M., et al. (1967). Metabolic effects of prolonged bed rest: their modification by simulated attitude. *Aerospace Medicine, 38,* 10–20.

Olson, E. (Ed.). (1967). The hazards of immobility. *American Journal of Nursing, 67*(4), 780–797.

Seiler, W. O., & Stahelin, H. B. (1986). Recent findings on decubitus ulcer pathology: Implications for care. *Geriatrics, 41*(1), 47.

Sklar, C. G. (1985). Pressure ulcer management in the neurologically impaired patient. *Journal of Neurosurgical Nursing, 17*(1), 30.

Tompkins, E. S. (1980). Effect of restricted mobility and dominance of perceived duration. *Nursing Research, 29,* 333–338.

Tyler, M. (1984). The respiratory effects of body positioning and immobilization, *Respiratory Care, 29*(5), 472–483.

Verhonick, P., Lewis, D., & Goller (1972). Thermography in the study of decubitus ulcers. *Nursing Research, 21*(3), 233–237.

Warren, R. (1977). Osteoporosis. *Journal of Oral Medicine, 32*(4), 113–119.

Winslow, E., & Weber, T. (1980). Progressive exercise to combat the hazards of bedrest. *American Journal of Nursing, 80*(3), 440–445.

Zubek, J., Bayer, L., Mitstein, S., & Shepard, J. (1969). Behavioral and physiologic changes during prolonged immobilization plus perceptual deprivation. *Journal of Abnormal Psychology, 74,* 230–236.

15 Alterations in Body Defenses

Sharon Dolce Manson, M.S., R.N.
Sylvia Elson, M.S., R.N.

The organs and tissues of the body work together to maintain the equilibrium of the internal environment. The maintenance of homeostasis requires the coordinated function of multiple body systems. The focus of this chapter is on alterations in body defenses, including disorders of the immune system, and coagulation.

The immune system protects the body against invasion by foreign substances. Innate immunity requires intact physical barriers, chemical barriers, and cells that protect against infection. The body also develops specific immunity, called acquired immunity, to protect against individual organisms. These two types of immunity are often compromised in critically ill patients because of a number of physiologic and environmental factors. The immune system and care of the immunocompromised patient is the focus of the first section of this chapter.

Hemostasis, or the prevention of blood loss, is vital to the surgical patient. Hemostasis is dependent on vessel-wall integrity, normal quantity and function of platelets, and an intact coagulation or clotting mechanism. Addressed in the second section of this chapter is care of the patient with a coagulapathy.

THE IMMUNOCOMPROMISED PATIENT

The potential for infection is a problem always faced by nurses caring for critically ill surgical patients. In immunocompromised patients, this problem is of particular concern. The risk for infection can be increased as a result of the surgical procedure, or the patient could be immunocompromised because of disease or medical management. This section is concerned with the care of immunosuppressed surgical patients.

To be able to understand the extent of the problems occurring with immunocompromised patients, it is important first to understand the normal immune response. The normal physiology of the immune system is reviewed in the first portion of this section.

Innate Immunity

Body's Defense Barriers

The body's defenses against invasion are its chemical and mechanical barriers. Acidic secretions and digestive enzymes in the stomach serve as a defense mechanism against ingested organisms (Vander, Sherman, & Luciano, 1990). Chemicals contained in skin-surface secretions, such as oil and sweat, are also effective in protecting against pathogens. Many anatomical structures serve as mechanical barriers against invasion by infectious organisms. The skin and mucous membranes are the major mechanical barriers, but many less evident barriers exist. The hair in the lining of the nose, the cough reflex, and the ciliary action in the respiratory tract are all mechanical barriers. Tears, saliva, and mucus remove potential invaders, thus providing additional protection (Thompson, McFarland, Hirsch, Tucker, & Bowers, 1986; Vander et al., 1990). The first-line defense mechanisms provided by the body's mechanical and chemical barriers are frequently compromised in critically ill patients.

The Inflammatory Response

Inflammation is the body's normal response to injury. After tissue damage resulting from invasion by microorganisms or other trauma, a complex sequence of events occurs. Cellular injury results in the release of a variety of substances, including histamine, bradykinin, and serotonin. These substances cause vasodilation in the affected area, as well as an increased vascular permeability. Large quantities of fluid and protein leak into the tissues, resulting in local edema and a delay in the systemic spread of the microorganisms present (Guyton, 1981).

Once the inflammatory response begins, the injured area is invaded by macrophages and neutrophils. These cells clear the area of infectious or toxic invaders. Tissue macrophages are the first line of defense and begin phagocytosis of foreign particles early in the defense process (Guyton, 1981; Thompson et al., 1986).

Inflamed tissue releases chemical substances, called leukocytosis-inducing factors, that cause the release of leukocytes from the bone marrow storage pool into the circulation. Neutrophils will be drawn to the damaged area and will stick to the damaged capillary walls. This process is called "margination" or "pavementing." Neutrophils then pass through the capillary walls into the tissue spaces (diapedesis). Once in the tissue spaces, chemicals released from damaged or necrotic cells attract the neutrophils to the area of the injury. This phenomenon of neutrophil attraction is known as chemotaxis.

Neutrophils are able to begin engulfing foreign matter upon arrival at the site of invasion (Guyton, 1981; Thompson et al., 1986).

Although neutrophils and macrophages are able to engulf large amounts of bacteria and necrotic tissue, most of them will eventually die during the scavenger process. A mixture of dead neutrophils, dead macrophages, and necrotic tissue, known as pus, will be formed. Pus formation usually continues until the infectious process is under control (Guyton, 1981).

Acquired Immunity

In addition to the nonspecific immunity previously described, the body has the ability to develop specific immunity against individual foreign invaders. This specific immunity is called *acquired or adaptive immunity*. These specific responses are often very strong and represent the principle behind vaccination (Guyton, 1981).

Two types of acquired immunity are available to protect against foreign invaders—humoral immunity and cellular immunity. Both humoral and cellular immunity are the products of the body's lymphoid tissue. Lymphoid tissue is composed primarily of the body's lymph nodes, spleen, submucosal area of the gastrointestinal tract, and bone marrow. Any deficiency in the lymphoid tissue, as a result of treatment, foreign invaders, or genetic mutation, will greatly immunocompromise an individual (Guyton, 1981). Two types of lymphocytes arise from lymphoid tissue: T lymphocytes and B lymphocytes. These two types of lymphocytes are responsible for the body's acquired immune responses.

Cellular Immunity   Cellular immunity is a function of sensitized T lymphocytes. An antigen is any foreign invader or toxin. When T lymphocytes are exposed to an antigen, a number of additional T lymphocytes will be formed and stored in the lymphoid tissue. On future exposure to the same antigen, these sensitized T cells will be released, producing a faster and stronger immune response.

Cellular immunity occurs most efficiently with slowly developing bacterial diseases, such as tuberculosis. It is also cellular immunity that battles against cancer cells, transplanted cells, fungal infections, and invasion by some viruses (Guyton, 1981).

Humoral Immunity   Humoral immunity can also be referred to as antibody-mediated immunity. B lymphocytes are the cells required for the production of this immune response. When stimulated by an antigen, B lymphocytes enlarge and divide into antibody-producing plasma cells or memory B cells. Memory B cells would be activated on subsequent exposure to the same antigen. Antibodies produced by the plasma cells will attach to the specific antigen for which they were produced, and stimulate destruction of the foreign invader by one of three methods. The first method is through direct attack and neutralization of the invader. A second option for destruction is through the activation of the complement system. This system is composed of enzymes that normally circulate inactively in the blood. When activated by antibodies, these enzymes attack the antigen directly, resulting in its destruction. These enzymes also promote inflammation and attract other leukocytes to the area. The final method through which antibodies stimulate destruction of foreign antigens is activation of the anaphylactic response. Inflammation secondary to this response localizes the antigen, thereby preventing further spread (Guyton, 1981; Thompson et al., 1986).

There are five general classes of antibody (immunoglobulin): IgG, IgM, IgA, IgE, and IgD. These classes of immunoglobulin have different actions, which are summarized in Table 15–1. IgG is the most abundant, comprising approximately 75% of the antibodies in the body (Guyton, 1981). Humoral immunity is usually a faster response during infection than cell-mediated immunity. Antibody-mediated immunity is more effective against acute bacterial infections than cell-mediated immunity, but sensitization is only maintained for a period of a few months to a few years. Cell-mediated immunity can persist almost indefinitely (Guyton, 1981).

Alterations in Physical Regulation

Causes of Immunodeficiencies

Immunodeficiency occurs when there is inadequate function of any part of the immune system. When the immune system is not intact, a person is susceptible to multiple foreign invaders. In addition, the delicate balance maintained over normal body flora can be tipped and the body can be over-

Table 15–1   Classes of Immunoglobulin

Class	Action
IgG	Engages complement system Crosses placenta Develops slowly, but lasts years
IgM	Activity the same as IgG Forms first during infection
IgA	Found in blood and body fluids
IgE	Active in allergic reactions Histamine release Found in tissue
IgD	Uncertain function Found in serum

Data from *Clinical Nursing* (p. 1475), by J. M. Thompson, G. K. McFarland, J. E. Hirsh, S. M. Tucker, & A. C. Bowers, 1986, St. Louis: The C. V. Mosby Co.

whelmed by organisms that are not problematic in an immunocompetent host.

Two basic categories of immunodeficiency exist: primary immunodeficiency and secondary immunodeficiency. This section will address these categories and provide examples of each type of immunodeficiency.

Primary Immunodeficiency

Primary immunodeficiencies can be subclassified into congenital and acquired immunodeficiency. Primary congenital immunodeficiencies are genetically transmitted traits, which result in a lack of substances or functions that are essential for intact immunity (Table 15–2). These genetically linked disorders in immune function can affect any component of the immune system, including humoral immunity, cellular immunity, or a combination of components, complement, or the phagocytic component. Primary acquired immunodeficiency is not apparent at birth but develops later in life. The cause of these changes in immune function is not known at the present time (Hamilton, 1985).

Secondary Immunodeficiency

Secondary immunodeficiencies develop as a result of some identifiable cause, including immune defects related to a disease process and those re-

---

Table 15–2 Primary Congenital Disorders

Cellular immune defects
  DiGeorge's syndrome
  Chronic mucocutaneous candidiasis
Combined defects
  Severe combined immunodeficiency (SCID)
  Wiskott–Aldrich syndrome
  Immunodeficiency with ataxia–telangiectasia
Complement system defects
  C1r, C3, C5 deficiencies
  Hereditary angioedema
Defective phagocytosis
  "Lazy leukocyte" syndrome
  Jobs/hyper IgE
  Chediak–Higashi syndrome
  Chronic granulomatous disease
Humoral immune defects
  Hypogammaglobulinemia
  Selective IgA deficiency

lated to treatment (also referred to as iatrogenic causes). Disorders resulting in an immunocompromised state can be malignant or nonmalignant processes. Malignant disorders can affect any component of the immune system, often by directly affecting production of the cell lines responsible for immunocompetence. Examples of malignancies associated with an immunodeficient state include the leukemias, the lymphomas, and multiple myeloma. Nonmalignant processes include an extensive list of disorders. Impaired immunity can result from a direct effect on some component of the immune system, such as in acquired immunodeficiency syndrome (AIDS), in which the responsible virus (HIV) invades and destroys T lymphocytes. In addition, some disorders affect the immune system indirectly. Malnutrition hinders lymphocyte production, resulting in immunodeficiency (see chapter 8) (DeVita, Hellman, & Rosenberg, 1985; Hamilton, 1985).

Iatrogenic causes of immunosuppression are immune disorders that result from medical treatment. Pharmacologic agents, such as chemotherapy, steroids, and antibiotics, can cause immunosuppression and predispose a patient to infections. Cyclosporine is an example of a drug used to prevent graft rejection in transplant recipients (see chapter 20). It acts by inhibiting one structural category of T lymphocytes, causing a deficit in cell-mediated immunity. Often those organ recipients are cared for by critical care nurses in surgical settings. Chemotherapeutic agents affect normal cells in addition to cancer cells. As a result of this activity, there may be a temporary decrease in the patient's white-cell counts. Corticosteroids have multiple effects, including decreases in phagocytic migration, poor wound healing, decreased T-cell effectiveness, and impaired immunoglobulin production. These combined effects greatly alter the immune status of the patient. Antibiotics alter normal bacterial flora, which can lead to the development of resistant strains of microbes (Hamilton, 1985).

Iatrogenic causes of immunosuppression are not limited to treatment with pharmacologic agents. Radiation therapy can also impair immune function. In the critical care setting many invasive procedures impair innate immune function. Any invasive procedure—surgery, intravenous lines, intramuscular injections, endotracheal intubation, chest tubes, drainage catheters, and intraarterial monitoring catheters—impairs immunity through the loss of normal mechanical barriers. Causes of secondary immunodeficiency are summarized in Table 15–3.

Nursing Assessment/Intervention

As a critical care nurse in a surgical setting, it is easy to identify immunodeficiency as a major problem. Many patients will have combinations of diseases and treatments that greatly compound their immunodeficient state. Through complete assessment of the patient's disease process, treatment plan, laboratory data, and physical condition, the critical care nurse can identify the severity of the problem and appropriate interventions for patient care. The physi-

Table 15–3 Causes of Secondary Immunodeficiency

Disease processes
  Malignant disorders
    Multiple myeloma
    Hodgkin's and non-Hodgkin's lymphomas
    Nonlymphoid malignancies
    Acute and chronic leukemias
  Nonmalignant disorders
    Prematurity
    Sickle-cell disease
    Protein-losing enteropathy
    Tuberculosis
    Acute viral infections
    Malnutrition
    Autoimmune diseases
    Crohn's disease
    Burns
    Chronic infections
    Diabetes mellitus
Iatrogenic causes
  Pharmacologic
    Cancer chemotherapeutic agents
    Corticosteroids
    Cyclosporine
    Antibiotics and antimicrobials
  Nonpharmacologic
    Surgery
    Splenectomy
    Radiation therapy
    Catheters, IVs, etc.

cal indicators and diagnostic tests used most often to assess immune status are summarized in Table 15–4.

Addressed in the following section are assessment and intervention guidelines for the nursing diagnoses relevant to care of the immunocompromised patient. These guidelines are organized according to the precipitating factor, site, and effects of the alteration on immune status.

Potential/Actual Infection Related to Alterations in Immune Regulation

Assessment begins with the nurse's obtaining a history to determine the causes of immunosuppression. Possible causes include drug therapy (chemotherapy, steroids, antibiotics), radiation therapy, disease processes, and/or

Table 15–4 Physical Indicators and Diagnostic Tests Commonly Used to Assess Immune Status

Test	Normal	Comments
Body temperature	36.3–37.1°C p.o.	Increases in these values may indicate infection. Values vary to some extent between adults and children.
Respiratory rate	12–20/min	
Pulse	60–90/min	
White-cell count	5,000–10,000/cm	
Differential white-cell count	Granulocytes, 60–70% lymphocytes, 30% monocytes, 5.3%	Indicates the percentage of specific cell types available.
Cultures	Fungal, bacterial viral, parasites	Cultures can be obtained from any body secretion.
Indicators of nutritional status		(see chapter 8)

nutritional status. Vital signs should also be obtained, as signs of immunocompromise may be detected. For example, a temperature higher than 38.3°C (100.4°F), unrelated to blood products or medications, may indicate infection, especially if it lasts more than 24 hours (Yasko, 1983). Tachycardia, tachypnea, and lower than usual blood pressure may indicate early sepsis.

The nurse should also assess the level of immunosuppression by reviewing laboratory data. Patients with a neutrophil count of less than 1,000/mm^3 are considered to be at risk for infection. The neutrophil count is determined by multiplying the total white-cell count by the percentage of neutrophils and dividing by 100.

Nursing interventions are designed to decrease further risks of immunocompromise. Good hand-washing technique is essential prior to contact with the patient, as is the use of strict aseptic technique when performing invasive procedures or treatments.

Nurses should avoid caring for infected patients in combination with immunocompromised patients in order to minimize the risk of inadvertent transmission of disease. Immunocompromised patients will frequently require a private room. Protective or reverse isolation may be used in some settings.

The nurse should encourage the patient to have a good, well-balanced nutritional intake. Consultation with a dietitian is recommended. Additionally, the nurse should work with the patient to identify sources of stress and to introduce stress-reduction interventions.

Potential/Actual Infection Related to Impaired Skin and Mucous Membrane Integrity

Assessment begins with the nurse's obtaining a history of infections and areas recently subjected to invasive procedures (IV sites, wounds, areas of radiation therapy). A physical examination should be performed, with emphasis on frequent sites of infection, including surgical incisions, IV sites, pressure points, skin folds, the oral cavity and the perirectal area. The nurse should monitor skin and mucous membranes for color, lesions, wounds, fissures, edema, and moisture. Remember that neutropenic patients may have a decreased or absent inflammatory response. If the patient becomes febrile, wounds should be cultured prior to beginning antibiotic therapy.

To maintain integrity of the skin and mucous membranes, the nurse should provide good body hygiene with attention directed toward high-risk areas. Thorough and consistent oral care should be a priority. Sitz baths may improve perineal care. Rectal exams, suppositories, enemas, and rectal temperature taking should be avoided, as should use of any substance that may irritate the skin, including tape, constrictive clothing, and abrasive towels. Invasive techniques should be done aseptically. Surgical and IV dressings should be kept dry and intact.

Potential/Actual Infection Related to Alterations in Respiratory Status

Assessment should begin by reviewing for the presence of factors that may predispose the patient to respiratory infections, including smoking, mechanical ventilation and other forms of respiratory therapy, chemotherapy, radiation therapy, and immobility. Actual signs of respiratory infection should also be assessed, noting the presence of a cough, sputum, altered lung sounds, dyspnea, and/or complaints of throat or pleural pain. Changes in the chest x-ray should also be monitored. If an infection is suspected, sputum and, if a sore throat is present, throat cultures should be obtained.

Interventions are designed to minimize or prevent alterations in respiratory functioning; these include using aseptic technique in suctioning, increasing mobility if possible, turning bedridden patients every 1-2 hours, and encouraging deep breathing and incentive spirometry, unless contraindicated. Chest physical therapy may help to mobilize secretions but may be contraindicated in some critically ill patients. Arterial blood gases can be monitored to assess the adequacy of oxygenation and ventilation in response to treatment. Use of noninvasive means of monitoring oxygen saturation using pulse oximetry and end tidal CO_2 using capnography may be preferred in the immunocompromised patient.

Potential/Actual Infection Related to Changes in the Urinary Tract

The nurse should assess the patient for predisposing factors to urinary tract infections, including catheterization, dehydration, and impaired renal function. The nurse should observe urine output for color, clarity, hematuria, and odor. The patient should be monitored for complaints of urgency and frequency.

Interventions are designed to minimize the risk or severity of urinary tract infections, and include the use of aseptic technique for catheterization and specimen collection, encouraging intake of fluids, unless contraindicated, and administering antibiotics after cultures are obtained.

Potential/Actual Complications Related to Systemic Infection (Sepsis)

The nurse should assess the patient for factors predisposing the patient to sepsis, including an immunocompromised state and positive cultures for gram-negative organisms (*Escherichia coli,* klebsiella species, pseudomonas species). The nurse should monitor for early signs of sepsis, including fever, chills, restlessness, confusion, coagulopathies, or vasoconstriction. Later signs include hypotension, cool, clammy skin, tachycardia, oliguria, and a decreased level of consciousness.

Interventions are designed to minimize the effects of sepsis, and include monitoring vital signs, providing respiratory assistance as indicated, and maintaining fluid status to normalize cardiac output. Intake and output data should be carefully recorded. Medications such as antibiotics, and/or steroids should be given as ordered. Hyperthermia should be treated with antipyretics and active cooling (see chapter 12).

Evaluation

The overall goal for the immunocompromised patient is the prevention of infection. If infection does occur, the goals of treatment become early detection and rapid initiation of therapy and resolution of the infection.

The goals of treatment can be considered to have been met when the patient (1) is able to remain afebrile while off antibiotics, (2) has normal laboratory values and vital signs, and (3) displays evidence that his or her immune function is returning to normal. All patients in the critical care setting are prone to infection. As nurses in this setting, it is important to identify what factors predispose a patient to infection and minimize the risks where possible.

Yannelli and Gurevich (1988) identify nosocomial pneumonia, catheter-associated bacteremia, and IV-line-related sepsis as the most commonly seen infection problems in the critical care setting. They emphasize that hand washing remains the most important infection control technique available. Consultation with the infection control practitioner should be sought in all cases of infection to be sure that all possible measures have been implemented to prevent transmission not only to other patients but also to health care workers (Gurevich, 1988, 1989).

Alterations in body defenses often result in multiple risks for the patient. While a patient may experience immunosuppression independent of a coagulopathy, frequently the two go hand in hand. A break in the mechanical barriers, resulting in bleeding, may permit pathogenic organisms to enter the body. Addressed in the following section is the care of a patient with a coagulopathy.

THE PATIENT WITH A COAGULOPATHY

Bleeding is a major complication in the surgical patient. Nursing management of this problem is of particular concern in the patient with a clotting disorder. Coagulopathies may develop from the surgical procedure or as a secondary complication. In addition, patients with previously existing coagulopathies often require surgical treatment.

Coagulation

Vascular injury activates a complex chain of reactions designed to prevent excessive blood loss. The primary hemostatic response to vascular injury is vasoconstriction. Constriction of the vessel wall lasts 10 to 20 minutes, depending on the size of the vessel (*Diagnostics,* 1983). During this time, circulating platelets collect at the site and adhere to the endothelium of the vessel. Platelets secrete adenosine diphosphate (ADP), which results in clumping and activation of greater numbers of platelets. This platelet aggregation results in the formation of a loose plug.

Once platelet aggregation has begun, coagulation or clotting is initiated. The coagulation cascade proceeds through the interaction of the intrinsic and extrinsic pathways (Figure 15–1). The intrinsic system is activated through procoagulants—substances in the blood that gather at the site of injury. Procoagulants initiate a series of reactions that result in the production of plasma thromboplastin. Tissue thromboplastin is released at the site of injury, which activates the extrinsic system. Plasma and tissue thromboplastin convert prothrombin to thrombin. Thrombin then interacts with fibrinogen to form fibrin strands. In this manner, a solid fibrin plug is formed at the site of injury. There are multiple clotting factors involved in the coagulation cascade.

To ensure homeostasis, a mechanism is provided for the breakdown of fibrin clots after their function has been served. This is known as fibrinolysis, or clot dissolution. Fibrinolysis (Figure 15–2) begins when thrombin, which is formed during coagulation, interacts with plasminogen to form plasmin. In the presence of plasmin, fibrinogen and fibrin are digested into fragments known as fibrin degradation products or fibrin split products. Further anticoagulation occurs as circulating fibrin split products interfere with clot formation and decrease platelet adhesiveness (Leavell & Thorup, 1976).

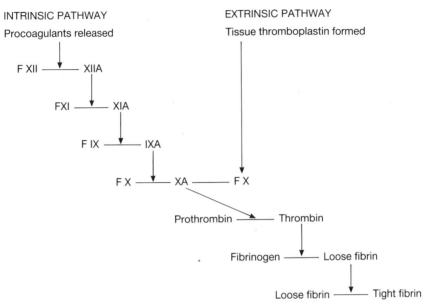

1) Vasoconstriction
2) Platelet Aggregation
3) Coagulation Cascade

INTRINSIC PATHWAY

Procoagulants released

EXTRINSIC PATHWAY

Tissue thromboplastin formed

F XII ——— XIIA

FXI ——— XIA

F IX ——— IXA

F X ——— XA ——— F X

Prothrombin ——— Thrombin

Fibrinogen ——— Loose fibrin

Loose fibrin ——— Tight fibrin

Figure 15–1. Hemostatic response to injury.

Normal hemostasis depends on the delicate balance between clot formation and clot dissolution. Any alteration in the system may result in uncontrolled bleeding and/or clot formation.

Alteration in Physical Regulation: Causes of Coagulopathies

Thrombocytopenia

Thrombocytopenia—an abnormally low number of platelets—places patients at high risk for bleeding. Thrombocytopenia may occur for a number of
reasons and with varying severity. Abnormal bleeding rarely occurs unless
the platelet count is less than 50,000/mm³ (normal, 150,000 to 400,000/mm³)
(Holguin & Caraveo, 1984). However, with trauma, bleeding may occur even
with a count greater than 50,000/mm³, and therefore a preoperative platelet
count of at least 75,000 to 80,000/mm³ is recommended (Berkman, 1986;
Beal, 1982). Spontaneous bleeding is usually not seen unless the platelet
count is below 10,000 to 20,000/mm³ (Williams, Beutler, & Erslev, 1983).
Causes of thrombocytopenia may be classified as decreased platelet production, increased platelet consumption, and platelet sequestration.

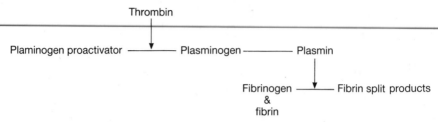

Figure 15–2. Fibrinolysis.

Decreased platelet production may be congenital, however it is more frequently an acquired phenomenon. Thrombocytopenia may occur as a result of a malignancy, as tumor infiltration of the bone marrow crowds out normal cell production; this is seen most commonly in leukemia. It may also be drug induced. Myelosuppressive chemotherapy has the most striking effect on platelet production. Other drugs that may cause platelet suppression include heparin, cimetidine, antibacterial agents, anticonvulsants, antihypertensives, antidysrhythmics, thiazide diuretics, estrogen, and alcohol (Holguin & Caraveo, 1984; Alspach & Williams, 1985). Aplastic anemia is a disease characterized by deficient production of blood cells: platelets, white cells, and red cells.

Increased platelet destruction is often immunologically mediated. Antibodies to surface antigens on platelets may be produced. This may be idiopathic, as in idiopathic thrombocytopenic purpura (ITP), or induced by the drugs previously mentioned. Bacterial, viral, and parasitic infections as well as fever may result in increased platelet destruction (Ersek, 1984). Consumption of platelets and clotting factors occur in disseminated intravascular coagulation (DIC).

Platelet sequestration, or abnormal pooling of platelets in the spleen, may also result in thrombocytopenia. The most common causes of sequestration are liver disease and congestive splenomegaly. Splenomegaly is often associated with hematologic malignancies.

Aspirin, aspirin-containing products, and nonsteroidal antiinflammatory agents (such as ibuprofen) have anticoagulant properties. Platelet function is altered with as little as one 650-mg dose of aspirin (Vandam, 1980). Patients receiving long-term therapy with these medications may be at higher risk for bleeding during surgical procedures.

Coagulation Defects

Coagulation defects that are addressed include congenital and acquired factor deficiencies, coagulopathies secondary to liver disease, and DIC. Deficiency of clotting factors I, II, VII, IX, X, and XII may be congenital or acquired. Acquired factor deficiency is often related to anticoagulant therapy, vitamin K deficiency, or hepatic disease. Factor VIII deficiency, seen in patients with hemophilia A and von Willebrand's disease, is congenital. Severe bleeding tendencies are greater with hemophilia A. Congenital deficiency of factor IX is known as hemophilia B. This results in a severe bleeding disorder. Hemophilia A, hemophilia B, and von Willebrand's disease are the most common hereditary coagulopathies (Green, 1984).

The liver is the major site of production of factors II, V, VII, IX, and X. Cirrhosis or any severe liver impairment may result in deficiencies of the named factors and thus coagulation defects. Vitamin K is required for the synthesis of factors II, VII, IX, and X. Vitamin K is normally ingested by diet and interacts with bacterial flora of the gastrointestinal tract. Alteration of dietary intake of vitamin K sources, malabsorption, antibiotic, or anticoagulant therapy may result in vitamin K deficiency and a subsequent decrease in vitamin K–dependent factors (Price & Wilson, 1982).

Disseminated intravascular coagulation (DIC) is a life-threatening complication most frequently seen in critically ill patients that results from overstimulation of normal coagulation mechanisms. It is a state of hypercoagulability that results in bleeding. DIC may result from numerous pathologic processes, including infection (especially gram-negative sepsis), obstetrical complications, malignancies (especially leukemia), vasculitis, hemolytic transfusion reactions, cardiopulmonary bypass surgery, shock, and cardiac arrest (Goldman, Brown, Levy, Slap, & Sussman, 1982; Rippe, Irwin, Alpert, & Dalen, 1985; Rooney & Haveley, 1985).

Disseminated intravascular coagulation is thought to be initiated by the intravascular invasion of foreign particles and/or by vascular endothelial injury, which trigger(s) systemic coagulation activity. As a result, an abnormal amount of thrombin is produced, which activates both clot formation and fibrinolysis. Clotting factors will be exhausted more quickly than they can be replaced because of the rapidity with which intravascular thrombin is formed. The availability of antithrombin III, an inhibitor, is greatly reduced because of the excessive amount of thrombin being generated.

Activation of coagulation causes activation of fibrinolysis. The fibrin degradation products that are formed interfere with platelet function and formation of a fibrin clot. Bleeding occurs, then, for two reasons: consumption of platelets and clotting factors used to form fibrin clots and the anticoagulant properties of fibrin split products produced during fibrinolysis. Compounding the situation is the simultaneous activation of the complement and kallikrein systems, which will further enhance clotting activity and increase vascular permeability, arteriolar vasoconstriction, and capillary dilatation. Blood will be trapped in the capillary beds, setting up a localized environment of procoagulation conditions (stagnation, acidosis, and concentration of clot-promoting substances). Arteriovenous shunts will form around the capillary beds. The ultimate result is a self-perpetuating cycle of simultaneous clotting and bleeding activity that occurs in response to the initiating event (Ives, 1990); this is depicted in Figure 15–3.

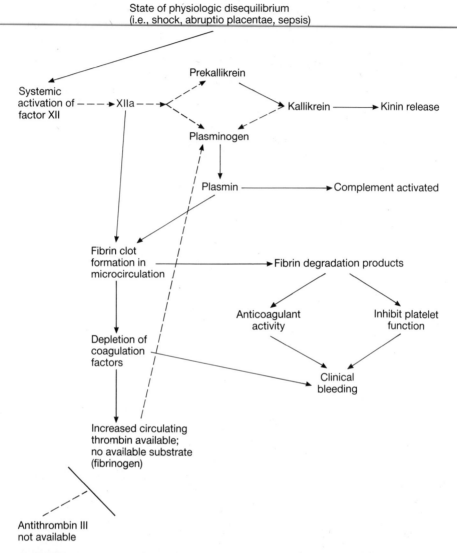

Figure 15–3. Self-perpetuating cycle of thrombosis and bleeding in DIC. From "Disseminated Intravascular Coagulation (DIC)" by J. Ives. In *Critical Care Nursing: A Holistic Approach* (5th ed.) (p. 819) edited by C. Hudak, B. Gallo, & J. Benz, Philadelphia: J. B. Lippincott. Copyright 1990 by J. B. Lippincott. Reprinted by permission.

The clinical manifestations of DIC are uncontrolled clotting and hemorrhage and organ system dysfunction due to ischemia secondary to deposition of platelet-fibrin thrombi in the microvasculature (Roberts, 1985). While any organ system may be involved, the kidneys, lungs, central nervous system, and gastrointestinal system are most often affected. Laboratory values will vary depending on the severity of DIC. A classic triad of findings can help to establish the diagnosis. These include a prolonged prothrombin time, a decreased number of circulating platelets, and a decreased plasma concentration of fibrinogen. Increased fibrin split products are also highly characteristic of DIC. Included in Table 15–5 are the laboratory findings seen as a result of DIC.

The severity of DIC varies, and correction of the coagulopathy depends on the elimination of the precipitating condition. Treatment is therefore geared toward the underlying disease. The cycle of thrombosis and bleeding can be controlled with the administration of heparin. By combining with antithrombin III, heparin inactivates thrombin and neutralizes activated factors IX, X, XI, and XII. Coagulation activity will be slowed, and restoration of clotting factors will be allowed.

Hemodilution

Dilution of platelets and clotting factors may occur during massive transfusion, intraoperatively or perioperatively. This results in a relative deficiency of coagulation components. During a bleeding episode, platelets and plasma with clotting factors are lost with red blood cells. Replacement transfusions with red blood cells result in dilution of remaining platelets and clotting factors, and bleeding may occur. In most patients, this will not occur until 10 or more units of red cells are transfused without platelet or factor replacement (Berkman, 1986; Beal, 1982; Hewson et al., 1985).

Nursing Assessment/Interventions

The patient with a coagulopathy must be monitored constantly for signs and symptoms of bleeding. Bleeding may be internal or external, mild or life-threatening. The nurse caring for such a patient must be alert to the potential

Table 15–5 Laboratory Findings in Acute Disseminated Intravascular Coagulation (DIC)

Test	Values
Prothrombin time	Prolonged
Partial thromboplastin time	Prolonged
Platelet count	Decreased
Fibrinogen level	Decreased
Antithrombin III level	Decreased
Thrombin time	Prolonged
Fibrin degradation products	Elevated
Plasminogen levels	Decreased
Plasmin levels	Present

From "Disseminated Intravascular Coagulation (DIC)" by J. Ives. In: *Critical Care Nursing: A Holistic Approach* (5th ed.) (p. 820) edited by C. Hudak, B. Gallo, & J. Benz, Philadelphia: J. B. Lippincott. Copyright 1990 by J. B. Lippincott. Reprinted by permission.

for bleeding and should investigate any patient complaints, such as weakness and/or pain, that may suggest bleeding. Laboratory tests that may be used to monitor or diagnose a patient with an actual or potential bleeding disorder are summarized in Table 15–6.

The relevant assessment and intervention guidelines for the nursing care of a patient with actual or potential impaired coagulation are outlined in the following text. These guidelines are organized according to the relevant precipitating factors, the possible site, and the effects of bleeding, should it occur.

Potential/Actual Bleeding Related to Alterations in Skin Integrity

Nursing assessment includes evaluating for the presence of bleeding, assessing surgical wounds for bleeding, assessing IV puncture sites for oozing, and

Table 15–6 Laboratory Assessment of Coagulation Status

Platelet count (normal, 150,000–350,000/mm^3)—This quantifies the number of circulating platelets.

Prothrombin time (PT) (normal patient/control activity, 70–130%)—This test bypasses the intrinsic pathway and platelets. It is an excellent screen for the function of the extrinsic pathway. The PT may be prolonged because of decreased factor I, II, V, VII, or X, hepatic disease, vitamin K deficiency, or warfarin therapy.

Activated partial thromboplastin time (aPTT) (normal, 21–31 sec)—aPTT evaluates all factors of the intrinsic pathway except for factor VII or XIII. aPTT may be prolonged because of heparin, fibrin split products, decreased factors other than factor VII or XIII, and antibodies to specific factors.

Thrombin time (normal, 10–15 sec)—This test estimates plasma fibrinogen levels. It is quick to perform but is not precise. Prolonged thrombin time may indicate effects of heparin, streptokinase, or urokinase therapy, hepatic disease, DIC, or fibrinogen deficiency.

Fibrinogen (normal, 200–400 mg/dl)—Plasma concentration of fibrinogen is quantified. Fibrinogen levels may be decreased because of congenital or acquired hypofibrinogenemia, DIC, fibrinolysis, severe hepatic disease, malignant processes, or obstetrical trauma. Fibrinogen levels may be increased in some malignant or inflammatory disorders.

Fibrin split products (FSP) (normal, <10 µg/ml)—This test quantifies the fragments or split products produced during fibrinolysis. FSP are increased during DIC and may differentiate DIC from other coagulation disorders.

Factor levels—Individual factors may be quantified. Deficiencies of individual factors or groups of factors may aid in the diagnosis of a bleeding disorder.

Bleeding time (normal, 3–9 min)—Bleeding time is the duration of bleeding after a standardized skin incision. This measures overall hemostatic response to injury. A prolonged bleeding time suggests decreased platelet number or function, or severe factor deficiency. Bleeding times are often done on patients with a history of a bleeding disorder before they undergo a surgical procedure.

assessing skin for petechiae (flat, round, nonpalpable hemorrhagic lesions about 1-4 mm in diameter), ecchymosis, and hematomas. Petechiae are characteristic of small vessel bleeding associated with thrombocytopenia. Ecchymosis may be associated with thrombocytopenia or coagulation defects. Hematomas are more commonly seen with severe coagulation defects, but may be found in patients with thrombocytopenia associated with trauma (Harrington, 1985).

Platelet counts may be drawn from a central line if in place. Coagulation studies may be affected by heparin in catheters that are capped off, and therefore should only be drawn through a catheter kept open with a continuous infusion (Almadrones, 1987). Accurate coagulation results have also been obtained following a 6 cc discard through an arterial line despite being kept open with 1,000 to 1,500 units of heparin/500 ml solution (Pryor, 1983).

Nursing interventions are directed toward minimizing additional disruptions in skin integrity. Subcutaneous and intramuscular injections should be avoided, as should the number of venipunctures. Pressure (5 to 15 minutes) should be applied to all venipuncture sites. Skin care is essential, with the use of paper tape recommended. The use of an electric razor will minimize injury. Any noted bleeding should be controlled and the amount of loss recorded.

Potential/Actual Bleeding Related to Alterations in Mucous Membranes

Nursing assessment includes evaluation of oral membranes for petechiae or gingival oozing. Nasal mucosa should be inspected for epistaxis (nosebleeds). Rectal bleeding should be monitored by performing guaiac tests on stools. Female patients should be monitored for vaginal bleeding.

Nursing interventions are directed toward preserving the integrity of mucous membranes. Oral care should be done with soft toothettes. Nosebleeds should be stopped with pressure. The patient should avoid blowing his or her nose forcefully. Rectal manipulation should be avoided, negating the use of rectal thermometers, medication, or tubes. Vaginal bleeding should be absorbed with a sanitary pad, and tampons should not be used.

Potential/Actual Bleeding Related to Alterations in Gastrointestinal Urinary Elimination Patterns

Nursing assessment will focus on monitoring bowel movements for the presence of blood, either overt or occult. Vomitus should also be inspected and/or tested for the presence of blood. Urine should be monitored for hematuria.

Interventions are directed toward minimizing gastrointestinal and urinary trauma. Measures should be implemented to prevent constipation, diarrhea, and vomiting. If a nasogastric tube is required, insertion should be done with a small, pliable, well-lubricated catheter. Hydration is important to prevent dehydration. If the patient must be catheterized, a small-lumen, well-lubricated catheter should be placed with aseptic technique. Indwelling catheters should be avoided.

Potential/Actual Deficit in Fluid Volume Related to Bleeding

Assessment is directed toward the awareness of the need to monitor the patient's intake (oral/IV) and output. Vital signs and vital sign stability will provide information about circulatory adequacy. Neurological assessment will provide information about the adequacy of perfusion and whether bleeding is occurring within the closed cranium leading to manifestation of increased intracranial pressure (see chapter 13). The blood urea nitrogen and serum creatinine levels will reflect the adequacy of renal function.

Interventions will be directed toward maintaining intake and output records, daily weights, hemodynamic monitoring (if available), and monitoring of electrolytes. Care is directed toward normalizing fluid balance and monitoring for symptoms of hypovolemia, including hypotension, tachycardia, and decreased mental status.

Alterations in Tissue Perfusion Related to Microvascular Thrombus Formation (DIC)

Nursing assessment will begin by observing the patient for pain or tenderness along vein pathways and for the presence of Homan's sign. Pulses should be assessed for presence and strength. Vital signs should be monitored for manifestations of organ system dysfunction secondary to embolism. Signs and symptoms of a pulmonary embolism include tachypnea, tachycardia, cyanosis, and chest pain. Signs and symptoms of cerebral embolism would include confusion, increased intracranial pressure, hypoxemia, and coma. Renal dysfunction will be reflected by decreased urine output and increased blood urea nitrogen and serum creatinine levels. Gastrointestinal dysfunction will be reflected by abdominal pain and absent or abnormal bowel sounds.

Interventions will include avoiding use of restrictive clothing and compression of extremities by positioning, and instructing the patient not to cross his or her legs, all of which are designed to minimize embolic events. Venous return should be promoted by bed exercises and increasing mobility levels and by the use of antiembolism stockings. Maintenance of intake and output is essential.

Patients with thrombocytopenia or coagulopathies should never receive aspirin or aspirin-containing products without serious consideration. Acetaminophen is a safe alternative, and most aspirin-containing products have an equivalent acetaminophen product.

Blood-product replacement therapy is important in the treatment of the patient with a bleeding disorder. Administration of the blood products summarized in Table 15–7, may become necessary in the treatment of a patient with a coagulopathy.

Table 15–7   Blood Products

Platelets

Indications—Platelet transfusions are given for the patient with bleeding secondary to thrombocytopenia or altered platelet function. Platelets may also be given to prevent bleeding in the patient with thrombocytopenia. In noncritical situations, a platelet count should be maintained over 20,000/mm^3. In some situations, platelets may be transfused to maintain the platelet count over 50,000/mm^3.

Types of Platelet Transfusions

Random-donor platelet concentrates are made from individual units of donated whole blood. Often 4 units of platelets are pooled in a pack, although occasionally individual units are provided.

Single-donor concentrates are collected from an individual donor during an apheresis procedure. A single-donor concentrate is equivalent to approximately 6 random-donor units. Single-donor platelets are given to patients who have a predicted long-term transfusion need. By exposing the patient to decreased numbers of antigens present on the platelet surface, the incidence of unresponsiveness to platelet transfusions is decreased.

HLA (human leukocyte antigen)—Matched platelets are given to patients who no longer respond to random-donor or single-donor platelets. These platelets are closely matched to the patient's own platelets and are less likely to be identified as foreign and destroyed. These products are often difficult to obtain.

Expected response—A 5,000–10,000/mm^3 increment in the platelet count is expected for each unit of transfused platelets in the 70-kg adult. As patients receive multiple platelet transfusions, it is common to see a smaller increment in the platelet count after transfusion.

Nursing considerations—Platelets should be infused rapidly to prevent clumping. Monitor the patient for febrile and allergic reactions. Premedication with diphenhydramine often reduces the risk of reaction. A platelet count should always be drawn 1 hour after transfusion to determine the patient's response to the transfusion. A low platelet count 24 hours later may reflect the patient's consumption of platelets.

Fresh Frozen Plasma (FFP)

Indications—FFP is indicated for patients with multiple factor deficiencies secondary to liver disease, DIC, or dilutional coagulopathies. This product is composed of plasma with all coagulation factors.

Nursing considerations—Patients receiving FFP should be monitored for evidence of allergic reactions and fluid overload, as plasma is a volume expander.

Clotting Factors

Indications—Individual clotting factor concentrate may be administered to the patient with a hereditary or acquired deficiency.

Evaluation

The desired outcome for the patient with a coagulopathy is the prevention of bleeding. If bleeding does occur, the goal of therapy becomes early recognition and promotion of hemostasis.

Evaluation of nursing and medical management of the bleeding disorder must be ongoing. Data that indicate the desired outcome has been achieved include physical assessment that fails to demonstrate evidence of bleeding; vital signs within normal limits; neurological signs within normal limits; no evidence of blood in vomitus, nasogastric contents, urine, or stool; and laboratory data maintained within normal limits.

SUMMARY

Infection and bleeding are serious threats to the recovery of any surgical patient. The critically ill surgical patient with altered body defenses is at risk for even greater disruption of physiologic homeostasis. Thorough, frequent assessment is imperative, and if complications related to impaired defenses arise, prompt, aggressive treatment is required if the patient is to recover.

BIBLIOGRAPHY

Alspach, J. G., & Williams, S. M. (1985). *Core Curriculum for Critical Care Nursing* (3rd ed.). Philadelphia: W. B. Saunders.

Beal, J. (Ed.) (1982). *Critical care for surgical patients.* New York: MacMillan.

Berkman, S. (1986). Hematologic care of the surgical patient. *Hospital Practice, 21*(2), 124-DD, 124GG–124HH, 124JJ.

DeVita, V. T., Hellman, S., & Rosenberg, S. A. (1985). *Cancer: Principles and practice of oncology* (2nd ed.). Philadelphia: J. B. Lippincott.

Diagnostics. (1983). Springhouse, PA: Intermed Communications.

Ersek, M. T. (1984). The adult leukemia patient in the intensive care unit. *Heart and Lung, 13*(2), 183–193.

Goldman, D. R., Brown, F. H., Levy, W. K., Slap, G. B., & Sussman, E. J. (1982). *Medical care of the surgical patient.* Philadelphia: J. B. Lippincott.

Green, J. B. (1984). Hereditary and acquired coagulation factor abnormalities. *Postgraduate Medicine, 76*(8), 118–127.

Gurevich, I. (1988). Transmissible infections in critical care. *Heart and Lung, 17*(4), 331–334.

Gurevich, I. (1989). Acquired immunodeficiency syndrome: Realistic concerns and appropriate precautions. *Heart and Lung, 18*(2), 107–12.

Guyton, A. C. (1981). *Textbook of medical physiology* (6th ed.). Toronto: W. B. Saunders.

Hamilton, H. K. (Ed.) (1985). *Immune disorders: Nurse's clinical library.* Springhouse, PA: Springhouse.

Hewson, J. R., Neame, P. B., Kumar, N., Ayrton, A., Gregor, P., Davis, C., & Skragge, W. (1985). Coagulopathy related to dilution and hypotension during massive transfusion. *Critical Care Medicine, 13*(5), 387–391.

Holguin, M., & Caraveo, J. (1984). Thrombocytopenia and granulocytopenia. *Postgraduate Medicine, 76*(8), 171–182.

Ives, J. (1990). Disseminated intravascular coagulation (DIC). In C. Hudak, B. Gallo, & J. Benz (Eds.) *Critical care nursing: A holistic approach* (5th ed.). Philadelphia: J. B. Lippincott.

Leavell, B., & Thorup, O. (1976). *Fundamentals of clinical hematology.* Philadelphia: W. B. Saunders.

Price, S. A., & Wilson, L. M. (Eds.) (1982). *Pathophysiology: Clinical concepts of disease processes* (2nd ed.). New York: Mc-Graw-Hill.

Rippe, J. M., Irwin, R. S., Alpert, J. S., & Dalen, J. E. (Eds.) (1985). *Intensive care medicine.* Boston: Little, Brown.

Roberts, S. L. (1985). *Physiological concepts and the critically ill patient.* Englewood Cliffs, NJ: Prentice-Hall.

Thompson, J. N., McFarland, G. K., Hirsch, S. E., Tucker, S. M., & Bowers, A. C. (1986). *Clinical nursing.* St. Louis: C. V. Mosby.

Vandam, L. (Ed.) (1980). *To make the patient ready for anaesthesia.* Reading, MA: Addison-Wesley.

Vander, A. J., Sherman, J. H., & Luciano, D. S. (1990). *Human physiology: The mechanisms of body function* (5th ed.). New York: McGraw-Hill.

Williams, W., Beutler, E., & Erslev, A. J. (Eds.) (1983). *Hematology* (3rd ed.). New York: McGraw-Hill.

Yannelli, B., & Gurevich, I. (1988). Infection control in critical care. *Heart and Lung, 17*(6), 596–600.

Yasko, J. M. (1983). *Guidelines for cancer care: Symptom management.* Reston, VA: Reston Publishing.

ADDITIONAL READINGS

Almadrones, L., Godbold, J., Raaf, J., & Ennis, J. (1987). Accuracy of activated partial thromboplastin time drawn through central venous catheters. *Oncology Nursing Forum, 14*(2), 15–18.

Ellerhorst-Ryan, J. M. (1985). Complications of the myeloproliferative system: Infection and sepsis. *Seminars in Oncology Nursing, 1*(4), 244–249.

Harrington, W. J. (1985). Generalized bleeding: Interpreting clinical findings. *Hospital Practice, 20*(1a), 75–90.

McNally, J. C., Stair, J. C., & Somerville, E. T. (Eds.) (1985). *Guidelines for cancer nursing practice.* New York: Grune & Stratton.

Pryor, A. C. (1983). The intra-arterial line: A site for obtaining coagulation studies. *Heart and Lung, 12*(6), 586–590.

Rooney, A., & Haveley, C. (1985). Nursing management of disseminated intravascular coagulation. *Oncology Nursing Forum, 12*(1), 15–22.

Snyder, E. E. (Ed.) (1987). *Blood transfusion therapy* (2nd ed.). Arlington, VA: American Association of Blood Banks.

SECTION IV

Surgical Procedures and Treatments: Responses and Interventions

16 Cardiac Surgery

Julie R. Marshall, M.S., R.N.

Cardiovascular disease remains the leading cause of death in the United States. The American Heart Association (1986) has reported that close to 5 million Americans have coronary artery disease and about 2 million suffer from rheumatic heart disease. In the future, many of these individuals will require coronary artery bypass graft (CABG) or valve-replacement surgery. While open heart surgical techniques have been available since 1954, the most rapid advances in cardiac surgery have been made in the past two decades. The number of cardiac operations has increased at a dramatic pace with the introduction of valve replacement in the early 1960s and of CABG in the late 1960s (McGoon, 1987). Advances in techniques of cardiopulmonary bypass, myocardial protection, medications, and support devices have significantly improved the morbidity and mortality rates of surgery (Sanderson & Kurth, 1983).

The advances in technology and the increase in the number of cardiac surgeries performed make it imperative that the critical care nurse maintain a high level of expertise in caring for these patients. In the future, more patients will be undergoing reoperation, and surgery in high-risk populations such as the elderly will place even greater demands on the skills of the critical care nurse. The intent of this chapter is to provide critical care nurses with current information about the care of open heart surgery patients in the early critical postoperative period. While the importance of the team approach to caring for these patients cannot be ignored, it is the critical care nurse at the bedside who must have the skills and knowledge to respond swiftly and competently to the needs of this patient population. Covered in this chapter are the indications for surgery in coronary artery disease and valvular heart disease, the operative procedure and nursing care in the immediate postoperative period. An overview of cardiac transplantation is provided in chapter 20.

INDICATIONS

Coronary Artery Disease

Coronary atherosclerosis is a disease process characterized by the accumulation of lipids, lipoproteins, smooth muscle cells, blood components, and other cellular deposits in the coronary vessels, causing loss of luminal and vessel-wall integrity, with the eventual reduction of myocardial blood flow (Lewicki, 1984; Kirklin & Barratt-Boyes, 1986). The pathogenesis of atherosclerosis is unknown. The incidence increases with age, and the three major known modifiable risk factors are hypertension, hyperlipidemia, and cigarette smoking (Cowan, 1982). The atherosclerotic process usually affects multiple coronary arteries. The proximal portion of the larger coronary arteries, at or just beyond the sites of branching, are usually affected by the disease. With extensive disease, the origins of more distal branches may be involved. The presence of diffuse severe distal disease is uncommon and renders the patient unsuitable for CABG (Kirklin & Barratt-Boyes, 1986).

The rate of progression of atherosclerosis in coronary arteries tends to be unpredictable. Once the disease process obstructs 65 to 70% of the vessel lumen, blood flow through the vessel is severely reduced, and when the myocardial demands exceed the oxygen supply, complications ensue. The heart at rest extracts the maximum amount of oxygen available from the circulating blood supply; therefore, there is no safety factor, and blood flow must be increased to meet oxygen demand in times of increased need. Myocardial ischemia results when the blood supply is insufficient, as in coronary atherosclerosis. Patients may experience symptoms such as angina, which can progress to myocardial infarction. Medical treatment for the patient experiencing angina is primarily aimed at improving blood flow to ischemic myocardium and reducing myocardial oxygen consumption.

The decision to choose surgical or medical therapy for the patient who has disabling coronary artery disease has been a controversial one. Based on a number of large-scale clinical trials (Christian, Mack, & Wetslein, 1985; Kirklin & Barratt-Boyes, 1986; Loop, 1985), the following general indications for surgery have been proposed:

1. Angina interfering with lifestyle
2. Left main coronary artery stenosis greater than 50%
3. Proximal anterior descending stenosis with angina or ischemia
4. Three-vessel disease
   a. with left ventricular dysfunction
   b. with a normal left ventricle at rest and with inducible ischemia and poor exercise capacity.

The nurse is in a key position to provide support to the patient and family as they make a decision. They will require candid, accurate information regarding long-term outcome after CABG surgery. When possible, arranging for the patient to meet someone who has recovered from CABG surgery can also provide support in the decision-making process.

Acquired Valvular Disease

Mitral Stenosis

Mitral stenosis is usually caused by rheumatic fever (Braunwald, 1984; Morgan, Davis, & Fraker, 1985). After the occurrence of rheumatic fever, 2 years may pass before mitral stenosis develops, and symptoms may not present for another decade (Braunwald, 1984). Commonly, symptoms appear in the third or fourth decade of life (Braunwald, 1984). Symptoms may be unrecognizable at first, and once they become severe, the life expectancy of the individual may be severely shortened. Common signs and symptoms are shortness of breath, orthopnea, paroxysmal nocturnal dyspnea, cough, hemoptysis, palpitations, atrial fibrillation, edema, and fatigue (Lewicki, 1984).

These symptoms occur because of the increased pressure gradient in the pulmonary vasculature that results when blood flow through the left side of the heart is obstructed by the stenotic valve. The orifice of the mitral valve becomes narrowed as a result of fusion of the junctional areas (commissures), scarring of the free margins of both the anterior and posterior leaflets, and shortening, fusion, and nodularity of the chordae tendineae (Sanderson & Kurth 1983, p. 49). Cardiac output may drop because of a decrease in flow across the valve. The increase in pulmonary vascular pressure is eventually transferred to the right heart, where hypertrophy and eventual systemic congestion occur. The usual causes of death associated with mitral stenosis are pulmonary edema, pulmonary hypertension with right-sided heart failure, systemic embolization, pulmonary embolization, and endocarditis (Morgan et al., 1985).

Because mitral stenosis is the only one of the four acquired valvular lesions in which the left ventricle is protected from hypertrophy, it is acceptable to defer surgery until the patient becomes severely symptomatic (Morgan et al., 1985). The exception to this is when systemic embolization occurs, or when a very tight stenosis is discovered during cardiac catheterization. In the former case, anticoagulation should be considered, to allow the patient to recover from the embolism prior to operation (Morgan et al., 1985).

Mitral Regurgitation

Mitral regurgitation may have many causes, including rheumatic fever, myocardial infarction, mitral-valve prolapse, and bacterial endocarditis (Morgan et al., 1985). Shortening of the valve leaflets occurs, resulting in backward flow during ventricular systole. The left atrial pressure rises, similar to the effects of mitral stenosis, and a chronic volume overload of the left ventricle occurs. The most frequent patient complaints are fatigue and decrease in

activity tolerance (Lewicki, 1984). The symptoms of pulmonary vascular congestion occur, along with the development of elevated left atrial pressures.
While the effects of the left atrial load are usually reversible, chronic left
ventricular distention may result in changes that do not improve after surgery. Patients with significant congestive heart failure on medical therapy
tend to develop an irreversible left ventricular dysfunction that is preventable
by an earlier operation. Therefore, the timing of surgery in mitral regurgitation is critical, and should be recommended for patients who are mildly
symptomatic but have a dilated left ventricle (Morgan et al., 1985).

Aortic Stenosis

Aortic stenosis is a progressive narrowing of the aortic-valve orifice and obstruction to left ventricular ejection. It may be caused by a congenital bicuspid
valve that is degenerating, rheumatic valvular scarring with adhesions and
fusion of the commissures, scarring and shortening of the leaflets, or fibrocal-
cific degeneration accompanying old age (Braunwald, 1984; Lewicki, 1984).
Atherosclerotic aortic valvular stenosis can also occur, and is particularly seen
in patients with severe hypercholesterolemia (Braunwald, 1984).

Significant aortic stenosis leads to a concentric left ventricular hypertrophy. Left ventricular failure can occur with resultant left ventricular and left
atrial enlargement and changes secondary to backward failure (Braunwald,
1984).

Symptoms that commonly occur as a result of aortic stenosis are syncope, angina, and congestive heart failure; however, symptoms usually appear
late in the course of aortic stenosis, and at this time the patient has a markedly
shortened life expectancy (Braunwald, 1984; Morgan et al., 1985). For this
reason surgery is recommended for all symptomatic patients, and medical
therapy is given only to stabilize the patient before surgery. Furthermore,
many patients with aortic stenosis will present with sudden death as their first
symptom. This supports the recommendation for early surgical intervention
in this patient population (Morgan et al., 1985).

Aortic Regurgitation

Causes of aortic regurgitation can include any of the following: rheumatic
disease, congenital abnormality, infective endocarditis, aortic dissection,
trauma, or Marfan's syndrome (Braunwald, 1984). Aortic regurgitation produces dilatation of the mitral-valve ring, and occasionally, hypertrophy and
dilatation of the left atrium (Braunwald, 1984). Patients may remain asymptomatic until the fourth or fifth decade after significant cardiomegaly and myocardial dysfunction have occurred. The principal symptoms are exertional
dyspnea, orthopnea and paroxysmal nocturnal dyspnea (Braunwald, 1984).
Surgical correction is indicated in symptomatic patients with chronic aortic
regurgitation. As with mitral regurgitation, every effort should be made to
operate on the patient before irreversible left ventricular dysfunction occurs.

PREOPERATIVE NURSING CARE

In elective, planned open heart procedures, preparation usually begins prior to hospitalization. Completion of the medical evaluation takes place, and data from tests such as the cardiac angiogram, graded exercise test, echocardiographic studies, and serial electrocardiograms (ECG) are compiled. The goal in the early preoperative period is to stabilize any other existing medical conditions and to optimize cardiac function by controlling arrhythmias and heart failure. Any potential sources of infection, such as periodontal disease, skin lesions, or stasis ulcer should be investigated and treated. Coumadin and aspirin should be discontinued at least one week prior to surgery when possible. Heparin therapy may be continued up until the time of surgery as its effects are easily reversed. Patients who are overweight or who smoke are advised to modify their diet and/or stop smoking.

With the advent of cost-containment measures in health care, open heart surgery patients are often admitted the night before or the morning of surgery, which poses a challenge for the nurse in terms of preoperative preparation time. In these situations, preoperative teaching must begin prior to hospitalization. Often patients receive their initial work-up in a community hospital, and are referred to a tertiary care center for surgery. In this case, nurses from the referring hospital should begin preoperative teaching. For the same-day-admission patient, the nurse should arrange a time for preoperative instruction when the patient comes to the hospital for preadmission testing. Changes in the patterns of hospital admission practices necessitate the identification of models for nurse–patient interaction to conduct preoperative teaching on an outpatient basis.

Preoperative Risk Factors

Several preoperative problems have the potential to affect postoperative outcome adversely, and are of special concern. The most important of these is pulmonary dysfunction (see chapter 7), as pulmonary complications are the most frequent cause of death and morbidity in the patient after anesthesia and operation. These complications may include pulmonary embolism, atelectasis, pneumonia, and acute respiratory failure (Horvath, 1984). Pulmonary function tests and arterial blood gases, as well as a detailed preoperative history and physical examination may help predict the patient's ability to tolerate anesthesia and cardiac surgery. The risk of respiratory complications is higher in cigarette smokers, and patients should be instructed to quit smoking at least a month before surgery to help decrease the risk (Horvath, 1984).

The patient with renal insufficiency is also at risk because of potential problems with fluid and electrolyte balance. This requires careful management postoperatively and will necessitate frequent assessment of the fluid intake and output and of serum electrolyte, the blood urea nitrogen, and creatinine levels.

Often patients presenting for coronary bypass surgery will have concomitant cerebrovascular or aortoiliac arteriosclerosis. Patients with severe carotid lesions are extremely prone to neurological insults during surgery, and should have angiographic studies and a neurological consultation done preoperatively. Elderly patients who have preexisting cerebrovascular disease or severe atherosclerosis of the ascending aorta, or who require extensive revascularization procedures, have a significantly increased risk of postoperative stroke (Gardner et al., 1985). The surgeon may elect to do a carotid endarterectomy before or simultaneously with the coronary bypass. Disease of the femoral or iliac arteries has implications in deciding on cannulation for cardiopulmonary bypass, insertion of an arterial line, or insertion of an intraaortic balloon pump.

Other preoperative conditions that may have an impact on postoperative outcome include hematologic disorders, nutritional deficits, or metabolic abnormalities such as diabetes. For the patient who undergoes planned, elective procedures, problems can be anticipated and optimally managed preoperatively. In emergency situations, this may not always be the case.

INTRAOPERATIVE PHASE

It is imperative that the critical care nurse have an understanding of the operative procedure, the anesthesia, and the mechanism of extracorporeal circulation. Many postoperative problems can be anticipated when one is aware of potential complications resulting from the surgical procedure itself.

Extracorporeal Circulation

Improvements in the technology of standard pump oxygenation have favorably affected the morbidity and mortality of patients undergoing open heart surgery (Weiland & Walker, 1986, p. 34). While most patients may demonstrate no lasting ill effects after cardiopulmonary bypass, in fact, some damage occurs temporarily in many patients. Clinical manifestations can include bleeding tendencies, increased capillary permeability and interstitial fluid loss, leukocytosis and fever, renal dysfunction, vasoconstriction, and destruction of red blood cells. The relatively low occurrence of severe complications such as pulmonary edema without elevated left heart pressures, severe bleeding, and neurological sequelae attests to the body's ability to compensate for the damaging effects of cardiopulmonary bypass (Kirklin & Barratt-Boyes, 1986; Kirklin & McGiffin, 1987).

The technique of cardiopulmonary bypass involves use of a mechanical apparatus to circulate and oxygenate the blood while it is diverted away from the heart and lungs. This allows the surgeon to operate in a dry field while the brain and tissues remain perfused (Weiland & Walker, 1986). The standard pump oxygenator became widely used in clinical operations in the 1950s.

Many types of open heart operations were performed before this time using living volunteers whose own hearts served as the pump oxygenator (McGoon, 1987).

The structural elements of current pump oxygenators are the pump itself to control circulation, the oxygenator, and the plastic circuitry (Weiland & Walker, 1986). A cannula placed in the right atrium drains venous blood into the cardiopulmonary bypass apparatus. Oxygenated (arterial) blood is returned to the patient via a cannula placed in the ascending aorta or in the femoral artery if the aorta is calcified, or in procedures involving the aortic arch. Besides oxygenation of the patient's blood, the apparatus also functions as a temperature-regulating and filtering device.

In order to offset some of the catastrophic consequences that can occur after cardiopulmonary bypass, several important principles are employed. Hemodilution of the patient's blood is accomplished by priming the pump circuitry with a crystalloid solution such as Ringer's lactate or normal saline. Priming with whole blood is no longer considered necessary or feasible because of the expense, risk of disease transmission, and other problems, such as hemolysis, experienced with whole blood. Systemic hypothermia (25 to 28°C) is made possible by a heat exchange unit in the pump. Hypothermia reduces tissue oxygen requirements, allowing some protection against ischemic injury (Shahian, 1985). Although higher blood viscosity can result, hemodilution compensates adequately for this effect (Heyman, 1985; Weiland & Walker, 1986).

Anticoagulation is used to prevent massive coagulation in the mechanical parts of the bypass system. Heparin sodium is given before the patient is placed on cardiopulmonary bypass and the coagulation status of the patient is monitored by measuring the activated clotting time. Protamine sulfate is given at the conclusion of the procedure to reverse anticoagulation (Heyman, 1985).

The probability of deleterious effects occurring in the acute postoperative period as a result of cardiopulmonary bypass are thought to be related to the duration of the bypass (especially when greater than 2.5 hours), age (very young or elderly), and preoperative patient condition. Technical aspects of the bypass, such as the type of oxygenator, composition of the perfusate, perfusion flow rate, presence or absence of pulsatile flow, and patient temperature may also contribute to clinical findings in the postoperative period. (Kirklin & McGiffin, 1987). An awareness of the "nonphysiologic" mechanism of cardiopulmonary bypass will help the critical care nurse anticipate potential clinical problems in the early hours after surgery.

Myocardial Preservation

The advances in cardiopulmonary bypass techniques have extended the safe period of myocardial ischemic time. The period of ischemic cardiac arrest is induced by cross-clamping the aorta, which interrupts blood flow to the myocardium (Seifert, 1983). A quiet, motionless heart and bloodless field is required for the surgeon to complete valve replacement or coronary revascularization.

Cardiac arrest is achieved by infusion of a cold cardioplegic solution. Development of the technique of cardioplegia has been an important contribution to the principle of myocardial preservation (Lazar & Roberts, 1985). The most widely used cardioplegic agent is a high-potassium solution, which when infused, quickly depolarizes the heart. Periodic infusion of cardioplegic solution is done throughout the period of cardiac standstill, at the discretion of the surgeon. Hypothermia as low as 20°C may be maintained to reduce myocardial oxygen consumption (Shahian, 1985). Evidence of injury to the myocardium presents during the period of reperfusion, as arrhythmias, decreased myocardial contractility, or ECG changes indicative of ischemia or injury (Shahian, 1985).

Surgical Approach

The most widely used surgical incision is the median sternotomy. With this approach, the anterior mediastinum is exposed without entry into either of the pleural cavities. The sternum is opened with use of a mechanical saw, and is secured at the conclusion of the surgery with wires or plastic sutures that are left permanently in place.

The pericardium is incised during surgery, and in most cases is left open at the conclusion of the procedure. The advantages of leaving the pericardium open are to promote drainage of accumulated blood and to help prevent retained blood, which can induce cardiac tamponade (Kirklin & Barratt-Boyes, 1986). Drainage tubes are placed in the anterior and posterior fields to facilitate drainage of the pericardial cavity and surgical site. If the pleural cavity was entered, a pleural tube may be placed. The mediastinal drainage tubes are brought out through skin incisions at the lower portion of the sternotomy incision.

Procedures for Coronary Artery Disease

The technique of aortocoronary bypass grafting involves procurement of a graft from the patient (usually the saphenous vein) and securing the proximal end to the aorta and the other distal to the coronary occlusion. This new vessel delivers blood flow to jeopardized myocardium. The surgeon is careful to reverse the saphenous-vein graft before sewing it to the coronary artery so that the venous valves will not obstruct blood flow. The internal mammary artery can also be used as a conduit, and it involves only one anastomosis.

In most patients multiple coronary arteries require vascularization and various graft techniques are employed to increase blood delivery to the myocardium (Figure 16–1). A single aortocoronary bypass graft (simple graft)

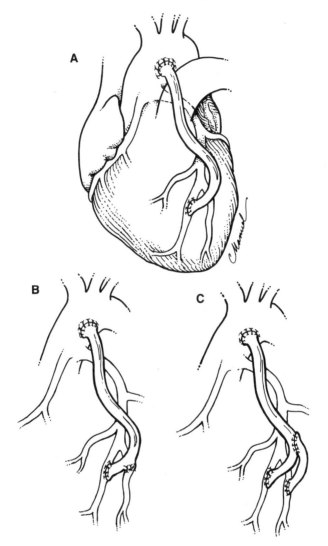

Figure 16–1. Types of coronary artery bypass grafts. (A) Simple graft. (B) Sequential graft. (C) Y graft. From *Techniques in Cardiac Surgery* (2nd ed.) (p. 234) by D. Cooley, 1984, Philadelphia: W. B. Saunders. Copyright 1984 by W. B. Saunders. Adapted by permission.

involves anastomosis of a single vein segment end-to-side to the aorta and a distal end-to-side anastomosis to the coronary artery beyond the site of stenosis. The sequential graft requires the above described anastomoses but also involves making an additional side-to-side anastomosis to one or more coronary branches, thereby bypassing multiple stenoses. The Y graft accomplishes the same goal, and also involves only one aortic anastomosis (Wulff & Hong, 1982).

The internal mammary artery (IMA) has been used widely for coronary artery bypass grafting in recent years. Although first introduced in 1968, the IMA graft has gained in popularity because of its superior early and late graft patency rates as compared with saphenous-vein grafts (Kern, 1986; Lewis & Dehmer, 1985; Loop et al., 1983; Loop et al., 1986; Ochsner, 1985; Tector, Schmahl, & Canino, 1986). While both the right and left IMA's can be used, the left is used more commonly because of its longer length and larger diameter. The left IMA is usually used to bypass proximal lesions in the anterior descending, diagonal, or marginal coronary arteries. The right IMA is used for obstructive lesions located proximally in the right coronary artery or in the osteum. Use of the IMA graft has several implications for postoperative nursing care, which will be discussed later.

Valvular Procedures

Replacement of degenerating heart valves can be accomplished using a variety of prosthetic devices. Presented in Figure 16–2 are some representative valve prostheses. Despite improvements in design and hemodynamics, commercially available prosthetic valves do not even approximate performance of the native heart valve (Morgan et al., 1985).

Valve prostheses can be grouped into two broad categories: biologic and mechanical (see Figure 16–2). Biological tissue valves are derived from animal cardiac tissues (xenografts) or may be human heart valves harvested from cadaver donors (homografts) (Weiland, 1983). Homografts perform well hemodynamically, but their use is limited by availability and their tendency toward early calcification (Weiland, 1983). Tissue-valve prostheses have a low incidence of thromboembolism, which obviates the need for lifelong anticoagulation (Weiland, 1983; Morgan et al., 1985). The disadvantage of tissue valves is early valve failure due to degeneration and calcification. Biological tissue valves have been in use since 1970. Commonly used tissue valves are the Hancock, Carpenter–Edwards (porcine), and the Ionescu–Shiley (bovine). Magillan, Lewis, Tilley, & Peterson (1985) have reported favorable survival results after 12 years of experience with the bioprosthetic valve. However, significant degeneration was noted in patients 35 years of age or younger. In another, larger, comparison series of valve performance over a 10-year period, analysis of morbidity and valve-related mortality favored biological valves in the first 5 years of the study and the mechanical valves in the second 5 years of the study. Overall, the 10-year results showed no significant difference between the two types of valves (Hammond, Geha, Kopf, & Hashim, 1987).

Mechanical valves are constructed of varying combinations of metal, plastic, and Dacron. These components make the valves highly durable (Weiland, 1983). Unfortunately, they are also associated with a high incidence of thromboembolism, necessitating lifelong anticoagulation. The functioning part of the artificial valve varies and may be a single caged ball (Starr–

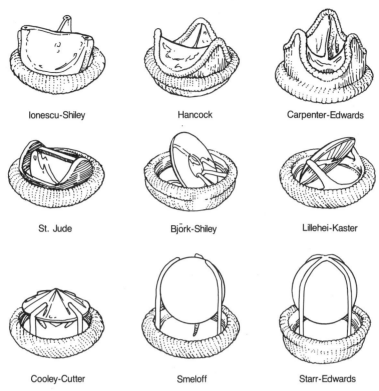

Figure 16–2. Prosthetic valve types in past and current clinical use. The biografts made from animal tissue have favorable hemodynamic flow characteristics and a low incidence of thromboembolic complications. Synthetic prostheses may also have these hemodynamic features but require anticoagulant treatment to control or prevent thromboembolism. The synthetic valves have a proven durability greater than that of the bioprostheses. From *Techniques in Cardiac Surgery* (2nd ed.) (p. 11) by D. Cooley, 1984, Philadelphia: W. B. Saunders. Copyright 1984 by W. B. Saunders. Adapted by permission.

Edwards, Smeloff), a caged disk (Cooley–Cutter), a tilting disk (Bjork–Shiley, Lillehei–Kaster, Omniscience, Medtronics–Hall), or a bileaflet mechanism (St. Jude) (Morgan et al., 1985; Sanderson, & Kurth, 1983, Weiland, 1983). The St. Jude valve is relatively new, but initial performance criteria appear promising (Aron, Nicoloff, Kerstein, Northrup, & Lindsay, 1985; Kinsley, Antunes, & Colsen, 1986).

Choosing a prosthetic valve for a particular patient involves an evaluation of the patient's cardiac anatomy and medical history, as well as life expectancy and lifestyle (Weiland, 1983). Lifelong anticoagulation may not be an ideal choice for an elderly person who is forgetful or prone to falls. Durability is an important consideration for a child or for an individual unable to undergo a reoperation in the case of a degenerating valve.

POSTOPERATIVE PHASE

Admission to the Critical Care Unit

Immediately after cardiac surgery, the goals of treatment center around maintenance of hemodynamic stability. Preparation of the intensive care unit is an important component of preadmission procedures. The exact protocols and equipment used vary between institutions. Ideally, the patient is admitted to the special care unit, where recovery can proceed for the first several days. The patient will return from surgery intubated and on a ventilator, with an arterial line, a central venous or pulmonary artery catheter (with or without mixed venous oxygen saturation monitoring capability), peripheral intravenous lines, two or three mediastinal chest drainage tubes, a nasogastric tube, and a urinary drainage catheter in place. Several nurses working together as a team can complete the admission assessment procedure. An important component of the admission procedure is the report given to the nurse by the surgeon and anesthesiologist regarding intraoperative events. Important data that the primary nurse needs to obtain include the following:

- Patient's medical history
- Preoperative medications, allergies
- Significant operative events
- Cardiopulmonary bypass and aortic cross-clamp time
- Heparin and protamine dosages administered
- Intake and output
- Anesthetic agents

This information is critical for the nurse to have when planning care for the next 24 hours.

Nursing Care during the Early Postoperative Phase

Nursing interventions in the first 24 to 48 hours postoperatively are aimed at promotion of physiologic and psychological stability. In most large cardiac surgical centers, the critical care nurse functions within a set of standardized postoperative orders. The nurse requires a high level of clinical knowledge in order to synthesize assessment data and act swiftly and accurately to restore physiologic stability. Nursing diagnoses for the cardiac surgical patient will be discussed in the next section, along with potential complications that may occur in the early postoperative period.

Potential for Decreased Cardiac Output and Tissue Perfusion

The primary goal in the postoperative period is to maintain sufficient cardiopulmonary function to provide an adequate flow of oxygen-enriched blood to meet the metabolic demands of the body. The amount of oxygen available for the tissues depends on oxygen delivery (cardiac output) and oxygen extraction. The determinants of cardiac output are preload, or end diastolic volume; contractility; afterload—systemic resistance or impedance to ejection of the left ventricle; and the heart rate. An awareness of these factors helps to organize assessment data and guide interventions. Alterations in cardiac output occur frequently in the postoperative period because of the disease state of the patient, surgery and anesthesia, and cardiopulmonary bypass. Cardiac performance in the early postoperative hours can be impaired by "incomplete repair at operation, an additional hemodynamic stress from valvular stenosis or incompetence, residual intracardiac shunting, or incomplete myocardial revascularization" (Kirklin and McGiffin, 1987, p. 327).

A decrease in circulating blood volume postoperatively decreases preload, and may result in low cardiac output and hypotension. Interstitial fluid shifts commonly occur after cardiopulmonary bypass as a result of increased capillary permeability, which allows plasma proteins to leak out of the intravascular space (Horvath, 1984; Weiland & Walker, 1986). Urinary diuresis immediately after surgery can occur because of transient hyperglycemia and as a result of the hemodilutional state during cardiopulmonary bypass. Decreases in preload also occur as vasodilation takes place during rewarming, resulting in peripheral venous pooling.

Excessive bleeding after cardiac surgery can also occur, and it has several possible origins, including clotting deficiencies, thrombocytopenia, heparin rebound, and/or ruptured suture or graft lines. Diffuse oozing from incisional sites accompanied by mediastinal oozing suggests a high probability of a coagulopathy (Conforti & Horvath, 1984). The precise source of the hematologic disorder should be identified through coagulation tests such as prothrombin time, partial thromboplastin time (PTT), clotting time, platelet count, and/or fibrinogen level analysis. The specific clotting factors can then be administered as needed for each patient (see chapter 15).

If the prothrombin time is prolonged, administration of phytonadione (Aquamephyton) (10 mg IV) given slowly is indicated. Infusion of 200 to 400 ml of fresh frozen plasma is an alternative that produces immediate correction. Prolonged PTT or activated clotting time may indicate inadequate heparin reversal, and the administration of additional protamine sulfate is required (DeLaria, Najafi, & Goldin, 1981). Heparin rebound in the early postoperative period can occur even after adequate reversal with protamine at the end of surgery. Heparin that has been sequestered in the interstitial fluid space shifts back into the circulating blood volume. Supplemental protamine should be administered after a determination of the activated clotting time (Heyman, 1985). Platelet infusions also may be indicated for treatment of thrombocytopenia.

Cardiac preload should be adjusted to maintain adequate filling pressures and cardiac output. Volume in the form of colloid or packed red cells is generally administered (Kirklin & McGiffin, 1987). Because the risk of disease transmission with homologous blood transfusion has increased, several blood-conservation techniques have been implemented in cardiac surgery (Frantz, 1987). Preoperation donation is perhaps the ideal technique, however, its use is limited because many individuals undergo urgent coronary revascularization. Another useful technique involves the collection and reinfusion of blood left in the cardiopulmonary bypass circuit at the end of the case. The blood is usually washed and packed before reinfusion, and has a hematocrit value in the range of 50 to 60%. Recently, there is renewed interest in reinfusion of shed mediastinal blood in the first 24 hours after surgery. There are many commercially available chest-tube drainage systems designed for autotransfusion. Mediastinal drainage must be reinfused with 4 hours of collection. This procedure is rarely employed beyond 24 hours because the drainage becomes primarily serum and lymph fluid (Frantz, 1987).

In cases of excessive postoperative bleeding, reoperation is indicated. This occurs in only about 1 to 2% of patients (Kirklin & Barratt-Boyes, 1986). Prompt reoperation is indicated in situations in which there is a sudden increase (300 ml or more) in chest-tube drainage. This usually indicates bleeding from an incision in the heart or great arteries (Kirklin & Barratt-Boyes, 1986).

Control of postoperative hypertension also helps to decrease bleeding. Positive end-expiratory pressure (PEEP) at low levels while the patient is on mechanical ventilation has been demonstrated in some cases to exert pressure on oozing mediastinal vessels and therefore to allow clot formation (Conforti & Horvath, 1984). This may not be indicated in all patients as PEEP can also result in an increased risk of cardiopulmonary complications, and consistent data supporting its effectiveness has not been reported (Banasik & Tyler, 1986).

Evidence of acute cardiac tamponade also requires emergency surgical intervention. Cardiac tamponade is described as compression of the heart by excessive fluid in the pericardium. The fluid exerts pressure that is transmitted across the myocardium, increasing ventricular end diastolic pressure and impairing ventricular filling during diastole. Other signs and symptoms include those of decreased tissue perfusion related to low cardiac output, hypotension, paradoxical pulse, and equalization of intracardic pressures. The cardiac silhouette, which appears widened on the chest film, nearly always indicates retention of some clots and blood in the pericardium (Kirklin & Barratt-Boyes, 1986).

Routine stripping of mediastinal chest tubes is no longer recommended in many institutions. This activity can cause transient rises in intrathoracic negative pressures in excess of the -20 cm H_2O commonly applied to chest-tube drainage systems (Duncan & Erickson, 1982). Theoretically, the elevation in negative pressures associated with stripping could cause injury to the tissues adjacent to chest-tube openings. Further investigation is needed to examine the relationship between stripping or milking techniques and the amount of mediastinal bleeding, as well as the effects of different types of suction (e.g., sump vs. continuous) on drainage (Isaacson, George, & Brewer, 1986; Duncan, Erickson, & Weigel, 1987).

Chest-tube stripping is indicated in situations in which there is excessive bleeding and clot formation. Maintenance of patency in this situation is crucial to prevent cardiac tamponade. Because use of the IMA graft requires more tissue dissection at the time of surgery, the patient with this graft may demonstrate more bleeding postoperatively. Jansen and McFadden (1986) reported a slightly greater incidence of transfusion requirements in IMA graft recipients when compared to saphenous-vein graft recipients. Furthermore, it is their recommendation that routine stripping of chest tubes be avoided because of the proximity of the IMA graft to chest-tube insertion. Because tube placement varies, the nurse should treat each case individually and check with the surgeon postoperatively to determine whether chest-tube manipulation is indicated.

Low cardiac output due to impaired contractility has many causes, including myocardial ischemia or infarction, congestive heart failure, electrolyte abnormalities, and/or acidosis (Conforti & Horvath, 1984). Heart failure is commonly present in patients undergoing valve-replacement procedures, and often contributes to a low output state in the postoperative period.

Fortunately, the incidence of myocardial ischemia and necrosis has decreased in recent years because of advances in myocardial protection during cardiopulmonary bypass and the use of cold cardioplegia (Buckberg, 1985; Kirklin & McGiffin, 1987; Val et al., 1983). The risk appears to increase with aortic cross-clamp times greater than 120 minutes (Kirklin & McGiffin, 1987). Diagnosis of perioperative myocardial infarction is difficult, as surgical trauma to the myocardium elevates serum cardiac enzymes. Goe (1987), in a summary of studies of enzyme activity in response to perioperative myocardial infarction, reported creatine kinase (CK) and creatine kinase isoenzyme (CK-MB) curves that tend to peak later and last longer than CK and CK-MB activity after uncomplicated cardiac surgery. After cardiac surgery CK-MB activity normally peaks in 4 to 7 hours and disappears rapidly. In the case of a perioperative infarction the CK-MB activity peaks at about 21 hours postoperatively and persists beyond 48 hours. A combination of diagnostic tests, including enzyme activity, persistent ECG changes, and radioisotope studies is recommended in making the diagnosis of perioperative myocardial infarction (Val et al., 1983).

Postoperative impaired contractility is suspected when cardiac output remains low despite adjustment of cardiac rate and ventricular preload and afterload (Kirklin & McGiffin, 1987). Administration of a specific catecholamine to improve contractility will depend on the clinical condition of the patient. Dobutamine and dopamine are commonly used agents, but isoproterenol is particularly useful when low cardiac output is associated with increases in pulmonary vascular resistance (Kirklin & McGiffin, 1987). The intraaortic balloon pump is the most widely used mechanical assist device. In the cardiac surgical patient it is employed intraoperatively and postoperatively when low cardiac output after surgery does not respond to moderate doses of inotropic support (Kirklin & McGiffin, 1987).

Elevation of cardiac afterload resulting in low cardiac output is effectively managed postoperatively with vasodilator therapy. Vasodilator therapy is most effective in situations of elevated pulmonary capillary wedge pressure, elevated systemic vascular resistance, depressed left ventricular function, and an increased or normal arterial blood pressure (Kirklin & McGiffin, 1987). Transient hypertension in the early postoperative period often is related to hypothermia and vasoconstriction (Weiland & Walker, 1986). As the patient rewarms, vasodilation occurs and the blood pressure normalizes or falls.

Agents commonly used to reduce afterload are nitroprusside and nitroglycerin. The theoretical advantage of the use of nitroglycerin is that it improves perfusion to ischemic myocardium. Excessive reduction of mean arterial pressure (less than 70 to 80 mm Hg) should be avoided, as this is likely to impair cardiac performance (Kirklin & McGiffin, 1987).

Rhythm disturbances are a potential cause of low cardiac output after cardiac surgery. The incidence of atrial and ventricular dysrhythmias is common, occurring in up to 25 to 30% of patients in the first 7 days after surgery (Guzzetta & Whitman, 1985). The usual causes of dysrhythmia include trauma caused by surgical manipulation, mechanical irritation from invasive hemodynamic monitoring lines, ischemia, metabolic or electrolyte imbalances, fear, anxiety, and pain. Treatment should be aimed at alleviating the cause. Immediately after cardiac surgery, it is common for patients to exhibit a sinus tachycardia (90 to 111 beats per minute). This is related to the effects of surgery and anesthesia, and does not warrant treatment unless it is greater than 110 beats per minute or persists beyond 4 to 6 hours (DeLaria et al., 1981). If the patient was on high doses of a beta blocker preoperatively, metoprolol, 25 mg or 50 mg b.i.d. IV or PO may be restarted to control the tachydysrhythmia. The short-acting beta blocker, esmolol, given as a continuous IV infusion, has been effective for control of tachycardias.

Hypothermia during the period immediately after cardiac surgery may be a cause of transient bradycardias (Weiland & Walker, 1986). Use of temporary atrial or ventricular wires placed epicardially at the time of operation may be employed to optimize cardiac output until the patient is rewarmed. Rewarming can be accomplished using both internal and external techniques (see chapter 12) (Phillips and Skov, 1988). Temporary pacing wires are placed routinely in valvular procedures because the incidence of heart block and dysrhythmias is greater than in routine coronary artery bypass operations. A recent investigation of the use of pacing wires after cardiac surgery revealed that the most common indication for pacing in the study group of CABG patients was to treat bradycardia in order to improve cardiac output. Additionally, epicardial pacing wires were used most often in older patients, in those who had recently sustained a myocardial infarction, and in those on preoperative diuretics (Vitello-Cicciu, Brown, Lazar, McCabe, McCormick, & Roberts, 1987). Atrial pacing wires can also be used in evaluation of certain supraventricular tachydysrhythmias (Kirklin & McGiffin, 1987).

Atrial arrhythmias may impair cardiac performance following cardiac surgery, and commonly occur in the first several days. The treatment of choice is intravenous digoxin. Verapamil and/or beta blockers are employed when digoxin is ineffective.

Ventricular arrhythmias commonly occur after cardiac surgery, often as a result of myocardial ischemia, hypokalemia, hypoxia, acid–base imbalance, or digoxin excess (Kirklin & McGiffin, 1987). Therapy is aimed at correction of precipitating factors. Overdrive pacing and pharmacologic therapy such as with lidocaine or procainamide can also assist in suppressing the ventricular arrhythmia.

Impaired Gas Exchange

Pulmonary dysfunction may occur after cardiac surgery because of the effects of prolonged anesthesia and cardiopulmonary bypass. Functional residual capacity, vital capacity, and total lung capacity are all reduced (see chapter 1). Lung and chest-wall compliance are diminished because of parenchymal damage, pulmonary interstitial edema, alveolar collapse, and the sternotomy incision. Nonventilated alveoli continue to be perfused, resulting in physiologic shunting of unoxygenated blood into the systemic circulation (Conforti & Horvath, 1984).

Although these significant changes in pulmonary physiology do occur, most patients are extubated within 24 hours after surgery (Kirklin & McGiffin, 1987). Ventilator weaning should be postponed in patients who demonstrate hemodynamic instability or neurological complications or when reoperation is likely (Kirklin & Barratt-Boyes, 1986).

Atelectasis is common after cardiac surgery, and reportedly occurs in about 50% of patients (Kirklin & McGiffin, 1987). After extubation, chest physiotherapy and use of incentive spirometry is instituted to help minimize the occurrence and extent of atelectasis and further pulmonary complications.

Pulmonary edema with a low atrial or pulmonary wedge pressure is a rare but potentially fatal complication after cardiopulmonary bypass and protamine administration. It is sometimes referred to as postperfusion syndrome, and is characterized by hemorrhagic pulmonary edema, accompanying cardiac dysfunction, generalized edema, renal dysfunction, and an elevated temperature (Kirklin & McGiffin, 1987). Treatment is aimed at prevention of hypoxemia until capillary integrity is gradually reestablished.

Potential Alteration in Consciousness/Mental Status

Assessment of neurological status after cardiac surgery is important, as patients may experience mild transient deficits that are considered normal postoperatively, or they may sustain permanent deficits due to hypoperfusion or embolization. In a series of 312 patients who underwent elective CABG surgery, the incidence of neurological complications was 61%, however, serious morbidity was rare, occurring in only 1.6% of the sample (Shaw, Bates, Cartlidge, Heaviside, Julian, & Shaw, 1985). Expected transitory abnormalities include mild mental confusion and mild hallucinations, thought to be due to fibrin, platelet, or other microemboli, and inability to focus the eyes appropriately. These symptoms usually subside rapidly during the postoperative period (Kirklin & Barratt-Boyes, 1986).

Uncommon symptoms are delirium, major hallucinatory and delusional experiences, and frank psychotic behavior (Kirklin & Barratt-Boyes, 1986). Appearance of these symptoms should alert the nurse to consider many causes, such as the intensive care unit environment, sleep deprivation, preoperative physical or mental state, as well as the effects of cardiopulmonary bypass.

Postcardiotomy psychosis or delirium is a syndrome characterized by typical behavioral responses in patients after cardiac surgery. Symptoms range from confusion and disorientation to more serious visual and auditory hallucinations, delusions, and paranoia (Quinless, Cassese, & Atherton, 1985). Associated factors include advanced age, severe cardiac disease, hypotension, hypothermia, prolonged cardiopulmonary bypass time, and microembolization (Quinless et al., 1985). This syndrome is discussed in more detail in chapter 5.

Localized neurological deficits, such as hemiplegia and visual-field deficits are thought to be due to embolic events (air, clots, or atheromas). Cerebral edema can occur in the cardiac surgery patient as a result of infarction, hypoxia, or altered metabolic states. The resultant increase in intracranial pressure can compromise cerebral blood flow. Cerebral edema can also occur in patients who have experienced prolonged cardiopulmonary bypass time. Several other physiologic changes that occur while on cardiopulmonary bypass can affect cerebrovascular activity. These changes include the institution of nonpulsatile flow, changes in cerebral venous pressure, dilutional anemia, anesthetic agents, hypothermia, and changes in arterial oxygen and carbon dioxide tensions (Horvath, 1984, p. 225). Recent investigations have focused on the monitoring of cerebral perfusion during the nonpulsatile flow state of cardiopulmonary bypass (Govier et al., 1984; Lundar et al., 1985). The marked changes in cerebral blood flow and hypoperfusional state are presumed responsible for many of the transient neurological symptoms observed postoperatively (Henriksen, 1984). Neurologic sequelae can appear postoperatively as seizure activity or as an alteration in level of consciousness. Once signs of abnormal behavior or increased intracranial pressure occur, the nurse should be prepared for the occurrence of seizures.

The elderly patient undergoing a valvular procedure and those who have preexisting cerebrovascular disease are at greatest risk for serious events such as a cerebrovascular accident. Gardner et al. (1985) reported a stroke rate after CABG of 0.57% in 1979, which rose to 2.4% in 1983. Age-adjusted data demonstrated that the risk of stroke increased because of the increase in mean age of patients undergoing CABG procedures.

Patients who remain unresponsive after cardiac surgery have a poor outcome, while those who demonstrate focal deficits or mental aberrations tend to resolve or improve significantly (Kirklin & Barratt-Boyes, 1986; Bojar, Najafi, DeLaria, Serry, & Goldin, 1983). It is imperative that the nurse assess the patient's neurological status on admission to the critical care unit. This initial assessment serves as the basis for assessments in the ensuing hours. As the patient awakens from anesthesia, frequent neurological checks should include assessment of gross motor movement, pupil reaction, orientation, and ability to follow commands. Any deviation from normal should be promptly reported to the physician. Documentation of neurological status and time of awakening from anesthesia should be included in routine charting. If neurological sequelae appear, a more complete neurological assessment should be incorporated into routine bedside documentation.

Potential for Infection

Antibiotic prophylaxis for cardiac surgery usually consists of administration of an agent such as cefazolin, cefuroxime, or vancomycin (for penicillin allergic patients) just prior to surgery. Therapy is continued for 48 hours or longer if the patient is on IABP therapy or has invasive hemodynamic lines. The protocol for antibiotic administration varies among institutions.

Fever commonly occurs after cardiac surgery, presumably due to the body's response to cardiopulmonary bypass, and should gradually subside over the first several postoperative days. Persistent fever above 101°F after the third or fourth postoperative day should be investigated by obtaining blood and urine cultures, Gram's stain and culture of the sputum, chest roentgenogram, white-cell count, and repeated examination of all surgical wounds (Kirklin & McGiffin, 1987).

Serious complications of the median sternotomy wound are uncommon, and occur in less than 1% of patients (Kirklin & McGiffin, 1987). More serious complications such as mediastinitis, sternal dehiscence, and retrosternal space infections require prompt, aggressive treatment. Once the infection is confirmed, intravenous antibiotics are begun for the specific organism involved. Generally, return to the operating room is necessary and the sternum is reopened and debrided. Drainage tubes are placed for continuous wound irrigation with either an antibiotic or dilute povidone-iodine solution. The tubes are attached to a closed drainage system and suction is applied. The irrigation is continued for 3 to 4 days, then the patient is returned to the operating room for removal of the tubes and wound closure (Kirklin & Barratt-Boyes, 1986). Minor complications such as localized subcutaneous collections of serum or necrotic fat occur in about 2% of all sternotomy patients, and do not necessarily suggest a wound infection (Kirklin & Barratt-Boyes, 1986).

The development of an infected median sternotomy wound is closely related to aseptic technique in the operating room. Prolonged operative time and faulty closure of the sternum also increase the incidence of significant sternal wound infections (Kirklin & Barratt-Boyes, 1986; Marshall & Conkey, 1985). Postoperative risk factors include complications such as low cardiac output, respiratory insufficiency, reoperation for bleeding, repeat median sternotomy, and triple valve replacement (Rutledge, Applebaum, & Kim, 1985).

Prosthetic-valve endocarditis is a serious complication after valve-replacement surgery. A recent analysis of bacterial infections after valve replacement and CABG procedures revealed the following as significant predictors of infection in patients after valve replacement: reoperation, duration of operation, IABP therapy, and replacement of more than 2500 ml of blood (Miholic et al., 1985).

Careful attention to aseptic technique intraoperatively and to wound and intravenous access sites postoperatively is critical, as the first-line body defense (skin) has been violated. The potential for infection exists throughout the postoperative stay.

Altered Fluid Volume and Composition

Metabolic acidosis, defined in the open heart patient as a base deficit of more than 2 mEq, may be present in the first few hours after cardiopulmonary bypass. This is usually attributed to reperfusion of areas of the microcirculation that were poorly perfused during cardiopulmonary bypass and so lactic acid is mobilized into the circulation during the recovery period. Persistence of a metabolic acidosis for more than 2 hours usually indicates inadequate tissue perfusion attributable to poor cardiac output (Kirklin & Barratt-Boyes, 1986, p. 146).

"Normal" postoperative changes that occur due to cardiopulmonary bypass include an increase in sodium and water retention, and a decrease in body potassium. The increase in extracellular body fluid may be reflected in a 5% increase in body weight, which should resolve within 5 days if renal function is normal (Kirklin & Barratt-Boyes, 1986). Large amounts of potassium may be lost through urinary diuresis in the first several hours after surgery. The serum potassium level should be monitored frequently and maintained at 4.0 mEq per liter to avoid myocardial irritability. Sodium and chloride levels should return to normal within hours after surgery (Weiland & Walker, 1986).

The incidence of acute renal failure after cardiac surgery is rare ($\leq 1\%$) and often is associated with a low cardiac output state (Kirklin & Barratt-Boyes, 1986; Kirklin & McGiffin, 1987). Acute renal failure can develop within 12 to 18 hours after surgery. It is characterized by oliguria resistant to treatment aimed at increasing urine output, such as with low-dose dopamine or furosemide (Kirklin & Barratt-Boyes, 1986, p. 152). The serum potassium level rises rapidly, followed by slowly rising blood urea nitrogen (BUN) and creatinine levels. Renal failure can also manifest itself in the later postoperative period (3 to 4 days); BUN and creatinine levels rise but usually oliguria and hyperkalemia do not develop. Spontaneous resolution often occurs.

Risk factors that should alert the nurse to the possible development of acute renal failure in the early postoperative period include preexisting renal impairment, prolonged cardiopulmonary bypass, high plasma hemoglobin level, use of aminoglycosides, and compromised cardiac output (Kirklin & Barratt-Boyes, 1986, p. 153). In patients with impaired preoperative renal function, mannitol (25% solution) or low-dose dopamine may be initiated after coming off cardiopulmonary bypass, as prophylaxis against renal failure (Kirklin & Barratt-Boyes, 1986).

Continuous accurate measurement of intake and output is initiated in the early postoperative period. Urine output and specific gravity should be assessed at least hourly in the early postoperative period and its appearance should be noted. Blood-tinged urine can be caused by hemolysis during cardiopulmonary bypass with a resultant rise in hemoglobin. Hemoglobinuria should clear with postoperative diuresis (Weiland & Walker, 1986). Serum electrolyte levels, including Na, Cl, K, and calcium, and the BUN and creatinine levels are assessed in the early postoperative period.

Altered Nutritional Status

Initially, the cardiac surgical patient may have a nasogastric tube in place to prevent gastric distention. This is usually removed along with the endotracheal tube and a liquid diet is begun, which is then advanced as tolerated. Patients with a history of peptic ulcer disease are given cimetidine or ranitidine either intravenously or by mouth. These high-risk patients should be carefully monitored for evidence of gastric bleeding.

Occasionally, abdominal distention due to the accumulation of gas in the intestinal tract may be present in the first 24 to 48 hours postoperatively. Bowel sounds may or may not be present. This condition responds to fasting, the use of glycerine suppositories, and the application of heat to the abdomen (Kirklin & Barratt-Boyes, 1986, p. 156). Unless the patient underwent an emergency operation, he or she generally receives an enema before surgery, which rules out fecal impaction.

More serious but rare gastrointestinal (GI) complications after cardiac surgery are acute pancreatitis, bowel infarction, GI bleeding, jaundice, and paralytic ileus (Kirklin & Barratt-Boyes, 1986; Haas, Warshaw, Daggett, & Aretz, 1985). Moneta, Misbach, and Ivey (1985) reported that bypass time approaching 100 minutes and the presence of postoperative cardiogenic shock are important risk factors in the development of GI complications in patients undergoing elective cardiac surgery.

Pain

A narcotic analgesic is usually given as part of the balanced anesthesia during cardiac surgery, which affords some pain relief in the early postoperative period. Once the patient has awakened and it is determined that the neurological status is normal, morphine sulfate can be administered intravenously to control pain and provide a sedative effect. Morphine, because of its vasodilatory effects, may cause a decrease in arterial blood pressure. This effect is beneficial in patients who have transient hypertension postoperatively, but caution should be exercised in patients who are hypotensive. Control of the cardiovascular consequences of pain is crucial in the early postoperative hours, as increased circulating catecholamines can increase myocardial oxygen consumption. Once the patient is extubated and tolerating intake by mouth, pain relief can be provided through regular administration of a medication such as acetaminophen with codeine. It is important for the critical care nurse to establish a regular routine of pain medication administration while the patient is still in the intensive care unit. This will encourage the patient to be aware of his or her care and to be an active participant in activities to help in convalesence. Patients who have had an IMA graft may experience more pain because of technical manipulation and electrocautery in dissecting the graft from the chest wall (Jansen & McFadden, 1986).

Recovery during the Remainder of Hospitalization

The average length of stay in the ICU for the patient recovering from open heart surgery is 2 or 3 days. The patient will be discharged to a step-down cardiac care unit once his or her cardiopulmonary status has stabilized and no complications are present requiring further intensive monitoring and follow-up. It is important for the critical care nurse to prepare the patient for transfer through education about the differences in the nurse–patient ratio, daily activities, and participation in self-care. Adequate preparation helps to reduce anxiety and fosters positive thinking about the steps to discharge.

The primary goals for nursing care during this late recovery period are to

1. Continue assessment of recovery and intervene as nursing diagnoses are identified.
2. Prepare the patient to assume self-care activities after discharge.

Because the stay in the step-down unit can be relatively brief (5 to 8 days) it is important for the nurse to begin discharge teaching as soon as the patient is ready. An assessment of expected teaching needs should be done during the preoperative instruction period. Usually it takes a day for the patient to adjust to the new environment once the transfer has been made.

Daily physical assessment data is collected, as well as routine laboratory studies in order to monitor electrolytes, hemoglobin, hematocrit, and white blood cell counts. Patients who have undergone valve replacements are started on anticoagulant therapy within several days after surgery. The dose is adjusted according to the daily prothrombin time determination. Continuous telemetry monitoring as well as 12-lead electrocardiograms provide information about cardiac electrical stability. Follow-up chest x-ray films are ordered to assess pulmonary status. Daily weights provide an indication of fluid balance. If signs and symptoms of fluid volume excess are detected, fluid restriction and/or diuretics may be ordered.

Progressive activity advancement initiated in the ICU is continued in the step-down unit. Recently, more attention has been focused on the description of Phase I Cardiac Rehabilitation protocols for the surgical patient (Dion et al., 1982; Marshall, 1985; Meiter, Pollock, & Graves, 1986). Instructions for activity progression should be individualized based on an assessment of the home environment, level of activity prior to surgery, and desired goals for activity. Stair climbing should be included if the home or work environment has stairs. Active range-of-motion and leg exercises begun in the ICU are still emphasized to promote muscle strengthening and prevent venous stasis.

Postoperative length of stay may be relatively brief, and planning for continuity of care after discharge is very important for the recovery of the patient. Perceived quality of life after cardiac surgery does not always correlate with success in the operating room (Flynn & Frantz, 1987). After discharge, many CABG patients lack confidence in their ability to tolerate physical activity, fearing return of angina. They may experience depression and difficulty in adjusting to home and work life. In planning for hospital discharge the nurse should assess the patient's and the family's expectations for recovery to determine if they are realistic. The patient and family need to understand the chronic nature of heart disease and the necessity of compliance with a healthy lifestyle. Follow-up care through nurse-initiated phone calls, referral to outpatient cardiac rehabilitation programs, and home health visits can lessen anxiety and alleviate problems early in the recovery process.

LONG-TERM OUTCOME

With the increased number of cardiac surgeries performed, there has been a concommitant decrease in operative mortality (Takaro, Ankeney, Laning, & Peduzzi, 1986). Major areas of technical advancement responsible for this improvement include myocardial protection, blood conservation, anesthetic management, pulmonary artery catheter monitoring, pharmacologic therapy, and IABP assistance (Kaiser, 1985). In the case of CABG, conduit selection (such as use of the IMA) and preservation have also had an impact. Because of these developments, many more individuals are experiencing improvements in lifestyle and longevity in some cases.

Long-term outcome after valve replacement surgery is closely related to the performance of the artifical valve with its associated problems of thromboembolism, thrombotic obstruction, periprosthetic leak, endocarditis, deterioration and failure, and the complications of anticoagulation. The development of less thrombogenic materials for mechanical valves is needed and the tissue failure problem in biological valves requires further study.

The majority of CABG patients will be angina-free after the first year; however, about 30% will have angina at 5 years and 38% at 10 years (Hollman, 1986). The return of angina is usually due to incomplete revascularization, progression of disease in ungrafted or grafted vessels, or graft failure. The incidence of reoperation for recurrent angina was 3% in the CASS registry population of 9,369 patients. Predictors of reoperation were young age, female sex, less extensive coronary artery disease, less left ventricular impairment, less evidence of congestive heart failure, and fewer coronary vessels bypassed at the first operation (Foster, Fisher, Kaiser, & Myers, 1984). Smoking, an elevated cholesterol level, and hypertension are other reported risk factors for reoperation, although they become nonsignificant in the setting of an IMA graft (Cosgrove et al., 1986).

The use of antiplatelet therapy, aspirin in combination with dipyridamole, instituted within 1 day after surgery has been found to influence graft patency favorably at 12 months (Chesebro et al., 1984). Studies in which antiplatelet therapy was instituted at 3 days or more after surgery did not demonstrate a significant effect on graft patency (Stein, Collins, & Kantrowitz, 1986). Antiplatelet therapy is not without risk, however, as one study demonstrated an increased incidence of late cardiac tamponade in patients receiving aspirin and dipyridamole (Brever, Rousou, Engleman, & Lameshaw, 1985). Repeat bypass surgery is a technically more difficult procedure, associated with higher rates of mortality and morbidity; greater use of donor blood transfusions and a higher incidence of perioperative myocardial infarction (Hollman, 1986). As an alternative to reoperation, the technique of percutaneous transluminal coronary angioplasty (PTCA) has been applied to patients with failed coronary bypass grafts (Hollman, 1986; Jones et al., 1983). The long-term results of this procedure and its comparability to a primary PTCA procedure are still being investigated.

SUMMARY

The first 48 hours after cardiac surgery are a critical time for the patient, and rapid changes in physiologic and psychological stability can occur. The nursing diagnoses identified in this chapter should serve as a guide for development of interventions and patient outcomes. In order to influence patient outcomes positively the critical care nurse must possess current knowledge regarding the pathophysiology of heart disease, indications for surgery, operative procedures, and postoperative care.

BIBLIOGRAPHY

American Heart Association (1986). *Heart facts.* Publication no. 55-005-J, 1985. Chicago: American Heart Association.

Aron, K. V., Nicoloff, D. M., Kerstein, T. E., Northrup, W. F., & Lindsay, W. G. (1985). Six years of experience with the St. Jude Medical valvular prosthesis. *Circulation, 72* (3, Part 2), II-153-II-158.

Banasik, J. L., & Tyler, M. L. (1986). The effect of prophylactic positive end-expiratory pressure on mediastinal bleeding after coronary revascularization surgery. *Heart and Lung, 15,* 43–48.

Bojar, R. M., Najafi, H., DeLaria, G. A., Serry, C., Goldin, M. D. (1983). Neurological complications of coronary revascularization. *Annals of Thoracic Surgery, 36,* 427–432.

Braunwald, E. (1984). Valvular heart disease. In E. Braunwald (Ed.). *Heart disease* (2nd ed.) (pp. 1063–1135). Philadelphia: W. B. Saunders.

Brever, R. H., Rousou, J. A., Engleman, R. M., & Lameshaw, S. (1985). Late postoperative tamponade following coronary artery bypass grafting in patients on antiplatelet therapy. *Annals of Thoracic Surgery, 39,* 27–29.

Buckberg, G. D. (1985). Progress in myocardial protection during cardiac operations. In A. J. Roberts (Ed.). *Difficult problems in cardiac surgery* (pp. 9–27). Chicago: Year Book Medical.

Chesebro, J. H., Fuster, V., Elveback, L. R., Clements, I. P., Smith, H. C., Holmes, D. R., Bardsley, W. T., Pluth, J. R., Wallace, R. B., Puga, F. J., Orszulak, T. A., Piehler, J. M., Danielson, G. K., Schaff, H. V., & Frye, R. L. (1984). Effect of dipyridamole and aspirin on late vein-graft patency after coronary bypass operations. *New England Journal of Medicine, 310,* 209–214.

Christian, C. B., Mack, J. W., & Wetslein, L. (1985). Current status of coronary artery bypass grafting for coronary artery artherosclerosis. *Surgical Clinics of North America, 65,* 509.

Conforti, C. G., & Horvath, P. T. (1984). Immediate postoperative nursing management and potential complications. In P. T. Horvath (Ed.). *Care of the adult cardiac surgery patient.* New York: John Wiley.

Cosgrove, D. M., Loop, F. D., Lytle, B. W., Gill, J. C., Golding, L. A., Gibson, C., Steward, R. W., Taylor, J. C., & Goormastic, M. (1986). Predictors of reoperation after mycardial revascularization. *Journal of Thoracic and Cardiovascular Surgery, 92,* 811–821.

Cowan, M. J. (1982). Pathogenesis of atherosclerosis. In S. L. Underhill, S. L. Woods, E. S. Sivarajan, & C. J. Halpenny (Eds.). *Cardiac nursing* (pp. 103–110). Philadelphia: J. B. Lippincott.

DeLaria, G. A., Najafi, H., & Goldin, M. D. (1981). Postoperative care of the open heart surgical patient. In M. Goldin (Ed.). *Intensive care of the surgical patient* (pp. 497–509). Chicago: Year Book.

Dion, W. F., Grevenow, P., Pollock, M. L., Squires, R. W., Foster, C., Johnson, W. D., & Schmidt, D. H. (1982). Medical problems and physiologic responses during supervised inpatient cardiac rehabilitation: The patient after coronary artery bypass grafting. *Heart and Lung, 11,* 248–255.

Duncan, C., & Erickson, R. (1982). Pressures associated with chest tube stripping. *Heart and Lung, 11,* 166–171.

Duncan, C. R., Erickson, R. S., & Weigel, R. M. (1987). Effect of chest tube management on drainage after cardiac surgery. *Heart and Lung, 16,* 1–9.

Flynn, M. K., & Frantz, R. (1987). Coronary artery bypass surgery: Quality of life during early convalescence. *Heart and Lung, 16,* 159–167.

Foster, E. D., Fisher, L. D., Kaiser, G. C., & Myers, W. O. (1984). Comparison of operative mortality and morbidity for initial and repeat coronary artery bypass grafting: The Coronary Artery Surgery Study (CASS) registry experience. *Annals of Thoracic Surgery, 38,* 563–570.

Frantz, P. T. (1987). Experience with autotransfusion following coronary bypass graft surgery. *Autotransfusion Update,* June, Series 1.

Gardner, T. J., Horneffer, P. J., Manolio, T. A., Pearson, T. A., Gott, V. L., Baumgartner, W. A., Borkon, A. M., Watkins, L., & Reitz, B. A. (1985). Stroke following coronary artery bypass grafting: A ten-year study. *Annals of Thoracic Surgery, 40,* 574–581.

Goe, M. R. (1987). Creatine kinase enzyme determination. *Progress in Cardiovascular Nursing, 2,* 44–52.

Govier, A. V., Reves, J. G., McKay, R. D., Karp, R. B., Zorn, G. L., Morawetz, R. B., Smith, L. R., Adams, M., & Freeman, A. M. (1984). Factors and their influence on regional blood flow during nonpulsatile cardiopulmonary bypass. *Annals of Thoracic Surgery, 38,* 592–600.

Guzzetta, C. E., & Whitman, G. R. (1985). Cardiac surgery. In C. V. Kenner, C. E. Guzzetta, & B. M. Dossey (Eds.). *Critical care nursing: Body–mind–spirit* (2nd ed.) (pp. 571–634). Boston: Little, Brown.

Haas, G. S., Warshaw, A. L., Daggett, W. M., & Aretz, H. T. (1985). Acute pancreatitis after cardiopulmonary bypass. *American Journal of Surgery, 149,* 508–515.

Hammond, G. L., Geha, A. S., Kopf, G. S., & Hashim, S. W. (1987). Biological versus mechanical valves. *Journal of Thoracic and Cardiovascular Surgery, 93,* 182–198.

Henriksen, L. (1984). Evidence suggestive of diffuse brain damage following cardiac operations. *Lancet, 1,* 816–820.

Heyman, S. (1985). Effects of cardiopulmonary bypass on coagulation. *Dimensions in Critical Care Nursing, 4,* 70–80.

Hollman, J. (1986). Percutaneous transluminal angioplasty in patients with failed coronary bypass graft. In G. D. Jang (Ed.). *Angioplasty* (pp. 346–356). New York: McGraw-Hill.

Horvath, P. T. (1984). Preoperative evaluation and preparation. In P. T. Horvath (Ed.). *Care of the adult cardiac surgery patient* (pp. 122–157). New York: John Wiley.

Isaacson, J. J., George, L. T., Brewer, M. J. (1986). The effect of chest tube manipulation on mediastinal drainage. *Heart and Lung, 15,* 601–605.

Jansen, K. J., & McFadden, M. (1986). Postoperative nursing management in patients undergoing myocardial revascularization with the internal mammary artery bypass. *Heart and Lung, 15,* 48–54.

Jones, E. L., Douglas, J. S., Gruentzig, A. R., Craver, J. M., King, S. B., Guyton, R. A., & Hatcher, C. R. (1983). Percutaneous saphenous vein angioplasty to avoid reoperative bypass surgery. *Annals of Thoracic Surgery, 36,* 389–394.

Kaiser, G. C. (1985). CABG 1984: Technical aspects of bypass surgery. *Circulation, 72*(6, Part 2), V46–V58.

Kern, L. S. (1986). Advances in the surgical treatment of coronary artery disease. *Journal of Cardiovascular Nursing, 1,* 1–14.

Kinsley, R. H., Antunes, M. J., & Colsen, P. R. (1986). St. Jude Medical valve replacement:

An evaluation of valve performance. *Journal of Thoracic and Cardiovascular Surgery, 92,* (3, Part 1), 349–360.

Kirklin, J. K., & McGiffin, D. C. (1987). Early complications following cardiac surgery. In D. C. McGoon & A. N. Brest (Eds.). *Cardiac surgery* (2nd ed.) (pp. 321–343). Philadelphia: F. A. Davis.

Kirklin, J. W., & Barratt-Boyes, B. G. (1986). *Cardiac surgery.* New York: John Wiley.

Lazar, H. L., & Roberts, A. J. (1985). Recent advances in cardiopulmonary bypass and the clinical application of myocardial protection. *Surgical Clinics of North America, 65,* 455–473.

Lewicki, L. J. (1984). Pathophysiology of acquired cardiac dysfunction. In P. T. Horvath (Ed.). *Care of the adult cardiac surgery patient* (pp. 90–121). New York: John Wiley.

Lewis, M. R., & Dehmer, G. J. (1985). Coronary bypass using the internal mammary artery. *American Journal of Cardiology, 56,* 480–482.

Loop, F. D. (1985). CASS continued. *Circulation 72* (Suppl. II), II-1.

Loop, F. D., Lytle, B. W., Cosgrove, D. M., Goormastic, M., Williams, G. W., Golding, L. A., Gill, C. C., Taylor, P. C., & Sheldon, W. C. (1986). Influence of the internal-mammary-artery graft on 10-year survival and other cardiac events. *New England Journal of Medicine, 314,* 1–6.

Loop, F. D., Lytle, B. W., Gill, C. C., Golding, L. A., Cosgrove, D. M., & Taylor, P. C. (1983). Trends in selection and results of coronary artery reoperations. *Annals of Thoracic Surgery, 36,* 380–388.

Lundar, T., Froysaker, T., Lindegaard, K. F., Wiberg, J., Lindberg, H., Rostad, H., & Normes, H. (1985). Some observations on cerebral perfusion during cardiopulmonary bypass. *Annals of Thoracic Surgery, 90,* 502–505.

Magillan, D. J., Jr., Lewis, J. W., Jr., Tilley, B., & Peterson, E. (1985). The porcine bioprosthetic valve: Twelve years later. *Journal of Thoracic and Cardiovascular Surgery, 89,* 499–507.

Marshall, J., & Conkey, C. (1985). Sternal wound complications: Nursing care for coronary surgery patients. *AORN Journal, 42,* 700–706.

Marshall, J. R. (1985). Rehabilitation of the coronary bypass patient. *Cardiovascular Nursing, 21,* 19–23.

McGoon, D. C. (1987). Prologue: From whence? In D. C. McGoon & A. N. Breast (Eds.). *Cardiac surgery* (2nd ed.). Philadelphia: F. A. Davis.

Meiter, C. P., Pollock, M. L., & Graves, J. E. (1986). Exercise prescription for the coronary artery bypass graft surgery patient. *Journal of Cardiopulmonary Rehabilitation, 6,* 85–103.

Miholic, J., Hudec, M., Domanig, E., Hiertz, H., Klepetko, W., Lacner, F., & Wolner, E. (1985). Risk factors for severe bacterial infections after valve replacement and aortocoronary bypass operations: Analysis of 246 cases by logistic regression. *Annals of Thoracic Surgery, 40,* 224–228.

Moneta, G. L., Misbach, G. A., & Ivey, T. D. (1985). Hyperfusion as a possible factor in the development of gastrointestinal complications after cardiac surgery. *American Journal of Surgery, 149,* 648–650.

Morgan, R. J., Davis, J. T., & Fraker, T. D. (1985). Current status of valve prostheses. *Surgical Clinics of North America, 65,* 699–720.

Ochsner, J. (1985). Technique in coronary artery bypass graft surgery: Saphenous vein on internal mammary artery. In A. J. Roberts (Ed.). *Difficult problems in adult cardiac surgery* (pp. 108–116). Chicago: Year Book.

Phillips, R., & Skov, P. (1988). Rewarming and cardiac surgery: A review. *Heart and Lung, 17,* 511–520.

Rutledge, R., Applebaum, R. F., and Kim, R. J. (1985). Mediastinal infection after open heart surgery. *Surgery, 97,* 88–92.

Sanderson, R. G., & Kurth, C. L. (1983). *The cardiac patient: A comprehensive approach* (2nd ed.). Philadelphia: W. B. Saunders.

Seifert, P. C. (1983). Protection of the myocardium during cardiac surgery. *Heart and Lung, 12,* 135–142.

Shahian, D. M. (1985). Concepts and techniques of myocardial protection for adult open heart surgery. *Surgical Clinics of North America, 65,* 323.

Shaw, P. J., Bates, D., Cartlidge, N. E., Heaviside, D., Julian, D. G., & Shaw, D. A. (1985). Early neurological complications of coronary artery bypass surgery. *British Medical Journal [Clinical Research Ed.]* 291, 1384–1387.

Stein, P. D., Collins, J. J., & Kantrowitz, A. (1986). Antithrombotic therapy in mechanical and biologic prosthetic heart valves and saphenous vein bypass grafts. *Chest, 89,* (Suppl.), 46–53.

Takaro, T., Ankeney, J. L., Laning, R. C., & Peduzzi, P. N. (1986). Quality control of cardiac surgery in the Veterans Administration. *Annals of Thoracic Surgery, 42,* 37–44.

Tector, A. J., Schmahl, T. M., & Canino, V. R. (1986). Expanding the use of the internal mammary artery to improve patency in coronary artery bypass grafting. *Journal of Thoracic and Cardiovascular Surgery, 91,* 9–16.

Val, P. G., Pelletier, L. C., Hernandez, M. G., Jais, J. M., Chaitman, B. R., Dupras, G., & Solymoss, B. C. (1983). Diagnostic criteria and prognosis of perioperative myocardial infarction following coronary bypass. *Journal of Thoracic and Cardiovascular Surgery, 86,* 878–886.

Vitello-Cicciu, J. M., Brown, M. M., Lazar, H. L., McCabe, C., McCormick, J. R., & Roberts, A. J. (1987). Profile of patients requiring the use of epicardial pacing wires after coronary artery bypass surgery. *Heart and Lung, 16,* 301–305.

Weiland, A. P. (1983). A review of cardiac valve prostheses and their selection. *Heart and Lung, 12,* 498–504.

Weiland, A. P., & Walker, W. E. (1986). Physiologic principles and clinical sequelae of cardiopulmonary bypass. *Heart and Lung, 15,* 34–39.

ADDITIONAL READINGS

Cohn, L. H., Allred, E. N., Cohn, L. A., et al. (1985). Early and late risk of mitral valve replacement: A 12 year concomitant comparison of the porcine bioprosthetic and prosthetic disc mitral valves. *Journal of Thoracic and Cardiovascular Surgery, 90,* 872–881.

Ernst, S. M., Van der Fletz, T. A., Ascoop, C. A., Bal, E. T., Vermeulen, F. E., Knaepen, P. J., Van Bogerijen, L. V., van den Berg, E. J., & Plokker, H. W. (1987). Percutaneous transluminal coronary angioplasty in patients with prior coronary artery bypass grafting. *Journal of Thoracic and Cardiovascular Surgery, 93,* 268–275.

Quinless, F. W., Cassese, M., & Atherton, N. (1985). The effect of selected preoperative, intraoperative, and postoperative variables on the development of postcardiotomy psychosis in patients undergoing open heart surgery. *Heart and Lung, 14,* 334–341.

17 Thoracic Surgery

Linda Bernard, M.S., R.N.

Surgery of the lung accounts for approximately 22% of all cardiothoracic procedures performed in the United States, at an approximate rate of over 70,000 operations on the lung and bronchus annually (Rutkow, 1986). The primary indication for thoracotomy and surgical resection is carcinoma of the lung. The American Cancer Society estimates a total of 155,000 newly diagnosed cases of lung cancer in 1989, with an increase in the incidence of lung cancer in both black and white females and in black males (American Cancer Society, 1989). To date, resection is the only hope for cure for lung cancer (Waldhausen & Pierce, 1985).

The majority of patients undergoing thoracic resection are 50 to 70 years of age (Shields, 1983). Of these surgical candidates a significant number have compromised preoperative functional status with concomitant cardiac or pulmonary pathology. These factors, in addition to the advanced technological practice of medicine, demand a high level of clinical expertise from the critical care nurse. Prompt recognition and timely assessment of real or potential patient care problems are essential elements in the care of such critically ill patients.

Addressed in this chapter are the major indications for the therapeutic thoracotomy and specific postoperative nursing care considerations. Major complications of thoracotomy, as well as their recognition and treatment, will be covered. The convalescent and rehabilitative aspects of thoracic surgery will conclude the chapter.

INDICATIONS

Primary neoplasia of the lung accounts for the majority of pulmonary resections. The types involved include squamous-cell carcinoma and adenocarcinoma. Squamous-cell is the most frequently seen carcinoma of the lung (Waldhausen & Pierce, 1985). In addition to the treatment of primary lung carcinoma, removal of granulomatous and metastatic lesions is a less frequent indication for thoracotomy.

Prior to the advent of modern antibiotic therapy, thoracotomy was often the treatment of choice for chronic infectious lung disease, primarily tuberculosis and postpneumonia abscess formation. Today, surgical treatment of chronic infectious diseases occurs predominantly in the setting of resistant empyemas and chronic fungal infections. Traumatic chest-wall injury may necessitate therapeutic thoracotomy. Bleb resection and treatment of resistant bronchiectasis may also be indications for thoracotomy.

PROCEDURES

Thoracic procedures may be divided into two major categories: diagnostic and therapeutic. Diagnostic thoracic procedures, which involve retrieval of tissue samples for pathologic analysis, include thoracentesis, closed-tube thoracostomy, needle biopsy, bronchoscopy, mediastinoscopy, and limited thoracotomy, i.e., open-lung biopsy (Kakos, 1983). Even though patients undergoing these procedures are not normally sent to an intensive care unit, the critical care nurse may have the opportunity to care for such patients, since respiratory and cardiac complications can complicate the postoperative course.

Therapeutic thoracotomy means the removal of some portion of the lung, mediastinum, and/or pleural contents. The goal of therapeutic thoracotomy is the removal of all of the lesion, while simultaneously minimizing the removal of healthy lung tissue (Brooks, 1979). There has been a shift toward more conservative resection for cancer of the lung, using the procedures of wedge resection, segmentectomy, and sleeve resection. This is similar to the conservatism that has occurred with cancer of the breast. If a neoplastic lesion is located peripherally and is well localized, a "wedge resection," removal of the diseased area, or segmentectomy, may be performed in conjunction with postoperative radiation. Lobectomy, removal of a lobe of the lung, is performed most often for primary and metastatic carcinoma and less often for bronchiectasis, tuberculosis, granulomas, fungal infections, and cystic diseases (Glenn, Liebow, & Lindskog, 1975). Pneumonectomy, the complete removal of a lung, is the treatment of choice for centrally located cancer of the bronchus or cancer involving the main-stem bronchus or the blood vessels of the hilum. Pneumonectomy may be performed in conjunction with exploration and resection of mediastinal lymph nodes, resections of chest wall and diaphragm, and removal of parietal pleura (Waldhausen & Pierce, 1985). Tuberculosis, bronchiectasis, and lung abscesses that are refractory to medical therapy may also be indications for pneumonectomy when the entire lung is diseased.

THE PREOPERATIVE EVALUATION

Information that is useful in determining a patient's tolerance for surgical resection includes the history and physical exam, electrolyte determinations, e.g., a biochemical profile and blood counts, a base-line arterial blood-gas determination, a chest roentgenogram, and pulmonary function tests. Patient data that may be significant for postoperative management include history of cardiac and pulmonary disorders, diabetes, age, concurrent infections, and smoking history. Preoperative physical exam information that is helpful postoperatively includes activity tolerance, history of sputum production, nutritional state, and base-line vital sign measurements. Thorough preoperative chest assessment provides an excellent data base for postoperative reassessment. Preoperative arterial blood gases will indicate levels of hypoxemia and hypercapnia that may preclude surgical intervention or can aid in postoperative management of these conditions. A chest x-ray film will localize the offending lesion. Diagnostic bronchoscopy is routinely performed. Brushings, washings, and biopsy will aid in diagnosing the lesion.

Well-documented alterations in pulmonary function occur after thoracic surgery. Vital capacity (VC) and forced expiratory volume in one second (FEV_1) are reduced by up to 50% for as long as 7 days after thoracotomy (Bryant, Preston, Houck, Mobin-Uddin, Trinkle, & Griffen, 1972). Functional residual capacity (FRC) is only 75% of normal for approximately 2 days postoperatively (Rea, Harris, Seelye, Whitlock, & Withy, 1978). Because of these and other physiologic alterations, it is necessary to screen patients with pulmonary pathology to determine their ability to tolerate resection. Impairment can be measured, postoperative morbidity and mortality can be estimated, and surgical intervention and postoperative care can be altered accordingly. Bronchospastic disease can also be diagnosed and treated prior to surgery.

In general, ventilatory volumes and timed expiratory flow rates are most predictive of pulmonary morbidity and mortality (Kakos, 1983). The FEV_1 is considered to be a respiratory parameter that can be used in combination with the forced vital capacity (FVC) to demonstrate both restrictive and obstructive components of lung disease (Burrow, Strauss, & Niden, 1965). An FEV_1 more than 0.8 to 1.0 liter is necessary to maintain a normal pCO_2 (Segalls & Butterworth, 1966). FEV_1, VC, and peak expiratory flow rates (PEFR) are considered by some authors to be the minimum preoperative examinations necessary for a smoking patient with a history of dyspnea and chronic sputum production (Gothard & Branthwaite, 1982).

Additionally, a ventilation–perfusion scan may be performed on an individual with abnormal pulmonary function tests. This screening test is most often performed in anticipation of a potential pneumonectomy and is helpful in determining the contribution that the diseased lung makes toward ventilation.

There may be circumstances that contraindicate therapeutic pulmonary resection in a given population. These include, but may not be limited to, the following: arterial blood-gas results on room air that demonstrate a PO_2 of less than 60 mm Hg and PCO_2 of more than 50 mm Hg, pulmonary hypertension, cor pulmonale, unstable angina, and recent myocardial infarction (Waldhausen & Pierce, 1985). Distant metastatic disease, superior vena cava syndrome, laryngeal nerve paralysis, positive pleural effusions, and regional lymph-node involvement may require radiation and chemotherapeutic intervention rather than surgery, since these disease processes are outside the boundary of surgical resection.

Well-documented risk factors in thoracic surgery include increased age, decrease in cardiopulmonary reserve, and need for pneumonectomy (Nagasaki, Flehinger, & Martini, 1982). Compromised nutritional status will also predispose the thoracic surgical patient to impaired wound healing.

PREOPERATIVE TEACHING

Preoperative teaching for thoracic patients includes information similar to the teaching done for any surgical patient. The anticipated surgical procedure, normal postoperative course, and the patient's participation in care should be discussed with the patient and family. Special emphasis is placed on demonstration of chest physical therapy, effective use of an incentive spirometer, coughing, and expansion exercises. It is important for the patient to practice these maneuvers and for the nurse to validate the patient's correct performance of them during the preoperative period. In addition, the chest-drainage apparatus and any other special postoperative respiratory equipment (e.g., supplemental oxygen and ultrasonic nebulizer) should be discussed. The patient should be taught incisional splinting maneuvers that may help to minimize postoperative discomfort during coughing and deep-breathing exercises. Postoperative arm and shoulder exercises should also be demonstrated to the patient. If the patient smokes he or she should be encouraged to stop smoking at least 1 to 2 weeks prior to thoracotomy, and more if possible. This should improve any existing bronchitis and bronchospastic disease and facilitate bronchial drainage during the entire convalescent period.

THE SURGICAL PROCEDURE

In general, most therapeutic thoracotomies are performed through a posterolateral or lateral incision. The posterolateral incision provides for excellent exposure of both the anterior and posterior surfaces of the lung, the blood vessels, hilum, and mediastinum. The incision is usually through the fifth intercostal space, while the patient is positioned in the lateral decubitus position. One should expect that this position will predispose the patient to the development of atelectasis on the unaffected, dependent side. In addition, if the patient is positioned improperly, peripheral-nerve injuries can occur in the dependent arm.

The median sternotomy has been advocated for thoracotomy by some authors, especially in patients with bilateral malignant or bullous disease, and those with particularly poor pulmonary function (Kakos, 1983). Advantages of this type of incision include reductions in the amount of postoperative pain, operative time, and length of hospital stay (Urschel & Razzuk, 1986). The disadvantages of this technique include poor surgical control and limited exposure of posterior, deep lateral, or basilar lesions. The use of this position is therefore limited (Kakos, 1983).

A unilateral endobronchial intubation by either a long tube or a double-lumen endotracheal tube may be used in order to isolate the operative lung field. This protects the nonoperative lung field from aspiration of bloody or purulent secretions or necrotic tumor (Brooks, 1979). Because the operative lung can be unilaterally collapsed this type of intubation also provides for excellent surgical exposure (Brooks, 1979). Frequent monitoring of arterial blood gases is necessary during thoracotomy, since the right-to-left shunt through the unventilated lung can cause systemic hypoxemia and hypercarbia.

Careful manipulation is critical to avoid tissue injury that can ultimately lead to infection, empyema, and bronchopleural fistula formation. Bronchial closure is assessed prior to chest closure. If an air leak is apparent the bronchial closure can be reinforced at this time.

During closure, drainage tubes are inserted to evacuate fluid and air from the pleural cavity. The tubes are tunneled subcutaneously, then through the skin, inferior to the incision. The subcutaneous tunnel protects the pleurae from direct atmospheric pressure when the chest tubes are removed.

POSTOPERATIVE PHASE

The patient is generally accompanied from the operating room to the critical care unit by the anesthesiologist and surgeon. Upon admission to the critical care unit, the priority treatment goals include maintenance of hemodynamic stability, adequate oxygenation and ventilation, and normal intrathoracic pressures. In most institutions, the thoracic patient will spend at least the first 24 hours in an intensive care unit for observation and institution of vigorous pulmonary hygiene. The patient may have several IV lines, an arterial line, and pleural tubes. Hemodynamic monitoring equipment, such as a pulmonary artery catheter, may be necessary, depending on the patient's condition.

A complete assessment of the patient including vital signs, level of consciousness, chest-tube drainage, and urine output is done on admission to the critical care unit. A chest examination is performed, including inspection for chest excursion, respiratory effort, and quality. The chest is auscultated for the presence of breath sounds in all areas of remaining lung tissue (Figure

17–1). In addition, the presence of adventitious sounds is noted. Continuous electrocardiographic (ECG) monitoring is initiated, and arterial blood gases and a chest x-ray film are also obtained upon admission. A thorough examination provides a basis for comparison of subsequent postoperative nursing assessments. Frequent observations and measurements of vital signs occur within the first several hours (e.g., every 15 minutes), until the patient is sufficiently recovered from anesthesia and is hemodynamically stable.

The following discussion outlines both actual and potential problems the critical care nurse may encounter in the early postoperative phase. The majority of complications in the early postoperative phase are cardiopulmonary in nature.

Potential Problem: Alteration in Cardiac Output: Dysrhythmias

Cardiac dysrhythmias occur with greatest frequency in older patients with preexisting heart or lung disease and after more extensive intrathoracic surgical intervention (Ellison, 1979). While the actual cause of postoperative dys-

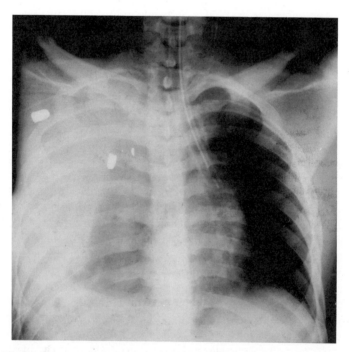

Figure 17–1. The endotracheal tube, as pictured, is inserted into the left main-stem bronchus. On physical examination, breath sounds were absent on the right chest. This tube must be pulled back into the trachea to allow ventilation of the right lung. Courtesy of Rush Presbyterian-St. Luke's Medical Center, Chicago.

rhythmias is unknown, their development is thought to be facilitated by a combination of factors—for example, postoperative mediastinal instability, increased vagal tone, hypoxemia, electrolyte imbalances, and the response to the stress of surgery and anesthesia. A local inflammatory reaction of the left atrium after ligation of large pulmonary veins is thought to contribute to dysrhythmia development in the pneumonectomy patient (Young & Perryman, 1979).

Sinus and supraventricular tachycardias, premature atrial and ventricular contractions, and atrial flutter and fibrillation, are the dysrhythmias that occur most frequently during the postoperative period. Mowry and Reynolds (1964), in a retrospective study of 574 patients, noted that 87% of dysrhythmias occurred between the third and sixth postoperative days. The incidence of dysrhythmias was also found to be higher in undigitalized patients undergoing pneumonectomy (Mowry & Reynolds, 1964). Atrial fibrillation occurs in approximately 30% of patients over age 60 (Kirsh, Rotman, Behrendt, Orringer, & Sloan, 1975). The nurse should carefully monitor the development and increase of premature atrial contractions, which frequently precede atrial flutter and fibrillation in this patient population.

Prophylactic digitalization to prevent atrial dysrhythmias may be routinely performed on pneumonectomy patients over age 60 with a history of cardiac problems (Young & Perryman, 1979), but its use is controversial in the preoperative care of other thoracic patients. Some physicians prefer to wait for the appearance of atrial dysrhythmias before treating with digoxin or with beta blockers, calcium antagonists, or cardioversion. If prophylactic digitalization is performed, the nurse should monitor for hypokalemia and hypoxemia, factors that may contribute to the development of digitalis toxicity.

If premature ventricular contractions occur in the postoperative period, hypokalemia, hypoxemia, and myocardial ischemia should be suspected and ruled out. If no contributory factor can be determined and the premature ventricular contractions (PVCs) are occasional and unifocal they will probably be monitored and will require no intervention. PVCs that are frequent, multifocal, and not part of the premorbid history are treated with lidocaine or other antiarrhythmic therapy to prevent deterioration to more lethal dysrhythmias. Continuous ECG monitoring and strict attention to electrolyte levels and arterial blood-gas results will assist in preventing and aid in the early detection of dysrhythmias.

Potential Problem: Fluid Volume, Alteration in: Excess

Generally, thoracic patients receive less fluid intravenously than nonthoracic patients in the early postoperative period to prevent the development of adult respiratory distress syndrome and pulmonary edema. Because the pneumonectomy reduces by 50% the vascular bed through which the right ventricle must pump, pulmonary artery pressure and right ventricular afterload increase significantly. This can lead to the development of pulmonary interstitial edema. The pneumonectomy patient will therefore be kept on a below-maintenance fluid restriction. The nurse should make hourly assessments of fluid status, including vital signs, urine output, urine specific gravity, and if available, other hemodynamic parameters, including central venous and pulmonary artery pressures. If a pulmonary artery catheter is available for fluid management in the pneumonectomy patient, it should not routinely be wedged, since rupture of the operative pulmonary artery stump is a possible consequence. Preoperative and daily postoperative weight measurements will also assist in assessment of fluid balance.

Potential Problem: Cardiac Output, Alteration in: Decreased Secondary to Myocardial Infarction

In patients over age 35 with no prior history of myocardial infarction, the postoperative incidence of myocardial infarction is approximately 1 to 3% (Ellison, 1979). The nurse should be especially vigilant in assessing any patient who has a prior history of coronary ischemic disease, hypertension, or diabetes for the potential development of myocardial ischemia. The nurse should suspect decreased myocardial function in any patient with hypotension and tachycardia that does not seem to be volume-related in the presence of chest pain, hypoxemia, and/or dysrhythmias. The pain of myocardial ischemia may be difficult to differentiate from normal thoracic postoperative pain. If there is any suspicion that an acute myocardial infarction has occurred, determination of serial cardiac enzymes and an electrocardiogram are indicated. The assessments and intervention at this point become those of a patient having a myocardial infarction, until proven otherwise. This will include maintenance of adequate oxygenation, blood pressure, and anxiety and pain control. Dysrhythmias should be monitored carefully and treated as ordered. A pulmonary artery catheter may be placed in order to determine cardiac output and stroke index measures and to assist with fluid administration and pharmacologic intervention.

Potential Problem: Decreased Cardiac Output Secondary to Cardiac Herniation

Rarely, death has occurred as a result of cardiac herniation through a pericardial defect into the pleural space after pneumonectomy (Gothard & Branthwaite, 1982). Hypotension, dysrhythmias, tachycardia, and cardiac arrest herald the onset of this event. In right-sided herniation, upper-body cyanosis and increased venous pressure are present secondary to vena caval obstruction (Young & Perryman, 1979). The nurse should suspect this rare complication if a patient's change in status is coincidental with position change and alert the physician immediately. A roentgenogram will confirm the diagnosis (Figure 17–2). This acute situation requires immediate thoracotomy to reduce the herniation and to repair the defect. Generally, large pericardial defects are covered with prosthetic material at the time of operation to prevent this rare complication.

Potential Problem: Alteration in Tissue Perfusion: Decreased Secondary to Hemorrhage

In the normal pleural space there is only about 20 ml of fluid. Complete drainage of intrapleural blood is necessary to prevent the coagulation of blood within the pleural space and monitor the amount of bleeding. To facilitate adequate drainage of fluid from the pleural space a large (28 French) pleural tube is usually placed in an adult.

Oozing of blood from raw parenchymal surfaces is one source of bleeding in the thoracic patient. These surfaces will usually stop bleeding with expansion of the lung as tissue surfaces become apposed. Complete lung expansion is the key to treatment in this type of bleeding.

Frank hemorrhage may occur with incomplete operative hemostasis or with tearing of the pulmonary artery or vein at the suture line. The patient rapidly deteriorates with this type of hemorrhage and immediate reoperation is necessary.

Serial measurement of vital signs and pleural drainage, hematocrit, and filling pressure is key to the timely determination of excessive bleeding. Initially, after lung resection, pleural tube output may be as high as 100 to 200 ml per hour but drainage volume should rapidly decrease over the first 4 postoperative hours. According to Brooks (1979), total drainage after lobectomy is seldom greater than 500 ml. Continued blood loss of 200 ml per hour for more than 4 to 6 hours would be an indication for reexploration of the thorax (Pairolero & Payne, 1983).

Hourly assessment of chest-tube drainage in the pneumonectomy patient is not possible, and assessment of tracheal position, serial vital signs, and hematocrits may be helpful in assessing hemorrhage. Filling-pressure measurements are not always helpful, since they may reflect changes in intrathoracic pressure and may not be indicative of decreasing intravascular volumes (Gothard & Branthwaite, 1982).

Tracheal position is assessed by placing the fingers just superior to the suprasternal notch. Normally, the trachea lies perpendicular to this notch. In the pneumonectomy patient, the trachea will lie either midline or deviate slightly to the operative side, due to the decreased pressure in the empty hemithorax relative to the normal side. As the pressure in the operative hemithorax increases in the bleeding pneumonectomy patient, the trachea will migrate from a midline position to that of deviation away from the operative site. In addition, the patient will begin experiencing respiratory distress. A chest roentgenogram will be ordered to determine fluid level in the hemitho-

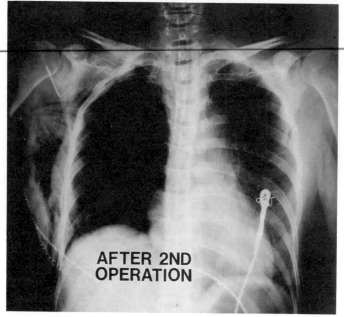

A

AFTER 2ND
OPERATION

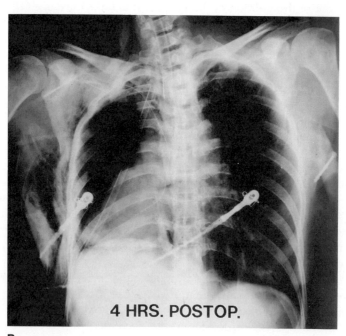

B

4 HRS. POSTOP.

Figure 17–2. Cardiac herniation. (A) This x-ray film was obtained after the patient experienced abrupt hypotension on turning to the right side after a right pneumonectomy. Note the position of the heart in the right hemithorax. (B) The x-ray film taken after emergency operation to reduce the cardiac herniation and to repair the pericardial defect. Courtesy of Rush Presbyterian-St. Luke's Medical Center, Chicago.

rax. A rapid rise in the fluid level of the operative hemithorax several hours after pneumonectomy indicates bleeding. Since the empty adult hemithorax has a capacity of 3 to 5 liters, significant blood loss can occur into this cavity.

Ineffective Breathing Pattern and Ineffective Airway Clearance

Clinically significant atelectasis is a frequent complication after thoracotomy (see chapter 1). Alveolar collapse and a corresponding decrease in compliance and reduction in lung volumes occurs secondary to ventilation at a constant tidal volume and the absence of periodic sigh or hyperventilation (Latimer, Dickman, Day, Gunn, & Schmidt, 1971). Decreased surfactant activity, potentiated by the loss of periodic deep sighing, results in premature airway closure and reductions in vital capacity and, consequently, functional residual capacity (Rehder, Sessler & Marsh, 1975). These factors, in addition to retained secretions secondary to edema in bronchial tissues, increased viscosity of secretions, inhibition of ciliary action, and depression of the cough mechanism cause atelectasis (Figure 17–3). Pain will also make the patient reluctant to deep breathe and cough and expand the injured thorax.

The immediate institution of a preventative respiratory therapy program is essential to postoperative treatment of the thoracic patient. In the intubated patient, maintaining adequate oxygen fractions and tidal volumes and maintaining clear airways by frequent suctioning and postural drainage are cornerstones of management. Ventilatory support is discontinued as soon as the awake patient has demonstrated the ability to maintain adequate spontaneous ventilation and airway clearance. Early extubation is important, since the positive pressure of mechanical ventilation promotes air leakage and could put additional strain on the healing closure sites. Surface air leaks after lobar or segmental resection are usually closed after 24 to 48 hours, but can be aggravated by positive-pressure ventilation. In addition, the trauma of repeated endotracheal suctioning could injure bronchial stump sutures in the pneumonectomy patient. However, some situations in which prolonged mechanical ventilation may be required include the following (Don, 1981):

- Impaired preoperative pulmonary function
- Preoperative hypercapnia
- Significantly impaired postoperative ventilatory mechanics
- Significantly impaired gas exchange
- Unstable hemodynamic or fluid status
- Continued blood loss
- Prolonged surgical procedure or complicated anesthesia
- Multiple blood transfusions
- Large doses of neuromuscular blocking agents or narcotics

If the patient is intubated, the nurse should initially check for proper position of the endotracheal tube by inspecting for excursion of the chest wall and by

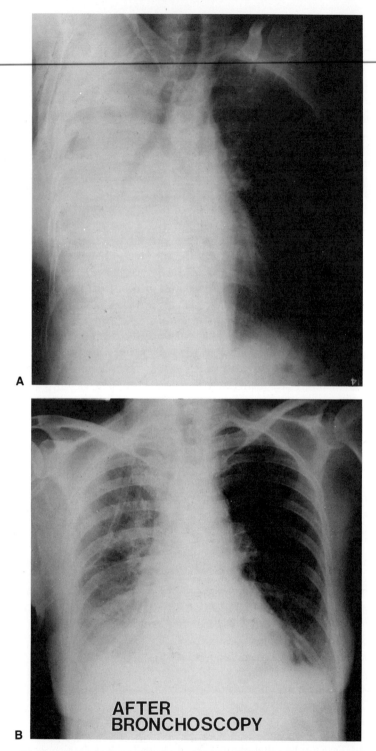

Figure 17–3. Postoperative atelectasis. (A) The x-ray film of a patient with diminished breath sounds and massive postoperative atelectasis. (B) The x-ray film postbronchoscopy. Courtesy of Rush Presbyterian-St. Luke's Medical Center, Chicago.

auscultating for the presence of bilateral breath sounds. In the extubated patient, the use of incentive spirometry, coughing, chest physical therapy, aerosol therapy, early ambulation, and exercise are critical for respiratory care. Continuous positive airway pressure (CPAP) delivered using a mask also is being evaluated as a therapy for the treatment of atelectasis (O'Donohue, 1985). Unless otherwise ordered, it is generally safe to place the thoracic patient in any postural drainage position, excluding the head-down position for lower lobar drainage. Contraindications to unlimited positioning are pneumonectomy and excessive pleural drainage.

Oxygen is routinely administered to a patient after thoracotomy. This is of help in the treatment of hypoxemia due to changes in pulmonary dynamics and ventilation–perfusion mismatching (Faber & Shepherd, 1981). Inspired humidity and mucolytic agents may be helpful in reducing the viscosity of secretions. Systemic hydration as a means of increasing mucociliary clearance should be used with caution, especially in the pneumonectomy patient, who because of pulmonary capillary bed reduction, is prone to the development of pulmonary interstitial edema.

If these measures fail to maintain airway clearance, nasotracheal suctioning or bronchoscopy may be employed. Nasotracheal suctioning should be performed carefully in patients who have had a pneumonectomy or bronchial resection, as trauma may disrupt the integrity of their suture lines. The nurse should be aware of the hazards of hypoxemia during nasotracheal suctioning, especially in the pneumonectomy patient. Interventions that should minimize hypoxemia are preoxygenation and limiting suction procedures to no longer than 15 seconds. In addition, the nurse should be alerted to the fact that bradycardia and hypotension may accompany an induced vagal response. If airway clearance is unachievable by the aforementioned interventions, bronchoscopy for the removal of secretions may be necessary.

Potential Problem: Impaired Gas Exchange Related to Respiratory Failure

Respiratory failure in the thoracotomy patient may result from a variety of causes, including pain, extensive resection, preexisting pulmonary and cardiac disease, marginal lung function, and fluid overload. After pneumonectomy the most common causes of respiratory failure include excessive fluid administration, pulmonary hypertension, preexisting ventilatory insufficiency, improper mediastinal position, and left ventricular failure (Young & Perryman, 1979). Additionally, atelectasis, pulmonary edema, pneumonia, and prolonged anesthesia and sedation may also be contributing factors. Inadequate alveolar exchange and oxygen delivery deficit results in ventilation–perfusion mismatching and, ultimately, tissue hypoxemia.

Nursing assessment of the adequacy of gas exchange includes observation of the patient's energy requirements for ventilation, chest assessment, serial blood gases, and monitoring of vital signs. The nurse should be prepared for the eventual intubation of the patient with deteriorating blood-gas levels, evidence of respiratory muscle fatigue, restlessness, confusion or deteriorating level of awareness, or tachypnea. Treatment of ventilatory failure is aimed at the identification of the cause of failure, oxygenation, intubation with positive-pressure ventilation, and the restabilization of fluid, electrolyte, and acid–base balances.

Pain

Pain control is a desirable and essential goal in the treatment of the patient who has undergone thoracic resection. Because of the pain, this type of patient finds pulmonary hygiene activities extremely difficult. The deep breathing and contraction of muscles necessary for a productive cough cannot effectively be performed. This impairment of cough and decreased expansion of the injured thoracic cage leads to hypoventilation, retention of secretions, and atelectasis. In addition, pain impairs early patient mobilization.

The recent popularity of continuous intermittent epidural analgesia in the treatment of postoperative pain has made a profound difference in pain control after thoracic surgery. While this method of analgesia is not without complications (e.g., possible respiratory depression, urinary retention, nausea, hypotension, pruritus, and infection), El-Baz and Ivankovich (1986) have reported benefits for pain control using continuous morphine via epidural infusion with minimal systemic risks. If epidural analgesia is not used, pain management may be achieved by judicious use of small doses of intravenous narcotics (Faber & Shepherd, 1981). However, the nurse should constantly monitor the patient for central nervous system depression. As with any surgical patient, timeliness of the administration of pain medication is essential.

If epidural analgesia is employed, it may be continued until the third or fourth postoperative day. The analgesic effect may persist for 12 to 24 hours after discontinuation of medication (Mehnert & Dupont, 1986). Most patients will then require only oral analgesics for pain control. The exception to this is the administration of intravenous or intramuscular analgesia prior to chest physical therapy maneuvers. Splinting the incision with a pillow, blanket, or the hands may help to provide support during movement and coughing.

Optimal surgical pleural-tube placement significantly aids in postoperative comfort. The exiting pleural tube must be positioned in such a way as to avoid a posterior location that would necessitate the patient's lying on it while recumbent. Likewise, arm motion is not impaired with an optimally placed pleural tube. In addition, the surgeon tries to prevent intercostal nerve pressure by placing the tube near the superior rib surface.

Adequate pain relief can be assessed by a patient's subjective statements as well as by observation of the ability to move the ipsilateral arm, willingness to increase activity, involvement in pulmonary hygiene activity, and by the improvement in tidal volume and vital capacity.

Impaired Tissue Integrity

Normally, after lung resection, the residual operative space fills with lung tissue. This occurs because of an overexpansion of the remaining lobes, migration of the mediastinum toward the operative side, narrowing of the intercostal spaces on the operative side, and elevation of the hemidiaphragm (Roe, 1981). Persistent air spaces in the pleural cavity can be a problem postoperatively in circumstances of extensive resection, decreased volume and compliance of remaining lung tissue, presence of underlying disease, or alveolar or bronchial leakage (Kirsh et al., 1975). Since atelectasis of remaining tissue can also cause residual spaces, nursing interventions to maintain an effective breathing pattern and adequate airway clearance and, therefore, full lung expansion can directly contribute to elimination of such spaces.

The pleural space is a potential residual space and should be nonexistent in the healthy lung. After thoracotomy, however, both air and fluid have been allowed to enter the pleural space, which may result in incomplete alveolar expansion, pneumothorax, and hemothorax. The objectives of postoperative pleural drainage are to remove air and fluid from the pleural space in order to facilitate complete apposition of the parietal and visceral pleural surfaces and to reestablish the negative pressure of the pleural space. This is accomplished by the use of a closed water-seal drainage system, which provides both a drainage chamber and a water seal that allows for expulsion of air from the pleural space, while at the same time providing protection from atmospheric pressure. Such a system can be set up for gravity drainage or can be attached to suction. In the closed water-seal drainage system, maximum suction is determined by the height of the column of water in the suction reservoir. Suction is regulated by raising or lowering the level of the column of water in the suction chamber. Obstruction of the atmospheric air vent in the suction chamber can cause an increase in the negative pressure generated in the system. For this reason, the atmospheric air vent should never be obstructed. The amount of suction necessary will be that which exceeds the intrapleural vacuum during inspiration (Fishman, 1983). For the adult patient, this is normally 20 cm H_2O pressure. There should be bubbling in the suction chamber during all phases of respiration. Large air leaks (e.g., stump leaks) may significantly increase the suction that is required to maintain full inflation and adequate pleural drainage. Atelectasis and airway obstruction also effect the ability to maintain full expansion at normal suction levels (Roe, 1981).

Small parenchymal air leaks are normal after surgery and will generally cease within hours if good apposition and sealing are present between the lung and the chest wall. Air may also leak intermittently for the first 24 to 48 hours with position changes and/or coughing. The nurse should observe the water-seal column when the system is removed from suction. The presence of bubbling in the water-seal chamber on end expiration without suction signals the presence of an air leak. The height of the water-seal column may help to determine whether or not an intermittent air leak is present. The nurse should suspect an intermittent air leak if the fluid in the water-seal compartment stays at the zero line. Since the water-seal column must return to the zero position after air has been expelled, it is unlikely that the patient has an intermittent air leak if the water-seal column is some distance from the zero point (Fishman, 1983).

The nurse must also monitor the color, quality, and quantity of drainage in the closed-chest drainage apparatus. Drainage tubing is assessed for patency. Chest tubes should not be stripped routinely. Clots can usually be dislodged by "milking" the chest tube. The nurse should also examine the pleural-tube drainage unit for dependent loops, since fluid in a dependent loop decreases the effectiveness of suction and requires that the patient generate a higher positive pressure to expel air and fluid. Kinking or accidental traction on tubes must also be avoided.

Pleural drainage is terminated when there is less than 100 ml of drainage in 24 hours, the lung is fully expanded, and no air leak is present. Chest tubes can be discontinued in the presence of a persistent space since, in the absence of an active air leak or bronchopleural fistula, such a space should decrease in 2 to 4 weeks (Kakos, 1983). In the normal postoperative thoracotomy patient the chest tube is removed in 3 to 7 days, and the site covered by an occlusive dressing. Some drainage should be expected after the tube is removed. If drainage is excessive, the dressing should be reinforced until 24 to 48 hours later, when it can be changed.

Air can also escape from the pleural space through the thoracotomy wound into the fascial and subcutanaeous tissue planes. In this situation, air spreads along the superficial tissue planes, distending the area, and producing crepitation or subcutaneous emphysema that is detectable on palpation. Subcutaneous emphysema is not harmful to the patient; however, progression of this condition must be carefully monitored since it may signal a perpetuating air leak. The nurse should mark the area where subcutaneous emphysema is palpated in order to document progression. Once in a tissue plane, air can spread easily. The presence of crepitations over a larger area does not necessarily mean an increase in the actual volume of air, but increasing tenseness of tissue, in combination with increasing margins of subcutaneous emphysema, are indications that the air leak is progressing. Should this occur, the physician should be notified of the increase in subcutaneous emphysema, as the potential for development of a tension pneumothorax exists. A chest film will be ordered to determine the adequacy of the present closed-chest drainage system. In the event that air is entering the pleural space faster than it can be removed by the pleural drainage apparatus, decompression will be necessary. This can be accomplished by repositioning the existing chest tube(s) or through insertion of an additional tube or tubes (Figure 17–4).

The postoperative management of the pneumonectomy space is considerably different from the management of the pleural space in less extensive

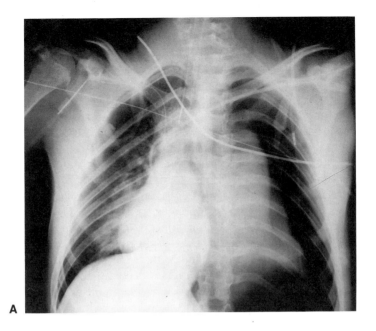

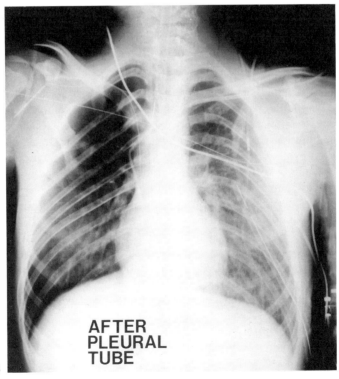

Figure 17—4. Tension pneumothorax. (A) Note the displacement of the mediastinum secondary to excessive pressure from air trapped in the pleural space. (B) After pleural tube placement, the mediastinum is again midline and the left lung is expanded. Courtesy of Rush Presbyterian-St. Luke's Medical Center, Chicago.

lung resection. Since evacuation of the pneumonectomy space would lead to mediastinal shift to the operative side, resulting in arrhythmias and respiratory and circulatory compromise, it is not drained. Medical management includes establishing and maintaining an appropriate volume of fluid and air in the pneumonectomy space in order to maintain the mediastinum near its preoperative position.

The fluid within the pneumonectomy space is the result of a serosanguineous effusion, and its level should reach the fourth thoracic vertebra within 48 hours postoperatively (Gothard & Branthwaite, 1982) (Figure 17–5A and B). It may be necessary either to remove or to add to the mediastinal contents during the initial postoperative period (Roe, 1981). Some surgeons used a closed drainage system, which is clamped after pneumonectomy. They may periodically release the clamped chest tube to remove air and fluid to reposition the mediastinum. Others may opt not to place a tube in this space, since the accumulating fluid may become contaminated through the tube tract and consequently lead to empyema. In this case, a needle can periodically be placed in the pneumonectomy space by the physician to alter air and fluid volumes. If a drainage tube is used, it will be removed after the risk of hemorrhage has passed and mediastinal position is stable. This usually occurs on the second or third postoperative day (Figure 17–5B). The serosanguineous effusion eventually clots and fibroses in the pneumonectomy space, resulting in permanent resolution of the mediastinal instability (Waldhausen & Pierce, 1985) (Figure 17–5C and D).

The nursing assessment of the postpneumonectomy space is done by palpating the trachea and point of maximal impulse. This point is normally palpated in the midclavicular line of the fifth intercostal space. Both of these assessments should be performed and documented in the postoperative admission assessment and repeated every shift. Any deviation from initial positions should be reported to the physician so that mediastinal position can be validated by chest film. The nurse should never unclamp a pneumonectomy tube without very specific orders from the surgeon. The postoperative pneumonectomy tube is *never* suctioned.

The most devastating complications of impaired wound healing in the thoracotomy patient are the formation of an empyema without bronchopleural fistula and bronchopleural fistula with empyema. In an empyema, the sequestration of fluid in a residual pleural space becomes infected. The patient presents with fever, and, if the chest tube is still in place, the drainage will be purulent. The patient will be placed on appropriate antibiotics and continue with pleural drainage. After the pleural surfaces have fused completely, the chest tube's water seal can be disconnected without fear of lung collapse and the pleural tube can become an open drainage system. If the empyema does not resolve with antibiotics and tube drainage, thoracotomy will be necessary to obliterate the space and release areas of loculation.

Bronchopleural fistula, or a fistula between the airway and the pleural space, usually occurs within the first 2 weeks postoperatively and is mani-

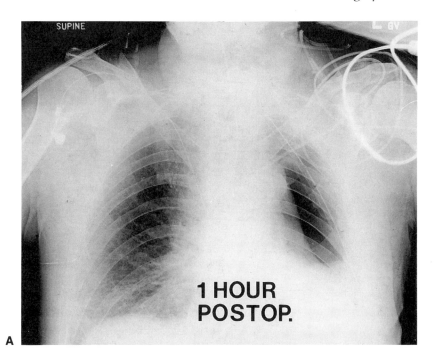

1 HOUR POSTOP.

A

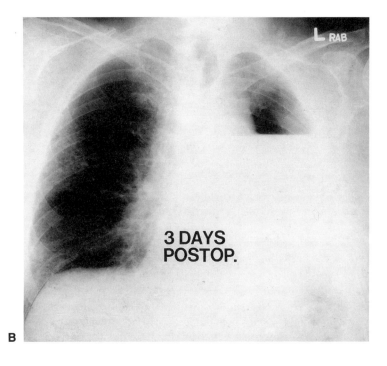

3 DAYS POSTOP.

B

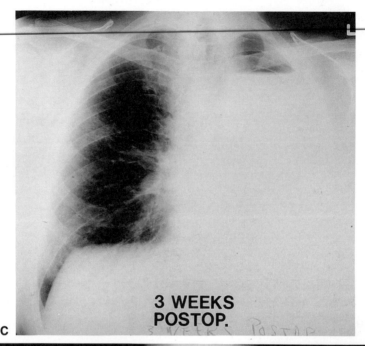

3 WEEKS POSTOP.

C

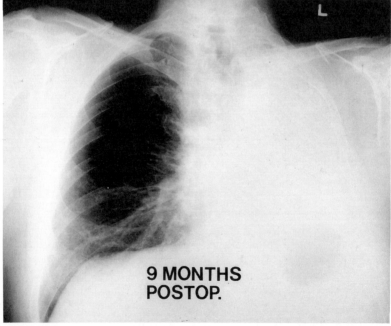

9 MONTHS POSTOP.

D

Figure 17–5. The resolution of the left hemothorax after pneumonectomy. Note the rising of the fluid line in the left hemithorax at (A) 1 hour postoperatively, (B) 3 days postoperatively, (C) 3 weeks postoperatively, and (D) 9 months postoperatively. Courtesy of Rush Presbyterian-St. Luke's Medical Center, Chicago.

fested by cough, hemoptysis, fever, contralateral pneumonia, and sepsis (Kakos, 1983). Impaired wound healing, residual tumor at suture line, bronchial stump length, method of closure, ischemic necrosis from extensive dissection, preoperative radiation, and trauma are all factors that may be associated with the development of bronchopleural fistula (Kirsh, 1975).

Bronchopleural fistula is most significant after pneumonectomy (Figure 17–6). The immediate danger to the patient is aspiration of the contents of the pneumonectomy space. The patient should be positioned with the operative site down until a chest drainage tube can be inserted. Bronchopleural fistulas are treated with tube thoracostomy for drainage, fluid replacement, and antibiotics. It should be noted that an empyema is always present (Kakos, 1983). Adequate antibiotic coverage and nutritional support are critical elements in the treatment of this devastating complication. If closure does not occur with more conservative measures, surgical closure will be necessary (e.g., muscle flap graft or thoracoplasty).

Bowel Elimination, Alteration in: Constipation

Almost all thoracic patients experience some degree of constipation postoperatively. Anesthesia, alteration in activity and diet, and large doses of narcotics contribute to this problem. It is an annoyance that patients and nurses sometimes overlook until the patient becomes quite uncomfortable. Constipation should be approached as a preventable condition. Administration of stool softeners, ensuring adequate fluid and fruit intake, providing increased fiber, and progressive ambulation should be included in the plan of care. Laxatives will be ordered if milder interventions fail to prevent or solve the problem.

Activity Intolerance

After an uncomplicated thoracic resection a patient's activity level progresses rapidly in the first few days postoperatively. Immediately after surgery a slight elevation of the head of the bed encourages the descent of abdominal organs that might otherwise impede diaphragmatic movement. Turning from side to side is encouraged in the early postoperative period in all except the pneumonectomy patient. The nurse should consult with the surgeon regarding turning restrictions in pneumonectomy patients. Turning onto the operative side in the pneumonectomy patient enhances expansion of the remaining lung. In addition, in the rare instance of bronchial stump rupture, this position prevents drainage of thoracic cavity contents into the remaining lung.

Most patients are encouraged to dangle their legs over the side of the bed the night after surgery and to proceed to sitting in a chair and then ambulation within the first 24 to 36 hours. Gradually increasing increments of activity are encouraged in the rehabilitative phase. Quite frequently, patients

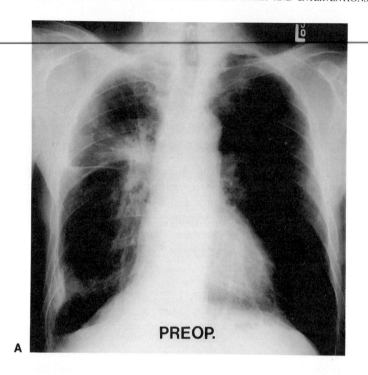

A   PREOP.

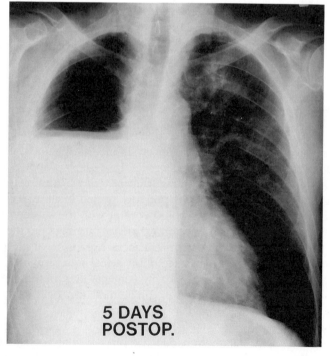

B   5 DAYS POSTOP.

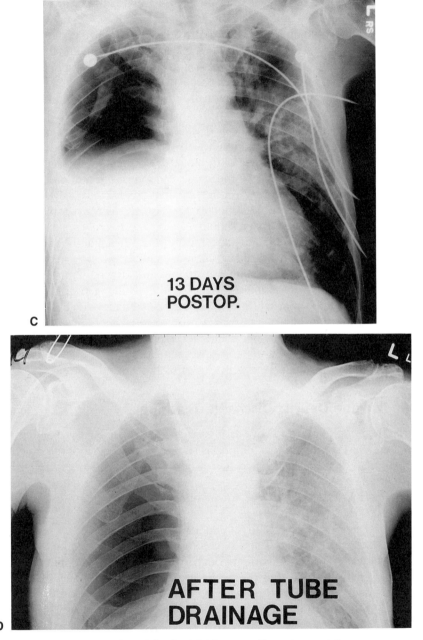

Figure 17–6. Bronchopleural fistula. (A) The x-ray film prior to right pneumonectomy. (B) Five days postoperatively. Note the fluid level in the right hemithorax. (C) Thirteen days postoperatively. Note the change in the fluid level and evidence of air in the right hemithorax, indicating a bronchopleural fistula. (D) A pleural tube is inserted to drain the contents of the hemithorax and begin treatment of the bronchopleural fistula. Courtesy of Rush Presbyterian-St. Luke's Medical Center, Chicago.

complain of increased fatigue level after discharge, usually because of greater activity at home. Fatigue should begin to resolve 48 to 72 hours after discharge. Stair climbing, walking, and activities of daily living should all be easily achievable activities if paced appropriately, that is, the patient ceases activity if excessive fatigue or dyspnea on exertion occurs. Dyspnea on exertion is related to a loss of functional parenchyma, pain, and decreased motion of the chest. It should improve gradually over the first several postoperative weeks.

Postoperative musculoskeletal disability, primarily of the shoulder girdle, can occur, since the patient tends to guard the incision and ipsilateral arm against movement. Early and frequent use of the arm on the operative side should be encouraged by the nurse. Motion of the arm and shoulder should begin in the recovery room. Frequent passive and active range-of-motion exercises will promote functional recovery, decrease pain, and prevent the development of frozen shoulder syndrome. Exercises, such as grasping a towel between the hands and raising it overhead, and "walking" the hand up a wall to an overhead position are encouraged to avoid shoulder stiffness. Active arm-strengthening exercises and driving a car should be avoided until recovery is more advanced. A 20-lb lifting restriction is also suggested for approximately 2 to 4 weeks to avoid the possibility of surgical wound disruption in patients with a posterolateral incision. Outcomes of musculoskeletal rehabilitation include full range of motion in the upper extremities, restoration of normal posture, return to base-line level of activity tolerance, and resumption of activities of daily living.

Knowledge Deficit: Discharge Teaching

The final step of postoperative care, discharge teaching, is begun on hospital admission. Prior to surgery, emphasis should be placed on development of pulmonary hygiene habits, and there should be a discussion of the activity progression and exercises to be performed throughout the entire convalescent period. Before discharge, a patient should be able to

1. Demonstrate arm and shoulder mobility.
2. Verbalize the signs and symptoms of infection, including fever above 100.5°F, persistent cough, change in chest pain, increased sputum production or change in sputum character, excessive fatigue, and redness or drainage from incision.
3. Describe side effects, dosage, and indication for prescribed medication.
4. State activity restriction and progression activity prescription. (*Note:* Patients should be forewarned of dyspnea that may occur with stair climbing and activity. This dyspnea should resolve in several weeks, as the pain decreases and the body adjusts to decreased pulmonary tissue.)

5. Describe the appropriate action if the patient experiences any problems (i.e., call the doctor/nurse, go to the emergency room).

SUMMARY

Presented in this chapter were the indications for thoracic surgery, an overview of different thoracic procedures, and the nursing diagnoses seen most frequently in thoracic surgical patients. The nursing care required by these responses to thoracic surgery is discussed in detail.

BIBLIOGRAPHY

American Cancer Society. (1989). *Cancer facts and figures.* New York: American Cancer Society.

Brooks, J. W. (1979). Complications following pulmonary lobectomy. In A. R. Cordell & R. G. Ellison (Eds.), *Complications of intrathoracic surgery* (pp. 235–245). Boston: Little, Brown.

Bryant, L., Preston, D., Houck, G., Mobin-Uddin, K., Trinkle, J. K., & Griffen, W. (1972). Lung perfusion scanning for estimation of postoperative function. *Archives of Surgery, 104,* 52–54.

Burrow, B., Strauss, R. N., & Niden, A. H. (1965). Chronic obstructive lung disease: III. Interrelationships of pulmonary function data. *American Review Respiratory Diseases, 91,* 861–868.

Don, H. (1981). Respiratory care. In B. B. Roe (Ed.). *Perioperative management in cardiothoracic surgery* (pp. 117–133). Boston: Little, Brown.

El-Baz, N. M., & Ivankovich, A. D. (1986). Management of postoperative thoracotomy pain: Continuous epidural infusion of morphine. In C. F. Kittle (Ed.). *Current controversies in thoracic surgery* (pp. 215–221). Philadelphia: W. B. Saunders.

Ellison, R. G. (1979). Cardiac complications of noncardiac intrathoracic surgery. In A. R. Cordell and R. G. Ellison (Eds.). *Complications of intrathoracic surgery* (pp. 93–100). Boston: Little, Brown.

Faber, L. P., & Shepherd, R. L. (1981). Thoracic surgery. In M. D. Goldin (Ed.). *Intensive care of the surgical patient* (pp. 472–496). Chicago: Year Book.

Fishman, N. H. (1983). *Thoracic drainage: A manual of procedures.* Chicago: Year Book.

Glenn, W. W. L., Liebow, A. A., & Lindskog, G. E. (1975). *Thoracic and cardiovascular surgery with related pathology* (3rd ed.). New York: Appleton-Century-Crofts.

Gothard, J. W. W., & Branthwaite, M. A. (1982). *Anesthesia for thoracic surgery.* Oxford: Blackwell Scientific.

Kakos, G. S. (1983). Complications of thoracic surgery: Avoidance and recognition. *Surgical Clinics of North America, 63,* 1259–1268.

Kirsh, M. M., Rotman, H., Behrendt, D. M., Orringer, M. B., & Sloan, H. (1975). Complications of pulmonary resection. *Annals of Thoracic Surgery, 20,* 215–236.

Latimer, R. G., Dickman, M., Day, W. C., Gunn, M. L., & Schmidt, C. D. (1971). Ventilatory patterns and pulmonary complications after upper abdominal surgery determined by preoperative and postoperative computerized spirometry and blood gas analysis. *American Journal of Surgery, 122,* 622–632.

Mehnert, J. H., & Dupont, T. (1986). Management of postoperative thoracotomy pain: Intermittent epidural infusion of morphine. In C. F. Kittle (Ed.). *Current controversies in thoracic surgery* (pp. 222–227). Philadelphia: W. B. Saunders.

Mowry, F. M., & Reynolds, E. W. (1964). Cardiac rhythm disturbances complicating resectional surgery of the lung. *Annals of Internal Medicine, 61,* 688–695.

Nagasaki, F., Flehinger, B. J., & Martini, N. (1982). Complications of surgery in the treatment of carcinoma of the lung. *Chest, 82,* 25–29.

O'Donohue, W. J. (1985). National survey of the usage of lung expansion modalities for the prevention and treatment of postoperative atelectasis following abdominal and thoracic surgery. *Chest, 87,* 76–80.

Pairolero, P. C., & Payne, W. S. (1983). Postoperative care and complications in the thoracic surgical patient. In W. W. L. Glenn (Ed.). *Thoracic and cardiovascular surgery* (pp. 338–351). Norwalk, CT: Appleton-Century-Crofts.

Rea, H., Harris, E., Seelye, E., Whitlock, R., & Withy, S. (1978). The effects of cardiopulmonary bypass upon pulmonary gas exchange. *Journal of Thoracic Cardiovascular Surgery, 75,* 104–120.

Rehder, K., Sessler, A. D., & Marsh, H. M. (1975). General anesthesia and the lung. *American Review of Respiratory Diseases, 112,* 541–563.

Roe, B. B. (1981). *Perioperative management in cardiothoracic surgery.* Boston: Little, Brown.

Rutkow, I. (1986). Thoracic and cardiovascular operations in the United States, 1979 to 1984. *Journal of Thoracic and Cardiovascular Surgery, 92,* 181–185.

Segalls, J. J., & Butterworth, B. A. (1966). Ventilatory capacity in chronic bronchitis in relation to carbon dioxide retention. *Scandanavian Journal of Respiratory Disease, 47,* 215–224.

Shields, T. W. (1983). *General thoracic surgery* (2nd ed.). Philadelphia: Lea & Febiger.

Tisi, G. M. (1979). Preoperative value of pulmonary function. *American Review of Respiratory Diseases, 119,* 293–310.

Urschel, H. C., & Razzuk, M. A. (1986). Median sternotomy as a standard approach for pulmonary resection. *Annals of Thoracic Surgery, 41,* 130–134.

Waldhausen, J. A., & Pierce, W. S. (1985). *Johnson's surgery of the chest* (5th ed.). Chicago: Year Book.

Young, W. G., & Perryman, R. A. (1979). Complications of pneumonectomy. In R. A. Cordell & R. G. Ellison (Eds.). *Complications of intrathoracic surgery* (pp. 257–266). Boston: Little, Brown.

ADDITIONAL READINGS

Bryant, L. R., Rams, J. J., Trinkle, J. K., & Malette, W. G. (1970). Present day risk of thoracotomy in patients with compromised pulmonary function. *Archives of Surgery, 101,* 140–144.

Bryne, N. (1978). Critical care of the thoracic surgical patient. *Cancer Nursing,* 135–141.

Finklemeier, B. A. (1986). Difficult problems in postoperative management. *Critical Care Quarterly, 9*(3), 59–70.

Gass, G. D., & Olsen, G. N. (1986). Preoperative pulmonary function testing to predict postoperative morbidity and mortality. *Chest, 89,* 127–135.

Lieb, R. A., & Hurtig, J. B. (1985). Epidural and intrathecal narcotics for pain management. *Heart and Lung, 14*(2), 164–173.

Mittman, C. (1961). Assessment of operative risk in thoracic surgery. *American Review of Respiratory Diseases, 84,* 197–207.

Neville, W. E. (1983). *Intensive care of the surgical cardiopulmonary patient* (2nd ed.). Chicago: Year Book.

O'Bryne, C. (1985). Postoperative care and complications in the thoracotomy patient. *Critical Care Quarterly, 8,* 53–58.

O'Donohue, W. J. (1985). Prevention and treatment of postoperative atelectasis. *Chest, 87,* 1–2.

O'Mara, S. R. (1986). Lung carcinoma. *Critical Care Quarterly, 9*(3), 1–11.

18

Gastrointestinal Surgery

Sally Brozenec, M.S., R.N.
Angie Z. Patras, M.S., R.N.

According to the National Center for Health Statistics, gastrointestinal disorders account for one out of three major surgeries in the United States (Given & Simmons, 1984). Increasing knowledge, surgical skill, and technology have resulted in an increase in the number of major operations to attempt to alleviate or cure such gastrointestinal problems as cancer, liver disease, and morbid obesity. Abdominal trauma is on the rise because of the unfortunate increase in violence in today's society. Care of the critically ill patient with a gastrointestinal problem is becoming an increasing challenge to the critical care nurse. Discussed in this chapter are the most common gastrointestinal problems encountered in surgical intensive care settings. Included are overviews of the procedures themselves, and the preoperative, intraoperative, and postoperative nursing care required.

PROCEDURES FOR MORBID OBESITY

Surgeries to correct morbid obesity were introduced in the late 1960s by Doctors Loren deWind and J. Howard Payne of the University of Southern California. After experimenting with a jejunocolic shunt, they developed and perfected the ileojejunal bypass. In this procedure, approximately 16 ft of small bowel is bypassed, as a section of the jejunum is anastomosed to the terminal ileum and the bypassed intestine is attached to the mesentery (Figure 18–1). The procedure reduces the absorptive surface of the intestine and therefore limits the amount of calories that enter the circulation. Although the patient experiences weight loss after this procedure, there are severe complications that result, primarily from the massive diarrhea that occurs (8 to 20

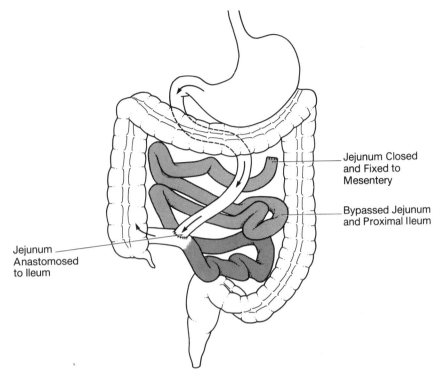

Jejunum Closed
and Fixed to
Mesentery

Bypassed Jejunum
and Proximal Ileum

Jejunum
Anastomosed
to Ileum

Figure 18–1.   Ileojejunal bypass. From *Gastroenterology in Clinical Nursing* (4th ed.) by
M. Givens and S. Simmons, 1984. St. Louis: The C. V. Mosby Co. Reproduced by permission.

stools per day) (Wastell, 1984). Complications include severe fluid and electrolyte imbalances that are difficult to control, hepatic abnormalities, and
renal failure. The bypass frequently needs to be reversed because of the
difficulty in managing these complications. According to Griffen, Bivins, and
Bell (1983), the procedure has a morbidity rate of 50% and a mortality rate of
10%. The literature indicates that newer procedures are safer and less complicated, but there are indications that the ileojejunal bypass is still considered a
viable option for individuals who may find the lifestyle changes in terms of
eating intolerable (Flint, 1986; Wastell, 1984).

At about the same time that the intestinal bypass was being studied, E. E.
Mason of the University of Iowa, while investigating patients with gastric resections for ulcers, noticed that these patients had difficulty gaining weight
postoperatively. He began experimenting with gastric bypass, rather than resection, and by 1965 had performed 300 procedures on obese patients, with a
3% mortality rate (Hornberger, 1976). Although a technically more difficult
procedure because of the location of the stomach in the upper abdomen, the
simpler alteration of normal anatomy results in fewer complications. With the
gastric procedures, the patient eats less, and therefore loses weight. What is

eaten is digested and absorbed in a manner only slightly different from nor-mal (Symmonds, 1983).

There have been several variations of gastric bypass procedures since Mason's original concept, and three methods appear to be most common. The gastric bypass or Roux-en-Y-gastrojejunostomy is Mason's technique, in which 85 to 90% of the stomach is excluded by stapling horizontally across the fundus leaving a 50-ml pouch (Figure 18–2A). The jejunum is looped up and anastomosed to this pouch. A nasogastric tube is inserted into the pouch to prevent pressure on the staple lines until healing occurs. Often, a gastros-

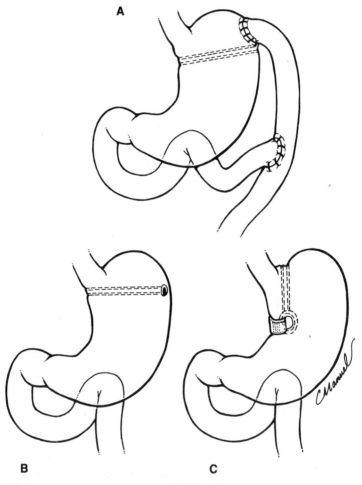

Figure 18–2. Gastric restrictive surgeries. (A) Gastric bypass with Roux-en-Y gastro-jejunostomy. (B) Greater curvature gastroplasty. (C) Vertical-band gastroplasty. From "Perioperative Complications of Gastric Restrictive Operations" by J. Buckwalter & C. Herbst, 1983, *American Journal of Surgery, 146,* p. A = 615, B = 616, C = 617. Copyright 1983 by Technical Publishers, New York. Adapted by permission.

tomy tube is placed in the distal stomach for decompression and for possible use for enteral feedings if warranted during the postoperative period. Complications of this procedure are usually related to the technique itself—anastomotic leaks, stomal obstruction, or bleeding.

With the gastroplasty (Figure 18–2B), the pouch is created in the same manner, but the intestine is not looped and anastomosed to the stomach. Rather, a small opening is left at the greater curvature end of the staple line. This opening is kept patent during the healing process by careful placement of a nasogastric tube. Food eaten is digested and absorbed in the normal manner. The small pouch creates a feeling of satiety after limited intake. Problems with this procedure are primarily related to breakdown of the staple line, often due to overeating and/or stomal obstruction.

The most recent variation of the gastric bypass is the vertical-band gastroplasty. Here, the pouch is created by a vertical, instead of horizontal staple line. A "window" is created and stapled, and a band is inserted, which prevents the stoma from enlarging over time (Figure 18–2C). This procedure takes less operating time, has fewer complications, lower operative mortality, and easier postoperative recovery than the other gastric procedures. The major disadvantage is that, because the banding process prevents the stoma from enlarging, there is a greater incidence of vomiting, and the patient remains on liquids longer than with the other procedures—usually for 3 to 6 months (Buckwalter & Herbst, 1983).

Because of their obesity, these patients are poor surgical risks and should be considered critically ill for the first 24 to 48 hours postoperatively. Obese persons often have abnormal circulatory, respiratory, metabolic, and hemostatic functions. The hours of immobility during and immediately after surgery add to the potential for complications in the postoperative period. Pulmonary hygiene, leg exercises and ambulation are essential in the first postoperative days (Pasulka, Bistrian, Benotti, & Blackburn, 1986). A potentially fatal early complication is pulmonary embolus; other potential complications include peritonitis from anastomotic leaks, wound infections, and ventral hernia development (Fakhry, Herbst, & Buckwalter, 1985).

Ultimately, patients are able to eat anything, but will find certain foods easier to manage. For example, heavy proteins might be difficult to digest, alcohol tolerance will be greatly reduced, and foods high in carbohydrates will cause the patient to feel full before adequate nutritional needs are met. These patients will need to adjust their eating habits so that several small meals are eaten each day to provide the essential food groups.

GASTROINTESTINAL TRANSPLANTATION

The development of cyclosporine as an immunosuppressant has made a significant difference in the outlook for organ transplantation. Liver transplants once carried a 25% 1-year and 20% 5-year survival rate; now the national figure is 70%. Unfortunately, liver transplantation has not been a break-through for patients with liver cancer, but is indicated primarily in adults with cirrhosis, fulminating hepatitis, or metabolic diseases, and in children with congenital abnormalities. Liver transplants are contraindicated in patients with portal-vein thrombosis, with active alcoholism, who are over 55 years old, and who lack strong psychosocial support (Smith, 1985). Liver transplan-tation is covered in detail in chapter 20.

Small-bowel transplantation (Figure 18–3) has also attracted renewed attention since the discovery of cyclosporine. There is limited documentation of these procedures, and insufficient data regarding the potential for a trans-planted intestine to take on the digestive and absorptive work of the normal small bowel. Rejection in these transplants is graft-versus-host disease (GVHD) rather than cell-mediated rejection, although cyclosporine can con-trol both types of rejection (Kirkman, 1984).

Most studies on intestinal transplantation have been done with animals, and recent work in Toronto, Canada, has demonstrated survival of a dog with a transplant for 550 days. However, these animals have had to be maintained

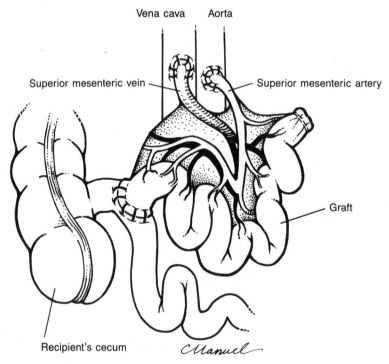

Figure 18–3. Small-bowel transplant. From "G. V. H. D. in Small Bowel Transplantation and Possibilities for Its Circumvention" by E. Deltz et al., 1986, *American Journal of Surgery, 151,* p. 380. Copyright 1986 by Technical Publishers, New York. Adapted by permission.

by artificial, intravenous nutrition (Cohen, Wassef, & Langer, 1986). The first small-bowel transplant on a human was attempted in 1967 at the University of Minnesota; the patient died 12 hours after operation. Longer survival rates have been documented (one patient lived 176 days after surgery) but there is no evidence that the transplanted bowel will function as a digestive organ. The commonest cause of failure of these transplants is arterial or venous thrombosis; as yet, the cause of this circulatory failure is not understood (Kirkman, 1984). Transplantation of the small intestine is indicated for patients with "short-bowel syndrome"—the lack of sufficient intestinal mucosa to maintain nutritional status—usually resulting from congenital malformations or frequent bowel resections, as in patients with Crohn's disease. Although these patients can be maintained by total parenteral nutrition, the long-term effects of this treatment, especially on the liver, indicate the need for a more permanent solution. Work in this area of gastrointestinal transplantation is expected to continue (Cohen et al., 1986).

Transplantation of the pancreas has been attempted in the treatment of diabetes mellitus for over 20 years. As with other transplant activity, the discovery of cyclosporine caused increased interest in pancreatic transplantation, and an improved success rate. Between 1977 and 1986, 716 transplants were performed at 69 institutions. Thirty-two percent of the 670 patients involved are insulin independent. The graft and survival rates at the University of Minnesota, which has the largest single institutional experience, are 43% and 88%, respectively. Segmental transplants of the body and tail may be used, or the entire organ can be transplanted (Figure 18–4). Researchers involved in pancreatic transplantation believe that it has the potential to be applied on as large a scale as renal transplantation. They believe that it is an effective treatment of diabetes and that early intervention can prevent the development of the severe complications of that disease (Sutherland, Kendall, Goetz, Najarian, 1986; Hanto & Sutherland, 1987).

SURGERIES FOR GASTROINTESTINAL CANCER

Gastrointestinal cancers are commonly tumor growths that metastasize very quickly because of the extensive lymphatic system of these organs. Unfortunately, the signs and symptoms of gastrointestinal cancers are very vague and nonspecific in the early stages when resection of the total neoplasm is possible. Often, the diagnosis is not determined until the tumor has begun to proliferate within the organ and/or other organs. There are extensive surgeries that are used to treat these more complicated gastrointestinal cancers. For example, a Whipple procedure (pancreatoduodenectomy or pancreaticoduodenal resection) will be performed for cancer of the head of the pancreas if there is no evidence of distant metastasis, especially to the liver. This operation involves the removal of the proximal pancreas, the duodenum, the

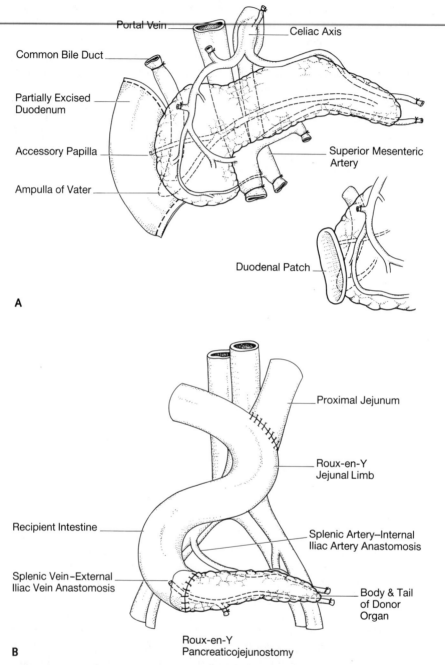

Figure 18–4. Pancreas transplantation. (A) Total pancreas transplant. (B) Segmental pancreas transplant. From "Pancreas Transplantation: Clinical Considerations" by D. Hanto & D. Sutherland, 1987, *Radiology Clinics of North America,* 25, p. A = 338, B = 337. Copyright 1987 by W. B. Saunders, Philadelphia. Reprinted by permission.

lower half of the stomach, the gallbladder, and the common bile duct (Figure 18–5). The pancreatic and hepatic ducts are implanted into the jejunum, and the remaining stomach is also connected to the jejunum. This allows gastric, hepatic, and pancreatic secretions to empty into the small intestine so that reasonably normal digestion may take place. The commonest complication from this procedure is anastomotic leakage and the resultant potential for abscess and fistula formation or peritonitis (Given & Simmons, 1984).

Esophagogastrectomy

The middle third of the esophagus is the most common site for squamous-cell carcinoma. This is followed closely by the lower third, which can include adenocarcinoma of the esophagogastric junction. Tumor masses in the esophagus are virulent and can extend up and down the submucosa. Since there is no limiting serosa, local extension and metastasis to regional lymph nodes is very common. Since cure is uncommon, surgery is performed to relieve dysphagia, the primary symptom.

There are many surgeries done for esophageal cancer. The most common and most successful procedure done for esophageal cancer in the lower

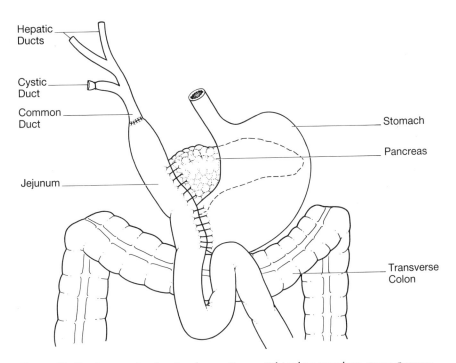

Figure 18–5. Pancreaticoduodenal resection or Whipple procedure. From *Gastroenterology in Clinical Nursing* (4th ed.) by M. Givens and S. Simmons, 1984. St. Louis: The C. V. Mosby Co. Reproduced by permission.

third of the esophagus is the esophagogastrectomy, otherwise known as gastric "pull-up." In this extensive procedure, the surgery is accomplished through a left thoracotomy incision. The tumor and distal esophagus are mobilized, and the tumor and the cardia of the stomach are removed. The cardia is sutured closed and the remaining part of the stomach is pulled up around the remaining esophagus. At the time of the esophagogastric anastomosis, a nasogastric tube is placed in the stomach and allowed to remain until peristalsis returns. The diaphragm is closed, and the chest is closed with water-seal chest drainage.

An anastomosis involving the esophagus and the stomach has a greater risk for leakage than does any other gastrointestinal surgery. The leakage is caused by tension on the suture line, poor healing, or impaired blood supply of the stomach, to which the esophagus is joined. The other complication with this surgery is pneumothorax. These two major complications can cause death (Schwartz, Lilleher, Shires, Spencer, & Stoner, 1974).

Hepatic Resection

Treatment for patients with tumors of the liver is usually only palliative. Surgical excision is the only effective treatment.

A single tumor may encompass a large portion of the liver or a significant portion of a single lobe. More common, however, is the multinodular or diffuse form, in which there are multiple nodules of tumor throughout both lobes of the liver. The liver is one of the few organs in which multiple gross tumors are commonly seen at the time that the disease is diagnosed. The treatment of choice is surgical removal of the tumor with an appropriate amount of surrounding tissue. Treatment of choice for malignant hepatoma is hepatic lobectomy. If the tumor masses are small a wedge resection of the liver may be performed.

In either case, resection of the liver is a difficult surgery to perform. The liver is very vascular and hemorrhage during this surgery is a common complication. The serum albumin level also falls significantly after resection and replacement is necessary for weeks after surgery. Resection of 50% of the liver can be carried out without fatal results as long as no other complications occur during the procedure. In many cases, the tumor masses are found to be obstructing the biliary system. This complicates the surgery, because decompression and rerouting of bile must be achieved. Overall, hepatic resection yields a small percentage of patients who survive to 5 years.

A thoracoabdominal incision is necessary for this procedure, and chest drainage is necessary during the postoperative period. The patient who has undergone liver resection should be watched for complications, which include hemorrhage, wound infection, subphrenic abscess, decreased albumin, and hepatic coma (Schwartz et al., 1974).

Cancer of the Colon

Cancer of the colon and rectum is an increasingly common health problem. Two thirds or more of malignant lesions occur in the rectosigmoid area of the bowel. Although this type of cancer has a good 5-year survival rate, it is often diagnosed too late for successful surgical intervention. Metastasis of the cancer occurs if the primary lesion is in close proximity to lymphatic circulation. By the time of surgery, most tumors have penetrated the bowel wall and spread to adjacent organs, such as the small intestine, liver, or uterus. The survival rate is proportional to the depth of the lesion and the number of lymph nodes involved (Given & Simmons, 1984).

Surgery is the primary treatment for colorectal cancer; alternative procedures are illustrated in Figure 18–6. The extensive abdominal–peritoneal resection is commonly required to ensure complete removal of the lesion and is the procedure most frequently seen in the critical care unit. This is a two-step procedure (Figure 18–6A). First, a colostomy is formed through an abdominal incision. Then, after closure of the abdomen, the lower colon, rectum, and anus are removed through a perineal incision, which is either left open or surgically closed. Common complications of this procedure are perineal wound infection, bowel obstruction, urinary problems, and impotence (Given & Simmons, 1984).

EMERGENCY SURGERIES

Abdominal trauma is often treated surgically, and usually these patients are critically ill from either the extent of the trauma or the operative procedure itself. Traumatic injuries to the abdomen are classified as blunt (commonly associated with sports injuries or motor vehicle accidents) or penetrating (stab or gunshot wounds). Blunt trauma used to predominate, however, changes in modern society have increased the incidence of penetrating wounds. Blunt trauma continues to have a higher mortality rate than penetrating wounds (Kennedy, Johnson, & Odling-Smee, 1981). The treatment of abdominal trauma is covered in detail in chapter 21.

Another reason for emergency surgery in the gastrointestinal tract is upper gastrointestinal bleeding. The commonest causes of this bleeding are the erosion of an artery by a penetrating peptic ulcer and the rupture of esophageal varices from increasing portal hypertension. Surgery is indicated in these situations when the bleeding cannot be controlled by lavage, tamponade, vasoconstriction, or vessel occlusion via endoscopy. Surgery should be considered despite the risk factors when a loss of 1000 to 1500 ml of blood can be estimated, the hematocrit falls and remains at 25 or less, after 24 to 48 hours of continued bleeding, or if the blood pressure and hematocrit cannot be stabilized with 1000 ml of blood replacement every 24 hours (Lamphier & Lamphier, 1981).

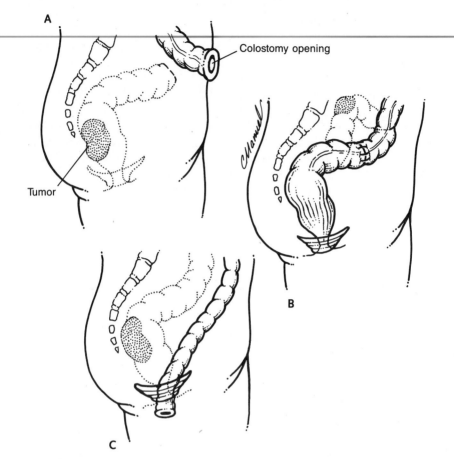

Figure 18–6. Diagrams illustrating the alternative approaches to resection of malignant tumors in the rectosigmoid segment. (A) Combined abdominoperineal resection
with permanent abdominal colostomy (Miles' operation). (B) Anterior resection with
primary anastomosis. (C) Proctosigmoidectomy with "pull through" and anastomosis
and preservation of external sphincter muscles. From "Malignant Tumors of the Colon and
Rectum. Part II. Surgical Treatment" by M. A. Block, 1976. In *Gastroenterology* (3rd ed., Vol. 2)
(p. 1050) edited by H. L. Bockus. Philadelphia: W. B. Saunders. Copyright 1976 by W. B. Saunders.
Adapted by permission.

If the bleeding is due to a perforating ulcer, an oversew of the ulcerated
area with ligation of the specific vessels may be performed. Vagotomy, or the
resection of part of the vagus nerve that controls gastric secretion, may be
done at the same time (Figure 18–7).

Although there are several shunting procedures to reduce the portal
pressure on the esophageal vasculature, the portacaval shunt is considered to
be the most useful in emergency situations because of its relative simplicity to
perform (American Gastroenterological Association, 1976). There are two

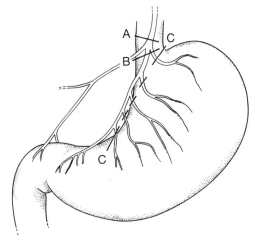

Figure 18–7.   Different types of vagotomies. (A) Truncal. (B) Selective. (C) Proximal. From "Interventions for persons with problems of digestion" by B. C. Long. In *Medical-Surgical Nursing: Concepts and Clinical Practice* (3rd ed.) (p. 1509) edited by W. J. Phipps, B. C. Long, and N. F. Woods, 1987. St. Louis: The C. V. Mosby Co. Reproduced by permission.

variations of this procedure: the end-to-side procedure shunts the portal vein into the inferior vena cava and totally bypasses the liver, while the side-to-side technique allows some portal blood to enter the liver (Figure 18–8). The decision as to which method to use is based on the amount of functioning liver tissue that exists.

OTHER FACTORS RESULTING IN CRITICAL STATUS

There are situations in which a patient is seen in the ICU for reasons other than the type of the surgical procedure. For example, some gastrointestinal procedures take longer than expected and the length of anesthesia is prolonged. After prolonged anesthesia (6 to 8 hours), changes occur in lung volume, pulmonary mechanics, and gas exchange. The reduction in vital capacity causes respiratory difficulty and the patient may require artificial ventilation for an extended period.

Another complication that can occur is extensive blood loss during surgery. For most of the procedures mentioned, extensive blood loss is a possibility. This complication may also necessitate that the patient remain in ICU until the hemodynamic status is stabilized. Although any form of shock may develop in the patient who has undergone gastrointestinal surgery, the most common type in the immediate postoperative period is hypovolemic shock. In this type of shock the loss of circulating volume may be a result of actual loss of blood and plasma during the procedure itself. Even though the blood has been replaced, observation of this patient in the ICU is necessary.

Vena cava

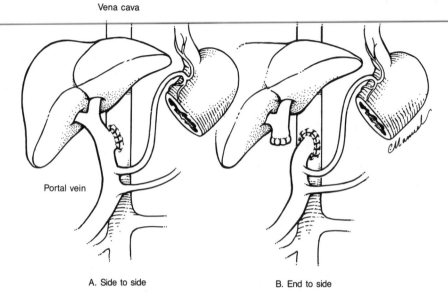

A. Side to side   B. End to side

Figure 18–8. Approaches to portacaval shunt. (A) Side-to-side. (B) End-to-side. From "Portal Hypertension and Bleeding Esophageal and Gastric Varices: A Surgical Approach to Treatment" by P. D. Ellis, 1977, *Heart and Lung,* 6(5), p. 794. Copyright 1977 by C. V. Mosby, St. Louis. Adapted by permission.

Other complicating circumstances, such as certain medical conditions, may also necessitate a patient going to the ICU postoperatively. A patient with brittle diabetes, hypertension, or chronic obstructive pulmonary disease may require close hourly monitoring of his or her medical status during the immediate postoperative period.

NURSING CARE

Preoperative Period

Since there is alteration in the gastrointestinal system with any major surgical procedure, preoperative assessment of this system is important for obtaining base-line data and for assisting in determining the extent of pathology. There are four major signs/symptoms related to gastrointestinal disorders—pain, vomiting, abdominal distension and changes in bowel activity.

Visceral pain arises from an abdominal organ, and is usually described as a deep, diffuse, aching sensation. It is poorly localized because the abdominal organs have few pain receptors. Pain is felt as a result of stretching or tension in an organ, and often is not perceived until a great deal of tissue damage has occurred.

Note the location, characteristics, frequency, onset, and duration of abdominal pain. Location: Because abdominal pain is often undifferentiated and poorly localized, the patient should be asked to point to the general area of discomfort. Characteristics: Although visceral pain is usually described as dull and aching, sharp burning pain may be felt when there is irritation to the peritoneum (parietal or somatic pain). This type of pain, which is more localized and thus, easier to pinpoint, could be indicative of a perforation and/or peritonitis. Frequency, onset, duration: Determine if the pain is intermittent or continuous, what factors aggravate or alleviate the pain, and relationships between the pain and meals, activity, bowel movements, and emotional stress.

The correlation between pain and nausea is important to know; the pain can cause nausea and must be differentiated from nausea originating from a problem in the gastrointestinal tract. If emesis occurs, note the presence or absence of blood, the amount of digested food, and the presence of bile. It is important to differentiate between vomiting and regurgitation.

Another nursing assessment is the determination of the presence of abdominal distention. The degree of distention will vary with the amount of vomiting that has occurred. Generally, patients will feel abdominal bloating when there is an obstruction of the tract below the ligament of Treitz in the jejunal area (Patras & Brozenec, 1984).

The patient should be asked about recent changes in bowel activity. With lower gastrointestinal tract obstruction, there usually is no bowel activity below the obstruction. With an obstruction higher in the gastrointestinal tract, loose, water stools may be passed even when other symptoms of obstruction are present. Dark brown or black tarry stools, called melena, denote bleeding in the lower tract. Because bilirubin in the bile makes the stools brown, any obstruction of the hepatobiliary system can result in light-colored stools. Fatty stools that appear greasy and frothy result from malabsorptive disorders such as pancreatitis, cystic fibrosis, or sprue (Given & Simmons, 1984).

Physical Examination of the Abdomen

The four quadrants of the abdomen are landmarks for physical assessment (Figure 18–9). An overview of potential findings and related problems seen on physical examination of the abdomen is presented in Table 18–1. First, inspect the abdomen for striae, scars, masses, contour, and symmetry. Previous abdominal surgeries can mean the development of adhesions, a common cause of bowel obstruction. Visible peristalsis may be seen in thin people and in children. Angiomata or vascularization of the abdomen, especially around the umbilicus, is indicative of liver disease or vena cava obstruction. Bulges of the abdomen can be a result of obesity, gas, or ascites. Percussion will differentiate between them.

The abdomen should be auscultated before percussion and palpation because these activities may cause increased peristalsis. Each of the four quadrants should be auscultated. The right lower quadrant is the best area for hearing bowel sounds without the interference of other organ noises. Bowel

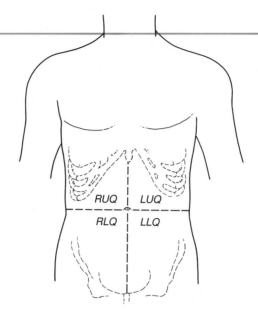

Figure 18–9. The four quadrants of the abdomen. The right upper quadrant (RUQ) contains the liver, gallbladder, duodenum, the head of the pancreas, the hepatic flex- ure of the colon, the transverse colon, a portion of the right kidney, and part of the ascending colon. The left upper quadrant (LUQ) holds part of the left lobe of the liver, the spleen, the body of the pancreas, the left kidney, the splenic flexure of the colon, and part of the descending colon. The right lower quadrant (RLQ) holds the cecum, the appendix, part of the ascending colon, the right ovary and uterus, and the right ureter. The left lower quadrant (LLQ) contains the sigmoid colon, part of the descend- ing colon, the left ureter, and the left ovary and uterus. Reprinted with permission from *AORN Journal,* Vol. 40, pp. 726–731, November 1984. Copyright AORN Inc, 10170 East Missis- sippi Avenue, Denver, CO 80231.

sounds, described as clicks and gurgles, are the result of intestinal peristalsis and they occur about 5 to 30 times per minute. For this reason, the abdomen should be auscultated for at least 2 to 5 minutes with the diaphragm of the stethoscope to obtain accurate information about peristaltic activity. Hyperac- tive sounds occur when there is increased peristalsis—for example, in the area above an obstruction, or when the patient has diarrhea. These noises are high-pitched and rushing. Hypoactive or absent sound means a reduction or cessation of intestinal activity, and is normal after any abdominal procedure. Normal activity should return to the small intestine within 48 to 72 hours, and to the colon in 3 to 5 days after surgery. Gastrointestinal activity ceases when- ever there is irritation of the peritoneum. It is therefore important to assess bowel sounds frequently on patients, since a change may be an early indica- tion of peritonitis.

The abdomen should also be auscultated for bruits (abnormal vascular sounds) at the epigastric area over the aorta and renal arteries. Venous hums

Table 18-1   Physical Examination of the Abdomen

Technique	Findings	Possible Problem
Inspection	Restricted abdominal movements	Peritoneal inflammation
	Generalized distention, umbilicus inverted	Obesity, gas
	Generalized distention, umbilicus everted	Ascites, tumor, umbilical hernia
	Lower half of abdomen distended	Ovarian tumor, pregnancy, bladder distention
	Upper half of abdomen distended	Gastric dilatation, pancreatic cyst/tumor
	Visible vasculature	Portal hypertension
	Dilated veins on abdomen	Vena caval obstruction
	Visible peristalsis	Intestinal obstruction May be normal in thin adult or in child
	Increased aortic pulsations	Aortic aneurysm or increased pulse pressure
Auscultation	Absent bowel sounds	Paralytic ileus, peritoneal irritation
	Hyperactive bowel sounds	Diarrhea, intestinal obstruction
	Arterial bruits	Obstructed vessel
	Venous hum above umbilicus	Portal circulation obstruction
	Friction rubs left upper quadrant	Splenic infarction or tumor
	Friction rubs right upper quadrant	Hepatic tumor or abscess
Percussion	Increased gastric tympany	Gastric dilitation
	Increased upper liver dullness	Right pleural effusion
	Decreased lower liver dullness	Gas in colon
	Dullness in left midaxillary line, below ninth rib	Enlarged spleen
	Shifting abdominal dullness	Free fluid—ascites
Palpation	Rebound tenderness	Peritoneal inflammation
	Right-upper-quadrant tenderness	Acute cholecystitis
	Epigastric tenderness	Acute pancreatitis
	Left-lower-quadrant tenderness	Diverticulitis
	Enlarged liver	Liver disease, emphysema
	Large, tender liver	Hepatitis, right-sided heart failure
	Large, irregular liver	Hepatic cancer
	Small, nodular liver	Late stage cirrhosis, cancer
	Palpable spleen	Splenic enlargement, almost always pathologic

451

indicating the development of collateral circulation between the portal and venous systems may rarely be heard in the right epigastric and umbilical area in the patient with cirrhosis. Another rare finding with auscultation is a friction rub—a grating sound heard with respiration in the right and left upper quadrants. These noises indicate inflammation of the peritoneal surface of an organ, as with a liver tumor or splenic infarct. The bell of the stethoscope should be used to auscultate bruits, hums, and friction rubs.

Percussion is done to identify tumors, size of solid viscera, and distention. The protuberant abdomen will sound tympanic if it is filled with gas, with the wall feeling thin and stretched. Obese abdomens have a thick, dull-sounding wall. Ascitic fluid will shift to the lowest point, and can be seen or felt moving as the patient is turned.

Basic percussion methods are used to define the liver, the gastric air bubble in the fundus, and the spleen. Beginning at the upper right chest area, percuss down the resonant area from the lung until dullness is heard. Mark the spot. Then percuss up from the tympanic area in the right lower quadrant until dullness is heard, then mark. These are the general boundaries of the liver. Normally, in an adult, the liver is 10 to 11 cm. A small ruler is invaluable in performing physical assessment of the abdomen.

The gastric air bubble can be percussed in the left lower, anterior rib cage, and will sound tympanic. The spleen is percussed down the midaxillary line to dullness below the costal margin. Because it is well hidden under the rib cage, the normal spleen cannot be percussed.

Light and deep palpation is done in all four quadrants to assist in the identification of organs, masses, and areas of tenderness. In light palpation, the pads of the fingers of one hand are "dipped" about 1 cm into the abdomen. Deep palpation is a bimanual technique in which the palmar surfaces of the fingers press into the abdomen about 4 to 5 cm. It is important to note that normal tenderness is usually felt over the aorta, cecum, and left sigmoid colon, so careful observation of the patient's verbal and nonverbal responses is essential. While palpating the patient's abdomen, determine the presence of rebound tenderness—pain felt after the palpating hands are quickly released from the abdomen. The pain is the result of displaced organs snapping back to the original position, and is indicative of peritoneal irritation as, for example, in peritonitis.

Deep palpation of the liver and spleen is done to determine further their size and texture. While supporting the patient's right side with your left hand, place your right hand on the abdomen just below the marked level of dullness. Ask the patient to take a deep breath while you press in and up with your right hand (Figure 18–10). Normally, the liver edge should feel regular and smooth, and the patient should not experience tenderness. An enlarged and/or tender liver may indicate cirrhosis or hepatitis. A hard or irregular surface may suggest tumor growth. Note that a patient with emphysema may have the liver displaced by the lowered diaphragm. The spleen is not palpable unless it is enlarged two to three times (Patras & Brozenec, 1984).

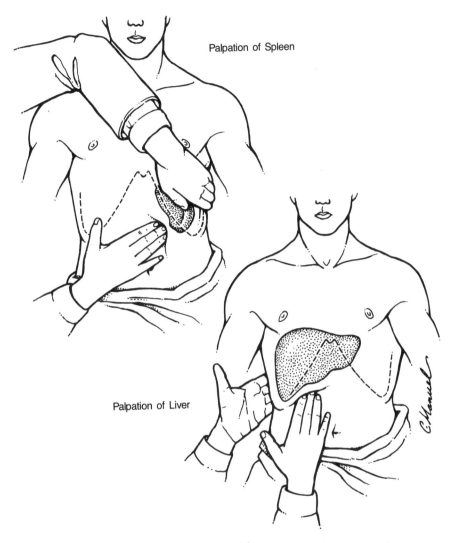

Figure 18–10. Palpation of the spleen and liver.

Another important assessment for the patient about to have major gastro-intestinal surgery is of nutritional status. Major surgery is a massive insult to the body, and surviving the procedure itself depends on the overall health of the patient. In many cases of gastrointestinal problems, the patient presents with nutritional deficits that must be corrected before surgery can be scheduled. Wound healing is largely dependent on nutritional status, especially in the patient's ability to spare proteins as energy sources. Proteins are essential for tissue regeneration, and the development and progression of such complications as fistulas, abscesses, and peritonitis can be retarded if the patient is satisfactorily nourished. The nursing assessment and treatment of alteration in nutrition: less than body requirements is discussed in chapter 8.

Finally, the teaching needs and learning levels of both the patient and significant others must be assessed. Not only can the actual surgery and hospitalization be complex and frightening, but often discharge involves complicated care at home. It is important to assess accurately the level at which learning can most effectively occur.

Preoperative teaching of patient and family includes the basic information for any surgical procedure (see chapter 1). It is also important that the family is prepared for what to expect after surgery. Major gastrointestinal surgery involves the insertion of any number of tubes and drains. The length of time under anesthesia may necessitate mechanical support of ventilation for hours to days after operation. Add to this the routine equipment and activity level of an intensive care unit, and it becomes clear the extent to which a visitor may be intimidated or frightened. Advanced preparation for the setting and for the appearances of the patient will help to alleviate the stress of the situation.

Intraoperative Period

Patients undergoing abdominal surgery may be placed in Trendelenburg or reverse Trendelenburg positions. During the excitement phase of general anesthesia, vomiting may occur, and care must be taken to prevent aspiration. The abdomen should be inspected for distention during the beginning of gas administration, as this can indicate a misplaced endotracheal tube.

The role of the nurse intraoperatively cannot be overemphasized. The nurse should make assessments during the entire surgical procedure, and note and report any spillage of feces or bile into the peritoneal cavity. Spillage into the peritoneum often causes chemical or bacterial peritonitis postoperatively.

Other nursing observations include noting the length of the surgical procedure and the extensiveness of the bowel resection. Patients who have undergone a long surgery (over 3 hours) and had an extensive gastrointestinal resection are prone to hypothermia during the procedure, and use of a hypothermia blanket may be necessary. If the surgery has been exploratory, and a great deal of bowel handling has taken place, prolonged paralytic ileus and distention may result.

Whenever the gastrointestinal tract is entered, "bowel technique" is used. Any instrument coming in contact with the mucosa or inner lining of the tract is not used again once the lumen has been reclosed. They are discarded in separate basins to avoid contact with other instruments. Some surgeons will request a new set of instruments, additional draping, and a change of gown and gloves for closure.

Irrigation solutions and/or moist laparotomy packs are frequently used during gastrointestinal procedures. The solution should always be warmed prior to use. Special instruments such as staplers are available in both reusable and disposable modes. It is important for the operating room nurse to be familiar with the equipment and its uses. The stapler has, in many settings, replaced conventional suturing since it can be used to divide, ligate, resect, and anastomose (Gruendemann, 1983).

Postoperative Period

The patient may be taken directly to the ICU or to a recovery room for immediate postoperative monitoring. In the first hours and days after complex gastrointestinal surgery frequent monitoring of vital signs, level of consciousness, urinary output and fluid status is essential. Other observations are also important. Addressed in the following sections are the usual responses to gastrointestinal surgery that require nursing intervention. Other responses that may occur and complicate the recovery process are also discussed.

Inspection of the abdomen for discoloration is necessary. A mottled, blue, or bruised appearance may indicate an intraperitoneal hemorrhage or hematoma. Postoperative hemorrhage may result from a suture sloughing off a vessel, movement of a clot from a vessel, or incomplete tying of a vessel. Any skin discoloration indicating possible hemorrhage must be reported immediately to the surgeon. The abdomen should also be observed for shape and size. Check for bilateral symmetry and look for abdominal distention. The abdomen may be tense, and the patient may complain of a feeling of fullness. Patients who have undergone gastrointestinal surgery frequently have a nasogastric tube or gastrostomy tube in place to prevent postoperative distention and accumulation of secretions in the stomach. Monitoring for distention and checking the patency of all drainage tubes should be done on a frequent basis (hourly and p.r.n.). Tubes are usually kept patent with irrigation and aspiration with normal saline as ordered by the physician. Even if irrigation is contraindicated, as when a delicate internal suture line exists, the nurse must ensure proper functioning of the suction equipment.

Potential for Fluid Volume Deficit: Hemorrhage

Incisional hemorrhage can occur during the first 24 to 48 hours after surgery, and the bleeding may be apparent or concealed. Inspection of the dressing for evidence of bright red blood should be done on an hourly basis. If bleeding is observed, the dressing should be marked with a pen at the time the drainage is observed. Continuous checking of the bedding under the patient for blood that has oozed under the dressing is also essential (Patras & Brozenec, 1984).

Wound drains such as the Penrose drain are often left in the incision for evacuation of blood, fluid, or pus. If drains are attached to drainage equipment or continuous suction, inspect all drainage equipment every hour for evidence of bleeding. Other types of drains such as T tubes, which drain bile, also need careful attention. Excessive drainage or bleeding from a T-tube drain indicates internal bleeding or a broken anastomosis (Patras & Brozenec, 1984).

Pain

The patient will experience alteration in comfort related to the operative procedure and the presence of tubes or drains. Postoperative incisional pain is localized along the abdominal or thoracotomy incision and can be managed with narcotic analgesics. Accurate assessment of postoperative incisional pain is sometimes difficult, as the patient will complain of severe pain only during conscious moments. Usually the dose given is half of the ordered dose with the remainder being administered after careful observation. In the later postoperative period, it is necessary to assess for pain every 1 to 2 hours because patients having abdominal surgery can experience fairly severe incisional pain for several days after surgery and may require high doses of narcotics.

Potential for Injury: Aspiration/Incisional Damage

Nausea and vomiting can also occur in the immediate postoperative period because of anesthetic drugs, pain, distention, or position changes. Vomiting usually does not occur in patients who have a patent and draining nasogastric or gastrostomy tube in place. If vomiting occurs in a patient without a decompression tube, the abdominal incision should be supported during the vomiting episode. Aspiration is a potential danger when gastric decompression is not used. Continuous retching and vomiting can severely increase intraabdominal pressure, causing strain on the suture line. Antiemetic medications are usually ordered to be given on a p.r.n. basis.

Impaired Skin and Tissue Integrity: Surgical Incision

Patients who have had extensive gastrointestinal surgeries may require special wound care. An example is the perineal wound created during an abdominal–perineal resection. The hollow space must heal from the inside, and this may take as long as 9 months to close completely. If the wound was closed surgically, drainage tubes that may be attached to suction are inserted on either side of the perineal incision. These are held in place with sutures, and are placed on continuous suction. When the drainage becomes minimal, usually 3 to 5 days after surgery, the drains are removed. Manual irrigation of the drain sites or sitz baths may be continued for several weeks to keep the area clean as well as to provide comfort.

The surgeon may decide to leave the perineal wound open, and this can be treated in a variety of ways. Numerous large Penrose drains can be inserted in the wound during surgery, which allows for profuse drainage in the immediate postoperative days. These drains may remain in place 5 days or longer and are shortened and finally removed as the drainage diminishes. Frequent dressing changes are required to maintain asepsis and control odor. When the drains are removed, warm packs or sitz baths will be ordered.

Sometimes the surgeon will pack the open wound with gauze dressings. In this case the packing is left in place for 3 to 5 days, after which the physician removes it. Wound care while the packing is in involves changing the outer dressing; after the packing is removed, wound irrigations with saline or peroxide are usually ordered. A bulb syringe, soft catheter, or spraying device must be used because the innermost area of the wound must be reached to provide healing from the inside out (Given & Simmons, 1984).

Many patients who have been diagnosed with cancer of the colon require the formation of a colostomy—the externalization of the colon to the abdominal wall. The colostomy may be temporary and replaced after a time, or it may be permanent, such as the colostomy developed when an abdominal–perineal resection is performed.

In the immediate postoperative period, the stoma should be assessed for color and condition. It should be deep pink to red in color, and slightly moist. If it appears dark purple or blue, there may be inadequate blood supply to the area. The surgeon should be notified immediately.

Although there will be no fecal output from the colostomy in the first days, there will be drainage of old blood and mucus. A clear, drainable colostomy appliance should be applied immediately after the initial dressing is changed. This provides visibility of the stoma and a receptacle for drainage until the colostomy begins to function 3 to 5 days after surgery.

Potential Complications

There are complications that may develop as responses to the gastrointestinal surgical procedure. These complications are serious, and can occur any time from the first to the seventh postoperative day.

Potential for Infection   The potential for infection of the surgical wound is common, despite the use of antibiotics. The wound infection rate increases as the length and complexity of the surgical procedure increases. Other factors that predispose a patient to infection include dehydration, anemia, altered nutritional status (malnutrition or obesity), the presence of wound drains, local hemorrhage, extensive wounds, and/or trauma (Patras, 1982).

It is the nurse's responsibility to prevent wound infection in the patient who has had abdominal surgery. During the first 12 hours after the operation, it is necessary to check all dressings every 1 to 2 hours. The original operating room dressing should be assessed for hemorrhage and/or excessive drainage. The drainage tubes and suction apparatus should be checked for patency and function at the same time. In most hospitals, the physician does the first dressing change, but it is important that the nurse be present at that time.

Orders for subsequent dressing changes may be written, but dressings should be changed and the wound inspected every 24 hours at the very least. The wound should be assessed for redness, swelling and unusual drainage, disruption of the suture or staple line, and approximation of the wound edges. All observations of the wound and drainage must be recorded and reported to establish a basis for comparison should changes occur. The entire abdomen should be inspected for distention or discoloration (Patras, 1982).

After complex abdominal surgery, the patient frequently has tubes and/ or drains in place (Figure 18–11). These sites are a source of potential infection, and must be assessed and kept clean on a continuing basis. To maintain skin integrity and patient comfort and to prevent infection, the drain insertion site should be cleaned with a half-strength peroxide solution every time the dressings are changed. Aseptic technique should be used, with gloves being worn and sterile cleansing solutions and dressings used (Brozenec, 1985).

Most wound infections develop within 3 to 4 days after surgery. Signs and symptoms of wound infections include redness and warmth along the incision, incisional tenderness, and temperature of 38°C (100.5°F) or above after the third postoperative day. During dressing changes, the nurse should check the amount, color, odor, and consistency of wound or tube drainage. Infected exudate can be thick, creamy yellow or greenish in color, and have a foul odor.

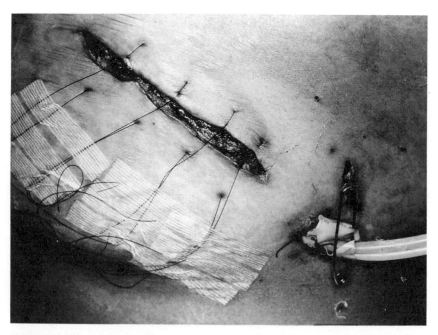

Figure 18–11. Wound with drain. Courtesy of Rush Presbyterian St. Luke's Medical Center, Chicago.

The infection must be resolved before tissue healing can occur. When a wound infection is suspected, a wound culture is taken to determine the causative organism, and appropriate antibiotic therapy is initiated. The usual method of wound care is adjusted so that debridement and irrigation of the infected wound tissue is done. Irrigation with saline and peroxide is the usual treatment. After irrigation, the wound is packed with wet–dry dressings, which are changed every 2 hours until the infection subsides (Patras, 1982).

Potential for Infection: Peritonitis   Peritonitis, or the inflammation of the lining of the peritoneum, may be the result of bacterial or chemical invasion of the peritoneal cavity. This complication can occur after any abdominal surgery. During the surgical procedure itself bacteria may be introduced into the peritoneal cavity, producing peritonitis. Other common causes of peritonitis include leaking anastomosis, spillage of intestinal contents during surgery, or a perforation of the intestine. The gastric or intestinal fluids that leak into the peritoneum cause irritation and infection.

Anastomotic leaks are a serious complication of any gastrointestinal surgery and usually occur when the stomach, esophagus, pancreas, or intestine are extensively incised and rerouted. The major causes of a leaking anastomosis include poor surgical technique, distal obstruction, poor nutritional status, and inadequate gastric or intestinal decompression during the postoperative period. The leak of intestinal or gastric fluid into the peritoneum can cause the development of peritonitis and/or subphrenic abscesses. Small localized leaks can sometimes be treated with intestinal decompression. Widespread leaks with extensive abscess formation can only be treated by further surgery, in which the areas of leakage are reanastomosed (Given & Simmons, 1984).

Symptoms of peritonitis include severe, sharp abdominal pain, and a sudden elevation in temperature. The abdomen becomes distended and there is tenderness and rigidity. A rising pulse rate is another common sign (Given & Simmons, 1984).

Impaired Wound Healing: Fistula Formation   Another complication frequently associated with gastrointestinal surgery is the formation of a fistula. A fistula is an abnormal passage leading from a body cavity or hollow organ to another cavity or to the surface of the skin (Figure 18–12). Fistulas usually develop in patients with abnormal wound healing capacity secondary to multiple abdominal surgeries in the past, poor nutrition, steroid use, or underlying pathologies such as diabetes mellitus or Crohn's disease. A fistula may also develop if an anastomotic leak occurs. A sinus tract forms between the leakage site and the abdominal skin. Fistulas usually develop along the edges or within the midline incision. The most common is the small-bowel fistula resulting from an anastomotic leak. Small-bowel fistulas are often called high-output fistulas because they can channel the loss of 1 to 2 liters of intestinal fluid in a 24-hour period (Patras & Brozenec, 1984).

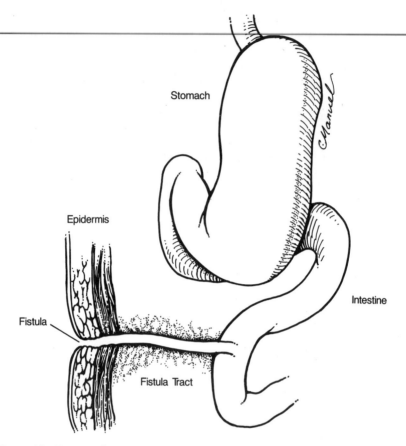

Stomach

Epidermis

Intestine

Fistula

Fistula Tract

Figure 18–12.   Fistula.

The nurse is usually the first to identify a fistula tract. Fistulas usually appear as small pinpoint openings along or near the incision or drain sites. The output is usually green or yellow, and will stain the abdominal dressing. As the tract becomes larger the fluid output can become large enough to necessitate the use of some type of drainage or suction apparatus. Because the enzyme content in small-bowel or pancreatic fistula secretions is so high, excoriation of normal tissue occurs. Wound and skin care around the fistula site must be performed meticulously to protect the patient's skin (Patras, 1982).

A potential complication of a small-bowel fistula is an alteration in fluid and electrolyte balance related to loss of secretions. The nurse must observe the patient for signs and symptoms of hypokalemia, hyponatremia, and dehydration. The character and amount of all secretions, as well as the amount of fluid intake, must be recorded accurately. Alterations in fluid, electrolyte, and acid–base status are discussed in detail in chapters 1 and 9.

Impaired Wound Healing: Disruption Wound dehiscence and evisceration (Figure 18–13) are also potential complications of gastrointestinal surgery. Wound dehiscence is a separation of the wound margins. The separation can be simple, involving only the skin and superficial tissue, or it can be severe, extending down into the fascia. The most frequent cause of wound dehiscence is a strain on the incision brought on by increasing intraabdominal pressure. This pressure can be a result of coughing, vomiting, or retching.

Evisceration is the separation of the wound through the entire fascia, causing abdominal contents to be externalized. This is considered a medical emergency—the patient must be treated for shock and the abdominal contents covered with sterile saline dressings. The patient is returned to the operating room immediately for surgical reclosure of the wound (Patras, 1982).

Knowledge Deficit: Discharge Teaching

It is necessary to formulate realistic teaching objectives during the postoperative period. A plan for the patient who has had gastrointestinal surgery will

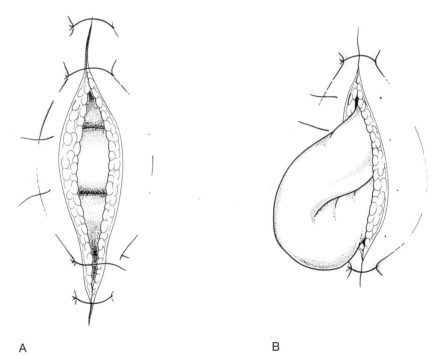

A   B

Figure 18–13. (A) Wound dehiscence, showing partial separation of incision edges. (B) Evisceration, showing protrusion of abdominal viscera through open incision. From *Gastroenterology in Clinical Nursing* (4th ed.) (p. 210) by M. Givens and S. Simmons, 1984. St. Louis: The C. V. Mosby Co. Reproduced by permission.

include preventive information on nutrition, exercise, medications, and post-operative wound- or skin-care instructions. Discharge teaching should be started as soon as possible, with the disease and surgery explained to the patient and his or her family at their level of understanding.

Wound care is often an essential part of postoperative teaching. If the patient has an ostomy or fistula, start with simple explanations and add a step at each teaching session. All teaching should be supplemented with models. Written material that the patient can take home should also be provided. This material should be assessed for its readability in light of the patient's level of literacy. Teaching interventions are successful when the patient can describe and perform the basics of wound, fistula, or ostomy care prior to discharge.

SUMMARY

There are many situations in which a patient with a gastrointestinal disorder may require intensive nursing care after surgery. Many procedures are complex and/or lengthy, and the compromised life functions may require extensive observation and nursing care during the first postoperative days. In this chapter, the specific procedures that most commonly require this kind of care have been described, along with the postoperative complications that have the greatest potential for occurring.

BIBLIOGRAPHY

American Gastroenterological Association. (1976). *Portal hypertension and ascites* (slides and tape). Baltimore: University of Maryland.

Block, M. A. (1976). Malignant tumors of the colon and rectum. Part II. Surgical treatment. In H. L. Bockus (Ed.) *Gastroenterology* (3rd ed., Vol. 2) (pp. 1045–1057). Philadelphia: W. B. Saunders.

Brozenec, S. (1985). Caring for the patient with an abdominal drain. *Nursing '85, 15*(4), 55–57.

Buckwalter, J., & Herbst, C. (1983). Perioperative complications of gastric restrictive operations. *American Journal of Surgery, 146*, 613–618.

Cohen, Z., Wassef, R., & Langer, B. (1986). Transplantation of the small intestine. *Surgical Clinics of North America, 66*, 583–587.

Deltz, E., Ulrichs, K., Schack, T., Freidrichs, B., Muller-Ruchholtz, W., Muller-Hermelink, H., Theide, A. (1986). G. V. H. D. in small bowel transplantation and possibilities for its circumvention. *American Journal of Surgery, 151*, 379–385.

Ellis, P. D. (1977). Portal hypertension and bleeding esophageal and gastric varices: A surgical approach to treatment. *Heart and Lung, 6*(5), 791–798.

Fakhry, S., Herbst, C., & Buckwalter, J. (1985). Complications requiring operative intervention after gastric bariatric surgery. *Southern Medical Journal, 78*, 536–538.

Flint, L. (1986). Dealing with failures of jejunoileal bypass for obesity. *American Journal of Surgery, 151*, 367.

Given, B., & Simmons, S. (1984). *Gastroenterology in clinical nursing.* St. Louis: C. V. Mosby.

Griffen, W., Bivins, B., & Bell, R. (1983). The decline and fall of the jejunoileal bypass. *Surgery, Gynecology and Obstetrics, 157,* 301–308.

Gruendemann, B. (1983). *Care of the patient in surgery.* St. Louis: C. V. Mosby.

Hanto, D., & Sutherland, D. (1987). Pancreas transplantation: Clinical considerations. *Radiologic Clinics of North America, 25,* 333–343.

Honesty, H. (1972). *Essentials of abdominal ostomy care.* New York: Springer Publishing.

Hornberger, H. (1976). Gastric bypass. *American Journal of Surgery, 131,* 415–420.

Kennedy, T., Johnson, G., & Odling-Smee, G. (1981). Abdominal injuries. In W. Odling-Smee & A. Crockard (Eds.), *Trauma Care.* New York: Grune & Stratton.

Kirkman, R. (1983). Small bowel transplantation. *Transplantation, 37,* 429–433.

Long, B. C. (1987). Interventions for persons with problems of digestion. In W. J. Phipps, B. C. Long & N. F. Woods (Eds.), *Medical-surgical nursing: Concepts and clinical practice* (3rd ed.) (pp. 1503–1524). St. Louis: C. V. Mosby.

Lamphier, T., & Lamphier, R. (1981). Upper GI hemorrhage: Emergency evaluation and management. *American Journal of Nursing, 81,* 1814–1820.

Pasulka, P., Bistrian, B., Benotti, P., & Blackburn, G. (1986). The risks of surgery in obese patients. *Annals of Internal Medicine, 104,* 340–346.

Patras, A. (1982). The operation's over, but the danger's not. *Nursing '82, 12,* 50–56.

Patras, A., & Brozenec, S. (1984). Gastrointestinal assessment. *AORN Journal, 40,* 726–731.

Schwartz, S., Lilleher, R., Shires, T., Spencer, F., & Stoner, E. (1974). *Principles of surgery.* New York: McGraw-Hill.

Smith, L. (1985). Liver transplantation: Implications for critical care nursing. *Heart and Lung, 14,* 617–628.

Sutherland, M., Kendall, B., Goetz, F., & Najarian, J. (1986). Pancreas transplantation. *Surgical Clinics of North America, 66,* 557–577.

Symmonds, R. (1983). Surgery for morbid obesity: Appraisal of old and new techniques. *Postgraduate Medicine, 74,* 183–190.

Wastell, C. (1984). The surgical treatment of obesity. *Postgraduate Medicine Journal, 60* (Suppl 3), 27–36.

ADDITIONAL READING

Honesty, H. (1972). *Essentials of abdominal ostomy care.* New York: Springer Publishing.

19

Neurosurgical Procedures

Janet M. Delgado, M.N., CNRN

Some of the commonly occurring neurological disorders can be treated effectively with surgery. Presented in this chapter are neurological conditions, diagnostic procedures related to neurosurgery, and the corresponding surgical interventions. Information regarding the preoperative, intraoperative, and postoperative nursing care of patients undergoing cranial, transsphenoidal, and spinal surgery is presented throughout this chapter.

NEURODIAGNOSTIC PROCEDURES

Besides routine preoperative diagnostic procedures, additional procedures may be necessary for the neurosurgical patient. Special neurodiagnostic procedures corresponding to the patient's problem and the planned surgery may be required. These procedures are reviewed in Table 19–1.

Preparation and teaching of the patient and family for diagnostic procedures is a component of the nurse's role. Some of the diagnostic procedures are done at the bedside and some in diagnostic units in which nurses are part of the staff; however, the majority of tests are done in procedure departments such as radiology, where a nurse is not usually present. Therefore, it is vital that the nurse prepare and educate the patient prior to the procedure in order to allay any anxiety and fears. The information that the nurse will provide and the teaching methods used will depend on the patient's level of consciousness, memory, and neurological stability.

If a patient's neurological status is rapidly deteriorating, persistent evaluation and care are required during the procedure and a nurse should supervise the patient throughout the procedure. A nurse who is familiar with the patient's status and problems can identify changes and prevent complications that may not be identified by a diagnostic technician.

Table 19–1 Neurodiagnostic Tests

Procedure	Objectives	Implications for Nursing
Radiographic films (skull and spine)	To visualize the integrity of the bones of the cranium and spine. To identify space-occupying lesions, abnormal calcifications, cerebral atrophy and vascular anomalies. To identify the integrity of the spinal canal, which encases the spinal cord.	If fractures are suspected, ensure proper body alignment at all times. Patient must not move once positioned. Inform radiologist if pregnancy is suspected, as abdominal shields can be used when taking skull films. If head trauma or loss of consciousness is present, monitor patient throughout procedure; sedation is contraindicated. To optimize visualization of films, remove metallic objects such as jewelry and dentures.
Magnetic resonance imaging (MRI)	To visualize cross sections of soft cranial and spinal tissues (tumors, edema, infarction, and vascular and congenital anomalies	Inform patient that he or she will lie inside a closed tunnel for 30 to 90 minutes. Unless contraindicated, sedate patients who may become claustrophobic. Prior to test, instruct patient in relaxation techniques (deep breathing and imagery). Inform patient that he or she will intermittently hear a loud rhythmic humming sound. Contraindicated in patients with metallic devices (foreign objects, implants, clips, or screws).
Computerized tomography (CT Scan)	To visualize three-dimensional cross-sectional view of head and spine. The radiologist is able to determine if a substance is soft tissue, bone, CSF, blood, air, or abnormal calcification. Enhanced visualization of areas of increased vascularity or of defective blood barrier may be obtained by injecting IV iodinated contrast dye.	Contrast medium is contraindicated if patient has allergy to iodine. Inform patient that head will be immobilized in a close-fitting rubber cap for about 30 minutes and that his or her face and body will be exposed. Patient should be told not to move during the procedure. May need sedation, unless contraindicated. If contrast medium is indicated, IV access must be obtained. Fasting for 4 hours prior to test may decrease the likelihood of nausea that is associated with the contrast medium. Unless on therapeutic fluid restriction, if contrast medium has been employed increase fluid intake to promote diuresis. Observe for evidence of allergic reaction to contrast medium.
Cerebral angiogram	To visualize the cerebral vascular system via the carotid or vertebral arterial systems. To detect vascular anomalies and to define the blood supply of a tumor.	If allergic to iodine, test is contraindicated, or extreme precautions must be taken. A long catheter is threaded up through a major artery, usually the femoral. Inform patient that a warm flushing sensation will be felt when contrast medium is injected. Observe for evidence of allergic reaction to contrast medium. After the procedure monitor vital signs, assess

Table 19–1   *(Continued)*

Procedure	Objectives	Implications for Nursing
		insertion site for swelling or other evidence of bleeding, and assess extremity distal to insertion site for color, temperature, and pulses. The puncture site is immobilized for 8 to 12 hours and the patient may be placed on bed rest for 24 hours.
Cerebral–blood-flow studies	To detect increased or deficient areas in the blood flow of the cerebral circulation. To identify presence of vasospasms, tumors, aneurysms, or arteriovenous malformations. To evaluate clinical brain death.	Inform the patient that a tracer will be administered, either by inhalation or intraarterial injection. The pathway of the tracer through the bloodstream is monitored using scalp electrodes. A computer display shows blood flow of both cerebral hemispheres.
Myelogram	To visualize the entire spinal column by injecting contrast medium into spinal subarachnoid space.	Approximately 10 ml of CSF is removed from the lumbar region, contrast medium is injected, and radiographs are taken. Precautions are determined by which of the two types of contrast medium is used. *Oil-based preparations:* Pantopaque, an iodine compound irritating to neural tissue, is removed via aspiration after the test is complete. The patient is maneuvered into various positions using a tilt table, as this allows the oily substance to flow. Headache after the procedure may be alleviated by lying in a horizontal position. *Water-based preparations:* Metrizamide, diffuses upward via the CSF regardless of the patient's position. It is absorbed by the body and excreted within 72 hours. After the procedure, the head is elevated to reduce upward flow of the contrast medium.
Electroencephalogram	To record the electrical activity of the brain. Can be used to identify diffuse or focal abnormalities.	Hair should be relatively clean prior to the procedure. Withhold dietary stimulants such as coffee and tea. Instruct the patient not to move during the procedure and that he or she may be asked to open and close his or her eyes, to look into a flashing light, to breathe rapidly, and to try to fall asleep. Wash the patient's hair thoroughly after the procedure.

Table 19–1   *(Continued)*

Procedure	Objectives	Implications for Nursing
Evoked responses (visual, auditory, somatosensory)	To evaluate the responses of the auditory, visual and somatosensory systems.	Inform the patient that he or she will receive specific stimuli, and the responses will be monitored via scalp electrodes. The patient may be shown checkerboard patterns (visual), asked to listen to clicking sounds (auditory), or have peripheral nerves stimulated (somatosensory). The procedure lasts 15 minutes and there are no risks to the patient.
Electromyography	To identify pathology of peripheral nerve and muscle. To identify the electrical characteristics of muscle.	Inform the patient that small needles will be inserted in specific muscles and that there may be a slight pricking sensation when the electrical stimulus is applied. The patient will also be asked to relax and contract certain muscles.
Lumbar puncture	To obtain CSF specimens, to measure CSF pressure, or to remove excess CSF volume.	Contraindicated in intracranial hypertension, sudden decrease in intracranial volume may cause downward displacement of the brain. Patient is positioned laterally, with knees drawn to chest, or to sit leaning forward, with back rounded and supported by an overbed table. A local anesthetic will be administered. The patient may be asked to cough or take deep breaths during the procedure. After the procedure, encourage hydration and lying flat to decrease headache, perform neurological assessments, note reports of leg pain, observe lumbar site for leakage of CSF or hematoma formation.

CSF = cerebrospinal fluid.

INTRACRANIAL PRESSURE MONITORING

Neurological conditions in which intracranial pressure monitoring would be of benefit, and the associated nursing interventions, are presented in chapter 13. An early sign of intracranial hypertension is deterioration of neurological status. However, once a patient's level of consciousness is severely affected, a more direct measure of intracranial pressure (ICP) is indicated. Intracranial pressure monitoring has been used in clinical practice since the 1950s (Lundberg, 1960) and is now an accepted tool for evaluation of critically ill patients with intracranial hypertension.

Monitoring Techniques

Intracranial pressure can be monitored directly or indirectly. The monitoring system is a closed one. Each monitoring system consists of a sensor, a transducer, and a recording apparatus. Intracranial pressure can be monitored using one of three routes: intraventricular, subarachnoid, or epidural (Figure 19–1). Each of these routes of access has clinical advantages and disadvantages, which will be presented in this section.

Ventricular Access

Ventricular fluid pressure is monitored via a polyethylene catheter placed in one of the lateral ventricles. It is the most direct measure of ICP available,

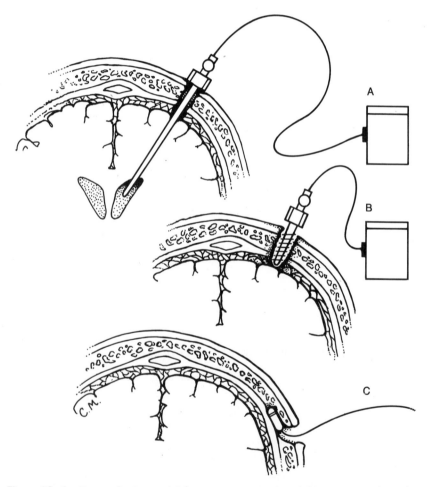

Figure 19–1. Routes for intracranial pressure monitoring. (A) Intraventricular catheter. (B) Subarachnoid screw or bolt. (C) Epidural sensor.

therefore the absolute ICP values are very reliable measures. The direct access to the ventricular system permits instillation of contrast media to visualize the ventricular system, test intracranial compliance, and therapeutically drain cerebrospinal fluid (CSF) and reduce ICP. However, the direct access to the ventricles could lead to inadvertent, excessive drainage of CSF and does pose a higher risk of infection. All connections and stopcocks must be sterile and securely sealed. If marked cerebral edema is present, lateral ventricles may be narrowed and therefore difficult to cannulate. Before insertion, a computerized tomographic (CT) scan is used to assess the size and shape of the lateral ventricles. The ventricle is accessed after the skull is penetrated with a burr hole. The transducer is leveled at the foramen of Monro and is recalibrated if the patient is repositioned. If a CSF collection device is connected to the system, it must remain stationary at a level no more than 10 mm below the foramen of Monro.

Subarachnoid Access

Subarachnoid monitoring via a bolt or screw is the most commonly used method of ICP monitoring. It is placed by first making a burr hole in the skull, usually in the frontal bone, and making a nick in the dura (Vires, Becker, & Young, 1973). The end of the screw or bolt lies in the subarachnoid space. Although not as invasive as ventricular monitoring, there is a risk of infection as a result of the penetration of the meninges. The transducer is leveled with the subarachnoid screw and must be recalibrated if the patient is repositioned. A major problem with this method is the possibility of upward herniation of brain tissue into the screw, which occurs when intracranial pressure is very high. The bolt becomes plugged, which can lead to inaccurate or dampened wave forms on the recording device.

Epidural Access

Epidural monitoring, the least invasive technique, also requires penetration of the skull via a burr hole. The sensor is placed on top of the dura and does not penetrate the meninges. This method predisposes the patient to less of a risk of infection. The transducers are calibrated prior to insertion and cannot be recalibrated once inserted. Using the indirect epidural route the absolute value of ICP is not a reliable measure; therefore, only the trends and patterns in ICP can be evaluated.

Implications

Trends in ICP must be evaluated in patients with intracranial hypertension. In addition, the ICP values may be used to evaluate perfusion of the cerebral hemispheres, which is done by calculating cerebral perfusion pressure (chapter 13).

When evaluating trends in ICP, the clinician must note the extent as well as the duration of any rise in pressure. In addition, the clinician needs to correlate trends in ICP with clinical signs. The early identification of intracranial hypertension will permit the clinician to intervene in a timely manner. In order to evaluate trends in ICP, a wave-form classification system consisting of A, B, and C waves is used (Figure 19–2). A waves, or plateau waves, indicate an extremely high rise in ICP, which can be sustained for up to 30 minutes. A waves are accompanied by sudden decreases in ICP that only last a few minutes; in addition, the level to which ICP decreases is still above normal. A waves are indicative of decreased cerebral perfusion and/or of impending cerebral herniation. Rudy (1984) notes that plateau waves above 20 mm Hg that are sustained longer than 30 minutes are indicative of malignant hypertension. B waves are sharp transient rises in ICP that have been associated with decreased wakefulness and alterations in the respiratory pattern (Langfitt, 1968). Frequent occurrence of B waves has been associated with the subsequent development of A waves. C waves are rhythmic periodic rises in ICP that are associated with changes in blood pressure. The clinical significance of C waves is not known.

The information gained from ICP monitoring and clinical observation can assist critical care clinicians in planning treatment strategies and in evaluating the effectiveness of interventions. In addition, this technology may be used to determine the patient's prognosis in relation to physiologic integrity, functional ability, and rehabilitation potential.

NEUROSURGICAL PROCEDURES

Managing the care of patients undergoing neurosurgery poses a challenge to the critical care nurse. Neurosurgical patients in critical care units most often

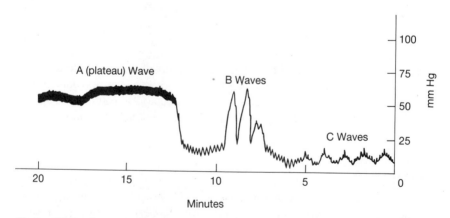

Figure 19–2. Intracranial pressure waves. Composite drawings of A (plateau) waves, B waves, and C waves. From *Nursing the Critically Ill Adult* (3rd ed.) by N. Meyer Holloway, 1988, Menlo Park, Calif.: Addison-Wesley. Copyright 1988 by Addison-Wesley Publishing Company. Adapted by permission.

have undergone a procedure to correct head trauma, for the diagnosis or treatment of a central nervous system lesion, or for implantation, revision, or removal of a shunt (Cunha & Tu, 1988). Although there are many surgical procedures that can be performed to correct or minimize neuropathology in the central nervous system, these procedures can be grouped into three categories: cranial, transsphenoidal, and spinal surgeries. Patients who undergo neurosurgery are at risk for all the complications associated with general surgery and for the added complication of residual neurological deficits. These risks and other nursing care considerations for neurosurgical patients are complex and numerous; therefore, only the patient management concerns most relevant to the intensive care nurse will be presented in the following three sections.

CRANIAL SURGERY

Cranial surgery is one of the treatments used to eliminate pathologic lesions that occupy precious space in the cranial cavity and can lead to the development of intracranial hypertension. If the lesion is a tumor, chemotherapy and/or radiation will be used in combination with surgery in a comprehensive treatment plan. In the following section, the preoperative, intraoperative, and postoperative phases of a general craniotomy will be presented. Particular neurological disorders that require cranial surgery, such as tumors, hematomas, arteriovenous malformations, and aneurysms will be described in the subsequent section.

Preoperative Care

The critical care nurse must perform an overall neurological assessment in the preoperative phase. Having preoperative base-line data is vital in evaluating the patient's progress or deterioration during and after cranial surgery. The neurological assessment should emphasize the areas of pathology or injury. The nurse must evaluate the impact that this pathology has had on the patient's functional status (see chapter 13 for neurologic assessment). Furthermore, depending on the pathology or surgery planned, the nurse must be aware of the potential of additional deficits precipitated by the surgical procedure.

Knowledge Deficit

Since cranial surgery is a major procedure, one can assume that definite concerns or symptoms caused the patient and his or her family to seek surgical treatment. The neurosurgeon and other members of the surgical team will provide the patient with information about the procedure and about risks and benefits involved with the surgery. Typically, a great deal of information is provided over a short period. This sudden overload of information can be overwhelming to the patient and family. The patient may have an altered cognitive status and may have difficulty understanding or remembering what was said. The nurse can allay many of the patient's anxieties and fears by clarifying and repeating information given to the patient and family.

The nurse should inform the patient and family about what to expect in the critical care unit after surgery. They should be told that the stay in the unit is for close observation and stabilization, and the length of that stay will depend on the surgical procedure and the patient's progress. They should also be told about the intravenous lines, respiratory equipment, indwelling urinary drainage catheter, monitoring equipment, and the drains and dressing(s) that can be expected. The patient should be told to expect a headache postoperatively and it should be emphasized that the nurse should be notified immediately at the onset of a headache, as the pain medication used is a mild analgesic. Analgesics strong enough to mask changes in neurological status or suppress vital functions will not be administered.

The physical preparation of the patient begins the evening before surgery. Since most cranial surgeries are 3 to 6 hours long, they are frequently scheduled as the first cases in the operating room. It is important that preparations be started early on the eve of surgery, as the patient must be provided with the optimal conditions for sleep that evening. Since infection in the central nervous system is very difficult to combat, precautions are taken to decrease surface bacteria preoperatively. An antibacterial shampoo is usually prescribed for the evening before surgery. It is common practice for the patient with severe facial acne to undergo intensive treatment with antibiotics over a period of several days. To decrease the psychological trauma to the patient and to maintain integrity of the scalp, the patient's hair is cut and shaved or clipped in the surgical suite. A child's hair is usually shaved and prepped after the anesthesia is administered. The morning of surgery, the patient routinely receives prophylactic broad-spectrum antibiotics and sedation and is then transferred to the surgical suite.

Intraoperative Care

A craniotomy is the most commonly performed cranial surgery. A craniotomy is a surgical opening of the skull consisting of incising a flap of scalp, bone, and dura to expose the surface of the brain. Surgical approaches can be classified as either *supratentorial* or *infratentorial*. The folding of the fibrous dura mater separating the cerebrum from the midbrain and cerebellum is the tentorium cerebelli. The cerebrum and other structures superior to the brain stem and cerebellum are considered supratentorial. Supratentorial structures are those that lie in the anterior and middle cranial fossa. Infratentorial structures such as the brain stem and cerebellum lie below the tentorium cerebelli. Infratentorial structures lie in the posterior cranial fossa. The relative positions of the cranial fossae are illustrated in Figure 19–3. There are different management strategies in the intraoperative and postoperative surgical

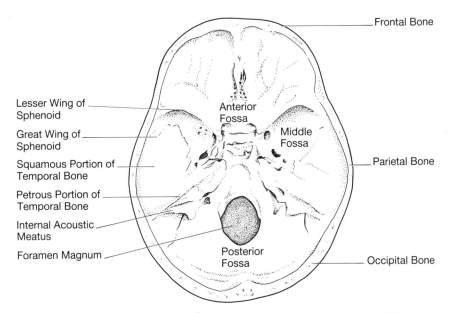

Figure 19–3. Base of skull as viewed from above, showing the location of the anterior, middle, and posterior fossae. From "Acoustic Neuromas: Nursing Management during the Acute Postoperative Period" by L. A. Gruppi, 1987, *Critical Care Nurse, 7*. Adapted from *Textbook of Anatomy* (4th ed.) (p. 868) by H. Hollinshead & C. Rosse, 1985, New York: Harper & Row. Copyright by 1985 by Harper & Row. Reprinted by permission.

phases for patients who have undergone supratentorial or infratentorial surgical approaches. The basic intraoperative cranial surgery positions are summarized in Table 19–2 according to their reference to the tentorium.

Once the patient is positioned using proper body-alignment techniques, the head is immobilized and stabilized in a headrest. The patient is draped, exposing the proposed craniotomy site. The scalp and muscles are incised and pulled aside. The cranial bone is either hinged or removed. If the bone is removed and will be replaced, it is placed in a basin of sterile saline. The dura mater is incised and the specific surgical procedure is performed. Throughout the procedure the dural tissue is moistened with saline. If needed, surgical drains are inserted. All incision sites are closed systematically and the surgical site is dressed.

Postoperative Care

During the postoperative phase the critical care nurse should maintain the patient's physiologic integrity, preventing or recognizing complications in a timely manner and promoting optimal function. In order to achieve these goals, the critical care nurse must develop a plan of care that is individualized to the patient's needs. The nursing diagnoses that may be identified postoper-

Table 19-2   Patient Positioning for Craniotomy

Position	Surgical Incision
SUPRATENTORIAL APPROACH	
Supine, head straight Supine, head rotated Lateral Sitting	For cosmetic reasons, attempts are made to position the surgical incision within the hairline. Incision is placed directly over the area of pathology.
INFRATENTORIAL APPROACH	
Lateral	Allows for transtentorial access to the posterior fossa.
Prone (contraindicated with intracranial hypertension) Sitting	Incision is made at the occiput, slightly superior to the point at which neck flexion occurs.

atively are discussed in the following text. The differences in prescribed nursing care after supratentorial and infratentorial surgery are summarized in Table 19–3.

Table 19-3   Postoperative Nursing Care: Supratentorial and Infratentorial Approaches

Goal of treatment	Supratentorial	Infratentorial
Promote venous return, prevent intracranial hypertension	Maintain the head of bed elevated 30 to 40 degrees at all times	Maintain the head of bed flat at all times
Maintain intact suture line, decrease likelihood of bleeding	Position laterally or supine, avoid pressure on operative site	Position laterally only. Avoid pressure on operative site (back of head).
Promote optimal level of activity	If stable, should be out of bed by second day after operation	Elevate the head of bed gradually over a period of several days, until sitting is tolerated by the patient
Promote optimal nutritional status	Start a clear liquid diet 24 hours after surgery. Advance diet as tolerated.	Start a clear liquid diet when able to tolerate without nausea and vomiting. Nausea is common. Progress diet to solid foods as tolerated.

Potential for Injury Related to Seizures

Unexpected postoperative seizures accompany cerebral edema. Some patients have seizures in the immediate postoperative phase because of brain swelling but may have no further problems throughout their recovery. However, since the surgery causes an irritable focal lesion, many neurosurgeons place patients on antiepileptic drugs for 2 to 5 years postoperatively. Information on the management of a patient who is experiencing seizures is provided in chapter 13. The pertinent observations that a clinician should note and record during a seizure are summarized in Table 19–4.

Alteration in Cerebral Tissue Perfusion

The onset of cerebral edema is a major postoperative concern. Nursing care measures to maximize optimal cerebral perfusion must be initiated, as uncontrolled cerebral edema may lead to decreased cerebral perfusion and herniation syndromes. For a summary of the nursing management of intracranial hypertension, refer to chapter 13. The overall control of cerebral edema may include the use of osmotic diuretics, corticosteroids, and fluid restriction.

Hydrocephalus can occur as a clinical syndrome that may be treated surgically or may develop as a postoperative complication. Hydrocephalus occurs when there is excessive CSF production, faulty reabsorption of CSF, or blockage of the CSF pathways to the arachnoid villi, which is where CSF is reabsorbed into the venous sinuses. Tumors of the choroid plexus (the area where CSF is manufactured) would cause an increased production of CSF, although such tumors are rare and occur most frequently in children. The normal reabsorption of the CSF could be prevented by the presence in the

Table 19–4   Clinical Observations of Seizure Activity

What events preceded the seizure?

Was an aura reported?

Was there an initial cry or sound?

In what part of the body did movements begin?

What was the sequence of the movements?

Were there separate tonic and clonic phases?

How long did each phase last?

Was there any incontinence?

Were there any changes in pulse, respiratory rate or pattern?

Were there any changes in pupillary reactivity?

What was the patient's level of consciousness during the seizure?

What was the patient's immediate postictal behavior?

subarachnoid space of an infectious exudate or blood after a subarachnoid hemorrhage or surgery. Blockage of the CSF pathways or obstructive hydrocephalus may be caused by mass lesions or by postoperative cerebral swelling. The patient will exhibit signs of increased intracranial pressure, and dilated ventricles will be apparent on a CT scan. For long-term management of this problem, a ventricular shunt is required. An acute build-up of large amounts of CSF can be rapidly controlled by placement of a temporary external drainage device, such as a lumbar drain or a ventriculostomy.

A ventricular shunt will divert the flow of CSF from the ventricles before reaching the point of obstruction to another body cavity where it can be reabsorbed into the bloodstream. The atrium of the heart and the peritoneum are the distal drainage points. The catheter is inserted to drain CSF from a lateral ventricle and is advanced to either the right atrium or the peritoneum (Figure 19–4). Valves are placed in the system to prevent CSF reflux and to allow flushing to assist in maintaining the patency of the system. Shunts will need to be revised if infection or blockage occurs and as patients who are children grow in height.

Ineffective Temperature Regulation

As with other surgeries, a transient increase in body temperature in the postoperative period is expected. However, an increase in body temperature could be indicative of wound infection, meningitis, or even central alteration of temperature control. The concepts related to temperature regulation and its management are presented in chapter 12. Wound infection, meningitis, posterior fossa syndrome, drug fever, IV-line sepsis, and nosocomial pneumonia are among the most common causes of temperature elevation in the neurosurgical patient (Cunha & Tu, 1988).

Central temperature control mechanisms are not easily altered. The hypothalamus is the central thermostat, and it would take severe cerebral swelling or manipulation and damage of the hypothalamus and surrounding structures to cause central temperature regulation problems. If such a condition occurs, fever would not be the only symptom, as the patient's temperature would vary dramatically between hyperthermia and hypothermia.

Potential for Infection

If a wound infection or meningitis develops, these complications must be treated immediately. All infections near the central nervous system must be identified early and aggressively managed (Cunha & Tu, 1988). The primary goal is to avoid involvement of brain tissue, since the majority of antibiotics do not effectively cross the blood–brain barrier. Nevertheless, an infection would take its toll on the neurosurgical patient; decreasing the level of optimal functioning and negatively affecting the chances for successful rehabilitation.

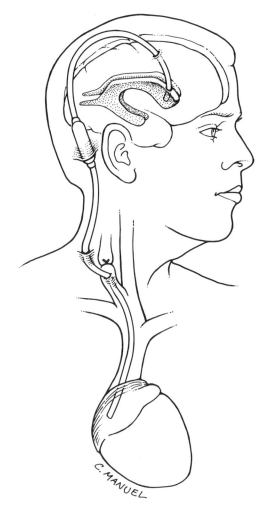

Figure 19–4. Ventriculoatrial shunt.

Altered Fluid Volume and Composition

Following cranial surgery, the patient is at risk for a potential alteration in fluid volume and composition due to disruption of the normal pattern of secretion of antidiuretic hormone (ADH). The normal function of ADH is discussed in chapter 9. Disruption of ADH secretion will be manifested by either the syndrome of inappropriate ADH secretion (SIADH) or diabetes insipidus. SIADH may occur postoperatively as a result of cerebral edema or manipulation of the pituitary gland. Removal of the pituitary gland will result in permanent diabetes insipidus. Transient forms of central diabetes insipidus can also occur. Other conditions that can cause diabetes insipidus include infections, tumors, vascular disease, trauma, or generalized cerebral edema.

SIADH is characterized by enhanced renal tubular reabsorption and re-tention of water due to the excessive and inappropriate secretion of ADH. This results in expansion of the extracellular volume, which is determined clinically by decreased serum osmolality, increased urine osmolality, and hyponatremia. The hyponatremia is the result of dilution of the extracellular fluid and excessive loss of sodium ions in the urine as aldosterone secretion is suppressed because of the increased fluid volume (Goldberger, 1980). Expansion of the intracellular fluid volume will also occur. The nurse should monitor the patient for a reduced volume of highly concentrated urine (with a high specific gravity) and signs and symptoms of water excess and hypona-tremia (see chapter 9). Treatment involves restricting the patient's daily fluid intake.

Central diabetes insipidus is characterized by loss of renal concentrating ability due to insufficient secretion of antidiuretic hormone. Polyuria and polydipsia (if the thirst mechanism is intact) are the presenting signs. The excreted urine will be extremely dilute, with a specific gravity of less than 1.010. A triphasic response typically follows intracranial surgery. Polyuria oc-curs during the first 4 to 5 postoperative days. This is followed by an antidiu-retic phase that lasts for 2 to 6 days. Either permanent central diabetes insipi-dus or normal water metabolism follows the antidiuretic phase (Goldberger, 1980; Groer & Shekleton, 1989). If diabetes insipidus is untreated, or if fluid replacement is inadequate, signs of water deficit may develop (see chapter 9). The polyuria of central diabetes insipidus is vasopressin responsive, which constitutes a basis for treatment (Table 19–5).

Table 19–5 Medications Used in the Treatment of Diabetes Insipidus

Drug	Dosage and Route	Nursing Implications
Aqueous vasopres-sin (Pitres-sin)	5–10 units, subcu-taneously, or 3 units per hour, intravenously	Duration of action is 3 to 6 hours. Used with transient cases of diabetes insipidus.
Vasopressin tannate in oil (Pitres-sin Tan-nate)	5 mg, deep intra-muscular	Prior to aspirating medication into syringe, must mix injectate well or dosage variations will occur. The injectate must be warmed prior to administration. Duration of action is 24 to 36 hours.
Lypressin (Diapid)	1–2 sprays per nostril; 3–4 times per day	If long-term therapy is needed, preferred to painful intramuscular injections. Drug is absorbed via nasal mucosa. If nasal mucosa is irritated, this will interfere with drug ab-sorption.
Desmopres-sin acetate (DDAVP)	0.1–0.4 ml, intra-nasally	Synthetic preparation similar to vasopressin. Slight mucosal irritation or vasoconstriction of nasal mucosa may occur. Duration of action is 12 to 24 hours.

Aside from participating in the prevention and treatment of all these potential postoperative complications, the critical care nurse can have a direct impact on the patient's prognosis and opportunities for rehabilitation. Early identification of normal neurological function and dysfunction is vital. The critical care nurse can encourage the patient to achieve maximal independence (as the patient's neuropathology permits) and work toward preventing additional functional deterioration. In addition to these early efforts at physical rehabilitation, the critical care nurse can have a great impact on the patient's family as well. The nurse can support the family as they learn about the patient's residual deficits and encourage them to ask questions and verbalize their feelings.

Presented in the previous section were the general concerns and possible complications associated with a nonspecific craniotomy. However, the varied intracranial neuropathologic disorders have specific attributes and clinical manifestations. The critical care nurse who is knowledgeable about the neuropathology and disease characteristics can effectively manage these disorders. In the following section, a few of the neurological disorders that necessitate performing a craniotomy will be presented.

Tumors

The majority of intracranial tumors can be classified into three major types: gliomas, metastatic neoplasms, and meningiomas.

Gliomas are tumors of the glial cells (the supportive tissue of the brain) that invade and interweave throughout the neurons and account for about 50% of all intracranial tumors. As in other parts of the body, malignancy occurs as tumor cells invade healthy tissue. While malignancy is a concern, in the tight compartment of the cranium, a space-occupying lesion is immediately life-threatening. The gliomas are described according to their origin, severity, and clinical prognosis in Table 19–6.

Metastatic neoplasms from extracranial sites are responsible for approximately 20% of all intracranial tumors. Primary sites that commonly metastasize to the brain include the lung and breast. Metastatic lesions in brain tissue may present as solitary or numerous widespread lesions, and these lesions may either be invasive or contained. Decisions about surgically excising metastatic lesions must be made carefully. Factors that must be examined closely include the presenting symptomatology, the extent of the primary cancer, the extent of the metastasis, and the impact the procedure may have on the patient's quality of life. Such a decision is a difficult one, as the empirical and clinical data as well as the wishes of the patient and family must be considered. A decision to undergo a major surgical procedure, such as a craniotomy, should be weighed carefully; particularly since most patients survive less than a year after metastasis is identified.

Meningiomas are slow-growing, well-contained tumors that originate from the meningeal layers that cover and protect the brain. Meningiomas are

Table 19-6   Description of Gliomas

Tumor Type	Source	Malignancy	Prognosis
Astrocytoma	Astrocytes in or near cerebrum, brain stem, optic nerve, and cerebellum	Initially benign and slow growing. Prone to malignant changes, becomes rapid growing in Grades III and IV.	Good in Grades I and II. Poor in grades III and IV.
Oligodendroglioma	Cerebral hemispheres. Common in the thalamus of children	Rare in adults. Slow growing. Usually benign; may become malignant.	Good while benign.
Ependymomas	Cells that line the ventricular system, particularly the fourth ventricle	Usually benign, may become malignant. Slow growing.	Poor. Death ensues due to intracranial hypertension (fourth ventricle is difficult to access).
Medulloblastoma	Cerebellum	Rapid Cerebellar Invasion. Spreads through entire central nervous system, often generating distant metastasis. Found in male children.	Very poor due to high level of metastasis.

classified as benign and account for approximately 15 to 16% of all intracranial tumors. Meningiomas are frequently vascular and can grow to a large size. They may erode adjacent bony structures as well as impinge on and compress healthy cerebral structures. The symptoms that are initially reported are focal, related to the anatomical placement of the meningioma or the structures upon which it is impinging. Meningiomas may be surgically resected. Since they are usually highly vascular, however, it is difficult and complicated to excise them completely. Meningiomas that are not completely excised can recur.

Hematomas

There are many causes of intracranial hematomas, however closed head injury is the most prevalent one. Three types of hematoma associated with a closed head injury are epidural, subdural, and intracerebral hematomas (Figure 19–5). Rapidly developing hematomas are a life-threatening emergency

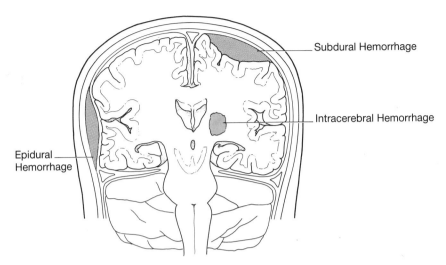

Figure 19–5. Types of traumatic intracranial hemorrhage. From *Clinical Neuroanatomy for Medical Students* by R. S. Snell, 1980, Boston: Little, Brown. Copyright 1980 by Little, Brown. Reprinted by permission.

since the brain's protective mechanisms cannot compensate for a large and rapid increase in volume. Hematomas are space-occupying lesions that frequently must be evacuated on an emergent basis in order to prevent cerebral herniation.

An *epidural hematoma* is a pooling of blood in the potential space between the dura and the inner table of the skull. If the hematoma is associated with a temporal or parietal skull fracture, the middle meningeal artery may be lacerated. Venous blood may also accumulate in the subdural space if one of the large venous sinuses is perforated. Epidural hematomas are sometimes characterized by a short period of unconsciousness followed by a short lucid interval. As the hemorrhage enlarges, the patient will exhibit progressive deterioration of consciousness and mentation. Clinical signs include ipsilateral oculomotor nerve paralysis, contralateral weakness, and the presence of a Babinski reflex. Signs of epidural hemorrhage are usually evident immediately after the cranial trauma and, if treatment is not initiated, herniation will occur within 24 hours. Emergency craniotomy to evacuate the hematoma must be performed as soon as the hematoma is diagnosed.

A *subdural hematoma* is the accumulation of blood between the dural and arachnoid meningeal layers. There are three types of subdural hematomas, which are classified according to their clinical presentation: acute, subacute, and chronic. An acute subdural hematoma presents with acute symptoms within 24 hours of the injury; the patient presents with a marked decrease in level of consciousness, ipsilateral pupil dilatation, and contralateral weakness. Two to 10 days after injury, a subacute subdural hematoma displays progressively worsening signs and symptoms; clinical manifestations include persistent headaches, lethargy, and other signs of depressed level of consciousness accompanied by focal neurological signs. To maintain intracranial integrity, acute and subacute hematomas should be surgically evacuated immediately. Signs or symptoms of a chronic subdural hematoma do not present until at least 10 days after injury. With a chronic subdural hematoma, slow progressive changes in mood, behavior, and affect are common. Additionally, the patient will report a persistent headache, demonstrate a decreased level of consciousness and mentation, report bowel and bladder dysfunction, and exhibit hemiparesis or paralysis. Chronic hematomas should be evacuated if the patient is symptomatic.

Intracerebral hemorrhage is the leakage of blood from a vessel into the parenchyma of the brain. This type of hematoma may develop from trauma or spontaneous hemorrhage (hypertensive). The patient will exhibit focal neurological deficits based on the location of the hematoma. If the hematoma impinges on vital structures or if there is evidence of a midline shift, immediate surgical evacuation is indicated.

In addition to closed head injury, cranial hematomas may develop when the integrity of the scalp and dura is impaired (open head injury). The prognosis for open head injuries is poor. The primary concern is the potential for infection, as the protective barriers of scalp, muscle, skull, and meninges have been penetrated. Crushed and contaminated bone fragments are removed via a craniectomy, and the surgical procedure focuses on debridement and repair. The patient is immediately started on an aggressive antibiotic and anticonvulsant regimen. Because of the direct mechanical damage applied to the cerebral cortex, individuals with intracerebral hematomas are likely to develop posttraumatic epilepsy, and as a result, may need to take anticonvulsant drugs for several years or for an entire lifetime.

The recovery period after suffering an intracranial hematoma can be difficult for the patient and family. The treatment of these patients is challenging and can frequently be frustrating to clinicians and to the patient and family. The patient and family must identify areas of concern and begin to cope with the consequences of the injury. They should receive information about the residual neurological deficits to which they will need to adapt. The deficits may be physical or psychosocial in nature. The family may have difficulty understanding why the patient, whom they have known for many years, is exhibiting highly aberrant behavior. The patient may appear irritable, display inappropriate emotional outbursts, use foul language, or show a sudden disinterest in his or her environment; the deficits demonstrated depend on the site of the injury. In addition, the patient may experience severe physical deficits such as hemiparesis, visual-field deficits, diplopia, anosmia, hearing loss, and problems with language. The critical care nurse repeatedly must reassure the family that these alterations in personality and residual deficits are characteristic responses to head trauma.

Individuals who have suffered minor head trauma, such as a slight blow to the head, may also have a difficult recovery process. One of the distressing problems that is associated with a minor head injury is the presence of *posttraumatic syndrome*. These patients report dizziness, headache, visual changes, and poor memory. Family members and friends will report changes in the patient's personality and a poor attention span. These symptoms can impose a severely negative impact on the patient's lifestyle and relationships with family and friends. The symptoms associated with posttraumatic syndrome may last from a few weeks to over a year.

Vascular Anomalies

Aneurysms are thin-walled weakened areas on an arterial vessel. Aneurysms are most common in the anterior circulation of the brain and tend to occur in multiple sites at vessel branches and bifurcations. When the vessel ruptures, the arterial blood rushes into the subarachnoid space, resulting in a subarachnoid hemorrhage. The aneurysm may rupture spontaneously, releasing a large amount of blood, or it may leak slowly over a period of time prior to its rupture.

To prevent further bleeding or rebleeding, the patient must be placed under aneurysm precautions. Aneurysm precautions decrease the likelihood of hypertension and increased intracranial pressure. The patient is placed in a cool, quiet, and dark private room. A totally quiet environment must be created, without a television or telephone. If the patient desires to listen to music, it must be calm and soothing.

The patient's chances for a good prognosis depend on the site and severity of the hemorrhage. Since the resulting subarachnoid hemorrhage is a mass lesion, these patients are at risk for developing intracranial hypertension and a herniation syndrome. The risk for developing such complications must be minimized. The patient is kept normotensive or slightly hypertensive if cerebral vasospasms develop, and is stabilized over a 7- to 10-day period. Antifibrinolytic agents such as epsilon aminocaproic acid (Amicar) may be administered prophylactically. It is thought that this drug will delay the normal lysis of the aneurysmal clot.

Once stabilized, the patient with slight alterations of consciousness, slight headache, slight nuchal rigidity, and no evidence of vasospasm is thought to be a good surgical candidate (Jennett & Galbraith, 1983). Aneurysms are isolated from the parent vessel by clamping the base of the aneurysm or by reinforcing the aneurysm by coating it with surgical epoxy. Aneurysms may also be treated by embolization of the affected vessel with silastic spheres.

Arteriovenous malformations (AVMs), or congenital vascular malformations, can occur throughout the central nervous system. An AVM is characterized by dilated and tortuous veins and arteries, which extend in a wedge-shaped pattern into the brain tissue. Because of the rapid, excessive high-pressured shunting of blood flow through the AVM, there are ischemic and necrotic areas on the surface of the adjacent cortex. Hemorrhage or leaking usually results from the more fragile venous vessels in the malformation.

The signs and symptoms that the patient experiences depend on the location and extent of the lesion. One of the first clinical signs the patient experiences is a focal seizure. The preoperative care of the patient with an AVM is similar to that of a patient experiencing an aneurysm. The surgical approach is to attempt to completely excise the AVM, clip the vessels feeding into it, or embolize the arterial vessels with silastic spheres.

TRANSSPHENOIDAL SURGERY

Historically, the pituitary gland has been accessed via an intracranial approach. However, the advent of surgical microscopes and microsurgical techniques has allowed the development of transsphenoidal surgery. The transsphenoidal approach is highly beneficial since the surgery has minimal risks and is reported to have a mortality rate of less than 0.5% (Randall, Laws, & Abboud, 1983). Transsphenoidal surgery is used to remove tumors of the sellar and parasellar regions. The sella turcica is a depression in the sphenoid bone in which the pituitary gland resides. Pituitary tumors are slow-growing and usually encapsulated and are most prevalent in childhood through middle age. The prognosis after pituitary surgery is good, and if the entire tumor cannot be resected the patient may be treated with radiation.

Pituitary gland removal has also been used to control metastatic bone pain and further metastasis that is associated with primary breast or prostate cancer. The mechanism by which this occurs is not clear but it is postulated that the lack of postoperative prolactin and growth-stimulating hormone secretion may be a factor.

Preoperative Care

Knowledge Deficit

The patient and family must understand that after removal of the entire pituitary (total hypophysectomy), a lifelong hormonal replacement therapy program must be followed. Teaching about medication will continue after surgery, but it should be initiated during the preoperative phase (Bell, 1972).

The patient will require long-term posterior pituitary hormone replacement. Such therapy related to ADH is discussed in detail in an earlier section of this chapter dealing with diabetes insipidus and the syndrome of inappropriate ADH secretion. Another hormone from the anterior pituitary lobe that will need to be replaced is adrenocorticotropic hormone (ACTH). The secretion of ACTH by the anterior lobe of the pituitary promotes the secretion of certain hormones by the adrenal cortex, including the glucocorticoids, mineralocorticoids, and sex hormones. The adrenal cortex may either be stimulated by ACTH replacement or the actual glucocorticoids such as cortisol can be replaced directly. Stimulation of the adrenal cortex or the replacement of glucocorticoids is vital, since adrenal insufficiency constitutes a life-threatening emergency.

Intraoperative Care

The patient is positioned in a semi-sitting position with the head secured in a head rest and rotated slightly toward the surgeon. Since a muscle or fat graft is obtained for closure, the anterior or lateral thigh must be exposed for easy access. The nasal cavity is accessed through an incision in the upper gums, the nasal septum is resected and a speculum is inserted. The floor of the sphenoid sinus is resected. The sella floor is removed and the dura mater is incised using a cruciate incision. Once the dural flaps are opened, the gland is resected or the tumor is squeezed from the gland and removed by aspiration. The muscle/fat graft is placed into the sella. The bones that were moved are rotated back into place. The gingival incision is closed. Lubricated dressings are packed into the nasal cavity, nasal drains may be inserted, and a mustache dressing is placed under the nose.

Throughout the surgery, the nurse must monitor for possible leaks of cerebrospinal fluid from the operative site. Any clear fluid that is present should be tested for the presence of glucose. If the presence of clear fluid is noted, and this fluid is mixed with blood, testing for the presence of glucose would be invalid, since both blood and CSF have high levels of glucose. Under such circumstances, an appropriate observation for the presence of CSF is the "halo sign." The presence of drainage noted to be in a circular pattern, with a yellowish ring surrounding the bloody drainage is considered highly suggestive of a CSF leak. Excessive leakage may require repacking of dressings in the operating room. Any suspicion of a CSF leak should be reported, as the patient is at risk for developing meningitis.

Postoperative Care

Sensory–Perceptual Alterations

Continual evaluation is vital during the postoperative phase. Because of surgical disruption of the nasal mucosa and the floor of the sphenoid sinus, the patient's sense of smell will probably be absent. The ability to smell and taste (since the sense of smell enhances the sense of taste) will return over a period of a few months.

Because of postoperative edema or surgical trauma the patient may experience visual-field deficits. Visual-field deficits are a potential complication in transsphenoidal surgery because of the close proximity of the optic nerves and the optic chiasm to the pituitary. As soon as the patient is alert, the nurse must obtain a base-line postoperative assessment of the patient's visual fields and compare the results to those obtained during preoperative assessment. Visual-field assessment must be performed as part of the standard ongoing evaluation of a patient who has undergone a hypophysectomy.

Altered Cerebral Tissue Perfusion

Because of the high vascularity of the surgical site, precautions must be taken to prevent hemorrhage. The patient should remain in a high Fowler's position at all times, even during sleep. Drainage from the nasal packing and mustache dressing should be carefully monitored. The nasal packing should not be manipulated, and excessive drainage (clear or sanguinous) should be reported immediately. The mustache dressing can be replaced as needed. Blowing of the nose or nasopharyngeal suctioning is contraindicated. Frequent mouth rinses and gentle mouth care can be done, but brushing of teeth should not be permitted.

Alteration in Fluid Volume and Composition

Complications such as transient diabetes insipidus or SIADH may occur postoperatively. If the entire pituitary gland has been removed, permanent diabetes insipidus will occur. In addition to these posterior pituitary complications, adrenal insufficiency may occur because of insufficient amounts of ACTH or glucocorticoid replacement (cortisol). Symptoms of acute adrenal insufficiency include orthostatic hypotension, weakness, and dizziness. If untreated, these symptoms can lead to circulatory collapse and death.

SPINAL SURGERY

Spinal surgery can be used to decompress or excise pathologic lesions and correct abnormalities of the vertebral column, meninges, and spinal cord. Some of the pathologic conditions that would require access to the spine include tumors, spinal column instability, and congenital anomalies. The major clinical concerns about spinal surgery contrast with those of cranial surgery. In cranial surgery, clinicians are concerned about the residual effects on a patient's functional status and, with a rapidly expanding space-occupying lesion, the prime concern is with the preservation of life. In spinal surgery, achieving physiologic stability is important; however, the major focus is to preserve existing function or prevent further deterioration of function. Spinal surgery may be indicated in the following pathologic states: disk disease, spondylosis, fractures/dislocations, tumors, syringomyelia, AVMs, aneurysms, hematomas, trauma, intractable pain, and congenital spinal anomalies. In the following section, the management of the preoperative, intraoperative, and postoperative phases of spinal surgery will be discussed. In-depth information about spinal trauma is presented in chapter 21.

Preoperative Care

In order to establish a base-line assessment of the patient's functional status, the critical care nurse must perform and analyze a comprehensive neurological exam. Although all components of the examination are essential, the clinician must focus on the implications of the spinal involvement. Using a specific framework such as that presented in chapter 13 (Mitchell, Cammermeyer, Ozuna, & Woods, 1984) will enable the clinician to develop a comprehensive spinal assessment that should focus on the body functions related to sensation, movement, and integrated regulation. Clinical evaluation should be done on a regularly scheduled basis as well as when sudden neurological changes are noted.

Knowledge Deficit

The patient and family need to be informed about the surgery, any possible complications, and the expected residual deficits, if any. For example, an individual with a herniated vertebral disk may expect no major complications from surgery; however, complete alleviation of back pain cannot be guaranteed. Likewise, a patient with a complete spinal cord transection must be informed that the purposes of surgery are to stabilize the spine and prevent further neurologic damage and not to restore the premorbid mobility status.

In addition to these long-term considerations, the patient and family need to know what to expect postoperatively. It is important to tell them about the postoperative environment and what routines to expect in the critical care setting. Helping them to understand the importance of frequent neurological checks may help to allay some of their concerns. If they receive verbal information and demonstrations about equipment such as dressings, braces, casts, tongs, and special beds, the patient and family may be less traumatized in the initial postoperative phase. Therapeutic restrictions on the patient's mobility may be a significant psychological stressor. This stress may be alleviated by teaching the patient preoperatively about mobility restrictions and how to participate in activities such as log rolling (turning a patient side-to-side while maintaining the patient in a straight plane—no twisting or bending). Pathology-specific preoperative teaching can have an impact on the patient and family's postoperative status and potential for rehabilitation.

Intraoperative Care

The basic principles of appropriate body alignment must be maintained throughout the surgery. Proper alignment and/or skeletal traction must be considered during transfers as well as during the surgery. Patients must be positioned appropriately to facilitate access via the anterior, posterior, and lateral approaches. Regardless of the position desired by the neurosurgeon, the patient should be positioned so that pressure within the abdomen and thorax is minimal. Ensuring that there is no compression or pressure on the chest or abdomen will decrease the engorgement of epidural veins and will therefore minimize meningeal bleeding.

Once the body is positioned, the patient's head is immobilized in a headrest. Anesthesia can be given by general, spinal, and/or local methods. Ventilatory intubation must be done with caution; the nasotracheal approach is preferred, as this will decrease flexion and extension of the neck.

Different spinal pathology will call for different highly specific surgical techniques; however, the basic opening and closing components are similar. The desired incision site is usually marked prior to draping the patient. The incision is made, hemostasis is achieved, the fascia is opened, and the muscles are dissected away from the surgical site. The required procedure is performed and the order of this process is reversed for surgical closure. At this time, any drains that have been inserted must be sutured in place.

Intraoperative assessment of spinal functioning is now commonly done using somatosensory evoked responses. Peripheral nerves, usually of the leg, are electrically stimulated and the response is visualized through the somatosensory pathways to the primary somatosensory cortex of the parietal lobe.

Although the assessment done in the operating room is sophisticated and complex, the nurse must coordinate a smooth and timely transfer to the recovery room or intensive care unit. If special equipment or a special bed will be needed postoperatively, it would be optimal for the patient to leave the surgical suite with such equipment. In order to assess alignment, spine films are routinely taken as soon as possible after the patient leaves the surgical suite.

Postoperative Care

During the postoperative phase, patients who have experienced spinal surgery are at risk for developing CSF leaks, infections, and hematomas. To allow for maximal visualization, the incision should be covered with a small dressing. The site should be observed for leaking cerebrospinal fluid or for areas of swelling that may indicate hemorrhage.

Sensory–Perceptual Alterations and Impaired Physical Mobility

As a result of surgery, additional sensory and motor losses may develop. These may be transient or permanent in nature. Transient losses may be due to postoperative edema, while permanent losses may be due to nerve damage. The critical care nurse must regularly assess both the sensory and mobility status. Sudden losses in mobility may indicate that emergency surgical intervention is required. Permanent losses must be discussed with the patient, and information given by the neurosurgeon should be reinforced.

Altered Tissue Perfusion

In addition to motor losses, a patient with spinal pathology may experience loss of vasomotor tone below the level of the lesion. The limbs should be examined for the presence of edema, moisture, coolness, and pallor. Extremities need to be elevated to decrease venous pooling, and additional clothing or covers may be applied.

Pain

Patients may experience incisional pain; however, narcotic analgesics are contraindicated if the patient has sustained head trauma. Under such circumstances, nonnarcotic analgesics should be administered. Patients who have undergone spinal fusions with a bone graft frequently report more pain from the graft site than from the spinal incision. It is important to evaluate this additional source of discomfort.

Altered Elimination Patterns

After spinal surgery, it is important to evaluate the patient's elimination status. Alterations in bowel and bladder elimination frequently occur in conjunction with spinal pathology, particularly that at the sacral level. A bladder disturbance due to a lesion in the nervous system is termed a *neurogenic bladder*. A pathologic lesion that leads to neurogenic bladder may be found in either the brain or the spinal cord. There are three types of neurogenic bladder: upper motor neuron, lower motor neuron, and mixed motor neuron. These varied types of neurogenic bladder dysfunction and the pathology involved are summarized in Table 19–7. In addition, problems with bowel elimination are also a common occurrence with spinal pathology. Both types of elimination problems (bowel and bladder) can be effectively managed, and the critical care nurse is in a position to identify such problems. These problems should be expected with spinal pathology, but may occur with any nervous system involvement. Bladder and bowel retraining programs should be started as soon as the patient is physiologically stable and alert enough to cooperate. Because of the complexity of neurogenic bowel and bladder dysfunction, the critical care nurse should consult a rehabilitation or neuroscience clinical nursing specialist in order to plan and evaluate a retraining program.

SUMMARY

Neurological problems often require swift and aggressive treatment. Presented in this chapter is information on the nursing care of a patient undergoing a neurological procedure. The surgical critical care nurse can have a

Table 19–7 Neurogenic Bladder Dysfunction

Name	Other Names Used	Sacral Reflex (S = 2, S = 3, S = 4)
Upper motor neuron bladder	Spastic, reflex, automatic, and central	Preserved: sensory and motor pathways to the sacral reflex are intact
Lower motor neuron disease	Atonic, flaccid, autonomous, peripheral, areflexic	Damaged: sensory input from the full bladder does not trigger the sacral reflex
Mixed motor neuron bladder	Any or all of the above	Diminished

Control of Higher Cortical Centers	Conditions Seen	Description
Loss of inhibitory influence	Spinal cord injury; cord lesions above the sacral reflex; can occur after spinal shock has resolved	Since the reflex arc is intact, the bladder empties, but without voluntary control.
		If spasticity is severe, the slightest stimulus such as straining, coughing, or a small amount of urine (15 to 25 ml) in the bladder can stimulate emptying of the bladder.
		If spasticity is minimal to moderate, the patient is instructed in recognizing signs associated with bladder fullness; he or she may then evacuate it by stimulating the sacral reflex— pressing on bladder (Credé method; stroking thigh).
Loss of sensation to cortical level	Spinal shock Sacral cord injury	Patient is unaware of bladder fullness and need to void. Bladder overdistends. Overflow incontinence, especially during coughing or transfer, often occurs.
		Autonomic hyperreflexia may be stimulated in a patient with high cord injury.
		Bladder is managed initially with an indwelling catheter, then intermittent catheterization.
		Bladder retraining is begun later.
Diminished	Stroke Brain tumor Multiple sclerosis Head injury	Patient often has urgency to void but is unable to control the urgency. Condition is associated with frontal lobe lesion or unconsciousness.
		Until patient is able and willing to cooperate, continence will not be achieved.
		Patient is good candidate for continence because perception of fullness and control are diminished, not lost.

From *The Clinical Practice of Neurological and Neurosurgical Nursing* (p. 198), by J. V. Hickey, 1986, Philadelphia: J. B. Lippincott. Copyright 1986 by J. B. Lippincott. Reprinted by permission.

significant impact on the patient's recovery during both the acute and rehabilitative phases of treatment. The provision of nursing care should be based on complete and accurate understanding of the principles underlying that care and the effect of treatment on the involved neurophysiology.

BIBLIOGRAPHY

Bell, M. (1972). Preoperative teaching and postoperative care of the hypophysectomy patient. *Journal of Neurosurgical Nursing, 4,* 165–170.

Cunha, B. A., & Tu, R. P. (1988). Fever in the neurosurgical patient. *Heart and Lung, 17*(6), Part 1, 608–611.

Goldberger, E. (1980). *A primer of water, electrolyte and acid–base syndromes* (6th ed.). Philadelphia: Lea & Febiger.

Groer, M. E., & Shekleton, M. (1989). *Basic pathophysiology: A holistic approach* (3rd ed.). St. Louis: C. V. Mosby.

Jennett, B., & Galbraith, S. (1983). *An introduction to neurosurgery.* Chicago: Year Book.

Langfitt, T. W. (1968). Increased intracranial pressure. *Clinical Neurosurgery, 16,* 436.

Lundberg, N. (1960). Continuous recording and control of ventricular fluid pressure in neurosurgical practice. *Acta Psychiatrica Et Neurologica Scandinavica, 149,* 1–193.

Mitchell, P. H., Cammermeyer, M., Ozuna, J., & Woods, N. (1984). *Neurological assessment for nursing practice.* Reston, VA: Reston Publishing.

Randall, R. V., Laws, E. R., & Abboud, C. F. (1983). Transsphenoidal microsurgical treatment of prolactin-producing adenomas: Results in 100 patients. *Mayo Clinic Proceedings, 58,* 108.

Rudy, E. (1984). *Advanced neurological and neurosurgical nursing.* St. Louis: C. V. Mosby.

Vires, J., Becker, D., & Young, H. (1973). A subarachnoid screw for monitoring intracranial pressure. *Journal of Neurosurgery, 39,* 416–419.

ADDITIONAL READINGS

American Association of Neuroscience Nurses (1980). *Core Curriculum for Neurosurgical Nursing in the Operating Room.* Chicago: American Association of Neurosurgical Nurses.

American Association of Neuroscience Nurses (1984). *Core Curriculum for Neuroscience Nursing.* Chicago: American Association of Neuroscience Nurses.

Anderson, B. (1979). Antidiuretic hormone: Balance and imbalance. *Journal of Neurosurgical Nursing, 11,* 71–73.

Chusid, J. G. (1982). *Correlative neuroanatomy and functional neurology.* Los Altos, CA: Lange Medical.

Conway-Rutkowski, B. L. (1982). *Carini and Owens' neurological and neurosurgical nursing.* St. Louis: C. V. Mosby.

Gruppi, L. A. (1987). Acoustic neuromas: Nursing management during the acute postoperative period. *Critical Care Nurse, 7,* 16–24.

Hardy, J. (1979). The transsphenoidal surgical approach to resection of pituitary tumors. *Hospital Practice, 6,* 81–89.

Hickey, J. V. (1986). *The clinical practice of neurological and neurosurgical nursing.* Philadelphia: J. B. Lippincott.

Isaacs, N. M. (1979). Intraspinal tumors: Meeting your patient's surgical needs. In J. Robinson (Ed.), *Coping with neurologic problems efficiently.* (pp. 139–148). Horsham, PA: Intermed Communications.

Krajewski, B. (1979). Head injury: Preventing life threatening complications. In J. Robinson (Ed.), *Coping with neurologic problems efficiently.* (pp. 85–98). Horsham, PA: Intermed Communications.

Langfitt, T. W. (1975). Pathophysiology of increased intracranial pressure. In M. Brock & H. Dietz (Eds.), *Intracranial pressure I.* New York: Springer-Verlag.

Mauss, N. K., & Mitchell, P. H. (1976). Increased intracranial pressure: an update. *Heart and Lung, 5,* 919–926.

Mayberry, C. L. (1979). Intracranial tumors: Giving expert pre- and postop care. In J. Robinson (Ed.), *Coping with neurologic problems proficiently.* Horsham, PA: Intermed Communications.

Miller, J. (1975). Volume and pressure in the craniospinal axis. *Clinical Neurosurgery, 22,* 76–105.

Mitchell, P. H. (1982). Neurological disorders. In M. R. Kinney, C. B. Dean, D. R. Packa, & D. M. Voorman (Eds.), *AACN's clinical reference for critical care nursing.* New York: McGraw-Hill.

Mitchell, P. H., & Mauss, N. K. (1978). Relationship of patient-nurse activity to intracranial pressure variations: A pilot study. *Nursing Research, 27,* 4–10.

Nikas, D. L. (1987). Prognostic indicators in patients with severe head injury. *Critical Care Nursing Quarterly, 10,* 25–34.

Nikas, D. L., & Konkoly, R. (1975). Nursing responsibilities in arterial and intracranial pressure monitoring. *Journal of Neurosurgical Nursing, 7,* 116–122.

Pallet, P. J., & O'Brien, M. T. (1985). *Textbook of neurological nursing.* Boston: Little, Brown.

Plum, F., & Posner, J. (1982). *The diagnosis of stupor and coma* (3rd ed.). Philadelphia: F. A. Davis.

Ropper, A., Kennedy, S., & Zervas, N. (1983). *Neurological and neurosurgical intensive care.* Baltimore: University Park Press.

Shalit, M. N., & Umansky, R. (1977). Effect of bedside procedures on intracranial pressure. *Israeli Journal of Medical Sciences, 13,* 881–886.

Shapiro, H. (1975). Intracranial hypertension: Therapeutic and anesthetic considerations. *Anesthesiology, 43,* 445–469.

Snyder, M. (1983). *A guide to neurological and neurosurgical nursing.* New York: John Wiley.

Snyder, M., & Jackle, M. (1981). *Neurologic problems: A critical care nursing focus.* Bowie, MD: Robert Brady.

Tindal, G., & Mauldin, B. (1981). Transsphenoidal hypophysectomy. *AORN Journal, 33,* 246.

Walleck, C. (1987). Intracranial hypertension: Interventions and outcomes. *Critical Care Nursing Quarterly, 10,* 45–57.

20 Transplantation

Linda Haggerty, M.S., R.N., C.C.T.C.

Organ and tissue transplantation has been advancing rapidly, and continues to do so, from the experimental to the therapeutic realm in the treatment of many forms of disease. Renal transplantation is an established therapeutic option for the treatment of end-stage renal failure. Liver and heart transplantation similarly offer great chance for life in the face of terminal organ failure. Pancreas, lung, and heart–lung transplants are being performed with increasing success. Bone and corneal tissue transplants are also established and offer viable therapeutic options for certain diseases. The potential for rehabilitation with all organ and tissue transplants is great, and remains a major goal of transplantation. Transplantation is an alternative to which many patients look with optimism.

The focus of this chapter is the clinical application of renal, liver, and heart transplantation. Emphasis will be placed on the immunology of transplantation, the transplant process, potential complications, and associated nursing care.

IMMUNOLOGY OF TRANSPLANTATION

Immunology has a vital, complex role in the transplant process. Studies of the function and modulation of the immune system, to prevent rejection and minimize the risk of infection, remain a major focus of transplantation research. Advances in understanding the role of cellular and humoral immunity, the application of the human leukocyte antigen system, mechanisms of immune regulation, and immune tolerance contribute to transplant success. Judicious control of chemical immunosuppression helps decrease the potential for infectious complications.

The Immune System

Specific immunologic responses in the transplant recipient can be categorized into cellular and humoral immune functions. Both the cellular (T-lymphocyte) and humoral (B-lymphocyte) systems are involved in the rejection process as well as in the body's natural fight against foreign invaders including bacterial, viral, and fungal organisms.

Cellular Immunity

In response to a certain foreign antigen, host T-lymphocytes proliferate. In transplantation, foreign antigen is presented on the donor organ. The proliferating T cells cause organ damage via two processes. They increase cytotoxicity, causing damage to graft cells via activity of the killer cells (cytotoxic T cells). T-lymphocytes also stimulate the release of lymphokines, which in turn activate a strong nonspecific inflammatory response causing graft damage (Solinger, 1985). Both effects, especially in combination, can initiate a rejection response.

Humoral Immunity

Also in response to a foreign antigen, B-lymphocytes will stimulate production of an antibody or antibodies against specific antigen(s). Antibodies themselves do not destroy the foreign antigen, but mark it for destruction by other parts of the immune system (Tonegawa, 1985). One such activity is formation of complement proteins that penetrate and destroy cells. They also combine with antigen–antibody complexes, which attract macrophages. It is the function of macrophages to engulf and destroy cells. The end result is cellular destruction of the graft.

Human Leukocyte Antigen (HLA) System

The recipient's ability to accept or reject a transplanted graft depends on the cellular and humoral responses to the antigens present on the donor organ. The human leukocyte antigens are the major targets of the transplant rejection reaction. These antigens are located on the sixth chromosome in an area termed the major histocompatibility complex (MHC). The MHC is divided into several loci. The loci involved in the transplant response are termed A, B, C, D (Class I antigens), and DR (Class II antigens). Greatest attention is paid to the A, B, and DR loci. The associated inherited antigens on each loci determine an individual's "tissue typing."

Each sixth chromosome contains one set of the A, B, and DR antigens, i.e., one haplotype. One haplotype is inherited maternally, one is inherited paternally, resulting in two of each A, B, and DR antigen per individual. There are a limited number of HLA antigens thus far defined; through worldwide histocompatibility organizations, the nomenclature for the HLA antigens has been standardized. Antigens are named by the letter of the loci in which they are located (A, B, etc.) and then further defined by numeric designations within that loci. Despite the limited number of identified antigens, it is apparent that there are many possible combinations. For this reason, cadaver donors have the potential of sharing antigen(s) with a potential recipient, but close matching is difficult on a random basis.

The importance of HLA matching for renal transplants is well appreciated in principle. When histocompatibility is maximized, the transplanted kidney is better accepted by the recipient's immune system. In fact, the overall differences in graft survival at 1 year are reported to be 10 to 15% between the best and poorest matches (Cecka, 1986). The effect of HLA matching is clearly demonstrated in transplants from living, related donors. HLA matching in transplants from cadaver donors, especially since the introduction of cyclosporin, remains controversial. Many centers choose not to wait for an HLA-matched cadaver kidney, citing satisfactory results independent of the degree of matching. Others report increased success in recipients who were not mismatched (Cecka, 1986; Sanfilippo, Vaughn, & Lefor, 1986). While the success rates of poorly matched recipients has increased since the use of cyclosporin, greater benefit has been reported with cyclosporin administration in combination with HLA matching (Sanfilippo et al., 1986). Additional

Table 20–1 Immunosuppressive Medications

Drug	Administration	Dosage
Azathioprine (Imuran)—antimetabolite; inhibits lymphoid differentiation	Generally oral; may be given intravenously	Preoperative: 2–5 mg/kg × 1–2 doses
		Intraoperative: —
		Postoperative: 2–5 mg/kg/day; dose adjustments if signs of toxicity develop
		Maintenance: 1.5–2.5 mg/kg/day
		During rejection: increased doses not recommended
Cyclophosphamide (Cytoxan)—alkalating agent; effective against lymphocytes	Oral; dose is one-half the azathioprine dose	Doses are given at one-half the azathioprine dose; dose adjustments if signs of toxicity develop
		During rejection: increased doses not recommended

data are needed regarding the long-term effects of matching, especially in comparison with other advances in transplant immunology, to determine which factors contribute the most to long-term graft success.

HLA matching is not required for liver or heart transplantation. No perceived benefit of matching has been clearly demonstrated in those populations. Additional data are needed to determine what effect, if any, matching may have.

Immunosuppression

Unless a transplant is performed between genetically identical twins, immunosuppressive therapy is necessary, or graft rejection is inevitable. The goals of immunosuppression are to prevent graft rejection while minimizing potential side effects, including infection. Current immunosuppressive regimens are safer now than in the past, due in part to more judicious use of immunosuppressive agents as well as to the development of agents more specifically targeted to the areas of the immune system involved in rejection. Patient education regarding rationale for administration, prevention of complications, and appearance of possible side effects is a vital part of immunosuppressive therapy.

Immunosuppression is attempted via a variety of pharmacologic agents administered at various doses with each organ transplant (Table 20–1). His-

Toxicity–Side effects	*Nursing Implications*
Decreased white-cell count (WBC) because of bone marrow depression	Monitor daily WBC; discontinue Azathioprine if WBC less than 2000/mm until normal WBC reestablished
Hepatotoxicity	Monitor liver function tests; substitute cyclophosphamide as ordered
Alopecia	Generally temporary
Decreased resistance to infection	Not generally used if cyclosporine is primary immunosuppressant
Bone marrow depression with decreased WBC	As above; incidence less than with azathioprine
Hemorrhagic cystitis	Often a substitute for patients unable to tolerate azathioprine
	Give medication in A.M.
	Adequate fluid intake

Table 20–1   *(Continued)*

Drug	Administration	Dosage
Prednisone— corticosteroid; inhibits synthesis of lymphocytes and depletes T-cell population; B-cell activity; antiinflammatory	Oral; intravenous equivalent is Solu-Medrol at 4/5 the oral prednisone dose	Preoperative: — Intraoperative: 500–1000 mg Solu-Medrol Postoperative: 2–3 mg/kg with taper to 0.5 mg/kg/day over several weeks Maintenance: 0.25 mg/kg/day with taper to 0.1–0.2 mg/kg/day over several months During rejection: 2–5 mg/kg/day with repeat taper, oral; three 500–1000 mg boluses of Solu-Medrol ("pulse" therapy)

Toxicity–Side effects	Nursing Implications
[Most side effects are dose-related.]	
Cushing's syndrome characterized by a round "moon face," truncal obesity, and a "buffalo hump"	Provide patient support and allow verbalization of feelings regarding body image; instruct patients to avoid excessive carbohydrates and weight gain as both may enhance a Cushing appearance
Salt and water retention	Avoid added salt in the diet; instruct patients that this may add to hypertension; teach patients to monitor own blood pressure; assess for edema.
Weight gain: secondary to salt and water retention and increased subjective feelings of hunger	Avoid salt, as described above; subjective feelings of hunger may remain unsatisfied; patients must be encouraged to eat a balanced diet without the excess caloric intake they may desire; instruct patients that obesity may contribute to hypertension, glucose intolerance, and stress on joints; instruct patients that obesity is easier to prevent than to treat.
Delayed wound healing	Incisional sutures are left in place for 10 to 14 days; injuries may take longer to heal, careful cleaning and assessment for infection is required.
Avascular necrosis; particularly of weight-bearing joints	Avoid obesity; avoid high-impact exercise; report symptoms of joint pain to health care team
Cataracts	Instruct patients to see an ophthalmologist every 6 to 12 months, or if visual changes occur; may require surgical removal
Steroid-induced diabetes	Avoid obesity; monitor for signs and symptoms of elevated blood sugar (polydipsia, polyphagia, polyuria); provide diabetic teaching as indicated; may require insulin therapy or oral hypoglycemic agents
Peptic ulcer formation; secondary to decreased synthesis of protective mucus by the gastric mucosa	Instruct patients on rationale for antacid prophylaxis, with or without such H_2 antagonists as ranitidine (Zantac); such prophylaxis is essential while prednisone dose is high,

Table 20–1   (Continued)

Drug	Administration	Dosage
Antilymphocyte globulin—depletes circulating T lymphocytes; used to treat rejection episodes; may be used as prophylaxis against rejection	Intravenous only; preferred route is through a central venous line, infused 4–6 hours, mix only with D$_5$W to avoid precipitation	Preoperative: — Intraoperative: — Postoperative: 10–20 mg/kg/day; dose adjustments if signs of toxicity or infection develop; may be given for up to 14 days
Cyclosporin—fungal metabolite; inhibits cytotoxic T cells; activates suppressor T cells; induces tolerance to alloantigens	Oral, mixed with juice, milk, etc. Intravenous at $\frac{1}{3}$ the oral dose. Infusion rates vary from 1 to 24 hr; may cause flushing, digital tingling, nausea	Preoperative: 10–15 mg/kg/day 1 day before surgery Intraoperative: — Postoperative: 5–15 mg/kg/day in divided doses with gradual taper; may be held if acute tubular necrosis or renal dysfunction exists Maintenance: varies depending on patient tolerance; Progressively lower doses required, probably because of tissue saturation

Toxicity–Side effects	Nursing Implications
	and required for extended periods of time if patient has an ulcer history and/or signs of gastritis or ulcer formation
Acne	Treat with thorough skin cleansing and benzoyl peroxide preparations
Muscle weakness	Strengthening exercises such as walking, swimming, stair climbing; avoid high-impact exercises
Mood swings	Provide support and education to patient and family; allow verbalization of feelings
Fever, chills, rash, pruritus	May require preinfusion administration of acetaminophen and diphenhydramine hydrochloride (Benadryl); obtain frequent vital signs
Thrombocytopenia	Monitor daily platelet count; dose adjustments may be required
Allergic reactions (anaphylaxis, arthralgias, myalgias)	Discontinue dose immediately; keep epinephrine and Benadryl at the bedside throughout administration.
Nephrotoxicity	Monitor daily serum electrolytes, BUN, and creatinine; monitor for signs of renal dysfunction, altered fluid volume status
Hypertension	Teach patients to monitor own blood pressure; monitor for signs of hypertension; administer antihypertensives as ordered
Hirsutism	Support patients and allow verbalization of feelings about body image
Fine hand tremors	Monitor for tremors, e.g., via changes in handwriting; may require decreased dose
Seizures	Monitor level of consciousness; monitor for drug interactions if anticonvulsants are given
Gum hyperplasia	Instruct patients on need for thorough dental hygiene

Table 20–1 *(Continued)*

Drug	Administration	Dosage
		During rejection: increased doses generally not given; may require dose reduction until BUN and creatinine return to acceptable levels
Monoclonal antibodies (OKT 3)—blocks function of T cells; blocks cell-mediated toxicity; reverses acute rejection	Intravenous Within 24 hours before first dose: 1. Chest film 2. Cannot be over usual dry weight without further evaluation	Preoperative: — Intraoperative: — Postoperative: experimental protocol

D₅W = 5% dextrose in water; BUN = blood urea nitrogen.

torically, azathioprine (Imuran) and prednisone were the stalwarts of immunosuppression, commonly termed "conventional therapy." Later, antilymphocyte globulin (ALG) was added, either as rejection prophylaxis or treatment. Cyclosporin has had a significant influence on transplantation, with its ability to inhibit T lymphocytes specifically and to improve transplant results greatly. Monoclonal antibodies are the most recent addition to therapy, being used most often to treat rejection episodes. Research continues also with other agents.

Complications of Immunosuppression

Potential for Infection

A variety of bacterial, fungal, viral, and protozoal organisms can be implicated in posttransplant infections. High doses of immunosuppressants, leukopenia, hyperglycemia, and preexisting uremia are predisposing factors to posttransplant infection (Anderson, Schafer, Olin, & Eickhoff, 1973). Many infections are short-lived and relatively benign, but life-threatening infectious episodes do occur. Careful prevention, diligent monitoring, rapid diagnosis and treatment, and patient education are required to decrease the incidence, morbidity, and mortality of infectious episodes. Figure 20–1 shows when various forms of infection are most likely to occur during the posttransplant course of the renal recipient. A similar picture is seen with other organ transplants. In the first month after a transplant, wound, pulmonary, and intravenous infections are the most frequently seen. The period from 1 to 6 months after

Toxicity–Side effects	Nursing Implications
Hepatotoxicity	Because of metabolism by the liver, monitor liver function tests; dose reduction may be required
Allergic reactions	Risk of anaphylaxis—often requires first dose to be given in a monitored setting
Shivering	Epinephrine and airway equipment at bedside
Fever, diarrhea, and *severe* flu-like symptoms (with first and second doses)	Frequently pretreated with diphenhydramine and aspirin
	Treat symptoms

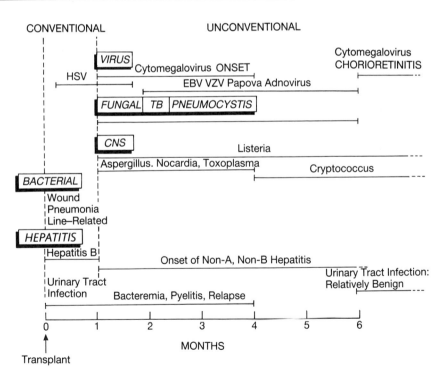

Figure 20–1. Timetable for the occurrence of infection in the renal transplant patient. HSV = herpes simplex virus; EBV = Epstein–Barr virus; VZV = varicella–zoster virus; TB = tuberculosis; CNS = central nervous system. From "Infection in the Renal Transplant Patient" by R. H. Rubin et al., 1981, *American Journal of Medicine, 70*, pp. 401–411. Reprinted with permission.

transplant is described as the critical risk period for life-threatening infections (Rubin, Wolfson, Cosimi, & Tolkoff-Rubin, 1981). At this time, the cumulative immunosuppressive effects of medication and cytomegalovirus as well as the development of opportunistic infections may all combine to present serious potential risk for the recipient. The common viral, fungal, and bacterial infections that affect transplant patients are summarized in Table 20–2.

Malignancy

Malignancy is a potential consequence of immunosuppression and various forms of cancers have been reported in the transplant population. Squamous cell carcinomas are the most common source of cancer in renal transplant

Table 20–2   Common Infections in the Transplant Patient

Type of Infection	Presenting Signs Symptoms
VIRAL INFECTIONS	
Cytomegalovirus (CMV)	Leukopenia
Present in 60–90% of renal transplant recipients	Anorexia
	Malaise
Increased incidence due to immunosuppression	Arthralgias
	Myalgias
	Fever
	↑ BUN/creatinine
	CMV hepatitis—abnormal liver function tests
	CMV pneumonia—hypoxia; tachypnea; changes on chest film
	CMV gastrointestinal—ulcers; hemorrhage; perforation
Herpes simplex	Herpes labialis
	Oral lesions
	Intraoral lesions
	Often painful
Herpes varicella–zoster	Pain and blisters along dermatome
FUNGAL INFECTIONS	
Candida	Whitish, plaque-like thrush on tongue
Oral	
Systemic	
BACTERIAL INFECTIONS	
Escherichia coli urinary tract infection	Urinary burning flank pain
	Urinary frequency

recipients (Penn, 1986). They have been reported with greater incidence in the transplant population than in the general population, with the degree of exposure to ultraviolet radiation greatly increasing incidence. Squamous cell carcinomas in renal transplant patients are most aggressive and form metastases more rapidly than in the general population (Boyle, Briggs, Mackie, Junor & Aitchison, 1984). Patient education regarding the use of sun-blocking agents and minimizing exposure to the sun is important in preventing this potentially serious problem. Compliance must be assessed. Patients should be instructed to notify the practitioner upon development of any skin changes or lesions. Continuous assessment is made throughout the long-term patient follow-up.

The incidence of other forms of cancer frequently seen, such as carci-

Treatment	Nursing Implications
↓ Immunosuppressive drug dosages Intravenous immune globulin Supportive care	5–10% mortality; CMV pneumonia most common form of serious morbidity; obtain sputum culture; test all stools for occult blood; good handwashing techniques necessary

Acyclovir (Zovirax)
  Oral
  Intravenous
	Daily assessment of lips, oral cavity, genitalia; patient education about cause, recognition, contamination, treatment

Pain medication, IV antiviral agents	3% incidence
Nystatin, oral, or chlortrimazole Amphotericin B flucytosine	Good oral hygiene, daily oral cavity assessment; ↑ risk with gastrointestinal damage and in patients on steroids; hemodialysis
IV antibiotics; pain medication; fluids	Infections may be asymptomatic and require routine culturing

noma of the lung, prostate, colon, and rectum, and female breast and invasive cervical cancers are not reported to be increased over the general population (Penn, 1986). However, certain tumors, such as those of the skin and lips, non-Hodgkin's lymphomas, Kaposi's sarcoma, in situ cervical cancer, and carcinomas of the vulva and perinium were found in significantly increased frequency (Penn, 1981, 1986). A history of risk factors for malignancy should be obtained from each patient. Early diagnosis is essential, and treatment via surgical excision, radiation, chemotherapy, and withdrawal of immunosuppression may be indicated. Mortality rates from malignancy, however, are higher in the transplant population than in the general population. Evidence is mounting, also, for a viral association with malignancy formation, particularly Epstein–Barr virus with the subsequent development of certain types of lymphomas (Hanto, Frizzera, Kazimiera, & Simmons, 1985; Yao, Rickinson, Gaston, & Epstein, 1985).

Rejection

Despite suppression of the immune system, graft rejection remains a major threat to the success of organ transplantation. Types of rejection are categorized as hyperacute, acute, and chronic. Severity, diagnosis, treatment, and prognosis of each category are summarized in Table 20–3.

Table 20–3 Graft Rejection

Type	Cause	Onset
Hyper-acute	Preformed antibodies present on the donor organ that stimulate a humoral immune response Presents in 5% renal transplant patients Not seen in liver transplant patients	Immediate or up to 24 hr postoperatively
Acceler-ated acute	Preformed antibodies, anamnestic response Rare—only seen in renal transplants	2–5 days postoperatively
Acute	Cell-mediated response with production of cytotoxic T cells against donor antigens	Usually in first 1–3 mo; may occur any time

RENAL TRANSPLANTATION

The story of renal transplantation has changed remarkably since 1952, when the first "successful" kidney transplants were performed by Hume, Merrill, and Miller. At that time, only three of six transplanted kidneys would continue to function for longer than 1 month. With improvements in technology and marked strides in medical science, particularly in the field of immunology, the frequency and severity of complications have decreased, and the chances for both patient and graft survival have increased. With 1-year graft survival rates of 70 to 85% for cadaver transplants and 90 to 95% for living, related donor transplants, and expected mortality rates of 5% or less, kidney transplantation offers distinct advantages over dialysis for most patients (Monaco, 1985; Sterioff, Engen, & Zincke, 1986). Human renal transplantation has become a viable and often preferred treatment for end-stage renal disease.

Renal transplantation is not a panacea. While the rehabilitation potential is significant, infection, graft rejection, and even death may occur. However, improved understanding of the immunologic basis of transplantation and posttransplant therapy, a thorough evaluation, and conscientious follow-up care all contribute to the current success of renal transplantation.

Signs and Symptoms	Histology	Treatment
Transplanted kidney does not function	Platelet thrombi, complement deposition, necrosis	Organ removal
Fever, leukocytosis or leukopenia, graft tenderness, increased BUN and creatinine, decreased renal blood flow on renal scan	As above	High-dose steroids or ALG may be attempted; transplant nephrectomy usually necessary
Renal: fever (temperature > 38.5°C), graft tenderness, decreased urine output, weight gain, malaise, edema, hypertension, elevated BUN and creatinine; renogram will demonstrate delayed excretion after	Presence of lymphocytes, vasculitis, fibrin deposits, complement, and/or interstitial nephritis	Increased oral steroid or IV Solu-Medrol ("pulse" therapy) or ALG or OKT3

Table 20–3 *(Continued)*

Type	Cause	Onset
		Usually in first months; may occur any time
		7–10 days
		In first 1–3 mo, may occur any time
Chronic	Humoral response with smaller contribution from cellular immunity	Weeks to years post transplant

Signs and Symptoms	Histology	Treatment
slow isotope intake; ultrasound may show parenchymal edema and increased vascular resistance		
Liver: Subclinical: intermittent changes in stool and/or urine color, increased abdominal girth, enlarged, tender liver, elevated SGOT, SGPT, and alkaline phosphatase, other liver function tests remain within normal limits		Supportive care, or may give increased oral steroids
Rejection crisis: rapid onset of symptoms; back, right flank, or right-upper-quadrant pain; severe jaundice; immediate changes in stool and urine color; cessation of bile flow; a swollen, hard, and tender graft; fever; tachycardia; abnormal liver function tests		One to three intravenous steroid boluses or ALG or OKT3
Heart: often clinically silent in early rejection; arrhythmias, hypotension, decreased cardiac output, congestive heart failure seen late in rejection process, symptoms such as weight gain, fever, tachycardia, pericardial rub, gallop, right axial deviation are vague, nondiagnostic and inconsistent	Cardiac cellular swelling, degeneration and necrosis, endothelial cellular swelling with sloughing, mononuclear cell infiltration; myocyte necrosis seen with advanced rejection	Steroids or ALG or OKT3
Renal: Slowly rising serum BUN and creatinine over months to years; proteinuria due to increased glomerular permeability; hypertension due to renal dysfunction and/or increased renin production	Vascular changes with obliteration of small arteries and arterioles, atrophic tubules, intimal thickening and complement deposition	Conservative management; may retransplant or return to dialysis when renal failure returns
Liver: difficult to identify; slow progressive decrease in liver function		May attempt ALG or steroids, generally requires retransplantation

Table 20–3   *(Continued)*

Type	Cause	Onset
		Weeks to years post transplant

BUN = blood urea nitrogen; ALG = antilymphocyte globulin; SGOT = serum glutamic oxaloacetic transaminase; SGPT = serum glutamic pyruvic transaminase.

Renal Functions

The kidneys play a vital part in the maintenance of body homeostasis through both excretory and regulatory functions. They are involved in the metabolism and excretion of metabolic waste products and the control of fluid and electrolyte balance. In addition, the renal system is critical in the regulation of blood pressure; the biosynthesis of various hormones such as erythropoietin factor, growth hormone, and prostaglandins; and the activation of vitamin D. Patients with renal dysfunction experience serious short- and long-term effects when these functions are compromised. Dialysis can maintain life and minimize some of the pathophysiologic changes of renal failure. It cannot, however, replace all of the compromised functions of the kidney. For this reason, renal transplantation is considered the best treatment for renal failure. In addition to physiologic factors, normal renal function allows the chance for an improved quality of life.

Recipient Selection

Patients with a wide variety of renal disease, and at various points along the health–illness continuum, present for renal transplantation. The most common forms of renal disease seen are glomerulonephritis, chronic pyelonephritis, interstitial nephritis, and renal involvement from systemic diseases such as diabetes mellitus and hypertension (Briggs, 1984). Certain patient categories may be considered high-risk, although many patient groups previously distinguished as such are now recognized as having significant potential for a successful outcome. Patients over the age of 55, for example, are reported to have no increased risk of death or graft loss when a steroid-sparing regimen is used in a carefully evaluated population (Jordan et al., 1985). Patients with diabetic nephropathy also undergo transplantation with success rates generally equal to those of patients without diabetes (Cook & Takiff, 1986). More and more frequently, patients are being referred for transplantation before the initiation of dialysis. This route is especially encouraged for

Signs and Symptoms	Histology	Treatment
Heart: atherosclerosis; generally clinically silent since the patient will not experience angina due to the effects of cardiac denervation		Empirical prophylaxis with dipyridamole and/or warfarin; may require balloon angioplasty, bypass, or retransplantation

children and patients with juvenile-onset diabetes, as the disadvantages of dialysis in these populations are even more significant than those of transplantation (Belzer, 1984). In any case, with every potential recipient, decisions about transplantation are based on the individual's own risk–benefit ratio.

Recipient selection is based on a thorough evaluation. The goal of this process is to identify and minimize the potential for posttransplant complications. First, a complete history and physical exam is obtained. Effort is made to obtain a formal or informal psychosocial assessment. A detailed description of the risks, benefits, procedures, and patient responsibilities relating to the pretransplant and posttransplant course is provided. Opportunities for the patients and significant others to learn and ask questions must always be available. It is essential that the patient and family have an understanding of the entire process and their respective roles in it. Information obtained during the history and physical may also guide the practitioner to other areas that require further evaluation.

The potential recipient undergoes a series of laboratory exams, radiologic studies, and consultations. Complete serologic studies are performed, including assessment of viral titers. The patients will undergo chest roentgenography to rule out chronic lung diseases such as tuberculosis. An upper gastrointestinal study is often performed, especially if the patient has a history of peptic ulcer disease, gastritis or upper gastrointestinal bleeding. This precaution is necessary because of the steroid side effect of decreased gastric mucosal protection, which could lead to ulcer formation, especially in a patient so predisposed. A prophylactic, highly selective, vagotomy with or without pyloroplasty may be performed. A lower gastrointestinal series is also performed on older patients or in patients who demonstrate occult blood in their stool or have a history of lower gastrointestinal bleeding or diverticulitis. Patients are evaluated via abdominal ultrasound for the presence of gallstones, which are a potentially dangerous posttransplant complication should cholecystitis later develop. A voiding cystourethrogram is often performed to assess for ureterovesical reflux or other urinary tract abnormalities that could predispose a transplant recipient to the dangers of urinary tract infections. Bladder capacity is also assessed.

The patients undergo a dental evaluation to assess for and treat sources of oral infection. They may also see an otolaryngologist to rule out related sources of infection. Other specialists, such as a cardiologist or urologist, are consulted as needed.

Pretransplant Surgical Procedures

In addition to the infrequent need for preliminary highly selective vagotomy and pyloroplasty, cholecystectomy, and colonic resection or colectomy, other surgical procedures may be considered in preparation for renal transplantation. In cases of intractable hypertension, significant ureterovesical reflux with frequent or chronic urinary tract infection, repeated infection or bleeding from polycystic kidneys, or renal tumors, a bilateral nephrectomy may be necessary. This is rarely done, however, especially in view of the surgical risk, subsequent anemia, and the stringent fluid and diet restrictions required for an anephric patient.

In the precyclosporin era, the role of a pretransplant splenectomy, while controversial, was considered. The idea was to improve tolerance to the immunosuppressant azathioprine or to reduce lymphoid mass and thereby diminish the rejection response (Stuart, Reckard, Ketel, & Schulak, 1980; Starzl, 1964). Because of the improved immunosuppression used currently, pretransplant splenectomy is no longer recommended (except perhaps in a severely leukopenic patient).

Pretransplant Blood Transfusions

Another aspect of pretransplant immune modulation is the administration of blood transfusions. Historically, transfusions were avoided or at least minimized in the dialysis patient awaiting transplantation. Opelz, Sengar, Mickey, and Terasaki (1973) found that patients who had received transfusions in the months prior to undergoing transplantation had significantly better success than patients who had not been transfused. The results were surprising but consistent. It subsequently became policy with many centers to administer 1 to 10 random blood transfusions to pretransplant patients. Since the introduction of cyclosporin as a successful immunosuppressant, the beneficial effect of random blood transfusions has not been so clearly demonstrated, although some centers continue to report significant benefit when cyclosporin and transfusions are used (Opelz, 1985; Klintmalm et al., 1985).

There are inherent risks in administering blood, such as the transmission of cytomegalovirus, hepatitis, human immunodeficiency virus, or other viruses, requiring careful screening of any blood products administered. Additionally, for reasons that are unclear as yet, a percentage of patients who are transfused will become "sensitized," i.e., will develop antibodies not only to the antigens present on the blood they receive, but to a wide spectrum of antigens, thus making it difficult to obtain a kidney to which they do not have antibodies.

Donor Sources

Human kidneys for transplantation can come from two sources, either living or cadaver donors.

Living Related Donors

There are significant advantages to receiving a living related donor kidney and, when available, such donors are preferred by many clinicians. It should be mentioned, however, that some clinicians prefer not to use living donors. Citing success rates with cadaver transplants, they choose not to jeopardize a living donor, no matter how slight the risk (Starzl, 1985). When available, the ideal living, related donor is an identical twin, for whom the recipient would require no immunosuppression. The next best option is an HLA-identical donor. However, even in HLA-disparate donor–recipient pairs, there is some degree of genetic histocompatibility as compared with that found with an unrelated cadaver donor. Advantages of a living, related donor transplant also include availability. There is a shortage of cadaver organs in comparison with the demand, and many patients must wait several months to years until an appropriate kidney is found. Elective scheduling is also possible, optimizing the health and convenience for both the recipient and donor. In addition, one can expect immediate function from a kidney transplanted from a living donor since preservation and ischemic time are minimized.

The potential living, related donor must meet strict medical and psychological criteria. They must be volunteers, and they must be perfectly healthy with normal renal function.

The donor evaluation is carried out in steps, from the least to the most invasive, proceeding to subsequent steps only when the previous tests are reported within normal limits. First, a complete history and physical exam is obtained. In addition to complete laboratory tests, the potential donor then collects a 24-hour urine specimen for creatinine clearance and protein analysis, a urinalysis, and a sterile urine for culture. If no abnormality is found, an intravenous pyelogram is performed to ascertain the presence of two normal kidneys. The donor also undergoes chest roentgenography and electrocardiography. A more extensive cardiac evaluation is often performed on an older donor. A renal arteriogram is performed, usually 48 hours before the donor nephrectomy, to assess renal vasculature and further rule out renal abnormalities. It is with these tests that there can be confidence that no long-term health compromises will occur. In fact, living donors have been found not to be at greater risk for health problems after donating (Vincenti et al., 1983). It is significant that most donors concur that donation did not adversely affect their health. This reaffirmed their decision to donate (Smith et al., 1986). A psychiatric evaluation is often performed to help assess motivation, underlying feelings, and concerns.

The decision to donate can be a difficult one for an individual or family and must be made on an informed basis and in confidence. If a potential recipient is not comfortable with accepting a kidney from a family member or has no family members psychologically or medically able to give, the individual is then placed on a list to await a suitable donor cadaver kidney.

Living Unrelated Donors

With equally careful medical evaluations, as well as scrutiny of ethical issues and motivation, transplants from living unrelated donors have been performed, with success rates reported to be equal to those involving living related donor transplants (Sollinger, Kalayoglu, & Belzer, 1986). Living unrelated donor–recipient combinations may include, for example, spouses, friends, and adoptive parents.

Certainly, the issue of living unrelated donors will generate further discussion, especially in light of the rapidly increasing numbers of patients waiting for kidneys, and a cadaveric supply unable to keep up with the demand. Additional data on the long-term effects on both recipient and donor, appropriate protocols, as well as important ethical issues must be addressed.

Cadaver Donors

Cadaver donors are previously healthy individuals who have sustained head trauma, cerebral hemorrhage, or other forms of brain injury causing permanent, irreversible brain and brain-stem nonfunction. When declared "brain dead" by the physician and/or neurologist, the issue of organ donation can be raised. With permission of the family, the organs can be removed and distributed to the appropriate recipients.

Any organ donor must meet strict medical criteria. For example, there are age limits for the various organs donated. They must be free of malignancy other than brain tumors, free of sepsis, diabetes, and longstanding hypertension, as well as have laboratory values within normal limits. Donor criteria are discussed in greater detail in a subsequent section of this chapter.

Tissue typing and ABO screening are performed on the donor. These results are then used to assist in organ placement, via a local and/or national computerized system, with the appropriate recipient, generally based on the degree of HLA matching.

The Operative Procedure

The surgical procedure for a renal transplant is quite standardized. The patient is prepped and draped in the operating room. An indwelling urinary catheter is placed in the bladder, through which an antibiotic solution is instilled to distend the bladder and to reduce the incidence of infection. An oblique or curvilinear incision is made in the lower abdomen from approximately the iliac crest to the symphysis pubis. The external oblique muscle and fascia are incised, as are the internal oblique and transverse abdominus muscles. The transversalis fascia is cut, with care not to cut the peritoneum, which is then retracted up. A pocket is thus made in the iliac fossa, extraperitoneally, for kidney placement. The vessels can then be isolated and dissected. The lymphatics that are divided during vessel exposure are ligated or tied off to prevent lymph drainage or potential lymphocele formation. Care is taken not to cut the spermatic cord in the male. The common iliac, external iliac, and hypogastric arteries are dissected free, as are the common and external iliac veins in preparation for placement of the donor kidney and revascularization.

The revascularization phase must be carried out quickly and efficiently in order to avoid a prolonged warm ischemic time, which could contribute to tubular damage and posttransplant acute tubular necrosis. The usual vascular anastomoses are end to end with the donor renal artery and recipient hypogastric artery or internal iliac artery. Occasionally, an end-to-side anastomosis of the renal artery to the external iliac artery is required. If the donor kidney has multiple arteries, they may be anastomosed together and then connected to the appropriate recipient artery, anastomosed on a patch, or anastomosed individually. After arterial anastomosis, the kidney is placed in the iliac fossa and the iliac vein is clamped. The renal vein is anastomosed to the iliac vein and the clamps are released. The kidney should now become firm and pink as blood flows through. Often, urine will begin to form immediately, and mannitol or furosemide may be given to promote diuresis.

The donor ureter is now ready to be connected to the recipient bladder, a ureteroneocystostomy. The ureter may be tunneled into the bladder submucosa before exiting into the bladder cavity itself. Thus, during micturition, the natural contraction of the bladder wall will collapse that tunneled segment of the ureter, preventing reflux. The entire wound is irrigated with saline and an antibiotic solution, and then closed in layers. The patient is then transferred to the intensive care unit.

LIVER TRANSPLANTATION

The first attempt at human liver transplantation was made in March 1963 at the University of Colorado. The recipient died, as did the next four on whom similar attempts were made. At that point, clinical trials were halted while trials on animal models continued. In 1966 and 1967, two additional human liver transplants were attempted, again unsuccessfully. Then, in June 1967, a $1\frac{1}{2}$-year-old child received a transplanted liver and lived for 13 months with a functioning liver before dying of metastatic disease (Starzl et al., 1982). Since that time, advances in immunosuppressant therapy have contributed to a decreased incidence of organ rejection and infection. Liver transplantation remains a technically difficult procedure with a challenging postoperative course, but with improved surgical technique, increased success rates, and significant rehabilitative potential, liver transplantation is a justifiable therapy for many patients suffering from chronic, irreversible, and progressive liver disease that cannot be treated medically.

Patient Selection

Liver transplantation is most often considered a last resort treatment, performed when no surgical or medical option exists to halt the progression of liver failure. Patients are at or near end-stage liver disease, with death as the inevitable outcome within 12 months. As advancements in the field continue at their current pace, however, the option of liver transplant is evolving into a more therapeutic one, considered as an acceptable treatment option prior to the onset of end-stage disease.

Before accepting a patient for liver transplantation, documentation of terminal disease must be made. It has been shown, however, that patients can be grouped in order of the severity of their illness at the time of their transplant, with outcomes predictable in each category. Williams, Vera, Peters, and VanVoorst (1986) have defined three patient groups and correlated them with 1-year success rates (Table 20–4). The authors also note differences in hospital course and cost of the transplant.

When evaluating a potential transplant candidate indications for liver transplantation must be assessed, as well as any contraindications, the expected and actual course of disease, current physical state, and medical and surgical history. Prognosis in comparison with the patient's expected course if he or she did not undergo transplantation must be considered. The contraindications to liver transplantation are identified in Table 20–5.

Patients present for liver transplantation with a variety of causes of end-stage liver failure. Table 20–6 provides a summary of potential disease categories, listed in relative order of incidence.

Table 20–4   Liver Transplant Success Rates

Patient Group	Definition	1 Year Success rates
Group 1	The patient can remain out of the hospital to await transplantation, and the patient has not had prior liver hilar surgery	90%
Group 2	The patient is confined to the hospital prior to transplantation but does not require intensive care	86%
Group 3	The patient is confined to the ICU prior to transplant, has had two hilar procedures previously, is constantly encephalopathic, and/or is on dialysis before the transplant	44%

Table 20–5   Contraindications to Liver Transplant

Relative	Absolute
Age greater than 60 years	Portal-vein thrombosis
Hepatitis B positive, particularly with positive hepatitis B antigenemia	Severe hypoxemia ($PaO_2 < 50$ mm Hg)
History of alcoholism	Extrahepatic sepsis
Intrahepatic or biliary sepsis	Extrahepatic malignancy
Irreversible renal disease	Active alcoholism
	Severe cardiopulmonary disease

Table 20–6   Transplantable Hepatic Disease

Chronic active hepatitis
Primary biliary cirrhosis
Sclerosing cholangitis
Acute fulminant hepatitis
Cryptogenic cirrhosis
Extrahepatic biliary atresia (most common cause in children)
Metabolic disorders
   Wilson's disease
   Hemochromatosis
   Alpha-1 antitrypsin deficiency
   Tyrosinemia
   Byler's disease
   Glycogen-storage disease
Primary hepatocellular carcinoma
Alcohol-related cirrhosis
Budd–Chiari syndrome
Autoimmune cirrhosis
Biliary tract carcinoma

Listed in relative order of incidence.

Liver Function

Patients present prior to transplant with various combinations of signs and symptoms of liver dysfunction. The healthy liver performs many vital functions that may be compromised in the presence of liver disease. Signs of liver dysfunction are identified in Table 20–7.

Evaluation Process

In assessing a patient's candidacy for liver transplantation, an extensive evaluation process is conducted. This process includes a variety of laboratory tests,

Table 20–7   Physical Signs of Liver Dysfunction

Increased	Decreased
Serum cholesterol	Albumin synthesis
Bleeding time	Phagocytic activity
Prothromin time/	Fat absorption
partial thromboplastin time	Serum calcium
Serum bilirubin	
Serum ammonia	
Jaundice	
Portal hypertension	

radiologic studies and consultations, which are summarized in Table 20–8. Based on this multidisciplinary evaluation, a determination of patient candidacy and transplant urgency is made. When deemed ready, the patient is placed on an active list to await a suitable donor organ.

The Donor Liver

Liver donors and recipients are matched for body size and ABO compatibility. Liver transplants have, however, been successfully performed across ABO blood groups in emergent situations (Gordon, Iwatsuki, Esquivel, Tsakis, Todo, & Starzl, 1986b). Since the transplanted liver appears to remove or neutralize circulating donor antibody, the existence of preformed antibodies and a pretransplant positive cross match has not been associated with decreased patient or graft survival, and is not measured (Gordon et al. 1986a). HLA matching is also not required.

The Operative Procedure

When an appropriate organ is found for a patient awaiting a liver, efficient patient preparation must be carried out quickly since the donated liver is viable for only a few hours.

1. Laboratory values are obtained immediately, including a chemistry profile, complete blood count, platelet counts, and coagulation studies. Severe coagulopathies may need to be adjusted with aminocaproic acid (Amicar) (a clotting agent) or fresh frozen plasma.
2. A clot is sent to the blood bank for an initial cross match of multiple units of packed red blood cells and fresh frozen plasma.
3. At least one large-bore IV line is placed peripherally. If the patient is unstable, the Swan–Ganz and arterial line catheters may be inserted and base-line hemodynamic parameters are established.

Table 20–8   Liver Transplant Evaluation

General

   Complete blood count, platelets
   Chemistry profile
   Coagulation profile
   Protein electrophoresis
   Amylase (to assess for pancreatic involvement)
   Fasting NH_4
   Arterial blood gases and pulmonary function tests
   Hepatitis B profile
   Cytomegalovirus, Epstein–Barr virus, and herpes titers
   HLA tissue typing
   ABO typing and antibody screen
   Immune deficiency profile

Special studies specific to the disease process and radiologic studies

   Chest roentgenogram (posteroanterior and lateral)
   Abdominal ultrasound (to assess for portal vein patency)
   Abdominal computerized tomagraphy scan (as needed to rule out malignant
     metastases)
   Angiography

Urine studies to assess renal function

   Urinalysis
   Urine culture and sensitivity
   24-hour urine collection for creatinine clearance and protein

Consultations

   Hepatology/gastroenterology (the patients may require endoscopy and/or scle-
     rosing of esophageal varices)
   Hematology
   Anesthesiology
   Social service
   Others (such as cardiology, pulmonary, neurology, endocrinology and nephrol-
     ogy as needed)

4. Either in the intensive care unit or in the operating room, two or three additional large-bore IV lines are inserted, including a central line and often a jugular line. These sites are necessary for administration of anesthetic agents and other medications, and are also available for the often required rapid infusions of fluid and blood products. Sterility in line placement is critical in order to prevent postoperative line sepsis.

Patient support during this time, including an explanation of the procedures, introduction of personnel, and the presence of a familiar care giver is beneficial for the patient and family. Anticipatory explanation of this process during the work-up phase will also help ease patient anxiety during this time. It is also important to keep the patient's family informed of the procedures and the patient's status.

The sterile prep is done in the operating room. The length of the operative procedure may range between 7 and 24 hours, with the average being 12 to 14 hours. The most difficult aspect of liver transplantation is removal of the recipient liver, which may take 4 to 5 hours or longer if the patient has had prior surgery, has severe coagulopathy or portal hypertension causing severe bleeding, or is otherwise unstable.

Blood loss can be great, with replacement of as few as 7 units of blood and blood products to, less commonly, 150 or more. Of benefit has been use of the venovenous bypass system, which is placed just prior to removal of the recipient liver. A heparin-bonded Gott shunt is inserted into both the left common femoral vein and the left axillary vein. During the anhepatic stage, the bypass pump assists venous return of blood from the lower portion of the body to the heart, as is seen in Figure 20–2. The use of venovenous bypass decreases venous hypertension and ideally helps limit operative blood loss (Griffith, Shaw, Hardesty, Iwatsuki, Bahnson, & Starzl, 1985). There is a significant operative mortality, although this varies between the groups of patients as described.

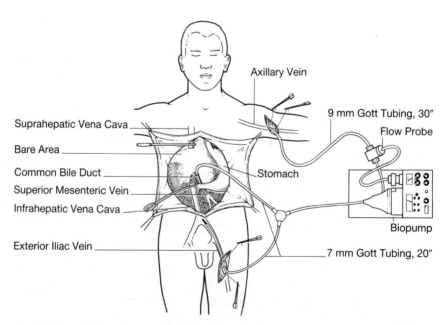

Figure 20–2. Venovenous bypass system used in liver transplantation. From "Venovenous bypass without systemic anticoagulation for transplantation of the human liver" by B. P. Griffith, 1985, *Surgery, Gynecology and Obstetrics, 160*, pp. 270–272. Reprinted by permission of Surgery, Gynecology and Obstetrics.

Surgery begins with a bilateral subcostal incision extending from the midline, with approximately 2 in. incised above the removed xiphoid. The hepatic artery and vein, portal vein, and common bile duct are isolated. The recipient liver is then ready to be removed, although no major vessels are ligated until the donor liver arrives, is reinspected, and is prepared. The patient is then placed on venovenous bypass, and the liver removed. A significant risk at this time is shock, with its concurrent potential for hypoperfusion of the kidneys and other organs, decreased oxygenation, acidosis, and even death. Control of blood loss and replacement of fluid and blood products is critical during this time.

The donor liver is first thoroughly flushed with lactated Ringer's solution. Flushing is an essential step to remove any air bubbles in the donor liver, thus minimizing the risk of an air embolus. It also serves to remove excess potassium in the liver, which arises from the preservation solution and lysed hepatic cells, thus preventing potentially fatal hyperkalemia.

Next, the suprahepatic vena cava is anastomosed, followed by anastomosis of the infrahepatic vena cava. The portal vein is then anastomosed and venous flow is established, followed by arterial anastomoses. The liver "pinks up" as blood flow is reestablished. Assessment for complete closure at all anastomosis sites is made. Any leaks could result in significant bleeding postoperatively, with the need for reexploration and repair. At this point, the healthy donor organ should begin to function and the patient's coagulation status should begin to return to normal, diminishing the risk of hemorrhage.

The next phase of the operative procedure entails the reconstruction of the bile ducts. This lengthy procedure is most often accomplished via an end-to-end anastomosis of donor and recipient bile ducts, stented with a T tube. For patients without bile ducts (as in biliary atresia) or with diseased bile ducts (as in sclerosing cholangitis), the donor common duct is anastomosed to a Roux-en-Y limb of the intestine (Starzl et al., 1982). Complete closure is critical, since bile leakage may contribute to development of peritonitis.

Finally, drains are placed in the abdomen and brought out through stab wounds and the incision is closed. Williams, Peters, Vera, Britt, VanVoorst, and Haggit (1985) have described a 2-in. incision left open at the xiphoid, through which the liver can be seen and easily biopsied. The patient is then transferred to the surgical intensive care unit and postoperative nursing care begins.

CARDIAC TRANSPLANTATION

Cardiac transplantation for various forms of end-stage disease, and heart/lung or lung transplants in cases of pulmonary hypertension or such diseases as Eisenmenger's syndrome, have also developed into therapeutic treatment options. The first heart transplants were performed experimentally on animals in the early 1900s, with poor successes because of a lack of immunosuppression. Transplantation in humans was not attempted until the 1960s, the most notable transplant being performed in 1967 by Dr. Christian Barnard. The recipient survived for 18 days before dying of pneumonia. An "explosion" of cardiac transplantation then followed (Griepp & Ergin, 1984). Unfortunately, overall success was limited and most centers abandoned attempts to perfect this procedure.

In recent years, cardiac transplantation has been as progressive as liver and renal transplantation, with 1-year survival rates now reaching 80%, with significant rehabilitation. As with other visceral-organ transplantation, improved surgical and immunosuppressive techniques have contributed to this success rate, providing hope and rehabilitation to another end-stage-disease patient population.

Recipient Selection

Recipients for cardiac transplantation are selected from a suitable patient population with end-stage cardiac disease for whom there exists no alternative medical or surgical therapy and who have an expected survival rate of less than 10% at 1 year. According to the registry of the International Society for Heart Transplantation, the most common causes for such end-stage disease are ischemic and idiopathic cardiomyopathy and coronary artery disease. Other causes include congenital heart diseases, rejection of a prior graft, viral myocarditis, postviral myopathy, postpartum cardiomyopathy and postoperative heart failure (Copeland et al., 1987). In any case, objective and subjective data regarding prognosis with or without transplantation are used in determining candidacy as summarized in Table 20–9.

Evaluation of a potential recipient includes the tests listed in Table 20–10. Additional tests are performed as indicated on an individual basis.

A clinical social worker and/or clinical psychologist is involved in the evaluation process. An assessment of past and present compliance patterns is done in order to determine the potential future compliance. The social support system of the candidate is assessed, since a long-term commitment to treatment and follow-up will be required. An evaluation of financial resources is conducted, since the posttransplant patient may face significant expenses for the transplant, long-term medications, and postoperative follow-up. Exploring a variety of potential financial resources is an important effort in the pretransplant phase.

In addition to information gathering, the pretransplant process must include several aspects of patient education. The patient must be provided with the information necessary for an informed decision. Discussion regarding the evaluation process, perioperative and postoperative periods, including the common use of strict isolation, posttransplant rehabilitation, administration of the required medications and their potential side effects, patient responsibilities, and financial issues must be open and complete.

Table 20–9 Selection Criteria for Cardiac Transplantation

Terminal cardiac disease with life expectancy of 12 mo or less

No other available medical or surgical therapy that may improve the patient's functional status or life expectancy

Normal function of other organ systems (if organ dysfunction exists secondary to compromised cardiac function, it must be reversible)

Absence of active infection

Age less than 50 yr. This is a relative requirement and each case is evaluated individually.

Absence of severe pulmonary hypertension, defined as greater than 6 Wood units. Pulmonary hypertension is a compensatory mechanism resulting from long-standing congestive heart failure that protects the lungs from increased pulmonary blood flow. The damaged recipient heart compensates for the elevated pulmonary pressure via right ventricular hypertrophy. The donor heart, however, is unable to adapt to the resulting sudden increase in workload. The resulting sequelae is early postoperative right-sided failure.

Absence of recent, unresolved pulmonary infarction with the associated risk of necrosis and infection

Absence of donor-specific antibodies or a positive cross match between recipient and donor. The presence of donor-specific antibodies, as described with renal transplantation, will result in hyperacute rejection of the donor heart.

Absence of significant peripheral or cerebral vascular disease

Absence of systemic disease, again evaluated individually

Evidence of the ability to comply with the treatment and adequate financial resources and social support. Rehabilitation from cardiac transplantation is a long-term, continuous endeavor with numerous patient responsibilities and the potential for taxing family relationships and financial resources.

As the evaluation is completed, the multidisciplinary team, including the cardiologist, transplant surgeon, nursing transplant coordinator, social worker, and/or clinical psychologist share information and determine if cardiac transplantation is the appropriate therapy for each individual patient. If a patient is deemed a suitable candidate, a determination of urgency is made and the patient is placed on the active list according to the degree of urgency. Changes in the patient's status are made as clinically indicated.

During the waiting period, intensive education continues for both the patient and family. Support during this period of fear and anxiety is critical. Frequent communication between members of the health care team should continue. During this time, the patient remains at risk for a variety of potential and actual nursing diagnoses, such as decreased cardiac output, altered tissue perfusion, impaired gas exchange, powerlessness related to the situation, sleep pattern disturbance, and impaired skin integrity (Futterman, 1988).

Table 20–10   Cardiac Transplantation Evaluation

Complete history and physical examination

Laboratory studies
   Complete blood count with differential
   Chemistry profile
   2-hour postprandial glucose
   Viral serology
      Cytomegalovirus
      Herpes simplex virus
      Epstein–Barr virus
      Hepatitis profile
      HTLV-3
      Toxoplasmosis

ABO typing

HLA tissue typing

Right and left cardiac catheterization, usually including left ventricular and coronary angiograms

Electrocardiogram

Chest roentgenogram

Pulmonary function tests

Evaluation of pulmonary vascular resistance

Urine studies
   Urine culture and sensitivity
   Microscopic urinalysis
   24-hour urine collection for creatinine clearance and protein studies

The Cardiac Donor

When the potential donor is identified, an appropriate recipient is found. Matching of a donor heart to a recipient is based on ABO compatibility, the existence of a negative lymphocyte cross match, and relative donor heart size to recipient body mass. The most critically ill recipients are given priority. Based on these criteria, the most suitable recipient is called into the hospital or, if already hospitalized, prepared for transplantation.

The Operative Procedure

The operative procedure for the recipient is quite standardized. First, a midline sternotomy is performed to expose the recipient heart. The patient is well heparinized and, after cannulation of the ascending aorta, superior vena cava, and inferior vena cava, cardiopulmonary bypass is initiated. The venae cavae are tied off and the aorta is cross clamped.

Next, the right and left atria are excised, leaving the atrial walls and their venous connection intact. Cold saline flushes are initiated to provide hypothermic protection to the remaining myocardial tissue.

The donor heart, which has been removed as a whole and placed in an iced saline solution, is trimmed to fit. Donor to recipient anastomoses are first made of the left then the right atria. The left atrium is flushed with cold saline, both to maintain hypothermic protection and to flush out any air remaining in the left ventricle. Suturing of the two aortic stumps follows. The aortic cross clamps are removed and the myocardium is reperfused. The pulmonary arteries will then be anastomosed.

Cardiopulmonary bypass continues for a short time until the new heart is able to control circulation. Temporary atrial or ventricular pacing wires are attached to the myocardium before chest closure. Chest tubes are often inserted into the mediastinum and right pleural space to promote adequate drainage. After being stabilized and taken off bypass, the patient is transported to the intensive care unit.

POSTOPERATIVE NURSING CARE OF THE TRANSPLANT PATIENT

Nursing care of the transplant patient is challenging and complex but also very rewarding. Successful rehabilitation of the recipient depends on careful nursing assessment, diagnosis, intervention, and evaluation of postoperative sequelae. The nursing diagnoses commonly seen in the transplant patient are presented in Table 20–11. Also identified are the related factors and nursing interventions associated with each diagnosis for the different types of transplants.

The major goal of nursing care in the immediate postoperative period is the stabilization of the patient as in any other type of surgery. The early identification of signs of postoperative complications is another nursing responsibility during the postoperative period. Potential postoperative complications specific to each type of organ transplant are summarized in Table 20–12.

A longer-term goal, which is the major focus of nursing care in the transplant patient, is the prevention of infection. The potential for infection due to immunosuppression was addressed in the first part of this chapter. Prevention of infection can be accomplished through strict adherence to aseptic technique and the use of protective isolation. Contact with persons with infection must be avoided, and visitors with colds or flu will have to be restricted from visiting. Should infection occur, early recognition and prompt, aggressive treatment is necessary if the patient is to recover. Before discharge, the patient and family must be taught to recognize the signs and symptoms of infection and what to do if infection develops.

Table 20–11 Common Nursing Diagnoses and Interventions for the Transplant Patient

	Related Factors

Nursing Diagnosis: Altered fluid volume, composition, and distribution

Renal	Postoperative diuresis
	Potential for dehydration
	Potential for overload with fluid replacement
	Risk of acute tubular necrosis

Hepatic	Postoperative hypotension due to third spacing and/or sepsis
	Blood products
	Incidence of postoperative renal dysfunction

Cardiac	Alterations in cardiac function
	Postoperative hypotension due to bleeding
	Postoperative overload due to renal insufficiency

Nursing Diagnosis: Potential for impaired gas exchange

Renal	Predisposition to CMV pneumonia

Hepatic	Mechanical ventilation for 2–3 days necessary because of pulmonary shunting or congestion due to hepatic failure
	↑ Administration of blood products
	↑ Risk of sepsis
	Pulmonary edema
	Hemodynamic instability
	Prolonged surgery

Interventions	Comments
Monitor intake/output Monitor vital signs Daily weight Auscultate lungs Fluid replacement ml/ml Monitor electrolytes Monitor hematocrit/hemoglobin Monitor central venous pressure Ensure catheter patency	Risk of acute tubular necrosis is ↑ with cadaveric kidneys stored more than 24 hr May require dialysis in presence of acute tubular necrosis—need is temporary and must be explained to patient Electrolyte imbalance may necessitate cardiac monitoring
Monitor Swan–Ganz readings Monitor electrolytes Strict intake/output 24-hour urine for creatinine clearance Monitor for signs/symptoms of dehydration/overload (skin turgor, edema, breath sounds, blood pressure, central venous pressure, intake/output, ascites) Daily weight	May require slow continuous ultrafiltration or dialysis Must treat hypotension promptly to protect body organs (may require blood, fluid vasopressors) Cyclosporin may contribute to renal dysfunction; monitor drug levels and renal function
Monitor electrocardiogram Daily weight Monitor vital signs Monitor Swan–Ganz readings Monitor intake/output Monitor for signs/symptoms of dehydration/overload Monitor electrolytes Administer blood/fluid as indicated	Renal failure may develop secondary to preexisting dysfunction, intraoperative hypoperfusion, and cyclosporin toxicity
Good respiratory assessment Good pulmonary hygiene Early ambulation Obtain sputum cultures Encourage coughing and deep breathing ↓	Prednisone may mask signs of infection May require serial chest films and bronchoscopy or open lung biopsy or both
Monitor electrocardiogram Monitor vital signs Monitor Swan–Ganz/central venous pressure Monitor for ARDS (see chapter 7) Strict pulmonary hygiene Obtain sputum cultures with ↑ temperature and/or secretions	Daily chest film Frequent finding—metabolic alkalosis with base excess of 15–20 mEq/liter Good patient education is mandatory regarding strict pulmonary hygiene

Table 20–11 *(Continued)*

	Related Factors

Cardiac	Mechanical ventilation for 8–12 hr
	Thoracic procedure
	Cardiopulmonary bypass

Nursing Diagnosis: Potential for infection*

Renal	Immunosuppression
	↑ Risk of viral/bacterial infections
	Multiple IVs/catheters

Hepatic	Multiple IVs/drains
	Multiple blood products
	Prolonged surgery
	Impaired liver function
	Multiple surgical dressings
	Immunosuppression
	Intubation
Cardiac	Multiple IVs
	Immunosuppression
	Catheters
	Preoperative physical status of patient

Nursing Diagnosis: Altered organ function

Renal	Postoperative diuresis
	Acute tubular necrosis
	Graft dysfunction
	Immunotherapy—toxicity from medications

Hepatic	Graft dysfunction
	Rejection
	Infection
	Ischemia
	Cholestasis
	Hepatotoxicity

Interventions	Comments
Monitor intake/output Monitor arterial blood gases	
	Weaning initiated as tolerated Cough and deep breathe after extubation

Sterile technique with line/catheter/
  dressing care
Monitor for signs/symptoms of infection
Strict pulmonary hygiene
Wound, urine, sputum, blood cultures
Monitor vital signs
Strict handwashing technique
Monitor white blood cell count
	Prednisone may mask signs of infection
	Chest film may be only early sign of
	  pulmonary infection

Strict pulmonary hygiene Obtain cultures p.r.n. Strict handwashing technique Sterile technique with line/drain care Monitor for signs/symptoms of infection Maintain skin integrity Monitor white blood cell count	Antibiotics may contribute to renal dys- function Monitor drug levels

Maintain strict protective isolation
Strict handwashing technique
Monitor for signs/symptoms of infection
Strict pulmonary hygiene
Monitor level of consciousness
Monitor white blood cell count
	May use laminar flow
	Room preparation essential (antimicro-
	  bial scrub/sterile supplies)
	Lungs are primary site of infection, fol-
	  lowed by urinary tract and central
	  nervous system
	Serial chest films

Monitor electrolytes Monitor BUN/CRT Monitor glucose Monitor white blood cell count Treat electrolyte disturbance promptly Monitor for cyclosporin toxicity Monitor intake/output Daily weight	Change in electrolytes may indicate dysfunction May require dialysis May need to decrease drug dosages
Monitor serum albumin	↓ Common finding with liver dysfunc- tion
Monitor alkaline phosphatase	↑ With rejection/obstruction/↓ bile se- cretion

Monitor liver enzymes	↑ With cell destruction, ischemia,
	  thrombosis, rejection, obstruction,
	  infection

Table 20–11   *(Continued)*

	Related Factors
Cardiac	Preservation of organ Reperfusion ischemic injury Surgical manipulation of heart Electrolyte imbalance Denervated transplanted heart Postoperative myocardial edema Cardiopulmonary bypass

Nursing Diagnosis: Potential for organ rejection†

Renal	Infection Cyclosporin nephrotoxicity Hypoperfusion Vascular thrombosis Urinary leaks
Hepatic	Infection Hepatic dysfunction Hepatic-vein thrombosis Hepatocyte necrosis Cholestasis Bile-duct obstruction
Cardiac	Infection Cardiac dysfunction Atherosclerosis Hyperlipidemia Hypercholesteremia

Nursing Diagnosis: Altered nutritional status

Renal	Tendency to retain fluids Tendency to retain potassium Lifting of dietary restrictions postoperatively ↑ Catabolism related to prednisone Preoperative electrolyte alterations

Interventions	*Comments*
Monitor bilirubin	↑ With cell destruction/obstruction
Monitor prothrombin time	↓ Synthesis by liver
Monitor for ↓ bile from T tube, change in color of bile	
Monitor for abdominal distention	
Monitor vital signs	
Monitor electrocardiogram	Bradycardia common; may require pacemaker
Monitor for dysrhythmias	
Treat dysrhythmias promptly	Remnant p-wave may be present, as recipient's own sinoatrial node is left in place; no clinical significance
Monitor for ↑ stress	
Allow for rest periods	
Monitor Swan–Ganz readings	Slow response to stress/cardiac work
Monitor for edema	May require inotropic support
Monitor renal function	Requires renal biopsy and histologic exam to diagnose; biopsy has associated risk of bleeding
Monitor intake/output	
Monitor vital signs	
Monitor electrolytes	
Monitor complete blood count/platelets	
Administer immunotherapeutic drugs	
Strict isolation	
Good handwashing technique	
↓	
Monitor hepatic function	Requires liver biopsy and histologic exam to diagnose
↓	
Monitor cardiac function	Major threat to successful transplantation
Monitor electrocardiogram	Requires cardiac biopsy and histologic exam to diagnose
Daily weight	
Nutritional consult geared to prevent weight gain	
Encourage good nutrition to promote wound healing	

Table 20–11 *(Continued)*

	Related Factors
Hepatic	Preoperative malnutrition ↓ Albumin Fat malabsorption Anorexia ↑ Metabolic demands ↑ Catabolism related to prednisone Liver dysfunction Electrolyte abnormalities Altered bowel elimination
Cardiac	Anorexia Fatigue Metabolic alterations from renal and/or hepatic dysfunction Infection Atherosclerosis Hyperlipidemia Glucose intolerance Hypertension

ATN = acute tubular necrosis; ARDS = adult respiratory distress syndrome; BUN = blood urea nitrogen; CRT = creatinine; TPN = total parenteral nutrition.
*See Table 20–2 for a summary of infections that may occur in the transplant patient.
†See Table 20–3 for summary of types of rejection; including causes, incidence, onset, signs and symptoms, histology, and treatment.

Table 20–12 Potential Postoperative Complications in the Transplant Patient

Postoperative Complications	Type/Source	Signs and Symptoms
Renal Urologic (uncommon)	Urine leaks from bladder, ureter, calyx	↓ Urine output; abdominal tenderness; pain; fever; distention; ↑ BUN; dysuria; ↑ CRT
	Obstruction from ureter	↓ Urine output; ↑ BUN; ↑ CRT
	Lymphocele	Genital edema; ipsilateral lower-extremity edema; ↓ U/O; ↑ BUN; ↑ CRT
Vascular (rare)	Renal-artery stenosis	Hypertension; renal dysfunction
	Venous thrombosis	Graft swelling; oliguria; proteinuria; lower-extremity edema

Interventions	Comments
Administer TPN Monitor intake/output Daily weight Monitor electrolytes Advance diet as tolerated Monitor for bowel sounds Encourage p.o. intake Monitor for abdominal distention, pain, constipation, nausea, vomiting	Goal is to maintain positive nitrogen balance, fluid and electrolyte balance, adequate caloric intake, and normal related laboratory values (for all types of transplants)
Encourage good nutrition to promote wound healing Monitor hepatic/renal function Monitor electrolytes Daily weight Maintain strict isolation Nutritionist consult geared toward low-fat/low-sodium diet	

Diagnosis	Treatment
Cystogram Nephrostogram	Surgical repair; promote drainage; promote healing; avoid bladder distention
Ultrasound	Retrograde stent placement; surgical repair
Ultrasound	Percutaneous drainage; surgical repair
Angiography	Balloon angioplasty; surgical repair
Venogram	Thrombectomy; anticoagulant therapy

Table 20–12   *(Continued)*

Postoperative Complications	Type/Source	Signs and Symptoms
Hypertension (common)	Cyclosporin Na^+/H_2O retention Obesity ↑ Renin secretion	Hypertension; ↑ weight
Hepatic Vascular	Hepatic-vein thrombosis (common)	Signs and symptoms liver failure; ↑ liver enzymes; sepsis; bile leak
	Portal-vein thrombosis (rare)	Abdominal distention; ↑ ascites; portal hypertension
Biliary	Obstruction (common)	↓ Bile production; jaundice; ↑ liver enzymes; fever
Cardiac	Atherosclerosis—related to humoral rejection	Hyperlipidemia; hypercholesterolemia; silent myocardial infarction (denervated heart); sudden death; arrhythmias; congestive heart failure

BUN = blood urea nitrogen; CRT = creatinine; U/O = urine output.

DONOR IDENTIFICATION

Another major part the critical care nurse can play in organ transplantation is in donor identification. For many patients, the option of transplantation is made available only through the donation of cadaver organs. Only a small percentage of appropriate donors are being identified and referred at the present time, however. Organ donation offers the family an opportunity to derive something positive from what is usually a very tragic situation. Skelley (1985) states that most families who have consented to organ donation report finding comfort in their decision and would donate again.

The critical care nurse is often the first person to identify a potential donor or to be approached by the family about the possibility of donating their loved one's organs. The critical care nurse may then initiate the donation process, participate in the assessment and care of the potential donor, and provide information and support to the family.

The usual organ donor is a previously healthy person who has sustained irreversible brain injury due to trauma, cerebral hemorrhage, a suicide attempt, or drowning. A careful medical history will be obtained, including the cause of injury and details of all resuscitation efforts. The potential donor should not have had trauma to the transplantable organs, prolonged cardiac arrest, or hypotension, and should have required only minimal inotropic

Diagnosis	Treatment
↑ BP	Salt restriction; weight loss; ↓ cyclosporin drug dose; patient education
Ultrasound Computerized tomography scan Arteriography	Retransplantation
Ultrasound Arteriography	Retransplantation
Percutaneous cholangiogram	Surgical placement of T tube or stent; surgical repair
Yearly cardiac catherization	Bypass surgery; angioplasty; retransplantation; dipyridamole; warfarin therapy; patient education about coronary artery disease

support. The potential donor should also be free of sepsis, transmissible disease, or malignancy (except primary brain tumor). Other criteria used in donor organ selection (which vary according to the organ being transplanted) are summarized in Table 20–13.

The certainty of brain death or the irreversible cessation of brain function, including that of both the brain stem and cerebrum, must be established. Determination of brain death is made by a neurologist who is not involved in any aspect of organ recovery or transplantation. Brain death is determined based on the criteria presented in Table 20–14.

When the possibility of brain death or organ donation is established, the potential donor is referred to the transplant coordinator of the regional organ procurement organization. The critical care nurse may initiate contact with the local organ procurement program as defined by hospital policy and procedures. A national 24-hour donor number (1-800-24-DONOR) may also be called to locate the appropriate contact center. The transplant coordinator may approach the families to request donation if this has not been done. Consent is always obtained from the next of kin even if the potential donor has signed an organ donor card. The coordinator will also provide support and information to both families and staff, answer questions, and assist in donor maintenance.

Table 20-13   Criteria for Donor Organ Selection

Organ	Age	Excluding diseases	Recovery time
Eyes	Any	Active hepatitis within 6 mo; damaged corneas; frontal eye neoplasms	Within 4 hr after death
Skin and bones	10–65 yr	Active hepatitis within 6 mo; untreated infection; untreated VD; cancer	Within 12 hr after death
Kidneys	5–50 yr	Active hepatitis within 6 mo; hypertension; untreated infection; neoplasm; poor renal function; diabetes; diseased or damaged kidneys	Must be recovered immediately on cessation of blood flow
Heart	Male: 15–35 yr Female: 15–40 yr	Active hepatitis within 6 mo History of MI; untreated infection; heart trauma; neoplasm; diseased heart	Must be recovered immediately on cessation of blood flow
Liver	6 mo to 45 yr	Active hepatitis; diseased or damaged liver; neoplasm; untreated infection	Must be recovered immediately on cessation of blood flow

VD = Veneral disease; MI = myocardial infarction.

From "Recognition and Nursing Care of Organ Donors" by C. L. Diggs, 1986, *Journal of Emergency Nursing, 12,* pp. 205–209. Reprinted by permission.

Care of the potential donor is similar to that of any patient on a ventilator, with the goal of preserving circulation and maintaining organ viability. Hemodynamic monitoring and the maintenance of fluid and electrolyte balances are required. If vasopressors are needed to maintain adequate blood pressure (generally greater than 90 mm Hg systolic), inotropic agents are preferred. Prolonged use, however, particularly at high doses, may impair organ function and preclude donation. Fluid and electrolyte replacement,

Table 20–14   Clinical Signs of Brain Death

No response to external stimuli, including response to deep pain and heat

No spontaneous movements, including respirations

    Absence of spontaneous respirations is determined by turning the ventilator off for 3 min and ascertaining that the patient is making no effort to breathe. Some muscle reflexes may exist but are short-lived spinal cord reflexes

Absence of cranial nerve reflexes

    Pupils are fixed, dilated, and unreactive to light. Absence of ocular movement as assessed with cold caloric testing and doll's eye maneuvers

    No corneal reflex

    No cough or gag reflex

    No response to plantar stimulation

    No response to noxious stimulation

Apnea in the presence of carbon dioxide stimulus

Two isoelectric (flat line) electroencephalograms taken at least 24 hr apart

Cerebral angiogram

---

especially in the face of the diabetes insipidus common in cases of head trauma, is essential to prevent dehydration and organ hypoperfusion. The use of sterile technique with all invasive procedures is critical in order to avoid sepsis.

SUMMARY

Nursing care of the transplant patient requires the integration of concepts of physiology—specifically, fluid balance, oxygenation, and cardiac output, immunology—specifically, related to rejection and immunosuppression, psychology—specifically, related to death and dying, crisis, and acute hospitalization, nutrition—specifically, related to wound healing, nitrogen balance, and hydration. In addition, the care is interdisciplinary, involving nursing, physicians, respiratory therapists, physical therapists, pharmacists, social workers, and chaplains. The care of the transplant patient is complex at best. However, the challenge can be a rewarding one, for both the patient and the critical care nurse.

BIBLIOGRAPHY

Anderson, R. J., Schafer, L. A., Olin, D. B., & Eickhoff, T. C. (1973). Infectious risk factors in the immunosuppressed host. *American Journal of Medicine, 54,* 453–460.

Belzer, F. O. (1984). Advances in renal transplantation. In R. L. Jamison (Ed.), *Transplantation in the 80's: Recent advances* (pp. 23–35). New York: Praeger.

Briggs, J. D. (1984). The recipient of a renal transplant. In P. J. Morris (Ed.), *Kidney transplantation: Principles and practice* (2nd ed.) (pp. 59–79). London: Grune & Stratton.

Cecka, J. M. (1986). The changing role of HLA matching. In P. I. Terasaki (Ed.), *Clinical transplants 1986*. (pp. 141–155). Los Angeles: UCLA Tissue Typing Laboratory.

Cook, D. J., & Takiff, H. (1986). Original disease of the recipient. In P. I. Terasaki (Ed.), *Clinical transplants 1986* (pp. 311–319). Los Angeles: UCLA Tissue Typing Laboratory.

Copeland, J. G., Emery, R. W., Levinson, M. M., Icenogle, T. B., Carrier, M., Ott, R. A., Copeland, J. A., McAleer-Rhenman, M. J., & Nicholson, S. M. (1987). Selection of patients for cardiac transplantation. *Circulation, 75,* 2–9.

Futterman, L. (1988). Cardiac transplantation: A comprehensive nursing perspective, Part 1. *Heart and Lung, 17,* 499–510.

Gordon, R. D., Fung, J. J., Markus, B., Fox, I., Iwatsuki, S., Esquivel, C. O., Tsakis, A., Todo, S., & Starzl, T. E. (1986a). The antibody crossmatch in liver transplantation. *Surgery, 100,* 705–715.

Gordon, R. D., Iwatsuki, S., Esquivel, C. O., Tsakis, A., Todo, S., & Starzl, T. E. (1986b). Liver transplantation across ABO blood groups. *Surgery, 100,* 342–348.

Griepp, R. B., & Ergin, M. A. (1984). The history of experimental heart transplantation. *Heart Transplantation, 3,* 145–151.

Griffith, B. P., Shaw, B. W., Jr., Hardesty, R. L., Iwatsuki, S., Bahnson, H. T., & Starzl, T. E. (1985). Veno-venous bypass without systemic anticoagulation for transplantation of the human liver. *Surgery, Gynecology and Obstetrics, 160,* 270–272.

Hanto, D. W., Frizzera, G., Kazimiera, J. G. P., & Simmons, R. L. (1985). Epstein–Barr virus, immunodeficiency, and B cell lymphoproliferation. *Transplantation, 39,* 461–472.

Hume, D. M., Merrill, J. P., & Miller, B. F. (1952). Homologous transplantation of human kidneys. *Journal of Clinical Investigation, 31,* 640–641.

Jordan, M. L., Novick, A. C., Steinmuller, D., Braun, W., Buszta, C., Mintz, D., Goormastic, M., & Streem, S. (1985). Renal transplantation in the older recipient. *Journal of Urology, 134,* 243–246.

Klintmalm, G., Brynger, H., Flatmark, A., Frodin, L., Husberg, B., Thorsby, E., & Groth, C. G. (1985). The blood transfusion, DR matching, and mixed lymphocyte culture effects are not seen in cyclosporine-treated renal transplant recipients. *Transplantation Proceedings, 17,* 1026–1031.

Monaco, A. P. (1985). Clinical kidney transplantation in 1984. *Transplantation Proceedings, 17,* 5–12.

Opelz, G. (1985). Current relevance of the transfusion effect in renal transplantation. *Transplantation Proceedings, 17,* 1015–1022.

Opelz, G., Sengar, D. P. S., Mickey, M. R., & Terasaki, P. I. (1973). Effects of blood transfusions on subsequent kidney transplants. *Transplantation Proceedings, 5,* 253–259.

Penn, I. (1981). The price of immunotherapy. *Current Problems in Surgery, 18,* 682–751.

Penn, I. (1986). Cancer is a complication of severe immunosuppression. *Surgery, Gynecology and Obstetrics, 162,* 603–610.

Rubin, R. H., Wolfson, J. S., Cosimi, A. B., & Tolkoff-Rubin, N. E. (1981). Infection in the renal transplant recipient. *American Journal of Medicine, 70,* 401–411.

Sanfilippo, F., Vaughn, W. K., & Lefor, W. M. (1986). HLA matching for cadaver renal transplantation in SEOPF: The impact of cyclosporine. In P. I. Terasaki (Ed.),

Clinical transplants 1986 (pp. 109–120). Los Angeles: UCLA Tissue Typing Laboratory.

Skelley, L. (1985). Practical issues in obtaining organs for transplant. *Law, Medicine, and Health Care, 13,* 35–37.

Smith, M. D., Kappell, D. F., Province, M. A., Hong, B. A., Robson, A. M., Dutton, S., Guzman, T., Hoff, J., Shelton, L., Cameron, E., Emerson, W., Glass, N., Hopkins, J., & Peterson, C. (1986). Living-related kidney donors: A multicenter study of donor education, socioeconomic adjustment, and rehabilitation. *American Journal of Kidney Diseases, 8,* 223–233.

Solinger, A. M. (1985). Organ transplantation and the immune response gene. *Medical Clinics of North America, 69,* (3), 565–584.

Sollinger, H. W., Kalayoglu, M., & Belzer, F. O. (1986). Use of the donor specific protocol in living unrelated donor-recipient combination. *Annals of Surgery, 204,* 315–321.

Starzl, T. E. (1964). Role of excision of lymphoid masses in attenuating the rejection process. In T. E. Starzl (Ed.), *Experiences in renal transplantation* (pp. 126–129). Philadelphia: W. B. Saunders.

Starzl, T. E. (1985). Will live organ donations no longer be justified? *Hastings Center Report, 15*(2), 5.

Starzl, T. E., Iwatsuki, S., Van Theil, D. H., Gartner, J. C., Zitelli, B. J., Malatack, J. J., Schade, R. R., Shaw, B. W., Hakala, T. R., Rosenthal, J. T., & Porter, K. A. (1982). Evolution of liver transplantation. *Hepatology, 2,* 614–636.

Sterioff, S., Engen, D. E., & Zincke, H. (1986). Current status of renal transplantation—1986. *Mayo Clinic Proceedings, 61,* 573–578.

Stuart, F. P., Reckard, C. R., Ketel, B. L., & Schulak, J. A. (1980). Effects of splenectomy on first cadaver kidney transplants. *Annals of Surgery, 192,* 553–561.

Tonegawa, S. (1985). The molecules of the immune system. *Scientific American, 253*(4), 122–131.

Vincenti, F., Amend, W. J. C., Kaysen, G., Feduska, N., Birnbaum, J., Duca, R., & Salvatierra, O. (1983). Long-term renal function in kidney donors. *Transplantation, 36,* 626–629.

Williams, J. W., Peters, T. G., Vera, S. R., Britt, L. G., VanVoorst, S. J., & Haggit, R. C. (1985). Biopsy directed immunosuppression following hepatic transplantation in man. *Transplantation, 39,* 589–596.

Williams, J. W., Vera, S. R., Peters, T. G., & VanVoorst, S. (1986). Survival following hepatic transplantation in the cyclosporine era. *American Surgeon, 52,* 291–293.

Yao, Q. Y., Rickinson, A. B., Gaston, J. S. H., & Epstein, M. A. (1985). In vitro analysis of the Epstein–Barr virus: Host balance in long-term renal allograft recipients. *International Journal of Cancer, 35,* 43–49.

ADDITIONAL READINGS

Anderson, C. B., Tyler, J. D., Sicard, G. A., Anderman, D. K., Rodey, G. E., & Etheredge, E. E. (1984). Pretreatment of renal allograft recipients with immunosuppression and donor-specific blood. *Transplantation, 38,* 664–668.

Baumgartner, W. M. (1983). Infections in cardiac transplantation. *Heart Transplantation, 3,* 75–80.

Betts, R. F., Freeman, R. B., Douglas, R. G., & Talley, T. E. (1977). Clinical manifestations of renal allograft-derived primary cytomegalovirus infection. *American Journal of Diseases in Children, 131,* 759–763.

Boyle, J., Briggs, J. D., MacKie, R. M., Junor, B. J. R., & Aitchison, T. C. (1984). Cancer, warts, and sunshine in renal transplant patients. *Lancet, 1,* 702–705.

Cosimi, A. B., Colvin, R. B., Burton, R. B., Rubin, R. H., Goldstein, G., Kung, P. C., Hansen, W. P., Delmonico, F. L., & Russell, P. S. (1981). Use of monoclonal antibodies to T-cell subsets for immunologic monitoring and treatment in recipients of renal allografts. *New England Journal of Medicine, 305,* 308–314.

Cuervas-Mons, V., Millan, I., Gavaler, J. S., Starzl, T. E., & Van Theil, D. H. (1986). Prognostic value of preoperatively obtained clinical and laboratory data in predicting survival following orthotopic liver transplantation. *Hepatology, 6,* 922–927.

Diggs, C. L. (1986). Recognition and nursing care of organ donors. *Journal of Emergency Nursing, 12,* 205–209.

Ehrlichman, R. J., Bettman, M., Kirkman, R. L., & Tilney, N. L. (1986). The use of percutaneous nephrostomy in patients with ureteric obstruction undergoing renal transplantation. *Surgery, Gynecology and Obstetrics, 162,* 121–125.

Glass, N. R., Miller, D. T., Sollinger, H. W., & Belzer, F. O. (1985). A four-year experience with donor blood transfusion protocols for living donor renal transplantation. *Transplantation Proceedings, 17,* 1023–1025.

Goldstein, G. (1987). Overview of the development of Orthoclone OKT3: Monoclonal antibody for therapeutic use in transplantation. *Transplantation Proceedings, 19,* 1–6.

Goldstein, L. I. (1986). Postoperative problems. In R. W. Busuttil, Moderator, Liver transplantation today (pp. 379–382). *Annals of Internal Medicine, 104,* 377–389.

Hannegan, L. (1987). Brain death: Diagnosis and dilemma. *Critical Care Nursing Quarterly, 10*(3), 83–91.

Hess, M. L., Hastillo, A., Mohanakumar, T., Cowley, M. J., Vetrovac, G., Szentpetery, S., Wolfgang, T. C., & Lower, R. R. (1983). Accelerated atherosclerosis in cardiac transplantation: Role of cytotoxic B-cell antibodies and hyperlipidemia. *Circulation,* Suppl II, II-94–II-101.

Hirsch, M. S., & Felsenstein, D. (1984). Cytomegalovirus-induced immunosuppression. *Annals of the New York Academy of Sciences, 437,* 8–15.

Hunt, S. A. (1983). Complications of heart transplantation. *Heart Transplantation, 3,* 70–74.

Iwaki, Y., Lau, M., Cook, D. J., Takemoto, S., & Terasaki, P. I. (1986). Crossmatching with B and T cells and flow cytometry. In P. I. Terasaki (Ed.), *Clinical transplants 1986* (pp. 277–284). Los Angeles: UCLA Tissue Typing Laboratory.

Iwaki, Y., & Terasaki, P. I. (1986). Donor-specific transfusion. In P. I. Terasaki (Ed.), *Clinical transplants 1986* (pp. 267–275). Los Angeles: UCLA Tissue Typing Laboratory.

Jamieson, S. W., Oyer, P., Baldwin, J., Billingham, M., Stinson, E., & Shumway, N. (1984). Heart transplantation for end-stage ischemic heart disease: The Stanford experience. *Heart Transplantation, 3,* 75–80.

Jenkins, R. L., Benotti, P., Bothe, A. A., & Rossi, R. L. (1985). Liver transplantation. *Surgical Clinics of North America, 65,* 103–123.

Kahan, B. D. (1987). Immunosuppressive therapy with cyclosporine for cardiac transplantation. *Circulation, 75,* 40–56.

Keith, J. S. (1985). Hepatic failure: Etiologies, manifestations, and management. *Critical Care Nurse, 5,* 60–86.

Kirby, R. M., McMaster, P., Clements, D., Hubscher, S. G., Angrisani, L., Sealy, M., Gunson, B. K., Salt, P. J., Buckels, A. C., Adams, H., Jurewicz, W. A. J., Jain, A. B., & Elias, E. (1987). Orthotopic liver transplantation: Postoperative complications and management. *British Journal of Surgery, 74,* 3–11.

Kupin, W. L., Venkatachalam, K. K., Oh, H. K., Dienst, S., & Levin, N. W. (1985). Sequential use of Minnesota antilymphoblast globulin and cyclosporine in cadaveric renal transplantation. *Transplantation, 40,* 601–604.

Lamb, J. (1980). Cardiac transplantation. *American Journal of Nursing, 80,* 1786–1787.

Leyden, J. J. (1985). Infection in the immunocompromised host. *Archives of Dermatology, 121,* 855–857.

Lieberman, R. P., Glass, N. R., Crummy, A. B., Sollinger, H. W., & Belzer, F. O. (1982). Nonoperative percutaneous management of urinary fistulas and strictures in renal transplantation. *Surgery, Gynecology and Obstetrics, 155,* 667–672.

Light, J. A., Metz, S. J., & Oddenino, K. (1983). Donor-specific transfusion with minimal sensitization. *Transplantation Proceedings, 15,* 917–923.

Mackintosh, A. F., Carmichael, D. J., Wren, C., Cory-Pearce, R., & English, T. A. H. (1982). Sinus node function in first three weeks after cardiac transplantation. *British Heart Journal, 48,* 584–588.

Malkowicz, S. B., & Perloff, L. J. (1985). Urologic considerations in renal transplantation. *Surgery, Gynecology and Obstetrics, 160,* 579–588.

Monaco, A., Goldstein, G., & Barnes, L. (1987). Use of Orthoclone OKT3 monoclonal antibody to reverse acute renal allograft rejection unresponsive to treatment with conventional immunosuppressive regimens. *Transplantation Proceedings, 19,* 28–31.

Morris, P. J. (1984). The immunology of rejection. In P. J. Morris (Ed.), *Kidney transplantation: Principles and practice* (2nd ed.). (pp. 15–32). London: Grune & Stratton.

Morris, P. J., French, M. E., Dunnill, M. S., Hunnisett, A. G. W., Ting, A., Thompson, J. F., & Wood, R. F. M. (1983). A controlled trial of cyclosporine in renal transplantation with conversion to azathioprine with prednisone after three months. *Transplantation, 36,* 273–277.

Painvin, G. A., Frazier, O. H., Chandler, L. B., Cooley, D. A., & Reece, I. J. (1985). Cardiac transplantation: indications, procurement, operation, and management. *Heart and Lung, 14,* 484–489.

Palmer, J. M., & Chatterjee, S. N. (1978). Urologic complications in renal transplantation. *Surgical Clinics of North America, 58,* 305–319.

Ponticelli, C., Rivolta, E., Tarantino, A., Egidi, F., Banfi, G., DeVecchi, A., Montagnino, G., & Vegato, A. (1987). Clinical experience with Orthoclone OKT3 in renal transplantation. *Transplantation Proceedings, 18,* 942–948.

Reece, I. J., Painvin, G. A., Zeluff, B., Chandler, L. B., Okereke, O. U. J., Gentry, L. O., Cooley, D. A., & Frazier, O. H. (1984). Infection in cyclosporine-immunosuppressed cardiac allograft recipients. *Heart Transplantation, 3,* 239–242.

Rubin, R. H., Russell, P. S., Levin, M., & Cohen, C. (1979). Summary of a workshop on cytomegalovirus infections. *Journal of Infectious Disease, 139,* 728–734.

Sigardson-Poor, K. M., & Haggerty, L. M. (Eds.) (1990). *Nursing care of the transplant recipient.* Philadelphia: W. B. Saunders.

Shinn, J. A. (1980). *Cardiac transplantation and the artificial heart.* New York: Appleton-Century-Crofts.

Starzl, T. E., & Fung, J. J. (1987). Orthoclone OKT3 in treatment of allografts rejected under cyclosporine-steroid therapy. *Transplantation Proceedings, 18,* 937–941.

Starzl, T. E., Koep, L. J., Haligrimson, C. G., Hood, J., Schroter, G. P. J., Porter, K. A., & Weil, R., III (1979). Fifteen years of clinical liver transplantation. *Gastroenterology, 77,* 375–388.

Starzl, T. E., Shaw, B. W., & Iwatsuki, S. (1984). The development of immunosuppression. In G. M. Abound (Ed.), *Current status of clinical organ transplantation* (pp. 39–48). Boston: Martinus Nijhoff.

Stinson, E. B., Bieber, C. P., Griepp, R. B. (1971). Infectious complications after cardiac transplantation in man. *Annals of Internal Medicine, 74,* 22–36.

Thistlethwaite, J. R., Cosimi, A. B., Delmonico, F. L., Rubin, R. H., Tolkoff-Rubin, N., Nelson, P. W., Fang, L., & Russell, P. S. (1984). Evolving use of OKT3 monoclonal antibody for treatment of renal allograft rejection. *Transplantation, 38,* 695–701.

Thistlethwaite, J. R., Haag, B. W., Jones, K. W., Stuart, J. K., & Stuart, F. P. (1985). Elective conversion from cyclosporine to azathioprine in recipients with stable renal function 6 months after kidney transplantation. *Human Immunobiology, 14,* 314–323.

Tsakis, A. G., Gordon, R. D., Shaw, B. W., Iwatsuki, S., & Starzl, T. E. (1985). Clinical presentation of hepatic artery thrombosis after liver transplantation in the cyclosporine era. *Transplantation, 40,* 667–671.

Wajszczuk, C. P., Dummer, J. S., Ho, M., Van Theil, D. M., Starzl, T. E., Iwatsuki, S., & Shaw, B., Jr. (1985). Fungal infections in liver transplant recipients. *Transplantation, 40,* 347–353.

Winearls, C. G., Lane, D. J., & Kurtz, J. (1984). Infectious complications after renal transplantation. In P. J. Morris (Ed.), *Kidney transplantation: Principles and practice* (2nd ed.). (pp. 427–467). London: Grune & Stratton.

Winston, D. J., Ho, W. G., Lin, C. H., Budinger, M. D., Champlin, R. E., & Gale, R. P. (1984). Intravenous immunoglobulin for modification of cytomegalovirus infections associated with bone marrow transplantation. *American Journal of Medicine, 76,* 128–133.

Wong, D. T., & Ogra, P. L. (1983). Viral infections in immunocompromised patients. *Medical Clinics of North America, 67,* 1075–1091.

Wozny, P., Zajko, A. B., Bron, K. M., Point, S., & Starzl, T. E. (1986). Vascular complications after liver transplantation: A 5-year experience. *American Journal of Radiology, 147,* 657–663.

21 Trauma

Jill Schoerger Walsh, M.S., R.N.

The morbidity and mortality associated with trauma is an important health issue in the United States today. Statistics show that traumatic injury is the leading cause of death in persons between the ages of 1 and 44 years. More than 140,000 Americans die from traumatic injury each year. Trauma care constitutes an expensive health problem, as approximately $75 to $100 billion is spent on it each year (National Research Council, 1985). Furthermore, such injuries cause the loss of more working-years than heart disease and all forms of cancer combined.

The availability of prehospital emergency care and the rapid transport of patients to acute care centers have increased the number of trauma patients who survive the initial injury and are subsequently admitted to a critical care unit. Care of the patient with multiple-systems injuries is complex and challenging. An understanding of trauma concepts can assist the critical care nurse in the ongoing assessment and management of the trauma patient and in the prevention of potential complications. This chapter will focus on the mechanisms and types of injuries usually seen in the trauma patient and discuss the related nursing diagnoses and interventions. The chapter includes a general section on multiple trauma, which is followed by sections on the effects of trauma in specific organ systems.

OVERVIEW: MULTIPLE TRAUMA

Multiple trauma causes pathophysiologic disruptions and adaptation in virtually every body system. In the initial resuscitation phase of care, the leading causes of death secondary to multiple trauma include airway/breathing disorders, uncontrolled hemorrhage, and massive head injury. Central nervous system injuries alone are responsible for 50% of trauma deaths in the hospital

(Bartkowski, 1984). Among the leading causes of trauma-related deaths that occur several days to weeks after the injury are sepsis (Carpenter, 1987) and multiple organ failure (See chapter 1). Recovery depends on the degree of injury experienced and on the continued presence of adequate oxygenation processes, central nervous system function, protein synthesis, immunologic and antibacterial functions, and wound healing. Other complications that occur secondary to trauma and that can lead to multiple organ failure include heart failure, adult respiratory distress syndrome (ARDS), disseminated intravascular coagulation (DIC), acute renal failure, cerebral edema, small-bowel obstruction, and immune dysfunction. The patient is also at risk for the development of fat embolism if orthopedic injuries are extensive and involve the long bones.

An early response to trauma is the "sick-cell" syndrome, in which aberrations in cellular function can lead to organ failure depending on the number of cells so affected in an organ system. Cellular dysfunction may include altered transport mechanisms, swelling, changes in the membrane potential, and altered excitation and secretion (Groer & Shekleton, 1989).

After a traumatic injury, the body will initially conserve oxygen, heat, and energy. However, 3 to 7 days after the injury a catabolic phase occurs in which hypermetabolism and an increase in oxygen consumption occur. Gluconeogenesis predominates and hyperglycemia, hyperglucagonemia, hypercortisolism, and insulin resistance will be present. Protein is broken down and protein synthesis and tissue repair are retarded as amino acids are used for gluconeogenesis. The caloric needs of the trauma patient are increased as a result: 25% in those patients who experience mild to moderate trauma and 50% in those who experience severe trauma (Groer & Shekleton, 1989). The difficulty meeting the nutritional needs of the trauma patient is discussed in chapter 8.

Another response to trauma is activation of the coagulation cascade, which may lead to the development of thromboemboli. The mechanism of cascade activation is thought to be exposure to tissue collagen. Decreased fibrinolysis occurs within 2 to 5 days after the injury and may contribute to the development of DIC, thrombosis and ARDS. ARDS may also occur in response to complement activation (see chapter 7). Any of these conditions can precipitate the multiple-organ-failure syndrome in the trauma patient.

Trauma patients are at risk for the development of sepsis because of the nature of the injury, which often involves impaired skin integrity and the introduction of pathogenic microorganisms. Additionally, many of the treatments are invasive and the potential for infection is as much a response to the treatment as well as to the actual trauma (Hoyt & Caplan, 1983). Immune system dysfunction, which may occur as a result of stress, the catabolic response to injury, and impaired nutritional status, also contributes to the development of sepsis by impeding the body's normal protective responses to infection. The development of sepsis with fever will further increase metabolic demands and can precipitate multiple organ failure.

INITIAL ASSESSMENT AND MANAGEMENT

It is essential that a rapid initial assessment of the trauma patient be performed. The purpose of the initial evaluation is to identify life-threatening injuries and to intervene rapidly to achieve immediate stabilization. The initial assessment includes the evaluation of the airway, cervical spine, ventilatory status, and circulatory status.

Once life-threatening conditions are under control, the secondary (head-to-toe) survey should be performed. The basic techniques of physical assessment, inspection, palpation, percussion, and auscultation are used to assess the body systems for injury.

The principal diagnostic studies done during the admission process are radiographic. Routine trauma roentgenograms include a portable, lateral cervical spine film (which includes C-7), upright chest film, and pelvic film. X-ray films of the extremities, skull, and abdomen will be ordered as indicated. Nursing responsibilities during radiographic examination include providing explanations of procedures to the patient and family, ensuring the safety of the patient during transfers and repositioning, and coordinating the timing of radiographic examinations and other procedures (Veise-Berry, 1983).

Initially, the full complement of laboratory tests, i.e., complete blood count, blood glucose, electrolytes, blood urea nitrogen, prothrombin time, partial thromboplastin time, amylase, and blood type and cross match should be done in order to establish base-lines for subsequent comparison. Many trauma centers have also established a protocol that includes a blood alcohol level, serum drug screen, and urine drug screen among the routine laboratory tests. The initial urinalysis should include a "dipstick" of the urine for the presence of microscopic hematuria prior to sending the specimen to the laboratory for analysis. Arterial blood gases should be drawn for base-line assessment of respiratory function.

The trauma patient should have a 12-lead electrocardiogram done and should be placed on a cardiac monitor. Dysrhythmias may be present secondary to hypoxia or cardiac injury.

Additional initial management procedures include the insertion of a nasogastric tube and a urinary drainage catheter. The nasogastric tube is necessary to prevent aspiration and abdominal distention. It is also useful for detecting blood in the stomach secondary to trauma. Massive head or facial injuries with a possible cribriform plate fracture are contraindications to the insertion of a nasogastric tube, as the tube may be placed inadvertently through the fracture site into the cranial vault. In these cases, placement of an orogastric tube may be necessary.

The placement of a urinary drainage catheter allows accurate assessment of urinary output, which will facilitate the monitoring of renal perfusion and the hemodynamic response to shock. Prior to the insertion of a urinary catheter a rectal exam must be performed in both male and female patients in order to rule out urethral damage. Insertion of an indwelling urinary catheter is contraindicated if the rectal exam reveals an abnormal or mobile prostate or if blood is present in the rectum or at the urethral meatus.

Open wounds should be cleansed and irrigated with sterile normal saline solution. Pressure dressings may be required in order to control bleeding. Tetanus prophylaxis may need to be administered if immunization has not been maintained or there is uncertainty about the history of immunization. Broad-spectrum antibiotic therapy may be initiated depending on the severity and degree of contamination of the wound.

The presence of gross or microscopic hematuria should be evaluated, requiring either an intravenous pyelogram (IVP) or a computerized tomography (CT) scan. In cases of abdominal trauma, an IVP is indicated for the unstable patient and a CT scan for the stable patient in order to identify the presence of injury and the functioning of the kidneys prior to surgery.

Depending on the type and location of the injury, various other procedures may need to be performed upon admission. These will be identified in the discussion of specific organ injuries in subsequent sections of this chapter.

NURSING DIAGNOSES AND INTERVENTION

The responses to trauma that the critical care nurse must diagnose and treat are both physiologic and psychological in nature. These responses can be overwhelming to both the patient and the family. The traumatic event is likely to have been catastrophic and unexpected, leading to responses of shock, disbelief, grief, and anger, depending on the circumstances. There will be profound physical and emotional stress, confusion, and family and social disruption. The patient's and family's coping abilities may be ineffective because of the complex and overwhelming nature of the event. Other nursing diagnoses that are likely to be present include anxiety, fear, and powerlessness. The assessment, diagnosis, and treatment of psychosocial responses to critical illness are discussed in detail in section II. The trauma patient also has the potential for developing any or all of the nursing diagnoses presented in Table 21–1. Priorities of care will vary over time. Therefore, the order in which these diagnoses are presented may not accurately reflect the priorities for an individual patient. Emergency care will always take precedence over any other patient problems.

HEAD INJURIES

The head is injured in about two thirds of all motor vehicle accidents. Furthermore, head injury is the cause of death in approximately half of the fatalities due to motor vehicle accidents (Bartowski, 1984). Head injury is the

Table 21–1   Nursing Diagnoses and Interventions Associated with Multiple Trauma

Assessment	Planning/Intervention	Expected Outcomes
Nursing Diagnoses: Potential for ineffective airway clearance, impaired gas exchange and ineffective breathing pattern		

Physical signs
  Airway obstruction: restlessness, confusion, apprehension, stridor, absent breath sounds
  Hypoxia: tachypnea, tachycardia, diaphoresis, restlessness, confusion
  Respiratory distress: use of accessory muscles, cyanosis, stridor, wheezing
 	
Laboratory data
  ABG's: increased $PaCO_2$, decreased PaO_2
 	
Subjective data
  Anxiety
  Air hunger
	Immediately after Trauma Nursing Care Aimed at Stabilization
	
	Patent airway
	  Perform jaw thrust maneuver to open airway
	  Prevent hyperextension of the neck
	  Provide finger sweep or suction for mechanical obstruction
	  Monitor for signs and symptoms of respiratory distress
	  Insert a nasopharyngeal airway in the conscious or semiconscious patient to maintain the airway
	  Insert an oropharyngeal airway in the unconscious patient and the patient who has been endotracheally intubated
	  Prepare to assist with endotracheal intubation as indicated
	  Prepare to assist with a criocothyroidotomy for the patient with glottic edema, fractured larynx, or lower maxillofacial trauma
	
	Adequate ventilation
	  Provide high-flow humidified oxygen
	  Monitor serial arterial blood-gas results
	
	Nursing Care after Stabilization
	
	Patent airway
	  Maintain an oropharyngeal airway in the unconscious patient and the unconscious patient who has been endotracheally intubated
	  Prevent airway obstruction due to retained secretions
	
	Adequate ventilation
	  Provide high-flow humidified oxygen
	  Assess respiratory status: note quality of respiration, auscultate chest every hour, check amount, color and consistency of secretions
	  Turn, cough, and/or deep breathe patient every 2 hr
	  Administer pain medication p.r.n. for more effective coughing and breathing
	  Monitor arterial blood-gas results and daily chest films
	  Preoxygenate patient before suctioning
	  Limit suctioning to 10–15 sec in the apneic patient to minimize hypoxia
	  Monitor the ventilator settings and delivered values at least hourly
		Alert and oriented
		
		Quiet respirations without evidence of stridor or wheezing
		
		Arterial blood-gas results within normal limits
		
		Respiratory rate 12–18 breaths/min
		
		Lung physical assessment normal
		
		Chest film normal or no worsening (i.e., patient with pulmonary contusion or pneumonitis—radiography may lag behind clinical improvement)

Nursing Diagnosis: Potential for alteration in tissue perfusion		

Physical signs
  Hypovolemic shock
  Vital signs: tachycardia, hypotension, narrowed pulse pressure
	Immediately after Trauma Nursing Care Aimed at Stabilization
	
	Control external hemorrhage
		Blood pressure, pulse, respiration within normal limits
		
		Skin warm/dry

Table 21–1   *(Continued)*

Assessment	*Planning/Intervention*	*Expected Outcomes*
Prolonged capillary refill (>2 sec) Pale, cool diaphoretic skin ↓ Mean arterial pressure ↓ PCWP or ↓ CVP ↓ Urinary output Laboratory data CBC: ↓ Hgb, ↓ Hct ↑ Urine specific gravity BUN, creatinine Electrolytes Subjective data Thirst, anxiety, nausea	Initiate two large-bore IV lines of crystalloid, replace at 3:1 ratio (3 ml crystalloid for every 1 ml blood loss) Establish base-line vital signs Anticipate order for fluid challenge Apply military antishock trousers (MAST), inflate to maintain a systolic blood pressure of 90 mm Hg Position patient in modified Trendelenburg position Establish base-line laboratory values Insert a Foley catheter to monitor renal perfusion and hourly urine output Assist physician with the insertion of an arterial line, central venous or pulmonary artery line to monitor hemodynamic pressures Administer blood transfusions as ordered **Nursing Care after Stabilization** Monitor vital signs every hour Monitor ECG continuously, document heart rate and rhythm on chart every 4 hr and p.r.n. Monitor CVP every 4 hr or PCWP every 2 hr or as necessary Monitor hourly urine output, maintain accurate records of intake and output Monitor laboratory values Administer fluids and blood products as ordered and assess patient response Administer antacids and/or cimetidine as ordered to prevent stress ulcer With Salem pump in place check pH of aspirate as ordered	Mean arterial pressure within normal limits for patient CVP or PCWP within normal limits for patient Urine output >30 ml/hr Arterial blood-gas values, serum electrolytes, PT, PTT, and platelet count within normal limits Capillary refill time <2 sec

Nursing Diagnosis: Potential for infection related to impaired skin integrity and altered immune and nutritional status secondary to stress

Physical signs Wound infection: redness, heat, tenderness, elevated temperature, swelling and/or induration of wound area, purulent drainage, unusual odor Respiratory infection: elevated temperature, increased amount of secretions, tachypnea Systemic infections: fever, tachycardia, fluctuating B/P, changes in level of consciousness, hyperpnea, oliguria	**Immediately after Trauma Nursing Care Aimed at Stabilization** Culture wounds before cleansing Cleanse wounds using sterile technique; irrigate with normal saline Apply sterile dressings to the wounds Administer prophylactic antibiotics as ordered Use sterile technique with suctioning and invasive procedures and treatments to avoid introducing bacteria into the patient Maintain NPO status to prevent aspiration during surgery	Afebrile Cultures negative Leukocyte count within normal limits Surgical wound is clean, dry, and healing properly

Table 21–1 *(Continued)*

Assessment	Planning/Intervention	Expected Outcomes

Laboratory data
  Positive wound culture
  Positive sputum culture
  Positive blood culture
  Elevated leukocyte count
  ↓ PaO$_2$ on arterial blood gases
 	
Subjective data
  Pain
  Apprehension, anxiety
  Dyspnea
	Nursing Care after Stabilization
	
	Monitor blood pressure and P–R interval every hour and temperature every 4 hr. If temperature is greater than 39.8°C (rectal) send wound, blood, urine, and sputum cultures for analysis
	
	Monitor leukocyte count daily
	
	Administer antibiotics as ordered
	
	Administer antipyretics as ordered
	
	Use strict aseptic technique when changing dressings
	
	Assess for signs of wound infection
	
	Use sterile technique with suctioning and fluid lines	

	Nursing Diagnosis: Impaired physical mobility	

Atelectasis
 	
Physical signs
  Restlessness, tachypnea, tachycardia, dullness on percussion, fever
  Chest film—patches of consolidation
Laboratory data
  Arterial blood gases: decreasing PaO$_2$
  Positive sputum cultures
  Elevated leukocyte count
Subjective data
  Apprehension
 	
Pulmonary embolus
 	
Physical signs
  Hypoxia: dyspnea, tachypnea, restlessness, irritability, fever
  Signs of acute right heart failure: atrial dysrhythmias, CVP readings, distended neck veins
Laboratory data
  Arterial blood gases: decreased PaO$_2$, decreased PaCO$_2$
Subjective data
  Chest pain
  Apprehension
 	
Impaired skin integrity
 	
Physical signs
  Small or large areas of redness
  Serous fluid, pus, or bleeding
  Raw appearance
Subjective data
  Aching pain, soreness
	Immediately after Trauma Nursing Care Aimed at Stabilization
	
	Reposition patient every 2 hr
	
	Nursing Care after Stabilization
	
	Perform ongoing assessment for signs and symptoms of atelectasis
	
	Turn, cough, deep breathe patient every 2 hr
	
	Position patient to facilitate lung expansion (↑ head of bed)
	
	Encourage oral fluids (is permitted)
	
	Perform chest physical therapy
	
	Encourage incentive spirometry
	
	Perform ongoing assessments for signs and symptoms of pulmonary embolism
	
	Apply antiembolism stockings postoperatively—remove for 1 hr of shift, if ordered
	
	Assist with range-of-motion exercises as ordered
	
	Assess bony prominences for evidence of skin breakdown
	
	Wash, apply lotion, and massage pressure points
	
	Place patient on sheepskin or silicone pad
	
	Change position frequently
	
	Apply heel protectors
	
	Use foot board to prevent foot drop
		Breath sounds normal
		
		Chest roentgenogram within normal limits
		
		No complaints of shortness of breath or chest pain
		
		Skin remains pink, warm and intact

Table 21–1   *(Continued)*

Assessment	Planning/Intervention	Expected Outcomes
	Nursing Diagnosis: Pain	
Subjective complaints of pain	Administer analgesics p.r.n.	Verbalizes absence of discomfort
Restlessness	Distraction and relaxation techniques	
Changes in vital signs	Repositioning	

PCWP = pulmonary capillary wedge pressure; CVP = central venous pressure; CBC = complete blood count; Hgb = hemoglobin; Hct = hematocrit; BUN = blood urea nitrogen; ECG = electrocardiogram; PT = prothrombin time; PTT = partial thromboplastin time

leading cause of death in the trauma patient (Carpenter, 1987). In addition, much of the disability that is experienced by the survivors of trauma results from brain injury.

Three mechanisms of injury can be identified: localized injury, crush injury, and acceleration/deceleration injury. Localized injury may be caused by either penetrating or blunt forces. Lacerations and contusions may result from minor and/or severe trauma. The severity of cerebral dysfunction and the manifestation of signs and symptoms is related to the site of impact and the area of the brain that has been affected.

A crush injury occurs as a result of the stationary head being compressed between opposing forces. Actual injury to the brain may or may not occur, as the skull acts as a shock absorber and dissipates the force.

The mechanism with the most diffuse injury is the acceleration/deceleration injury, which may occur as a result of a motor vehicle accident or the striking of the head. This mechanism causes a coup–contre coup pattern of brain trauma. That is to say, when a sudden impact sets the brain in motion against the bony structure within the skull, injury results at the point of impact (coup phenomenon) as well as at the point opposite the impact (contre coup phenomenon). Furthermore, the motion of the brain on rebound is rotary. Therefore, there is a torsion effect that occurs on impact; the main site of this torsion is the brain stem. The resultant brain-stem contusion causes a disruption of the electrical activity in the reticular activating system, with the result of transient loss of consciousness. Generally, there is little damage to the scalp or skull; however, the brain can be seriously injured as a result of tissue disruption and/or hemorrhage.

Trauma to the head can injure the scalp, skull, and/or brain. Frequently, the type of injury is described solely by the presence or absence of injury to the skull. The prognosis for recovery, however, is directly related to the presence or absence of injury to the brain. Trauma to the head may produce two types of injury. The primary injury (i.e., laceration, fracture) is generally self limited. The secondary injury, that resulting from the development of cerebral edema and/or increased intracranial pressure, represents the physiologic response of the brain to the primary injury. The secondary injury to the brain occurs as a result of the initial force, and is due to hypoxia, edema, an altered blood–brain barrier, or infection. In many cases the secondary injury can be far more serious than the primary injury. The pathophysiology of the secondary injury related to the presence of cerebral edema and/or increased intracranial pressure is discussed in detail in chapter 13.

Primary head injuries include closed head injury, open head injury, and injuries to the brain. Most patients with closed head injuries will require hospitalization. Closed head injuries can be classified as mild, moderate, or severe depending on the amount of neurological changes. Serious brain injury is more common when no skull fracture is present. If a major skull fracture is present, there is less brain-tissue damage because the energy has been dissipated.

Open head injuries involve a break in the skull or dura. The cerebral dysfunction that results from this injury will depend on the site of trauma. A basilar skull fracture is difficult to recognize on skull roentgenograms. Diagnosis is usually made clinically or from the CT scan. Clinical signs include rhinorrhea or otorrhea, which contains cerebrospinal fluid, hematotympanum (blood behind the eardrum), Battle's sign (bruising over the mastoid bone), and Raccoon's sign (periorbital ecchymosis).

Injuries to the brain are classified as either diffuse brain injury or focal brain injury. Focal brain injuries refer to cerebral contusion, epidural hematoma, subdural hematoma, and intracerebral hemorrhage.

A cerebral contusion is present when bruising or edema occurs in the brain as a result of intracranial trauma. The contused frontotemporal area is particularly likely to swell from edema formation. Brain swelling in association with a cerebral contusion is a leading cause of death from head injury in the first 24 hours (Clark, 1985).

Blood that accumulates between the skull and the dura mater is referred to as an epidural hematoma (Figure 21–1). This type of injury is commonly associated with an accompanying linear skull fracture and tearing of the middle meningeal artery. Signs and symptoms may include a short period of unconsciousness followed by a lucid interval. The patient may then again become unresponsive as intracranial pressure rises. The presence of a lucid interval, while frequently diagnostic of an epidural hematoma, may not always occur. The patient may not lose consciousness immediately after the injury, or conversely, may not regain consciousness after an initial period of unconsciousness. Relying on the presence or absence of the lucid interval is one of the pitfalls of early diagnosis of epidural hemorrhage. The mortality rate associated with this injury is about 20% (Clark, 1985).

The most serious hemorrhage in closed head injuries is an acute subdural hematoma, which results from venous bleeding into the space between the dura mater and the arachnoid space (Figure 21–2). The mortality rate is about 70% (Clark, 1985). If the patient is identified early and the hematoma is evacuated within 4 hours of injury, the prognosis for recovery is significantly improved. In other words, the time from identification to drainage or evacua-

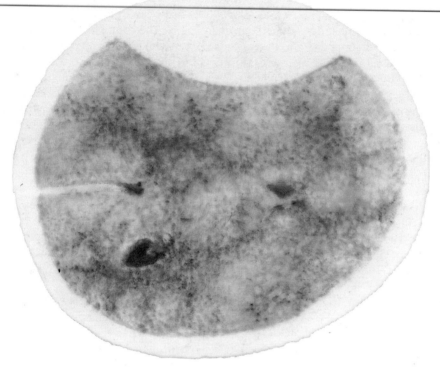

Figure 21–1. Computerized tomography (CT) scan demonstrating a left epidural hematoma characterized by the lens (biconvex) configuration associated with a shift of the ventricles.

tion is the key in determining outcome. Death in patients with an acute subdural hematoma is due to a sudden rise in intracranial pressure, with a loss of cerebral perfusion pressure.

Diffuse brain injury includes cerebral concussion and diffuse axonal injury. A cerebral concussion causes a temporary disturbance of neurological function, most likely as a result of transient ischemia. Symptoms of a concussion include a temporary loss of consciousness and evidence of retrograde amnesia. Classic concussion refers to a period of unconsciousness of usually less than five minutes and no longer than six hours.

The most severe form of diffuse brain injury is diffuse axonal injury (DAI). This injury differs from concussion in the degree of injury. The hallmark of DAI is immediate and prolonged coma, greater than six hours in duration. This prolonged coma is caused by severe widespread damage of the conducting white matter. Since the damage is microscopic in nature, radiographic studies are not useful in diagnosing DAI. The severity of DAI is diagnosed by the patient's clinical characteristics and the duration of the coma.

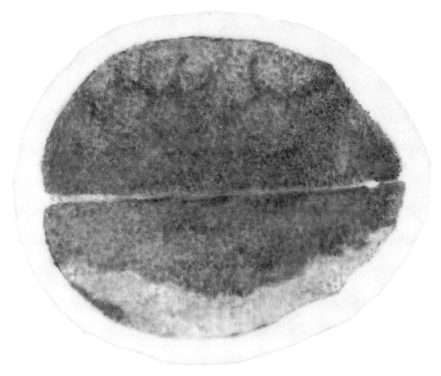

Figure 21–2. Computerized tomography (CT) scan demonstrating a right subdural hematoma. This type of hematoma resembles a smudge mark.

Diagnostic Procedures and Definitive Care

The use of skull x-ray films in the initial management of the head-injured patient is somewhat controversial. While there may be a low yield of positive findings, skull x-ray films may be very valuable in diagnosing significant fractures.

Computerized tomography has literally revolutionized the treatment of the head-injured patient. Intracranial bone, air, hematomas, and edema can be detected. Computerized tomography can determine the need for surgical decompression and can be useful in predicting outcome. The use of angiography has been markedly reduced since the advent of computerized tomography. Angiography still is valuable, however, in a patient with a penetrating injury of the head and/or neck.

The leading cause of death in head-injured patients during the first 24 hours is cerebral edema and increased intracranial pressure. All patients with severe head injury, i.e., Glasgow coma score of 8 or less (Table 21–2), should be intubated and hyperventilated as soon as possible. Arterial blood

Table 21–2   Glasgow Coma Scale

Reaction	Stimulus	Score
Eye opening	Spontaneous	4
	Voice	3
	Pain	2
	None	1
Verbal response	Oriented	5
	Confused	4
	Inappropriate words	3
	Incomprehensible words	2
	None	1
Motor response	Obeys command	6
	Localizes pain	5
	Withdraw (pain)	4
	Flexion (pain)	3
	Extension (pain)	2
	None	1
	Best Possible Total =	15

gases should be drawn and the $PaCO_2$ reduced to 25 to 28 torr. Hyperventilation rapidly produces venous vascular constriction and causes a reduction in intracranial bulk. The FiO_2 (fraction of inspired oxygen) on the ventilator should be set at 100%. Drainage of cerebrospinal fluid (CSF) is an effective method of controlling intracranial pressure (ICP) in patients with large or at least normal ventricles. An intraventricular catheter (Figure 21–3) allows for the immediate drainage of CSF and therefore immediate reduction of ICP. However, as CSF is produced at a rate of 20 ml/hr, this may be only a temporary reduction of ICP. ICP monitoring is indicated for patients with severe closed head trauma, a Glasgow coma score of 8 or less, patients with significant intracranial hemorrhage or edema, or those with a shift of the ventricular system as shown on CT scan (Clark, 1985). Additional information regarding the procedure for intracranial pressure monitoring is included in chapter 19.

Osmotic diuretic agents are the most commonly used drugs for lowering intracranial pressure. Osmotic diuretic agents such as mannitol are frequently used for removal of extracellular fluid within the brain. While the mechanism of action of these agents is complex and not completely understood, it appears that mannitol has its effect on cerebral edema by removing fluid from the normal brain tissue. In effect, the edema in the traumatized tissue is

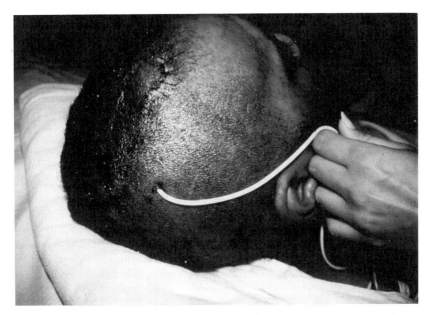

Figure 21–3. Placement of an external ventricular drainage catheter. The scalp incision and underlying burr hole are positioned over the anterior horn of the right lateral ventricle. In order to avoid a direct route for pathogens to invade the cerebral tissue, the catheter is tunneled subcutaneously to an exit site some distance from the entrance site. Courtesy of Foster G. McGaw Hospital, Loyola University Medical Center, Maywood, IL.

untouched. Moreover, the administration of mannitol improves the microcirculation around the areas of brain injury, and in fact this may be its most beneficial effect (Clark, 1985). Marked diuresis follows administration of these agents. Loop diuretics such as furosemide (Lasix), which are less widely used, appear to remove the fluid from the edematous, injured tissue as well as the normal brain tissue.

Craniotomy may be indicated for patients with skull fractures in order to debride bone fragments and necrotic tissue from normal brain tissue and to elevate and realign bone fragments. Intracranial bleeds may be surgically evacuated through burr holes or a craniotomy may need to be performed. As a last resort, surgical decompression may also be used in the management of cerebral edema.

Barbiturate coma can be a valuable adjunct in the management of patients whose ICP cannot be controlled by conventional therapy. High doses of barbiturates decrease intracranial pressure by effecting a reduction in cerebral metabolic rate and cerebral blood flow. Systemic blood pressure is also reduced. This helps to reduce cerebral edema through a reduction in hydrostatic pressure.

Nursing Diagnoses

In addition to the nursing diagnoses for the multiple trauma patient, the head-injured patient requires the nursing assessment and interventions presented in Table 21–3.

THORACIC TRAUMA

Trauma to the thorax occurs in 50% of all fatal accidents and is the cause of death in 25% (Trunkey, 1984a). Blunt trauma to the chest occurs more frequently than penetrating chest trauma in all but urban areas.

Three mechanisms of injury can be identified as causes of blunt trauma to the chest. Direct blows to the thorax may result in chest-wall injury. Deceleration injuries may result in a pulmonary contusion, cardiac contusion, aortic tear, and/or tracheobronchial tear. Compression injuries of the chest include aortic tear, cardiac rupture, diaphragm rupture, and membranous tracheal blowout.

Stab wounds and gunshot wounds are examples of penetrating trauma. Stab wounds generally cause less destruction than bullet wounds. The extent of injury is based on several factors. The location of the wound as well as the length of the object used to inflict the wound must be considered in the case of a stabbing injury. It is also important to determine if the weapon was manipulated once the victim was stabbed. If the penetrating object is still protruding through the chest wall at the time of evaluation, it should not be removed until the patient is in the operating room.

Factors that affect the extent of tissue injury in gunshot wounds include the velocity, the trajectory, the mass of the bullet, and the firing distance. The magnitude of the injury is proportional to the amount of kinetic energy imparted by the bullet to the victim. For example, handguns, which cause low-velocity injuries, transfer little kinetic energy to the tissue along the bullet's path. Therefore the wound generally involves tissue destruction approximately the same diameter as that of the bullet.

High-velocity missiles, in contrast, impart tremendous amounts of kinetic energy in the form of shock waves. A temporary cavity of up to 20 to 30 times the diameter of the bullet may be formed. Therefore, tissue that is not directly in the area along the bullet track may be disrupted. In addition, high-velocity missiles often have an erratic trajectory through the tissue as they may bounce and ricochet, thereby causing more extensive tissue damage.

Injuries to the chest may be subdivided into two categories: immediately life-threatening and potentially life-threatening. The immediately life-threatening injuries include airway obstruction, open "sucking" pneumothorax, tension pneumothorax, massive hemothorax, flail chest, and cardiac tamponade. The potentially life-threatening injuries include pulmonary contusion,

Table 21–3 Nursing Diagnoses and Interventions Associated with Head Injury

Assessment	Planning/Intervention	Expected Outcomes
Nursing Diagnoses: Potential for ineffective breathing patterns and impaired gas exchange		
Abnormal respiratory patterns: Cheyne–Stokes respiration, central neurogenic hyperventilation, apneusis, cluster breathing, ataxic breathing ↓ PaO_2 and ↑ $PaCO_2$ levels	Intracranial pressure is highly sensitive to arterial PaO_2, $PaCO_2$, pH. Cerebral vasodilation, occurs when PaO_2 drops below 50 mm Hg. **Immediately after Trauma Nursing Care Aimed at Stabilization** Administer paralyzing agents as ordered Monitor the ventilator settings and delivered values at least hourly Monitor arterial blood-gas results **Nursing Care after Stabilization** Administer paralyzing agents as ordered Monitor the ventilator settings and delivered values at least hourly Monitor arterial blood-gas results	Patient not struggling against the ventilator Arterial blood gases within desired limits for patient, usually PaO_2, 80–100 mm Hg, and $PaCO_2$, 25–30 mm Hg
Nursing Diagnosis: Potential for hemodynamic instability		

Physical signs
  Hypovolemic shock
  See Table 21–1
 	
Diabetes Insipidus
 	
Physical signs
  Polyuria
 	
Laboratory data
  Urine specific gravity, 1.001 to 1.005
  Slightly elevated hematocrit and serum sodium levels
 	
Subjective data
  Excessive thirst in the alert patient
	A normotensive state should be maintained in order to promote autoregulation of cerebral blood flow.
	
	Immediately after Trauma Nursing Care Aimed at Stabilization and Cardiovascular Support
	
	Assist physician with the insertion of an arterial pressure line
	
	Monitor arterial blood pressure in order to assess cerebral perfusion pressure
	
	Administer fluids as ordered to maintain a systolic blood pressure of at least 100 mm Hg
	
	Administer vasoactive agents as ordered to maintain a systolic blood pressure between 100 and 180 mm Hg
	
	Nursing Care after Stabilization—Cardiovascular Support
	
	Monitor arterial blood pressure at least hourly
	
	Administer fluids as ordered to maintain a systolic blood pressure of at least 100 mm Hg
	
	Administer vasoactive agents as ordered to maintain a systolic blood pressure between 100 and 180 mm Hg
	
	Monitor response to osmotic diuretic agents and diuretics
	
	Monitor urine specific gravity to distinguish between induced diuresis and diabetes insipidus
	
	Monitor serum electrolytes
	
	Administer vasopressin as ordered to treat diabetes insipidus
		Blood pressure, pulse within normal limits
		
		Mean arterial pressure within normal limits
		
		Pulmonary capillary wedge pressure within normal limits
		
		Urinary output within normal limits

Table 21–3 *(Continued)*

Assessment	Planning/Intervention	Expected Outcomes
	Prepare to assist the physician in inserting a pulmonary artery line to monitor hemodynamic pressures in the patient in barbiturate coma	
	Prepare to administer vasopressor and/or colloids to the patient in barbiturate coma	

Nursing Diagnosis: Altered level of consciousness

Physical signs
  Level of consciousness:
    Glasgow coma scale
  Pupils
  Cranial nerves
  Motor: skeletal muscle,
    reflexes
	Immediately after Trauma Nursing Care Aimed at Stabilization
	
	Decrease intracranial pressure
	  Administer osmotic diuretic agents (mannitol) and diuretics as ordered
	  Prepare to assist with endotracheal intubation
	  Monitor arterial blood gases to maintain a $PaCO_2$ of 25–30 torr, as ordered
	  Monitor vital and neurological signs
	  Keep head in midline, neutral position to avoid jugular venous compression
	  Place head of bed at 30–60 degrees
	  Prevent Valsalva maneuvers
	  Prevent flexion and hyperextension of the neck
	  Monitor patients being mechanically ventilated and on PEEP closely, since PEEP may cause an increase in ICP
	  Administer lidocaine, 50 mg IV push, as ordered to prevent an increase in ICP when certain procedures such as suctioning are performed
	  Space out nursing activities known to increase ICP (suctioning, positioning)
	
	Decrease cerebral edema
	  Maintain fluid restriction as ordered
	  Monitor hourly intake–output
	  Maintain IV fluid rate as ordered
	  Maintain normothermia with acetaminophen
	  Place patient on cooling mattress, as ordered
	  Administer corticosteroids if ordered (controversial)
	
	Nursing Care after Stabilization
	
	Decrease intracranial pressure
	  Administer osmotic diuretic agents (mannitol), diuretics, or barbiturates as ordered
	  Monitor arterial blood-gases to maintain a $PaCO_2$ of 25–35 torr as ordered
	  Monitor vital and neurological signs, mean arterial pressure
	  Monitor ICP readings and wave forms
	  Drain CSF from intraventricular catheter, as ordered
	  Keep head in midline, neutral position, avoid flexion of the neck
	  Place head of bed at 30–60 degrees
	  Prevent Valsalva maneuvers
		Alert and oriented
		
		Pupils will be equal and reactive to light
		
		Deep tendon reflexes will be normal
		
		High Glasgow coma score

Table 21–3   *(Continued)*

Assessment	Planning/Intervention	Expected Outcomes
	Administer lidocaine, 50 mg IV push, as ordered Monitor patients being mechanically ventilated and on PEEP closely since PEEP may cause an increase in ICP Space out nursing activities known to increase ICP (suctioning, positioning) Administer phenytoin as ordered to prevent seizure activity Administer codeine as ordered for relief of headache Decrease cerebral edema Maintain fluid restrictions to produce mild dehydration as ordered Monitor hourly intake–output Maintain IV fluid rate to prevent hypotension Maintain normothermia with acetaminophen, cooling mattress Administer corticosteroids if ordered (controversial)	

Nursing Diagnosis: Potential for infection—Meningitis

Assessment	Planning/Intervention	Expected Outcomes

Physical signs
  Deterioration in level of consciousness
  Nuchal rigidity
  Fever
  Seizures
  Photophobia, nystagmus
  Vomiting
  Tachycardia
  Positive Kernig's signs
Laboratory data
  Positive wound culture
  Elevated serum white-cell count
  CSF findings
    White-cell count 10,000–20,000/mm³
    Cell type—mostly polymorphonuclear cells
    ↑ Protein, ↓ glucose, ↓ chloride
Subjective data
  Pain
  Violent headache
	Immediately after Trauma Nursing Care Aimed at Stabilization
	Cleanse scalp wounds thoroughly
	Use aseptic technique to dress wounds
	Administer antibiotics as ordered
	
	Nursing Care after Stabilization
	Use sterile technique with ICP monitoring device
	Administer antibiotics as ordered
	Monitor patients on steroids closely for signs of masked infection
	Check head dressing frequently for signs of drainage
	Check wound drains (note amount and kind of drainage)
	Change dressings every 24–48 hr
	Monitor for signs of further infection (osteomyelitis, meningitis, or brain abscess)
		Afebrile
		Cultures negative
		White-cell count within normal limits

Nursing Diagnosis: Potential for physical injury related to seizure activity

Assessment	Planning/Intervention	Expected Outcomes

Physical signs
  Twitching at the corner of the mouth or eye
  Grand mal tonic–clonic seizure activity
Laboratory data
  Phenytoin and phenobarbital levels
	Immediately after Trauma Nursing Care Aimed at Stabilization
	Administer anticonvulsants as ordered
	Maintain normothermia through use of antipyretics, cooling blanket or sponging
	Pad side rails
		Absence of seizure activity
		Absence of injury secondary to seizure activity
		Phenytoin and phenobarbital levels within therapeutic range

Table 21–3   *(Continued)*

Assessment	Planning/Intervention	Expected Outcomes
	Nursing Care Post Stabilization	
Subjective data	Administer anticonvulsants as ordered	
Patient may describe an "aura" prior to seizure activity	Monitor laboratory results for therapeutic levels of anticonvulsants	
	Maintain normothermia	
	Pad side rails	
	Maintain quiet environment	
	Monitor patient for respiratory depression, cardiac dysrhythmias, and hypotension with use of IV phenytoin and diazepam	

PEEP = positive end expiratory pressure; ICP = intracranial pressure; CSF = cerebrospinal fluid.

myocardial contusion, aortic rupture or tear, tracheobronchial tear injury, rupture of the diaphragm, and esophageal rupture.

An airway obstruction is the most common cause of inadequate ventilation. Foreign material such as blood, vomitus, or displaced teeth may obstruct the airway. In the unconscious patient, relaxation of the soft tissues of the pharynx and the patient's tongue may occlude the airway. Another cause may be edema of the soft tissue. Signs and symptoms of an airway obstruction include restlessness, confusion, apprehension, or air hunger; stridor or wheezing; an inability to speak; sonorous respirations; cyanosis; or absent breath sounds. In order to open and maintain the airway initially, suctioning, use of the jaw-thrust maneuver, and the insertion of a nasopharyngeal airway may be necessary. An oropharyngeal airway is generally contraindicated in the conscious or semiconscious trauma patient since it may stimulate the gag reflex and cause vomiting and possible aspiration of gastric contents. Definitive care may include endotracheal intubation or cricothyroidotomy.

An open "sucking" pneumothorax generally results from penetrating injury to the chest. As a result of the negative, subatmospheric pressure in the chest, the positive-pressure atmospheric air rushes in through the wound, thereby creating a "sucking" effect. Signs and symptoms include a "sucking" noise, bleeding from the wound, cyanosis, respiratory distress, and decreased or absent breath sounds. Arterial blood gases will show an increased $PaCO_2$ and a decreased PaO_2. Treatment includes immediate covering of the hole with a sterile three-sided vaseline dressing, which is applied at the time of forced end expiration. This allows the fourth side to act as a flutter valve. As soon as possible, a chest tube should be inserted through a separate incision in order to reexpand the affected lung.

A tension pneumothorax may be caused by either blunt or penetrating forces. By definition, a tension pneumothorax refers to a collapsed lung under pressure (see Figure 17–4). A tear in the lung or pleura acts as a one-way valve. Air enters the intrapleural space on inspiration but cannot exit on expiration. As pressure increases, the lung tissue collapses. If the tension pneumothorax is severe enough, it can compress the lung on the unaffected side as well as the trachea, the heart, and the great vessels. Signs and symptoms of a tension pneumothorax include respiratory distress, cyanosis, decreased or absent breath sounds on the affected side, jugular venous distention, hypotension, deviated trachea, and hyperresonance to percussion. The immediate lifesaving intervention is the insertion of a large-bore needle into the second intercostal space along the midclavicular line to relieve the tension. Decompression is followed by insertion of a chest tube.

Blunt trauma with a penetrating rib fracture can cause the accumulation of a large volume of blood within the pleural space. A massive hemothorax may be caused by pulmonary lacerations from rib fractures, laceration of an intercostal artery, or a ruptured bronchus. Signs and symptoms of a massive hemothorax include cyanosis, respiratory distress, decreased or absent breath sounds, dullness to percussion, hypovolemic shock, and flat neck veins. Autotransfusion or rapid volume replacement is needed to stabilize the vital signs before chest-tube insertion (Figure 21–4).

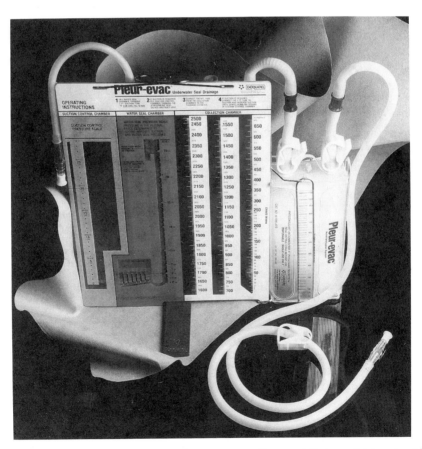

Figure 21–4. Pleur-evac Autotransfusion system allows reinfusion of the patient's own blood, which has been lost as a result of a massive hemothorax. Courtesy of DEKNATEL, Fall River, Mass.

A flail chest refers to three or more continuous ribs broken in two or more places. This segment of the chest wall no longer has integrity with the rest of the bony thorax and therefore moves independently from the rest of the thorax. This results in paradoxical breathing, since on inspiration, as negative intrathoracic pressure increases, the flail segment collapses inward and on expiration, as negative pressure decreases, the flail segment expands outward. Therefore, minimal or no ventilation occurs on the affected side of the chest. Initially, muscular guarding may prevent the development of paradoxical breathing. Later though, when lung compliance decreases as a result of pulmonary contusion and pain control, the flail becomes obvious. Signs and symptoms of a flail chest, and the inevitable underlying lung contusion, include rapid, shallow respirations; cyanosis; chest-wall pain; and asymmetrical chest-wall movement. Arterial blood gases will show hypoventilation. Endotracheal intubation and positive-pressure ventilation in conjunction with adequate analgesia may be required to assist respiratory exchange.

Cardiac tamponade can be caused by either blunt or penetrating trauma, although most commonly it is caused by penetrating injury (Trunkey, 1984a). Blood accumulates in the pericardial sac and exerts pressure on the heart. Diastolic filling and systolic output are both affected. Signs and symptoms include Beck's triad (classic signs of cardiac tamponade, including hypotension, neck-vein distention and distant muffled heart sounds), narrowed pulse pressure, elevated central venous pressure, pulsus paradoxus, anxiety, apprehension, and respiratory distress. Initially, a pericardiocentesis may be necessary to relieve the pressure. Generally, prompt thoracotomy, pericardial decompression and repair of the myocardial wound is the treatment of choice for most patients (Trunkey, 1984a).

Pulmonary contusion is a potentially life-threatening injury that typically progresses in size and density for 24 to 48 hours (Shin, 1987). A pulmonary contusion, or bruise of the lung, is usually associated with rib fractures and occurs in a large number of patients with chest injury. Overhydration must be avoided to prevent the development of the adult respiratory distress syndrome.

A myocardial contusion refers to a bruise or intramural hematoma of the myocardial wall as a result of blunt trauma to the chest. An elevated creatine kinase (CK) MB isoenzyme of more than 5% is generally considered indicative of myocardial contusion. The 12-lead electrocardiogram often reveals nonspecific ST–T-wave changes. In addition, dysrhythmias, most commonly sinus tachycardia, frequently are present. Ventricular dysrhythmias as a result of myocardial contusion should be treated with standard antiarrhythmic agents. Serial electrocardiograms and cardiac isoenzymes are obtained for the first three days post injury. It should be noted that suspicion or evidence of myocardial contusion is not a contraindication for surgical intervention for other traumatic injuries.

Aortic injury may occur as a result of severe deceleration injuries or penetrating injuries. Before the establishment of prehospital emergency care systems, most patients with an aortic rupture or tear died before arriving at the hospital. Today, however, because of prehospital stabilization and rapid transportation to an emergency care facility, more of these patients are surviving this life-threatening injury. On chest roentgenography, rupture of the thoracic aorta secondary to blunt trauma may be identified by either a widened mediastinum or obliteration of the aortic knob. Immediate thoracotomy and repair of the injured vessel are required.

Tracheobronchial tear injury is most often the result of penetrating trauma, but may occur as a result of a compression injury such as hitting the chest against the steering wheel. Signs and symptoms include respiratory distress, the presence of subcutaneous emphysema, and hemoptysis. Endotracheal intubation, chest-tube insertion, and thoracotomy may be necessary.

A ruptured diaphragm occurs secondary to penetrating or blunt trauma. The left hemidiaphragm is more frequently injured, as the right diaphragm is protected by the liver. Bowel obstruction or strangulation may occur if the lesion goes undetected or untreated. Signs and symptoms include respiratory distress, bowel sounds audible in the left lower chest, ipsilateral hemothorax, and referred shoulder pain.

Esophageal rupture may be caused by both blunt and penetrating forces. In blunt trauma, rupture occurs just above the diaphragm, whereas in cases of penetrating trauma, the rupture is often at the pharyngoesophageal junction. Signs and symptoms include the sudden onset of severe chest or upper abdominal pain, increased respirations, subcutaneous emphysema, pneumothorax, pain on swallowing, and the presence of gastric contents in the chest tube.

Diagnostic Procedures and Definitive Care

The highest priority of patient care is always the establishment of an adequate airway. Endotracheal intubation and mechanical ventilation may be necessary to gain control over the airway and to provide for adequate ventilation. Unconscious patients are best treated with an invasive airway. Multiple rib fractures and flail chest require aggressive airway management if ventilatory difficulty is present.

An initial chest x-ray film can be valuable in identifying rib fractures, pneumothorax, atelectasis, and great-vessel injury. Whether due to blunt or penetrating trauma, 80 to 90% of all chest injuries are adequately treated by insertion of one or more chest tubes and do not require open thoracotomy (Trunkey, 1984a). In order to drain both fluid and air effectively, a large-bore siliconized tube (32 to 40 French) should be inserted in the midaxillary line at the level of the nipple or higher.

Emergency department thoracotomy offers the only chance of successful resuscitation for the injured patient who has sustained or is about to sustain cardiac arrest. This surgical procedure succeeds most often in patients with penetrating cardiac thoracic injury (Trunkey, 1984a). In cases in which the patient with a penetrating cardiac or thoracic injury or blunt chest injury presents with absence of vital signs and is in asystole, successful resuscitation is unlikely; therefore it may not be appropriate to perform a thoracotomy in the resuscitation area.

Nursing Diagnoses

In addition to the nursing diagnoses for the multiple trauma patient, the patient with a thoracic injury requires the nursing assessment and interventions presented in Table 21–4.

ABDOMINAL TRAUMA

Abdominal trauma is often treated surgically. These patients are usually critically ill, either because of the extent of the trauma or the operative procedure required to repair the effects of the traumatic injury. Mortality rates depend not only on the organ injured and the extent of the injury to that organ but also on the extent of injury to other systems. The severity of injury may be masked by drug or alcohol intoxication, head and spinal cord injuries, or decreased cerebral perfusion due to hypovolemia.

Traumatic injury to the abdomen can be classified as either blunt or penetrating. Penetrating trauma is usually the result of stabbing or gunshot injuries, while blunt trauma is most often associated with sports injuries or motor vehicle accidents. Blunt trauma results in a higher mortality rate than penetrating injuries (Flint, 1987). Epidemiologic reviews suggest that the combined effects of the use of restraints and slower speeds have contributed to a redistribution of injuries, with fewer fatal head injuries but more chest and abdominal trauma (Flint, 1987).

Blunt trauma tends to cause multiple organ injuries, with the spleen and liver most commonly involved, followed closely by the duodenum and pancreas (Flint, 1987). Injury is the result of both the direct blow itself and the crushing of organs against the harder surface of the vertebrae. Blunt trauma to the abdomen can cause a life-threatening situation even without obvious external signs of injury and should be suspected in patients involved in falls, fights, possible physical abuse, or motor vehicle accidents, and when a decreased level of consciousness is present.

As stated previously, penetrating trauma is usually the result of either stab or gunshot injuries. Of the two, stab wounds are generally less destructive, with fewer complications; the incidence of visceral injury as a result of stab wounds is 30 to 40% while the incidence of visceral injury due to gunshot wounds is as high as 80 to 90% (Marx, 1983).

There are two types of organs in the abdomen: solid (encapsulated) and hollow. The solid, encapsulated organs are usually injured as a result of blunt trauma. The major complication of injury to solid organs such as the spleen and liver is hemorrhage. Hollow organs such as the stomach and intestines

Table 21–4 Nursing Diagnoses and Interventions Associated with Thoracic Injury

Assessment	Planning/Intervention	Expected Outcomes
Nursing Diagnoses: Potential for ineffective breathing patterns and impaired gas exchange		

Physical signs:
  Respiratory distress
  Subcutaneous emphysema
  Decreased or absent breath sounds
  Chest wound
  Distended neck veins with hypotension
Laboratory data
  Arterial blood gases demonstrate hypoxemia and/or carbon dioxide retention
	Immediately after Trauma Nursing Care Aimed at Stabilization
	Prepare to assist with chest-tube insertion
	Monitor chest-tube drainage system for large amount of bubbling (not in suction side) and amount of blood loss
	Nursing Care after Stabilization
	Monitor chest-tube drainage system for large amount of bubbling (not in suction side) and amount of blood loss
	Provide analgesics as ordered to promote deep breathing
	Monitor the patient closely for the development of ARDS
	 • Usually occurs 18–36 hr after injury
	 • Marked hypoxemia (inability of the lungs to maintain a $PaO_2 <$ 50 mm Hg despite an increasing FiO_2)
	 • Respiratory distress and cyanosis
	 • Reduction in functional residual capacity
	 • Decrease in lung compliance
	 • Patient requires increasing levels of PEEP
	 • Bilateral alveolar infiltrates on roentgenography
		Alert and oriented
		Arterial blood gases within normal limits
		Respiratory rate 12–18 breaths/min
		Lung physical exam normal
		Chest film normal (or no worse—radiography may lag)

FiO_2 = fraction of inspired oxygen; PEEP = positive end expiratory pressure.

are usually injured as a result of penetrating trauma. The complication of injury to these organs is the development of peritonitis.

The intrathoracic abdomen is protected by the bony thorax and includes the spleen, liver, and stomach. Injury to the spleen is frequently associated with left-lower-rib fractures. Signs and symptoms include left upper quadrant tenderness and rigidity, Kehr's sign (referred left shoulder pain), signs of hypovolemic shock, and a rapid rise in the white-cell count, which may go as high as 20,000 to 30,000/mm^3.

An attempt is made to repair the spleen or to perform a partial splenectomy as opposed to a total splenectomy, as the spleen is an important organ of the immune system. The spleen functions to present antigen to the immune system and is necessary for antibody and opsonin production.

The liver is also commonly injured as a result of blunt trauma. Lacerations of the liver are a common result of the high acceleration/deceleration steering wheel mechanism of injury. Liver injury should be suspected when right-lower-rib fractures are detected. Signs and symptoms include right upper quadrant tenderness and guarding, referred right shoulder pain, peritonitis, and signs of hypovolemic shock. Severe liver injuries have a high intraoperative death rate. Most liver injuries, however, are successfully treated by observation, compression, packing, suturing, or a combination of these techniques.

The stomach is usually injured as a result of penetrating trauma. The leaking of gastric juices into the abdominal cavity will cause a rapid inflammatory response. Signs and symptoms include evidence of blood in the nasogastric tube, fever, and abdominal rigidity.

The true abdomen is not protected by the bony thorax and includes the small and large intestine, urinary bladder, uterus, and ovaries. The small intestine is injured most commonly as a result of penetrating trauma. Signs and symptoms include peritonitis, rebound tenderness with small-bowel injury, and with duodenal injury, vomiting of bile.

The urinary bladder has a high incidence of injury when distended, otherwise it is well protected in the pelvis. The usual mechanism of injury is a seat-belt injury upon rapid deceleration. Signs and symptoms may include hematuria, ecchymosis on the lower abdomen, and peritonitis.

The retroperitoneal abdomen refers to the organs that lie behind the peritoneum, inside the posterior walls of the abdominal cavity, and includes the pancreas, kidneys, ureters, and urethra. Injury to the pancreas is frequently associated with a T-11 to L-2 vertebral body fracture. The pancreas is rarely injured in isolation, and when it is injured it is often the result of steering wheel trauma. Signs and symptoms include left upper quadrant, epigastric and/or back pain, Grey Turner's sign (ecchymosis on left flank), elevated white-cell count, and elevated serum amylase.

Injury to the kidneys is frequently associated with injuries of the lower ribs. Because it is displaced by the liver to a lower position in the abdomen, the right kidney is injured more frequently than the left. Injury to the ureters is uncommon; however, this may occur in conjunction with kidney injuries. Eighty to ninety percent of all renal injuries are treated conservatively with bed rest (Marx, 1983). Signs and symptoms of renal injury include hematuria (although absence of hematuria may mean injury to the renal pedicle or a renal vascular thrombosis), anuria, flank pain, Grey Turner's sign, and costal vertebral angle tenderness.

Urethral trauma in the male patient is commonly associated with pelvic fractures and with straddle-type injuries, in which the urethra gets caught between the inferior border of the pelvic arch and an external force. Treatment should include a suprapubic cystostomy and drains if needed, followed by a secondary surgical reconstruction several months later. A primary surgical reconstruction should be avoided since there is a higher incidence of impotence after such repair. Signs and symptoms include blood at the urethral meatus, an inability to void, perineal bruising (butterfly hematoma), and a high-riding prostate gland on rectal exam. Urethral trauma is a rare injury in females, although when present it is frequently associated with vaginal tears. Treatment consists of primary surgical exploration, reapproximation of the urethra to the bladder, and closure of the vaginal laceration (Gurriero, 1984).

Diagnostic Procedures and Definitive Care

A surgical abdominal series of x-ray films includes the following views: flat plate of the abdomen, anteroposterior upright abdomen, posteroanterior chest, and left lateral decubitus. The flat plate of the abdomen is used to visualize fractures of the lower ribs, pelvis, and spine; the position of abdominal organs; and the presence of psoas muscle shadows. The anteroposterior upright abdomen is used to detect free air under the diaphragm. This film may not be appropriate in the less stable patient since it may take 10 minutes for the free air to rise. The upright chest is used to visualize the thoracic structures, the width of the mediastinum, and intestinal herniation into the chest. The left lateral decubitus is used to visualize free air above the liver (pneumoperitoneum).

Computerized tomography is extremely accurate in identifying intraabdominal injury, as hematomas, free blood, and urine can be detected. CT scans can be extremely valuable in evaluating retroperitoneal injuries of the pancreas and duodenum. In fact, CT scans of the abdomen have replaced peritoneal lavage in some institutions as the diagnostic tool of choice for the assessment of intraabdominal injury.

A cystogram is indicated for the patient with a fracture of the symphysis in order to rule out extravasation from the bladder. An intravenous pyelogram (IVP) is indicated for patients with gross or microscopic hematuria and for penetrating abdominal trauma victims. The IVP demonstrates the nature and location of injury to the kidney. A retrograde urethrogram is indicated for the patient with frank or dried blood at the urethral meatus to rule out extravasation from the urethra.

The decision to operate on a patient with a blunt abdominal injury presents a dilemma to the surgeon since the procedure itself may be dangerous to the patient. Absolute indications for exploration are evidence of hemorrhage, free gas in the peritoneum, abdominal rigidity, and increasing abdominal distention. Careful and continual abdominal assessment is essential, especially in questionable cases. An excellent aid to diagnosis in blunt trauma is the peritoneal tap and lavage (Figure 21–5). Aspirant obtained with a large-bore needle or a peritoneal dialysis catheter can provide essential data that will assist in the decision-making process. Indicators favoring surgery are the presence of frank blood, a red-cell count greater than 100,000, an amylase level greater than 200 units, or the presence of bile, fecal matter, or bacteria. Peritoneal aspiration should not be instituted until shock is controlled and abdominal films are obtained. In general, there is agreement in the literature that a high level of suspicion is valuable in deciding about operating and that exploration should be done if there is any possibility of serious intraabdominal lesion, since undue delay could be fatal (Flint, 1987).

The use of peritoneal lavage is controversial in the management of gunshot wounds, since patients with possible penetration are generally explored because of the high incidence of intraabdominal injury. Repairs on gunshot wounds can be extensive, with the surgeon working against time if the patient is severely injured. Complete repair is sometimes not feasible and these procedures are always considered to be contaminated cases.

Postoperative complications can be numerous after repair of a gunshot wound. The incidence of wound infection is high. The number of anastomoses that may be required increases the incidence of peritonitis, or abscess and fistula formation. Furthermore, the patient may have sustained other major

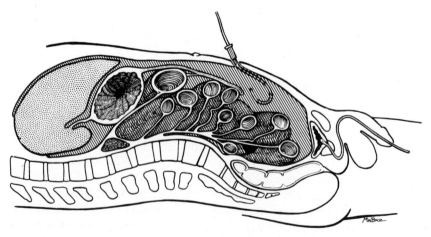

Figure 21–5. Diagnostic peritoneal lavage. The trocar is inserted into the peritoneum. The shaded area illustrates the intraperitoneal structures. A urethral catheter is in place in order to decompress the bladder prior to the procedure.

injuries or episodes of shock as part of the traumatic event, which increases the critical nature of the injury.

Regarding stab wounds, an exploratory laparotomy is indicated for unstable vital signs, peritoneal irritation, bowel protrusion or evisceration, free intraperitoneal air, significant gastrointestinal bleeding, evidence of diaphragmatic rupture, and positive peritoneal lavage (Marx, 1983). In many cases, surgery can be deferred if the peritoneum is believed to be intact or the degree of visceral injury is believed to be minor. Depending on the injuring weapon, these minor wounds may heal with just nutritional and antibiotic support.

Nursing Diagnoses

In addition to the nursing diagnoses for the multiple trauma patient, the patient with abdominal injury requires the nursing assessment and interventions presented in Table 21–5.

ORTHOPEDIC INJURIES

Approximately 75% of all accidents involve the extremities. Extremity injuries rarely are life-threatening unless they cause massive blood loss. Even with prompt attention, however, the morbidity associated with injuries of the ex-

Table 21–5 Nursing Diagnoses and Interventions Associated with Abdominal Injury

Assessment	Planning/Intervention	Expected Outcomes
Nursing Diagnoses: Alteration in fluid volume and distribution and potential for decreased tissue perfusion		
Hypovolemic shock (see Table 21–1)	After stabilization	Blood pressure, respiration within normal limits
Third-space loss	Measure and record all gastrointestinal losses (nasogastric, sump, wound drainage, etc.)	Central venous pressure and/or pulmonary capillary wedge pressure within normal limits
Loss phase—first 48–72 hr after surgery or trauma		
Decreased urinary output	Check surgical dressing for heavy bleeding; notify M.D.	Capillary refill < 2 sec
Reabsorption phase	Intake: output, 3:1 ratio (3 ml crystalloid for every 1 ml of urinary output) during loss phase	Urine output > 30 ml/hr
↑ Urinary output (200 ml/hr)		Hematocrit and hemoglobin within normal limits
Generalized edema		
Laboratory data		
Hemoconcentration: ↑ hematocrit, ↑ hemoglobin		

tremities may be significant. Permanent disability can often be prevented with prompt temporary measures such as immobilization until the life-threatening injuries have been cared for and definitive management for the injury can be performed.

Direct injury refers to the mechanism of injury in which the bone is broken at the point of impact. An indirect injury refers to a fracture at some distance from impact. In a twisting injury there is torsion on a joint with the distal part of the limb fixed.

Fractures can be subdivided into two categories: closed (simple) and open (compound). A fracture is said to be a "closed" fracture when the overlying skin remains intact. When a fracture is present and an open wound of the overlying skin is also present, the fracture is referred to as an open fracture. Open fractures can be categorized according to the amount of damage. A Grade I open fracture refers to an open fracture with a small wound and minimal soft-tissue damage. Grade II refers to skin and muscle contusions at the fracture site. Grade III refers to moderate or massive wounds and trauma to muscle, blood vessels, and possibly nerves.

Pelvic fractures can be life-threatening emergencies. Each fracture site can cause up to 1,000 ml of blood loss. Associated injury to the genitourinary system is common. A stable fracture of the pelvis, such as a unilateral fracture of the superior and inferior pubic rami, can be treated with bed rest and progressive weight bearing.

External fixation is usually the treatment of choice for unstable fractures, such as bilateral fractures to the superior and inferior pubic rami, and is often used in the treatment of trauma. In addition to pelvic fractures, indications for external fixation include open and/or infected lower extremity fractures, certain closed fractures of both the lower and upper extremities, some rare joint injuries, and arthrodeses. The primary and secondary indications for external fixation are included in Table 21–6. The advantages of this form of treatment over others requiring casting include ready access to wounds for additional treatments, greater early mobility for the patient with unencumbered motion of adjacent joints, a greater margin for making adjustments, and stabilization away from any soft- or bone-tissue lesions. The potential for infection exists because the pins are inserted through the skin, and pin care must be performed once or twice a day. Discharge teaching may need to include pin care, since the patient may be discharged with the fixator in place. Further impairment of physical mobility can be prevented through elevation of the extremity to prevent edema formation, splinting of the joints to maintain anatomic position, muscle-strengthening exercises to minimize atrophy and weakness, and early ambulation as the patient's total condition allows, as many patients are able to walk with a pelvic or lower extremity fixator in place (Searls, Heichel, Niemuth, & Behrens, 1983). An external fixation system is illustrated in Figure 21–6.

A great deal of force is required to fracture the femur, and this injury can be life threatening, since up to 2 liters of blood can be lost because of a

Table 21–6 Primary and Secondary Indications for Use of External Fixation

Injury	Benefits of External Fixation
Primary	
Open fractures	
Large lacerations and/or damage to muscle, nerves, or vessels	Stabilization at a distance from bony and soft-tissue lesion
	Free access for debridement and secondary procedures
Skeletal infections	
Osteomyelitis; infected joints requiring arthrodesis	Rigid immobilization
	Free wound access
Limb lengthening	Distraction of osteotomized bone
	Preservation of alignment
Secondary	
Multiple injuries	Avoids cutaneous and pulmonary complications associated with traction
	Early ambulation
	Early joint rehabilitation
Fractures plus burns or other serious soft-tissue problems	Free wound access with fracture management
Severely comminuted closed fractures	Limb length maintained
	No devascularized fracture fragments
Periarticular and intraarticular fractures; fracture line into joint, often with ligamentous injury	Fracture alignment through longitudinal distraction
Extensive soft-tissue injury without fracture	Free access for reconstructive procedures
	Less cumbersome than most other methods

Adapted from *Critical Care Nursing Quarterly* (formerly *Critical Care Quarterly*), 6(1), pp. 46–47. Copyright June 1983 by Aspen Publishers, Inc. Reproduced with permission.

closed femur fracture. For over a century, the association between long-bone or pelvic fractures and respiratory distress has been recognized. The patient with these types of injuries must be monitored for the development of *fat embolism syndrome,* which may present with restlessness, disorientation, and the appearance of petechiae on the anterior trunk and axillae. Other signs and symptoms depend on the system in which the embolus lodges. Most often, pulmonary involvement occurs and the patient develops dyspnea, wheezing, and rales. The adult respiratory distress syndrome may also develop. The leading hypothesis to explain the development of fat embolism syndrome is that fat globules from the marrow of the injured bone enter the

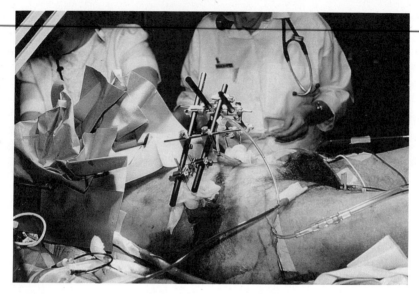

Figure 21–6. Use of the external fixator in the management of an unstable pelvic fracture. Courtesy of Foster G. McGaw Hospital, Loyola University Medical Center, Maywood, IL.

circulation through disrupted blood vessels at the fracture site and then become lodged in the capillary beds (Flint, 1987).

The major potential complication of a tibial fracture is the development of a *compartment syndrome.* Cardona (1985) describes compartment syndrome as "a common cause of neuromuscular functional deficiency precipitated by an ischemic–edema cycle; increased pressure within the compartment [which] compromises the circulation to the contents of that space" (p. 294). As a result, permanent damage to the sensory and motor functions of the patient's peripheral nerves may occur. Compartment syndrome may arise suddenly or gradually over several days. The primary causes include forearm, elbow, and lower leg fractures; crush injuries; and soft-tissue injuries with hemorrhage and edema. Direct tissue-pressure monitoring and emergency fasciotomy to relieve pressure may be required (Burg, 1983).

The patient with a humeral fracture may require external fixation in order to maintain alignment and stabilization of the fracture. Volkmann's ischemic contracture, which is the end result of an ischemic injury to the muscles and nerves of a limb, may develop.

Diagnostic Procedures and Definitive Care

Assessment of the extremities should include an assessment of the "5 Ps"— pain, pulse, paresthesia, pallor, and paralysis. A physician should be notified when the patient is experiencing pain out of proportion to the injury, absence of a previously present pulse, sensations of paresthesia, a pale extremity, or evidence of paralysis. Roentgenograms will be necessary to confirm the injury. Arteriograms may be necessary to confirm vascular damage.

Closed femoral shaft fractures can be managed by several methods (Robinson & Marx, 1985). Each method has advantages and disadvantages. Skeletal traction with the use of a Steinmann pin through the proximal tibia is a universally accepted procedure. The major disadvantage is that this method requires three months of bed rest and traction.

Closed reduction and internal fixation by intramedullary nailing allows for partial weight bearing 2 to 5 days postoperatively. Since only a short incision is made at the greater trochanter, the risk of infection is significantly reduced as compared with open reduction. The disadvantage to this method is that the nail does not stabilize the fracture as rigidly as a plate does.

Open reduction and internal fixation by intramedullary nailing requires a long incision from the greater trochanter to the fracture site. This method allows for partial weight bearing 5 days postoperatively. However, since the fracture site has been opened there is an increased risk of infection.

Open reduction and internal fixation by plating has a higher incidence of infection and is indicated for salvage of a limb that may otherwise be amputated. This method requires 2 to 3 months of no weight bearing and has an increased incidence of nonunion.

Rehabilitation begins with diagnosis and early treatment of orthopedic injuries. Passive/active range of motion exercises should begin early in the hospital course. Muscles become weakened by injury and inactivity and will require exercise to regain their strength. Well-directed rehabilitation efforts frequently contribute more to the outcome than the medical fracture management.

Nursing Diagnoses

In addition to the nursing diagnoses for the multiple trauma patient, the patient with orthopedic injuries also requires the nursing assessment and interventions presented in Table 21–7.

SPINAL CORD INJURY

Over 10,000 persons in the United States are involved each year in accidents that result in spinal cord injury. Motor vehicle accidents are the leading cause of injury, followed by falls and diving accidents. In general, young male adults most often incur spinal cord injury. Statistics from one spinal cord center showed a higher incidence among males than females by approximately 82%, with a mean age of 33 years (Richmond, 1985). This study also showed that 53% of the cases of spinal cord injury result in quadriplegia and 47% result in paraplegia.

Table 21–7 Nursing Diagnoses and Interventions Associated with Orthopedic Injury

Assessment	Planning/Intervention	Expected Outcomes
Nursing Diagnosis: Potential for impaired gas exchange related to fat embolism syndrome		
Physical signs Tachycardia Slight hypertension Fever Tachypnea and dyspnea Bibasilar rales Inspiratory crowing and expiratory wheezing Restlessness and confusion Petechiae in the axillary folds and the root of the neck Laboratory data Arterial blood gases: decreased PaO_2 with increased $PaCO_2$, slight respiratory acidosis Free fat in urine Elevated lipase level Elevated sedimentation rate Subjective data Apprehension Feeling of "smothering" Dyspnea	**Nursing Care Immediately after Trauma Aimed at Stabilization** Immobilize all long-bone fractures (single most important nursing intervention in reducing possibility of fat embolism) Elevate injured extremity **Nursing Care after Stabilization** Monitor vital signs Monitor serial arterial blood-gas results Monitor urine for the presence of fat Monitor serum lipase levels Assess patient for development of petechiae If patient develops signs and symptoms of a fat embolism • Provide high-flow humidified oxygen to maintain the PaO_2 • Prepare to assist physician with endotracheal intubation as needed • Start a large-bore IV for fluid and drug administration • Monitor intake and output • Administer steroids as ordered • Assess for signs and symptoms of pulmonary edema • Assess for signs and symptoms of adult respiratory distress syndrome	Vital signs within normal limits Arterial blood gases within normal limits Absence of respiratory distress
Nursing Diagnosis: Potential for infection		
Physical signs Wound Redness Elevated temperature Heat Tenderness Swelling and/or induration of wound area Purulent drainage Unusual odor Osteomyelitis Fever Vomiting Local area is swollen, warm Extremities tender to touch Drainage from the wound Laboratory data Positive wound cultures Elevated leukocyte count with a shift Elevated sedimentation rate	**Immediately after Trauma Nursing Care Aimed at Stabilization** Culture wounds before cleansing Cleanse wounds using sterile technique, irrigate with normal saline Apply sterile dressings to the wounds Administer prophylactic antibiotics as ordered Maintain NPO to prevent aspiration during surgery **Nursing Care after Stabilization** Monitor blood pressure, temperature, and pulse and respiratory rates Monitor leukocyte count daily Administer antibiotics as ordered Administer antipyretics as ordered Use strict sterile procedure for wound care Obtain blood and wound cultures as ordered Use sterile technique with fluid lines and suctioning	Afebrile Normal white-cell count Negative wound cultures Absence of swelling, pain, redness, drainage and odor at wound site

Table 21–7 *(Continued)*

Assessment	Planning/Intervention	Expected Outcomes

Subjective data
  Pain
  Severe, constant, pulsating pain
	Observe patient for signs of systemic infection
	
	Provide pin and wound care as per protocol
	
	Instruct patient regarding antibiotic therapy since the patient probably will go home on antibiotics	

Nursing Diagnosis: Potential for impaired physical mobility related to compartment syndrome		

Physical signs
  Paresis
  Paralysis
  Edema
  Pallor
  Lack of pulse (late finding)
Subjective data
  Intense pain in the injured limb progressive
  Numbness, tingling or loss of sensation in the web space between the first and second toes (leg muscle compartment swelling)
  Paresthesias of the medial and ulnar surfaces of the hand (forearm superficial flexor compartment swelling)
	Immediately after Trauma Nursing Care Aimed at Stabilization
	
	Assess circulation, color, sensation, and movement of extremity
	
	Nursing Care after Stabilization
	
	Perform ongoing assessment of extremity color, sensation, movement and distal pulses every 2 hr
		Absence of signs of compartment syndrome

Types of Injury

Severe traumatic injury to the spinal cord can result in one of three types of injury and may or may not involve the bony vertebrae. The first type of injury involves vertebral column injury with no spinal cord injury. In this case the patient is neurologically intact. There may be varying degrees of bony instability so this patient must be properly immobilized in order to prevent the intact spinal cord from being damaged. The second type of injury involves an intact vertebral column with spinal cord injury. This type of injury most commonly results from penetrating trauma. The third type of injury involves a combination of a vertebral injury and injury to the spinal cord. This type of injury is the most common of the three.

Consequences of Injury

A complete spinal cord lesion, that is to say total loss of sensation and voluntary motor activity below the level of the lesion, may result from a fractured spine or a penetrating injury. An incomplete spinal cord lesion may result from an interruption of blood supply to the spinal cord, trauma to the cord, disk degeneration, or direct pressure on the cord as a result of hematoma, tumor, or abscess. This condition involves a loss of voluntary motor activity and sensation below the level of the lesion, with a partial interruption of spinal cord function. Varying sensory and/or motor tracts can remain intact.

The patient with an incomplete spinal cord lesion will have a variable amount of return of neurofunction over time. The hallmark of an incomplete spinal cord lesion is the presence of "sacral sparing." Because the fibers from the sacral segment travel along the outermost, more protected portion of the white matter, the presence of sacral sensation during the acute stage is clear evidence that the injury is incomplete.

Four incomplete spinal cord syndromes may result, including the anterior cord syndrome, posterior cord syndrome, central cord syndrome, and Brown–Séquard syndrome (Zejdlik, 1983). It is unusual to see the syndromes in pure form in clinical practice.

The *anterior cord syndrome,* which is the most commonly occurring syndrome, is caused by injury to the anterior aspect of the spinal cord, usually as a result of a flexion injury. Clinically, the patient usually has complete motor paralysis below the level of the injury (corticospinal tracts) and loss of pain, temperature, and touch sensation (spinothalamic tracts). The posterior columns are spared. Therefore, the patient will maintain the position sense, proprioception, and light-touch sensation. Dramatic motor recovery is not expected with this syndrome.

The *posterior cord syndrome* is a rare injury, which when it occurs results from extension injuries. In this syndrome the posterior aspect of the spinal cord is damaged. The clinical presentation is one in which the patient experiences a disruption in the position, vibration, and touch senses but is able to exhibit motor function below the level of the lesion.

The *central cord syndrome* results from an insult to the central portion of the spinal cord, usually secondary to hyperextension of the cervical spine. The greatest damage is to the cervical tracts supplying the arms. The clinical presentation is one in which the patient presents with paralyzed arms but with no deficit in the legs. Prognosis for recovery is good if the lesion is not converted to a complete lesion.

The *Brown–Séquard syndrome* results from hemisection of the spinal cord. Clinically, the patient usually has either increased or decreased cutaneous sensation of pain, temperature, and touch below the level of the lesion on the same side as the lesion. The ability to sense pain and temperature is lost on the opposite side of injury below the level of the lesion because the spinothalamic tracts cross soon after entering the cord. Below the level of the lesion, on the same side as the injury, there is complete motor paralysis and loss of the ability to perceive vibration and light touch.

The neurological level of spinal cord injury will determine the extent of respiratory compromise. The normal muscles of respiration include the accessory muscles, the diaphragm, the intercostal muscles, and the abdominal muscles. Lesions above C-4 may result in respiratory arrest if the injury is complete, since the intercostal muscles and diaphragm are paralyzed. These patients will require mechanical ventilation. Lesions above T-1 may result in respiratory distress secondary to posttraumatic ascending edema of the spinal cord, intestinal paralysis, or gastric dilatation. The patient with a C-4 or lower spinal cord injury should be able to be weaned from the ventilator (Richmond, 1985).

When injury to the spinal cord occurs, the patient often presents in spinal shock. Spinal shock may develop within 30 to 60 minutes after injury and may last for 3 weeks to 2 years, although resolution within 3 months is average.

Spinal shock results from a complete loss of neural function below the level of the lesion. Loss of sympathetic innervation causes peripheral vasodilatation, venous pooling, and decreased cardiac output. Therefore, the patient in spinal shock presents with hypotension, bradycardia (as a result of dominance of parasympathetic nervous system innervation) and with warm, dry extremities. There is a complete loss of motor, sensory, reflex, and autonomic activity below the level of the lesion during this phase. Many spinal cord centers use vasopressors such as dopamine, rather than large amounts of colloids or crystalloids (which could overload the heart and lungs) to manage spinal shock (Ducker, 1987).

Autonomic dysreflexia is a syndrome that sometimes occurs in patients with a spinal cord lesion above T-6 and constitutes a medical emergency. Once the patient has recovered from spinal shock, the potential for autonomic dysreflexia exists. Stimuli such as a distended bladder or bowel, spasms, or decubitus ulcers may trigger this syndrome. These stimuli produce a massive sympathetic discharge that causes a reflex vasoconstriction of the blood vessels in the skin and splanchnic bed below the level of the injury. The body attempts to reduce the hypertension, but the spinal cord injury interrupts transmission of the vasodilatation message below the level of the lesion. Clinically, the patient presents with a pounding headache, severe hypertension, reflex bradycardia, and diaphoresis above the level of the lesion.

The emergency treatment of autonomic dysreflexia is to remove the triggering stimulus. The nurse should check for a kinked urinary catheter or may need to perform an intermittent catherization before it is scheduled. If the urinary system does not seem to be the cause, a digital examination is required to rule out a bowel impaction. Dibucaine (Nupercaine) or lidocaine (Xylocaine) should be used to anesthetize the rectum to prevent further noxious stimulation. The impaction should not be removed until the symptoms subside.

Diagnostic Procedures and Definitive Care

Neurological assessment includes in-depth muscle and sensory testing performed every 2 hours. Each muscle group is graded for strength on a 5-point scale: 0 = no movement to 5 = movement against full resistance. Key muscle functions to assess include the ability to raise and extend arms (spinal level C-5/C-7), open and close hand (C-7/T-1), raise legs (L-2/L-4), wiggle toes (L-3/S-1), and tighten anus (S-3/S-5).

The patient should also be assessed for the ability to differentiate dull and sharp pin prick or pain as well as deep-touch sensation. This should be done systematically and should progress from the area of deficit to the neurologically intact area. Sensory alterations should be documented according to the dermatomes. Sensory levels with which the critical care nurse should be familiar include top of shoulder (C-4 spinal nerve level), thumb (C-6), middle and ring fingers (C-7), little finger (C-8), nipple line (T-4), umbilicus (T-10), great toe (L-4), and top of little toe (S-1). Early recognition of worsening neurological status is the essential first step to effective intervention.

Immobilization and stabilization of the spine are of paramount importance in the management of the patient with a suspected or diagnosed spinal cord injury. The primary goal of care is to prevent further neurological damage. Initially, the patient should be immobilized on a long backboard. A hard cervical collar should be applied and sandbags placed on either side of the patient's neck and head.

Nonsurgical management of cervical injuries involves stabilization through use of skull tongs, halo traction, or a halo brace. If traction for realignment of the spinal column is necessary, Trippe–Wells tongs have the advantage over Gardner–Wells tongs in that they allow for placement of a halo brace without having to remove the tongs once realignment of the spine has been established. Stryker frames that allow the patient to turn from supine to prone and Roto-Rest beds that constantly rotate in a 60 to 60-degree arc are the two most commonly used beds to manage spinal-cord-injured patients in traction. A halo brace, which has the advantage of earlier mobilization may be applied once the injury is stable (Figure 21–7).

Surgical intervention is indicated if there is spinal cord compression by bone, vertebrae, or disk; penetrating injury; or a spinal fracture that cannot be reduced any other way. Surgical stabilization involves placement of Harrington rods by laminectomy and fusion and/or wiring.

Radiographic studies are necessary to determine the presence of fractures, to determine if the fracture is stable or unstable, and to determine proper alignment of the fracture. On admission to the trauma resuscitation area, cross-table lateral cervical spine and anterior posterior views should be done. Standard tomograms, which are multidirectional, may be necessary to localize bony fragments. CT scans may be necessary to rule out or confirm a fracture. The role of magnetic resonance imaging in spinal cord injury has not yet been established, although its use in the acute phase may be promising.

Pharmacologic intervention in the acute phase remains controversial. The exact efficacy of steroids has yet to be determined, although several studies have demonstrated that steroids enhance the recovery index of injured animals (Ducker, 1987). Most spinal cord centers have a protocol that involves the administration of steroids, although the exact regimen varies.

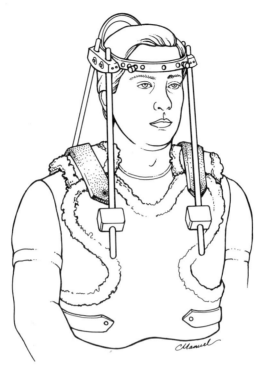

Figure 21–7. Halo system for immobilization of cervical spine fractures.

Naloxone is the only other drug that so far has been identified as a potential treatment for spinal cord injury. Naloxone (an opiate antagonist), when given in large doses, e.g., 5 to 10 mg/kg, appears to improve recovery of function and spinal cord blood flow (Ducker, 1987).

Rehabilitation efforts must begin during the acute care phase in order to facilitate the patient's transition from dependence to the maximum level of independence possible. Bowel and bladder programs should be initiated by the critical care nurse. Once the period of spinal shock has resolved, a bowel program can be established. An intermittent bladder catheterization program should be initiated as soon as possible in order to minimize the risk of infection.

Strict attention must be paid to pressure points in order to maintain skin integrity. The spinal-cord-injured patient is at risk for all the effects of impaired physical mobility, which are discussed in detail in chapter 14.

Nursing Diagnoses

In addition to the nursing diagnoses for the multiple trauma patient, the patient with spinal cord injury requires the nursing assessment and interventions presented in Table 21–8.

Table 21–8   Nursing Diagnoses and Interventions Associated with Spinal Cord Injury

Assessment	Planning/Intervention	Expected Outcomes
Nursing Diagnoses: Potential for ineffective breathing patterns and impaired gas exchange		
Physical signs Assess for level of cord injury Motor: reflexes Sensory: pain, pressure, proprioception Respiratory rate Use of diaphragm Use of intercostal muscles Decreased vital capacity Laboratory data Arterial blood gases: ↓ PaO_2, ↑ $PaCO_2$ Subjective data Anxiety, apprehension	**Immediately after Trauma Nursing Care Aimed at Stabilization** Establish base-line motor and sensory levels Anticipate ascending lesions associated with spinal shock: prepare to assist physician with intubation Provide patient with high-flow humidified oxygen, as the spinal cord is very sensitive to hypoxemia Have suction equipment available Position patient to prevent aspiration Insert nasogastric tube to prevent abdominal distention, which can impair respiratory function **Nursing Care after Stabilization** Administer humidified oxygen as ordered Measure vital capacity every 4–8 hr Monitor quality of respirations Monitor arterial blood-gas results Assist patient to clear secretions with "quad-assist coughing" every 2–4 hr (compress or "punch" the diaphragm during exhalation) Provide nasotracheal suctioning to clear secretions (*Caution:* may cause severe bradycardia secondary to vagal stimulation) Prepare to assist physician with intubation if respiratory failure occurs Provide intermittent positive pressure breathing every 4–6 hr as the condition of the patient warrants Provide incentive spirometry exercises every 1–2 hr while awake Tape a wrench to the cross bar on the front side of the Halo vest (if applied) so that it can be quickly removed if the need for cardiopulmonary resuscitation arises	Absence of respiratory distress Respiratory rate is within normal limits Arterial blood gases within normal limits Effective cough Lungs clear on auscultation and/or chest film
Nursing Diagnosis: Potential for decreased tissue perfusion		
Physical signs Spinal shock Hypotension Bradycardia Warm, dry extremities Hypothermia Poikilothermia (patient assumes the temperature of his or her environment) Decreased cardiac output	**Immediately after Trauma Nursing Care Aimed at Stabilization** Establish base-line vital signs Monitor vital signs every hour and p.r.n. Initiate two large-bore IVs of crystalloid—infuse at rate to maintain systolic blood pressure ≥ 100 mm Hg Insert urinary catheter Monitor hourly urine output Maintain normothermia	Hemodynamic stability Blood pressure and pulse rate within normal limits Urine output greater than 30 ml/hr Temperature within normal limits

Table 21–8 *(Continued)*

Assessment	Planning/Intervention	Expected Outcomes

Decreased urinary output
Orthostatic hypotension (hypotension upon change of position)
Autonomic dysreflexia (in patient who has recovered from spinal shock)
Severe hypertension
Reflex bradycardia
Diaphoresis above the level of the lesion
Reddened face
Subjective data
  Pounding headache
  Nasal congestion
	Administer vasopressors such as dopamine, as ordered
	Administer dexamethasone as ordered to prevent spinal cord edema
	Administer atropine, 0.5 mg, for heart rates less than 60/min as ordered
	Assist physician with insertion of intraarterial catheter and pulmonary artery catheter in order to monitor hemodynamic status
	
	Nursing Care after Stabilization
	Monitor vital signs every hour and p.r.n.
	Infuse IV fluids at a rate to maintain systolic blood pressure ≥ 100 mm Hg
	Monitor hourly urine output
	Maintain normothermia
	Administer vasopressors such as dopamine, as ordered
	Administer dexamethasone as ordered to prevent spinal cord edema
	Administer atropine 0.5 mg for heart rates less than 60/min
	Monitor arterial pressures and pulmonary artery pressures as ordered
	Apply abdominal binder and antiembolic stockings to reduce the amount of blood that pools in the abdomen and the extremities
	Elevate the head of the bed gradually
	Make all position changes slowly
	Autonomic dysreflexia
	  Elevate head of bed
	  Remove the cause of autonomic dysreflexia
	  • Check for a kinked urinary catheter
	  • Perform intermittent catheterization prior to schedule
	  • Check for distended rectum
	  • Administer antihypertensive drugs as ordered	

	Nursing Diagnosis: Impaired physical mobility	

Atelectasis
Physical signs
  Restlessness
  Tachypnea
  Tachycardia
  Dullness on percussion
  Chest film—patches of consolidation
Laboratory data
  Arterial blood gases: decreasing PaO$_2$
  Possible sputum cultures
  Elevated leukocyte count
	Immediately after Trauma Nursing Care Aimed at Stabilization
	Reposition patient every 2 hr
	
	Nursing Care after Stabilization
	Perform an ongoing assessment for signs and symptoms of atelectasis
	Turn, cough, deep breathe patient every 2 hr
	Position patient to facilitate lung expansion (↑ head of bed)
	Encourage oral fluids (if permitted)
		Absence of signs of respiratory impairment
		Arterial blood gases within normal limits
		Circulation to all extremities intact—pulses present and strong
		Skin intact, pink and warm at all pressure points

Table 21–8 *(Continued)*

Assessment	Planning/Intervention	Expected Outcomes
Subjective data Apprehension	Perform chest physical therapy Encourage incentive spirometry	
Deep-vein thrombosis	Apply antiembolic stockings	

Physical signs
  Increasing calf and/or
   thigh measurements
	Assist with range-of-motion exercises as
	  ordered
	Administer low-dose heparin as ordered	

Subjective data
  Tenderness and pain on
   dorsiflexion of the
   foot are eliminated in
   this population
	Assess bony prominences for evidence of
	  skin breakdown
	Wash, apply lotion, and massage pressure
	  areas every shift	

Impaired skin integrity	Place patient on sheepskin or silicone bed	

Physical signs
  Small or large area of
   redness
  Serous fluid, pus, or
   bleeding
  Raw appearance
	Change position frequently (Stryker frame
	  or Roto-Rest bed)
	Apply head protectors
	Teach patient how to do weight shifts
	  when up in wheelchair	

Subjective data
  Pain may not be present
   below the level of the
   lesion		

Nursing Diagnosis: Potential for infection

Physical findings
  Redness, swelling, heat
  Wound drainage
  Elevated body tempera-
   ture
	**Immediately after Trauma Nursing Care
	Aimed at Stabilization**
	Cleanse the wounds using sterile tech-
	  niques
	Apply sterile dressing to wounds
		Afebrile
		Normal white-cell count
		Urine, sputum, wound cul-
		  tures negative

Laboratory data
  Positive urine cultures
  Positive wound cultures
  Elevated white-cell count
	Use sterile technique with urinary catheter
	  insertion
	Use sterile technique with suctioning and
	  fluid lines	

Subjective data
  May not feel pain de-
   pending on level of
   spinal cord lesion
	Use sterile technique with insertion of
	  tongs or Halo device
	Nursing Care after Stabilization
	Monitor vital signs every hour; monitor
	  temperature every 2 hr
	Cleanse insertion sites of immobilization
	  device as per protocol
	Start patient on intermittent catheterization
	  as soon as possible
	Monitor white-cell count daily
	Administer antipyretics as ordered
	Administer antibiotics as ordered
	Assist patient with "quad-assist coughing"
	  to clear secretions and prevent respira-
	  tory infection	

REHABILITATION OF THE TRAUMA PATIENT

In the concern regarding the immediately life-threatening problems of the trauma patient, it is easy to overlook the long-term goals of care. As soon as the immediate life-threatening crises have been resolved, however, interventions to promote recovery and rehabilitation should be initiated.

Discharge planning should begin on admission. Plans for recovery and rehabilitation should be initiated early in the hospital stay to promote complete recovery and rehabilitation of the trauma patient.

SUMMARY

Patients who sustain injuries of multiple systems require complex nursing care during the acute phase. Stabilization may take hours to weeks, necessitating continual assessment and changes in priorities of care as the patient's condition progresses toward the rehabilitation phase.

In addition to the primary traumatic injuries, the nurse must be aware of the possible severe hidden injuries and/or complications that may accompany trauma. Astute nursing care is critical in reducing the morbidity and mortality associated with multiple trauma.

BIBLIOGRAPHY

Bartowski, H. M. (1984). Neurologic injury. In D. D. Trunkey & F. R. Lewis (Eds.), *Current therapy of trauma—1984–1985* (pp. 47–52). St. Louis: C. V. Mosby.
Burg, M. E. (1983). Compartment syndrome. *Critical Care Quarterly, 6*(1), 27–32.
Cardona, V. D. (Ed.) (1985). *Trauma reference manual.* Bowie, MD: Brady Communications.
Carpenter, R. (1987). Infections and head injury: A potentially lethal combination. *Critical Care Nursing Quarterly, 10*(3), 1–11.
Clark, K. (1985). Trauma to the nervous system. In G. T. Shires (Ed.), *Principles of trauma care* (pp. 232–266). New York: McGraw-Hill.
Ducker, T. (1987). New techniques of spinal injury management. In R. Cowley, A. Conn, C. Dunham (Eds.), *Trauma care—Surgical management.* (pp. 213–222). Philadelphia: J. B. Lippincott.
Flint, L. (1987). Abdominal injuries. In J. Richardson, H. Polk, & L. Flint (Eds.), *Trauma—Clinical care and pathophysiology* (pp. 353–395). Chicago: Year Book Medical.
Groer, M., & Shekleton, M. (1989). Basic pathophysiology: A holistic approach. (3rd Ed.) St. Louis: C. V. Mosby.
Gurriero, W. (1984). Management of urologic injuries. *Trauma Quarterly, 1*(1), 52–66.
Harley, D. P., Mena, I., Miranda, R., and Nelson, R. (1983). Myocardial dysfunction following blunt chest trauma. *Archives of Surgery, 118,* 1384–1387.

Hoyt, N. J., & Caplan, E. S. (1983). Identification and prevention of infections in the critically ill trauma population. *Critical Care Quarterly, 6*(1), 17–26.

Marx, J. A. (1983). Abdominal trauma. In P. Rosen (Ed.), *Emergency medicine: Concepts and clinical practice* (pp. 380–404). St. Louis: C. V. Mosby.

National Research Council and the Institute of Medicine, Committee on Trauma Research, Commission of Life Sciences (1985). *Injury in America: A continuing health problem.* Washington, DC: National Academy Press.

Richmond, T. (1985). The patient with a cervical spinal cord injury. *Focus on Critical Care, 12*(2), 23–33.

Robinson, J., & Marx, L. (1985). Fail-safe method. *American Journal of Nursing, 85*(2), 158–161.

Searls, K., Heichel, S., Niemuth, P., & Behrens, F. (1983). External fixation: General principles of patient management. *Critical Care Quarterly, 6*(1), 45–54.

Shin, B. (1987). Lung contusion. In R. Cowley, A. Conn, & C. Dunham (Eds.), Philadelphia: J. B. Lippincott.

Trunkey, D. D. (1984a). Thoracic trauma. In D. D. Trunkey & F. R. Lewis (Eds.), *Current therapy of trauma—1984–1985* (pp. 85–91). St. Louis: C. V. Mosby.

Veise-Berry, S. W. (1983). Nursing considerations during radiologic examination of the massively injured trauma patient. *Critical Care Quarterly, 6*(1), 55–65.

Zejdlik, C. (1983). *Management of spinal cord injury.* Monterey, CA: Wadsworth.

ADDITIONAL READINGS

Baker, J. P., O'Neill, B., & Karpf, R. S. (1984). *The injury fact book.* Lexington, MA: Lexington Books.

Bires, B. A. (1987). Head trauma: Nursing implications from prehospital through emergency department. *Critical Care Nursing Quarterly, 10*(1), 1–18.

Carpenito, L. (1983). *Nursing diagnosis—Application to practice.* Philadelphia: J. B. Lippincott.

Hoppe, M. C. (1983). Nutritional management of the trauma patient. *Critical Care Quarterly, 6*(1), 1–16.

Manifold, S. (1986). Craniocerebral trauma: A review of primary and secondary injury and therapeutic modalities. *Focus on Critical Care, 13*(2), 22–35.

Mullins, R. Respiratory pathophysiology. In J. Richardson, H. Polk, & L. Flint (Eds.), *Trauma—Clinical care and pathophysiology* (pp. 167–212). Chicago: Year Book.

Nikas, D. (1987). Critical aspects of head trauma. *Critical Care Nursing Quarterly, 10*(1), 19–44.

Nikas, D. (1987). Prognostic indicators in patients with severe head injury. *Critical Care Nursing Quarterly, 10*(3), 25–34.

Staller, A. G. (1987). Systemic effects of severe head trauma. *Critical Care Nursing Quarterly, 10*(1), 58–68.

Summey, L. B. (1985). Orthopaedic trauma. In V. D. Cardona (Ed.), *Trauma nursing* (pp. 69–85). Ordall, NJ: Medical Economics.

Trunkey, D. D. (1984b). Abdominal trauma. In D. D. Trunkey & F. R. Lewis (Eds.), *Current therapy of trauma—1984–1985* (pp. 93–100). St. Louis: C. V. Mosby.

22 Thermal Injury

Deborah Goldenberg Klein, M.S.N., R.N., CCRN, C.S.

EPIDEMIOLOGY AND ETIOLOGY

A burn injury is in many respects the worst tragedy an individual can experience. With a major burn there is an overwhelming insult to the patient, both physically and psychologically. Burns are catastrophic in the cost of care required and in the suffering experienced by the patient and family.

It has been estimated that 1% of the population of the United States (over 2 million people) is burned or scalded each year (American Burn Association, 1984). Of these victims, 500,000 seek medical attention and 6,000 die as a direct result of the burn injury (Maley, 1982). Burns are caused by dry or moist heat, chemical exposure, electrical currents, and radiation. The most common cause of burns is fire, with an estimated 75,000 hospitalizations for a prolonged period and 12,000 deaths annually (Trunkey, 1983). Because of the systemic effects of the burn injury, psychological implications and prolonged hospitalization, comprehensive nursing care is required during the acute and long-term phases.

CLASSIFICATION OF BURNS

Traditionally, burns have been classified as first-, second-, third-, or fourth-degree. These terms are not descriptive of the injury because they are based only on the visual characteristics of the burn wound. The injury of a burn extends beyond what can be seen. More accurate descriptions are superficial, partial-thickness, and full-thickness, which graphically describe the burn and indicate depth and severity of the tissue injury (Figure 22–1).

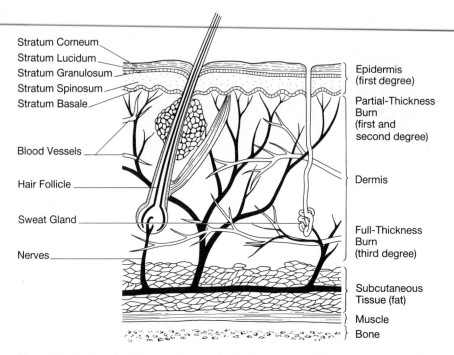

Figure 22–1. Levels of human skin involved in burns. From "The Patient with Burns" by D. G. Klein in *Medical-Surgical Nursing: A Nursing Process Approach,* 2nd ed., edited by B. C. Long and W. J. Phipps, 1989, St. Louis, The C. V. Mosby Co. Reproduced with permission.

Superficial burn wounds are frequently the result of either prolonged exposure to low-intensity heat (e.g., sunburn) or to a short-duration flash exposure to a high-intensity heat source. The wounds are erythematous, dry, and do not blister. These injuries are painful because sensitive nerve endings remain intact. These wounds heal within 5 to 10 days without leaving a scar.

Partial-thickness burns are the result of either increased exposure time or higher-intensity flash exposure. They are characterized by destruction in varying depths from the epidermis to the dermis. The depth of tissue injury is described further as superficial partial-thickness, which involves only the epidermis, or deep partial-thickness, which involves the entire epidermis and part of the dermis. The stratum basale provides the line of demarcation; it is not totally destroyed in the superficial partial-thickness injury. The vascular response occurring within the dermis results in edema formation at the dermal–epidermal junction. As fluid accumulates, the junction separates, forming a blister that may increase in size as the result of continuous exudation and collection of tissue fluid.

Superficial partial-thickness burns are moist and are painful because of irritation of nerve endings. Healing occurs in 10 days to 2 weeks. During the healing phase, dryness and itching are common and are caused by increased vascularization of sebaceous glands, reduction of secretions, and decreased perspiration.

Deep partial-thickness burns consist of a wound with complete disruption of the epidermis and destruction of most of the stratum basale. Edema fluid infiltrates the dermal–epidermal junction, resulting in blister formation. Black networks of coagulated capillaries may be seen, caused by the coagulation of the dermis. Dermal appendages such as hair follicles and sweat glands may be spared, potentially allowing the wound to regenerate. Eschar, a leathery covering comprised of denatured protein, may form as the result of surface dehydration. Sensation is diminished because of actual destruction of nerve endings in the stratum basale.

The significant difference between these deeper burns and superficial burns is the loss of the cellular barrier that protects against bacterial invasion and wound sepsis. Deep partial-thickness burns may take more than 30 days to heal. With good nutrition and the absence of infection, these burns heal spontaneously but may result in poor-quality skin that is prone to breakdown and scar formation.

Full-thickness burns result from prolonged contact with the flaming environment and are often associated with inhalation injuries. The epidermis is destroyed along with dermal appendages and supporting structures. Coagulation necrosis of the entire dermis results in an avascular wound. Thrombosis of vessels may be visible, giving a "cracked pot" appearance. Edema and cellular infiltrates occur only at the edges of the wound. Often a deep partial-thickness burn may convert to a full-thickness burn as a result of infection, trauma, or decreased blood supply. A thick, leathery eschar forms that allows copious fluid losses and fails to prevent bacterial invasion and wound sepsis. Granulation tissue consisting of new fibroblasts and endothelial tissue develops as the result of an inflammatory response at the margin of the wound (edges and undersurface of the eschar). The eschar becomes loosened and will eventually slough. Because of the lack of skin appendages, the wound will heal by contraction and epithelial growth from the edges. The result is a contracture deformity and scarring. In clinical practice, skin grafts are applied to seal the wound and speed the healing process.

The fourth-degree burn represents the extreme full-thickness wound, in which the level of injury extends well beyond the skin. The terminology from the traditional classification is retained. In these injuries, subcutaneous tissue, muscle, fascia, and even bone can be destroyed. Coagulation necrosis of the tissue occurs and cellular inflammation is absent except at the periphery. Because of massive muscle destruction, myoglobinuria can be come a significant problem and may lead to renal failure in the poorly hydrated patient.

THE NATURE OF THERMAL INJURY

The mechanisms by which thermal energy injures body tissue are denaturation of cellular protein, inhibition of cellular metabolism, and secondary interference with local vascular supply. The factors that determine the extent of thermal injury are the heat intensity, the duration of exposure, the conductance of the tissue involved, and the type of burning agent.

TISSUE RESPONSE TO THERMAL INJURY

Thermal injury is the result of denaturation of cellular proteins and disruption of the cellular metabolic processes and vascular supply, which leads to cellular necrosis. Some cells are instantly destroyed, others are irreversibly injured, and others are injured but are capable of survival under certain conditions. Jackson (1953) described three concentric zones of thermal injury. The inner zone of coagulation represents the longest thermal contact and is characterized by coagulation necrosis. This area is surrounded by a zone of stasis, which may or may not survive based on what happens in the 24 to 48 hours following the burn injury. The outer layer is called the zone of hyperemia. This is an area of minimal injury and will heal in 7 to 10 days. Additional trauma, edema, ischemia, desiccation, or bacterial invasion will irreversibly damage cells that survived the initial thermal insult.

If the zone of coagulation lies above the level of the dermal appendages, the wound will be a partial-thickness one and have the potential for spontaneous healing. If the zone of coagulation extends below this level, a full-thickness wound is produced.

PHYSIOLOGIC RESPONSE TO THERMAL INJURY

As a result of burn injury, normal skin function is diminished, resulting in physiologic alterations. These include loss of protective barriers against infection, escape of body fluids, lack of temperature control, destroyed sweat and sebaceous glands, and a diminished number of sensory receptors. The severity of these alterations will depend on the extent and depth of the burn.

Numerous physiologic changes occur as a result of a major burn injury. Patients may present with acidosis, hypovolemia, hypoxemia, and organ failure. Summarized in Figure 22–2 are the pathophysiologic changes seen in major burns. Alterations in fluid volume, distribution, and composition occur in two stages after the burn injury: the immediate hypovolemic stage and the diuretic stage. Summarized in Table 22–1 are the specific fluid, electrolyte, and metabolic alterations by stage.

After the period of fluid shifts, the patient remains acutely ill. This subsequent period is characterized by anemia and malnutrition. Anemia develops from the loss of red blood cells. Negative nitrogen balance begins at the onset of the burn as the result of tissue destruction, protein loss, and the stress response. It continues throughout the acute period and is secondary to continued loss of protein from the wound, from tissue catabolism resulting from immobility, and from decreased protein intake. Special attention to the nutri-

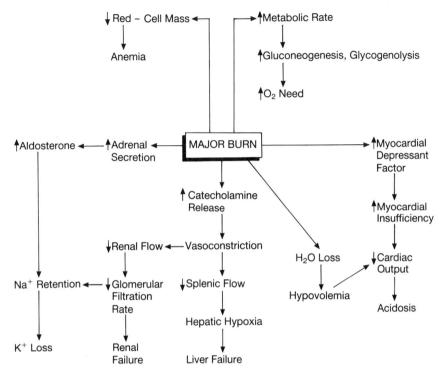

Figure 22–2. Overview of pathophysiology of major burn. From "The Patient with Burns" by D. G. Klein in *Medical-Surgical Nursing: A Nursing Process Approach,* 2nd ed., edited by B. C. Long and W. J. Phipps, 1989, St. Louis, The C. V. Mosby Co. Reproduced with permission.

tional needs of the patient is an integral part of the comprehensive care during this time. Increased metabolism, loss of fluid during diuresis, and catabolism during tissue breakdown contribute to weight loss.

Complications of the gastrointestinal system frequently occur after severe thermal injury. Gastric and duodenal ulceration (Curling's ulcer) has been reported in 66% of severely burned patients, with significant ulceration in nearly 20% (Pruitt & Goodwin, 1981). Bleeding is the major clinical problem from these lesions. Treatment is aimed at prevention and is best accomplished by antacids and enteral feedings. Cholecystitis, pancreatitis, and hepatic dysfunction may also be seen as the result of tissue ischemia from hypoperfusion.

PATHOPHYSIOLOGY OF INHALATION INJURY

Inhalation injuries are caused by both the heat of inhaled smoke and by toxic chemicals inhaled into the respiratory tract. Heat and inhaled chemicals cause injury through different mechanisms.

Table 22–1 Physiologic Changes with Burns

HYPOVOLEMIC STAGE		
Change	*Mechanism*	*Result*
Extracellular fluid shift	Vascular to interstitial	Hemoconcentration Edema at burn site
Renal function	Decreased renal blood flow from decreased blood pressure and decreased cardiac output	Oliguria
Sodium level	Na^+ reabsorbed by kidneys but Na^+ lost in exudate and trapped in edema fluid	Sodium deficit
Potassium level	K^+ released as result of tissue and red blood cell injury; decreased K^+ excretion from decreased renal function	Hyperkalemia
Protein level	Protein lost into tissues by increased capillary permeability	Hypoproteinemia
Nitrogen balance	Tissue catabolism; protein loss in tissues; more nitrogen lost than taken in	Negative nitrogen balance
Acid–base balance	Anaerobic metabolism from decreased tissue perfusion; increased acid end products; decreased renal function (causing retention of acid end products); loss of serum bicarbonate	Metabolic acidosis
Stress response	Occurs because of trauma	Decreased renal blood flow

Heat causes direct damage to the respiratory epithelium, resulting in cellular necrosis and surrounding inflammation. Airway obstruction generally develops in the first 24 to 48 hours as a result of the inflammation and swelling of the upper respiratory tract. Heat damage is limited to the upper airway, especially the supraglottic area, because inhaled smoke cools as it moves down the airway. When steam is present, however, the heat-carrying capacity is increased and more severe injury may result further down the airway.

Toxic chemicals are produced in fires as a result of incomplete combustion of burning materials. Commonly produced toxic chemicals include nitrous oxide, sulfur dioxide, hydrochloric acid, and hydrocyanic acid. With the

DIURETIC STAGE	
Mechanism	*Result*
Interstitial to vascular	Hemodilution
Increased renal blood flow from increased blood volume	Diuresis
Na$^+$ loss with diuresis (becomes normal in 1 wk)	Sodium deficit
K$^+$ moves back into cells; K$^+$ lost by diuresis (begins 4–5 days after the burn)	Hypokalemia
Loss of protein during continued catabolism	Hypoproteinemia
Tissue catabolism, protein loss, immobility	Negative nitrogen balance
Sodium bicarbonate lost in diuresis; hypermetabolism with increased metabolic end products	Metabolic acidosis
Occurs because of prolonged nature of injury and psychological threat to self	Stress ulcers

From "The Patient with Burns" by D. G. Klein in *Medical–Surgical Nursing: A Nursing Process Approach,* 2nd ed., edited by B. C. Long and W. J. Phipps, 1989, St. Louis: The C. V. Mosby Co. Reproduced with permission.

inhalation of toxic chemicals, there is an immediate loss of bronchial epithelial cilia, preventing the mobilization of secretions and necrotic pulmonary debris. Laryngeal occlusion occurs as edema increases. Lower airway obstruction occurs because of the loss of surfactant and the presence of pulmonary exudate, which interferes with adequate oxygen exchange. Wheezing and dyspnea will be experienced and atelectasis frequently develops. After the initial injury, tracheal and bronchial epithelium begin to slough and a hemorrhagic tracheobronchitis may develop.

Inhalation injury is suspected when a patient has burns to the face and neck, singed facial or nasal hairs, hoarseness, intraoral charcoal (especially on the teeth and gums), brassy cough, and a history of a burn injury in a closed space. Treatment includes the administration of humidified oxygen, intermittent positive-pressure breathing, suctioning, administration of bronchodilators, postural drainage, and bronchoscopy to remove secretions. Symptoms of impending airway obstruction include dyspnea, cyanosis, tachycardia, tachypnea, copious amounts of carbonaceous sputum, increased respiratory effort (sternal retractions and abdominal breathing), restlessness, and/or an altered level of consciousness. If respiratory distress is present, an airway must be established before the airway narrows. Endotracheal intubation is preferred over tracheostomy because of the increased risk of infection associated with a surgical procedure.

A frequent early complication of burn injury, especially with smoke inhalation, is pulmonary edema. Increased pressure in the pulmonary vascular bed causes transudation of fluid first into the interstitial space and then into alveoli. Pulmonary edema is often related to the amount of fluid given immediately after the initial burn injury as well as to the patient's cardiopulmonary status. The patient with left ventricular pump failure who has received aggressive fluid administration is at risk for the development of pulmonary edema and later may develop a typical presentation of adult respiratory distress syndrome. With the onset of the diuretic phase, pulmonary edema will begin to subside.

Carbon Monoxide Poisoning

Carbon monoxide poisoning results from prolonged inhalation of smoke and other noxious products of combustion. It is an odorless, colorless, tasteless, nonirritating gas with an affinity for hemoglobin (210 times that of oxygen). It displaces oxygen to form carboxyhemoglobin. The displacement of oxygen leads to tissue hypoxia. Carbon monoxide also binds myoglobin, decreasing oxygen transport, particularly to cardiac muscle. Signs and symptoms of carbon monoxide intoxication are related to the degree of exposure and the amount of carboxyhemoglobin present. The diagnosis of carbon monoxide poisoning can only be made by serum measurement of carboxyhemoglobin concentrations. As the level of carboxyhemoglobin increases, the symptoms become more severe. A patient with a carboxyhemoglobin level of 20% may present with headache, dizziness, and nausea. As the level approaches 50%, symptoms may include agitation, vomiting, convulsive seizures, loss of consciousness, shortness of breath, tachycardia, and tachypnea. Cherry-pink skin is a late sign. Carboxyhemoglobin levels of 80% are usually fatal.

Treatment of carbon monoxide poisoning includes the administration of high-flow, 100% oxygen by face mask or by ventilatory support. Blood samples are monitored for a decrease in carboxyhemoglobin concentration.

TREATMENT OF THERMAL INJURY

Three periods of treatment can be identified in the care of the seriously burned patient. These are the emergent, the acute, and the rehabilitative periods.

The emergent period refers to the first 48 to 72 hours after the burn. When the patient is admitted, the severity of the injury is determined, and first aid and wound care are given. The acute period of treatment begins at the end of the emergent period and lasts until all of the full-thickness wounds are covered with skin grafts or partial-thickness wounds are healed. The rehabilitation period focuses on returning the patient to a state of optimal function. There are two areas of concern during this phase: (1) the restoration of function over joint surfaces that were scarred and (2) the emotional assistance that the patient and family will need. The rehabilitation of the patient actually begins early during hospitalization and is addressed throughout the hospitalization. After the initial discharge, the patient may require emotional assistance and counseling, and many readmissions may be necessary for reconstructive procedures. Each of these treatment periods is discussed in greater detail below.

It is important to state that comprehensive care of the burn patient can best be provided through a multidisciplinary team approach. The physician, nurse, social worker, physical and occupational therapists, teacher, registered dietitian, vocational counselor, and others all must work together to address the complex and varied needs of the patient. The nurse's role in the team is to coordinate the interactions of the various disciplines and to incorporate the team's suggestions and approaches into an effective plan of care.

Emergent Period

The emergent period of therapy is defined as the time required to resolve the immediate problems resulting from the burn injury. First aid measures are directed to treating the systemic response to trauma, concurrent injuries, and the burn wound. The first step is assessment of the patient and the severity of the burn injury.

Assessment

Knowledge of the circumstances surrounding the burn injury is extremely valuable in the treatment of a burn victim. This information can be obtained from either the burn victim or witnesses to the event and should include the following:

1. How the burn injury occurred
2. When the injury occurred
3. Duration of contact with the burning agent

4. Location (enclosed space suggests possibility of smoke inhalation and/or carbon monoxide poisoning)
5. Presence of an explosion (suggests possibility of other injuries)

The nurse has the responsibility to learn as much as possible about the patient, as the state of health and age of the burn victim are important factors that may modify treatment. The elderly and very young have a higher rate of mortality than a young adult with the same percentage burn. Infants under 2 years of age and adults over 60 years of age have a higher rate of mortality than persons in other age groups with a similar-size injury. The infant has a weak antibody response to infection, and in older victims the serious burns may aggravate the degenerative processes or exacerbate a preexisting health problem.

Preexisting endocrine, pulmonary, cardiovascular, or renal disease or a history of drug use will decrease a victim's ability to cope with severe burns. Since most of these patients will require topical and systemic therapy with a number of drugs, allergies and drug sensitivities must be determined and documented.

The severity of the burn is categorized as major, moderate, or minor. This categorization is made on the basis of size, depth, and location of the burn and the presence of complicating factors (Table 22–2).

Table 22–2   Classification of Severity of Burns

Major Burn Injuries

Greater than 25% body-surface area (BSA) (greater than 20% in children under 10 yr and adults over 40 yr)
Greater than 10% BSA, full-thickness
Involvement of face, eyes, ears, hands, feet, perineum
Electrical burns
Burns complicated by inhalation injury or major trauma
Burns in patients with preexisting disease (diabetes, congestive heart failure, or chronic renal failure)

Moderate Burn Injuries

15–25% BSA in adults, partial thickness (10–20% BSA in children under 10 yr and adults over 40 yr)
Less than 10% BSA, full-thickness
Burns with no concurrent injury
Burns in patients with no preexisting disease

Minor Burn Injuries

Less than 15% BSA in adults (10% in children or the elderly)
Less than 2% BSA, full-thickness injury
Burns in patients with no preexisting disease

The percentage of body surface area burned is estimated by using charts that depict anterior and posterior drawings of the body. In adults, the body is divided into areas equal to multiples of 9% as depicted in Figure 22–3 ("Rule of Nines"). The burned area is marked on the drawings and the amount of body surface area burned is calculated from the shaded areas. Calculations are modified for infants and children under 10 years of age because of the relatively larger head and smaller body sizes.

The depth of the burn injury is determined by the cause of the burn and the appearance, color, and degree of sensation present in the burned area. Summarized in Table 22–3 are the assessment factors related to the various possible depths of a burn injury.

The anatomical part of the body burned must also be considered when estimating the severity of the burn: a 3% burn of the anterior surface of the

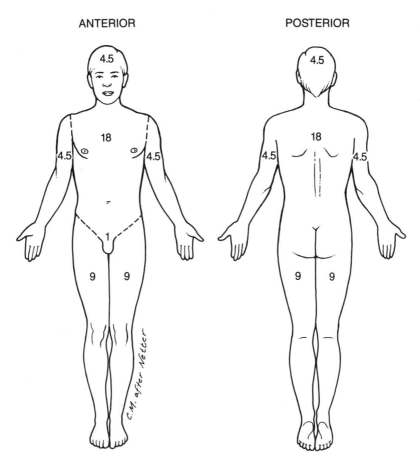

Figure 22–3.   Rule of nines for estimating the area of body surface burned.

Table 22–3   Causes and Factors Determining Depth of Burn Injury

Depth	Cause	Appearance	Color	Sensa-tion
Superficial (First-Degree)	Flash flame, Ultraviolet light (sun burn)	Dry, no blisters Minimal or no edema Blanches with finger-tip pressure and refills when pressure removed	Increased redness	Painful
Partial-Thickness (Second-Degree)	Contact with hot liquids or solids Flash flame to clothing Direct flame Chemicals Ultraviolet light	Large, moist blisters that will increase in size Blanches with finger-tip pressure and refills when pressure removed	Mottled with dull white, tan, pink, or cherry-red areas	Very painful
Full-Thickness (Third-Degree)	Contact with hot liquids or solids Flame Chemicals Electrical contact	Dry with leathery eschar Charred vessels visible under eschar Blisters rare but may be present as thin-walled that do not increase in size No blanching with pressure	White, charred, dark tan Black Red	Little or no pain Hair pulls out easily

thigh will probably not be as serious as a 3% burn of the neck, face, or perineum. Injuries that involve cosmetic and functional areas of the body warrant a prognosis of long-term morbidity and mortality. A burn of the face, hands, and feet will require extensive meticulous care. A burn of the head, neck, and chest may also involve injury to the respiratory tract and may result in severe respiratory difficulty. Burns of the perineum are difficult to treat because of the high risk of infection due to potential contamination with fecal material. The circumferential or encircling burn of a limb, the neck, or the chest can have serious consequences. This type of burn will cause constrictive contraction of the skin and produce a tourniquet effect that may impair breathing and/or circulation.

The identification of the causative agent of the burn injury is of primary importance because the nature of the agent has a direct effect on prognosis and treatment. Thermal burns are the most common, and occur as the result of the transfer of energy from a heat source to the body (flame, hot surfaces, sunburn, hot metals, and hot grease). The flame is a highly concentrated heat that affects a localized area and burns deeply. In contrast, scald injuries or moist burns are caused by steam or boiling water, which conducts heat to a larger, widespread area.

Chemical burns, commonly seen in industry, are caused by strong acids or alkali, such as hydrochloric acid and lye. Household chemical burns frequently occur from accidental exposure to drain cleaners, paint removers, and disinfectants. Burns to the eye occur when a chemical splashes onto the face, and burns to the upper gastrointestinal tract occur upon ingestion of the noxious chemical. The severity of chemical burns is directly proportional to the duration of exposure. Chemicals cause deep burns over a rather limited surface. The agent should be identified and treatment initiated quickly. The first priority is removal of the chemical agent, which is accomplished by copious flushing with water for as long as 20 to 30 minutes to ensure complete removal of the destructive agent. Although specific chemical agents have known antidotes, it is best to flood the exposed area with water to ensure removal and to transport the victim to the nearest medical facility. Burns occurring about the eyes should be lavaged continuously with copious amount of cool, clean water for up to 30 minutes.

Electrical burns are caused by electrical sparks and arcs or by an electrical current passing directly through the body. The duration of contact and the intensity of the current are the primary factors determining the severity of injury. Tissue with the highest water content has the least resistance to electrical current and, consequently, suffers the most damage. Blood, muscles, skin, tendons, fat, and bones are affected in decreasing order of resistance. Further, calloused skin is more resistant to current flow than is thin skin, and dry skin is more resistant than sweaty skin. Tissue damage may appear minor at the entrance and exit points, making electrical burns difficult to evaluate. The burn typically appears as a central, charred black area, surrounded by a gray-white region of coagulation necrosis with another outer ring of bright erythema. The visual damage is referred to as the "tip of the iceberg" and does not reflect underlying tissue destruction generated by the passage of electrical current though the body. Victims of electrical burns must be monitored closely for signs and symptoms of hemorrhage, intestinal perforation, and/or cardiac arrhythmias. The passage of electrical current may cause a cardiac arrest at the time of injury.

The nursing diagnoses relevant to the emergent-period care of a patient who has sustained thermal injury are summarized in Table 22–4. Related factors and desired patient outcomes are included. Interventions related to each diagnosis are discussed below.

Intervention

Intensive nursing care of the burned patient will begin in the emergency room, where the patient will be stabilized before transfer to a burn unit or

Table 22–4   Relevant Diagnoses During the Emergent Period

Nursing Diagnoses	Related Factors	Expected Outcomes
Airway clearance, ineffective	Laryngeal, edema, obstruction, secretions	*The patient will:* Maintain a patent airway and adequate ventilation and gas exchange
Anxiety	Threat of death, threat to self-concept, threat to/ changes in health status	Exhibit control of anxiety
Comfort, alteration in: acute pain	Exposed nerve endings from burn injury, trauma	Experience minimal pain
Fluid volume deficit, actual	Movement of fluid from intravascular to interstitial space (hypovolemic stage), evaporation	Regain optimal fluid and electrolyte balance.
Fluid volume excess, actual	Movement of fluid from interstitial to intravascular space (diuretic stage)	Same as above
Hypothermia	Environmental exposure of burn wounds	Demonstrate normal body termperature
Potential for infection	Loss of protection created by damage to skin	Remain free of infection
Impaired skin and tissue integrity	Loss of skin from burn injury	Experience no further skin loss
Tissue perfusion, alterations in: cerebral, cardiopulmonary renal, gastrointestinal, peripheral	Hypovolemia	Demonstrate adequate perfusion of vital organs

critical care unit. In many emergency rooms, the nurse directs prehospital emergency care in the field through radio communication. The immediate treatment of a burn patient is summarized in Table 22–5.

Alteration in Fluid Volume and Tissue Perfusion   Replacement of fluids and electrolytes is an essential part of the treatment of the burn victim, and is instituted as soon as the severity of the burn and the patient's condition is known. Ideally, fluid therapy is started within an hour after a severe burn to prevent hypovolemic shock. Insertion of two large peripheral catheters or one large central venous catheter and one large peripheral catheter permits the rapid administration of fluids and electrolytes. Placement of these catheters is through an unburned site to prevent the introduction of infection. An indwelling urinary catheter is inserted to monitor urine output measurements adequately, as these are used as a guide to volume replacement.

Fluids administered during the first 48 hours are given to maintain circulating blood volume. Additional fluids and electrolytes are added to replace losses from vomiting or from nasogastric drainage.

Three types of fluid are considered in calculating the needs of the patient: colloids, including plasma and plasma expanders such as Dextran; electrolytes, such as a physiologic solution of sodium chloride and Ringer's solution; and nonelectrolyte fluids, such as water with 5% glucose. Medical authorities do not agree about the proportion of colloids and electrolyte fluids needed. Several formulas are described in the medical literature to

Table 22–5   Initial Treament of Major Burns

Field

1. Remove victim from source of burn.
2. Douse with water and remove nonadherent smoldering clothing.
3. If chemical burn, carefully remove clothing and flush wound with large amounts of water.
4. If electrical burn and victim still in contact with electrical source, do *not* touch victim. Remove electrical source with dry nonconductive object (e.g., rope).
5. Establish patent airway and assess for inhalation injury. Give oxygen if available.
6. Assess and initiate treatment for injuries requiring immediate attention.
7. Remove tight-fitting jewelry or clothing.
8. Cover burn with moist sterile or clean cover.
9. Cover victim with warm, dry cover to prevent heat loss.
10. Transport victim to nearest medical facility.

Emergency Room

1. Establish airway.
2. Initiate intravenous fluid therapy.
3. Insert indwelling catheter for hourly urine measurement.
4. Insert nasogastric tube to remove stomach contents and prevent aspiration.
5. Insert central intravenous catheter, if appropriate.
6. Treat pain by intravenous narcotic in small frequent doses.
7. Provide tetanus prophylaxis.

From *Medical-Surgical Nursing: Concepts and Clinical Practice,* 3rd ed., edited by W. Phipps, B. Long, and N. F. Woods, 1987, St. Louis: The C. V. Mosby Co.

guide clinicians in determining the type and amount of fluids to be administered based on the patient's weight, age, and the percentage of the body burned (Jelenko, 1981). The present trend is to administer balanced salt solutions (lactated Ringer's), water, and plasma and to use whole blood only if a large number of red cells are destroyed or if anemia develops. Colloids are not usually used in the first 24 hours because capillary changes allow leakage of the protein-rich fluid into the interstitial space, causing edema. Indications for fluid resuscitation are summarized in Table 22–6.

Fluids are administered in three time periods of 8 hours each. The time is calculated from the time of injury, not from the time emergency care was started. In the first three 8-hour periods (24 hours) Ringer's lactate solution (RL) is administered according to the following formula:

4 ml RL × weight (kg) × % BSA burned = ml RL to be infused during the first 24 hours after burn injury

(BSA = body-surface area.) Because blood volume falls most rapidly and edema increases fastest in the first 8 hours, intravenous replacement is at a rapid rate and one half of the total amount (50%) is given in the first 8 hours after the injury. In the second 8-hour period, one fourth (25%) of the total amount of calculated Ringer's lactate solution is given, and in the third 8-hour period, the remaining one fourth (25%) is given.

Patients may complain of moderate to severe thirst during this period. Almost every patient who is burned over 15% of the body develops thirst and an ileus. Oral fluids will not pass beyond the stomach and, if taken, create a threat of regurgitation and aspiration. A nasogastric tube is inserted and the stomach kept empty by suction to prevent gastric distention. Aggressive oral hygiene may alleviate discomfort. If oral fluids are permitted, accurate recording of intake is important. Unlimited oral intake and failure to measure and record it may result in water intoxication.

During the second 24 hours after the burn, one half to two thirds of the initial 24-hour volume will be required. It is also during this second 24-hour period that colloid solutions are used to replace intravascular volume once capillary permeability significantly decreases.

During fluid resuscitation, the adequacy of volume replacement is assessed by monitoring mental status, vital signs, peripheral perfusion, body

Table 22–6   Indications for Fluid Resuscitation

Burns greater than 20% body surface area (BSA) in adults

Burns greater than 10% BSA in children

Patient older that 65 or younger than 2 yr of age

Patient with preexisting disease that would reduce normal compensatory responses to minor hypovolemia (cardiac or pulmonary disease, diabetes)

weight, and urine output. A 15 to 20% weight gain in the first 72 hours of resuscitation is anticipated. Important laboratory tests are serum and urine electrolytes, serum and urine osmolality, and hematocrit. Hourly urine output is generally the most reliable index of adequate fluid replacement. Fluid should be given to ensure an output of 30 to 50 ml/hr in the adult. A drop in urine output below 30 ml/hr may indicate insufficient fluid replacement. The most common reasons for this are that the calculated amount of fluid is behind schedule and the severity of the burn has been underestimated. The urine is observed for color and checked for the presence of blood. The physician is notified if hematuria or a positive Hemastix reaction is present. Criteria that indicate adequate fluid resuscitation include a pulse rate of 120/min or less in the adult, a central venous pressure in the low to normal range; a pulmonary artery and diastolic pressure in the low to normal range, mental alertness, and a urine output of 30 to 50 ml/hr.

After the first 48 to 72 hours, the patient enters the diuretic phase, as edema reabsorption occurs. The urinary output increases dramatically and it is no longer a reliable guide to fluid needs. Fluid needs are assessed by measuring serum and urine electrolyte levels, and replacement is based on individual assessment using 5% dextrose in water (D_5W). If dehydration occurs from diuresis, fluid replacement therapy is continued until blood volume is stabilized. Potassium may be added to the intravenous fluid because of potassium losses through the urine. The patient is monitored closely for signs of water intoxication or pulmonary edema.

An early complication of thermal injury is the constricting effect of a circumferential eschar of the trunk or extremities. Eschar is a crust or scab that forms over a burn wound within 24 hours of the burn. Edema forming rapidly under the constricting eschar of a full-thickness wound on the arms or legs will produce enough pressure to cause occlusion of venous and arterial circulation and may result in ischemic necrosis, especially if the unburned areas are distal to the constrictive eschar. Clinical signs include cyanosis, decreased capillary filling, and complaints of pain, numbness, and tingling distal to the constricting eschar. Peripheral pulses are checked every 15 minutes with Doppler ultrasonography to ensure uninterrupted vascular flow to the extremities. Use of the Doppler has been noted to be more sensitive to early compression than clinical judgment alone (Aucher & Martinez, 1985).

It is possible to have intact pulses and severe muscle ischemia. Therefore, the most sensitive and objective method of assessing the burned limb is tissue pressure measurements. A wick catheter is inserted into a muscular compartment (or beneath the eschar) and the line is filled with fluid and connected to a transducer or manometer. Readings are taken every 1 to 2 hours during the first 36 hours. Two sequential readings above 30 mm Hg indicate that escharotomy is necessary.

An escharotomy consists of surgically cutting the eschar linearly or into squares to alleviate stricture (Figure 22–4). This is a painless procedure in a full-thickness burn because the nerve endings have already been damaged.

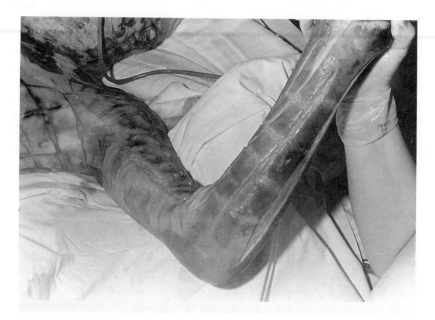

Figure 22–4.   Escharotomy used to alleviate circulatory and pulmonary constriction. Courtesy of Burn Center, MetroHealth Medical Center, Cleveland, Ohio.

The effectiveness of an escharotomy can be documented with the tissue pressure measurements described above.

Circumferential burns of the neck and chest not only occlude circulation but may result in pressure on the trachea or rib cage, causing respiratory distress. If circumferential burns of the neck and chest are accompanied by decreased chest-wall motion and/or respiratory difficulty, an escharotomy needs to be performed.

Impaired Skin Integrity and Potential for Infection   Care of the burn wound can be delayed until all first-aid measures have been initiated. Wound care should be carried out carefully and with as little discomfort to the patient as possible. One of the most important factors to be considered in wound care is that the patient has lost the ability to withstand infection in the area where the skin is damaged or destroyed.

The goals of the initial wound care are to

1. Cleanse the wound to eliminate or decrease the dead tissue and debris that serve as the media for bacterial growth.
2. Prevent further destruction of viable skin.
3. Provide for patient comfort.

During the admission procedure, the burn wound and entire body are washed to remove dirt and debris from the accident and loose dead tissue on the burned areas. Detergent (Dreft) or antiseptic preparations such as povidone-iodine (Betadine) are effective cleansing agents. Gentle cleansing with gauze is effective in removing dead tissue without causing further tissue damage. All hair in and around the burn wound is shaved and wiped away because hair attracts and shelters bacteria. Singed hair is clipped short to avoid bacterial contamination of the wound. Firm, intact blisters should be left undisturbed because they are a natural protective, pain-free dressing. If the blisters are broken and the epidermis is separated, loose tissue must be debrided.

After the wound is cleaned and before a dressing is applied, cultures of the wound are obtained. Prophylactic systemic antibiotics are usually not indicated. However, base-line wound cultures are obtained to determine which organisms are present in the wounds at the time of admission.

Photographs are taken on admission and at intervals during the patient's hospitalization. They provide a graphic record of the appearance of the burn wound on admission, before the application of topical therapy, and during the healing process.

Hypothermia   The maintenance of body temperature is a critical factor during cleansing because the severely burned patient has lost some of the ability to regulate body temperature. The environment must be heat controlled and kept warmer than usual. Drafts should be eliminated. A heat lamp or warming lights should be available. Prolonged exposure to air should be avoided. Exposed areas of the body should be covered with sterile sheets and blankets while other areas of the burn are being cleansed.

Acute Pain   Pain in extensive burns is best controlled by gentle and minimal handling and by the application of dressings to exclude air from the burned surfaces. The degree of pain is usually inversely proportional to the depth of the burn injury—full-thickness burns are usually painless because nerve endings have been destroyed. In small partial-thickness burns, cool (not cold) compresses on the burn site may provide some relief as long as the victim is kept warm. Ice packs are contraindicated because they may cause further skin injury and hypothermia.

Morphine sulfate is the drug of choice for pain relief and is given in small increments intravenously (2 to 4 mg). A morphine sulfate drip can be used during wound care (15 mg in 250 ml of D_5W) and titrated according to the patient's pain. The intravenous route is used because of inadequate absorption at peripheral sites. No medication of any kind should be given intramuscularly or subcutaneously. Inadequate tissue perfusion due to decreased cardiac output and low blood pressure can cause medication given by intramuscular or subcutaneous injection not to be absorbed immediately but later when adequate cardiac output and blood pressure are restored. Large doses of sedatives and analgesics are avoided because of the danger of respiratory depression and the potential masking of other symptoms.

Anxiety   Patients with a significant burn have received a profound insult to their body and self-image. They are fearful and anxious about possible scarring and disfigurement. They are also aware that they may not survive and this increases feelings of fear and helplessness. The shock and pain of the accident, the chaos and rush to the hospital, and the unknown surroundings and people all intensify emotional stress.

The nurse spends the most time with the patient and has considerable influence on the patient's psychological adjustment. Interventions that can be used to reassure the patient and alleviate his or her anxiety include the following:

1. Identifying self to the patient.
2. Orienting the patient to the surroundings.
3. Describing the reasons for the physical symptoms (skin loss, pain, cold).
4. Explaining the equipment and procedures to used in treatment.

Acute Period

The acute period of treatment begins at the end of the emergent period and lasts until the burn wound is healed. The length of this period varies for each individual patient. If the burn is a partial-thickness injury, the acute period is over within 10 to 20 days; if the burn is a full-thickness injury over a large percentage of the body and requiring surgery for skin grafting, the acute period can last for months.

During the acute period there are two main principles of management: treatment of the burn wound; and avoidance, detection, and treatment of complications. The most common complications are infection (septicemia, pneumonia), renal disease, and heart failure.

Assessment

Burn patients are often frightened and anxious about the burns and the associated treatments. These responses can be compounded by the ICU environment and the pain associated with dressing changes.

During every 8-hour period an assessment of mental status, vital signs, breath sounds, bowel sounds, dietary intake, motor ability, intake and output, weight pattern, circulatory adequacy, and the burn wound (or dressings), grafts, and donor sites is done. Abnormalities in any of these parameters or purulent drainage, abnormal color, foul odor, redness, or swelling in the burn wound and surrounding normal skin, or the presence of healing, should be noted. Changes in these parameters make further investigation necessary.

Metabolism is increased after moderate to severe burns as a result of stress, fluid loss, fever, infection, increased tissue catabolism, and immobility.

Wound healing may be prolonged if adequate nutritional support is not initiated on admission. A nutritional assessment is performed during the first days after burn injury and includes anthropometric measurements (to determine actual weight loss as compared with ideal weight), serum electrolytes, liver-function tests, and urinalysis. (See chapter 8 for greater detail.)

The nursing diagnoses relevant to the acute-period care of a patient who has sustained a thermal injury are summarized in Table 22–7. Related factors and desired patient outcomes are included. Interventions related to each diagnosis are discussed below.

Table 22–7   Relevant Diagnoses During the Acute Period

Nursing Diagnoses	Related Factors	Expected Outcomes
Anxiety	Threat to self-concept, threat to change in health status/role function, situational crisis	The patient will: Verbalize anxiety
Alteration in comfort; acute pain	Treatment of burn wounds: (dressings, surgery)	Obtain pain relief
Fear	Long-term illness, death, pain, treatment, life-style changes	Not be fearful; establish a trusting relationship with primary nurse
Hypothermia	Environmental exposure of burn wounds	Demonstrate normal body temperature
Infection, potential for	Decreased nutrition, burn wound, treatment (dressing, surgery)	Remain free of infection
Knowledge deficit	Lack of familiarity with routines and treatments	Verbalize understanding of treatments and surgical procedures and participate appropriately in care
Nutrition, alteration in, less than body requirements	Increased metabolic requirements and protein loss	Demonstrate optimal nutritional status
Impaired skin and tissue integrity	Burn wounds	Exhibit clean, small open wounds Demonstrate a majority of closed wounds
Social isolation	Alteration in physical appearance, physical isolation (wound, skin)	Be free from withdrawal and depression

Intervention

Potential for Infection   Measures to prevent infection begin at the time the patient is admitted to the hospital and continue until there is complete healing of the burn wound. Local and systemic infections (septicemia) are the most common complications of burns and are the major cause of death, particularly in burns covering more than 25% of the body. Autogenous sources are the primary sources of infection initially due to bacteria that survive in the hair follicles and sweat glands beneath the burned tissue. However, the patient is also susceptible to infection from exogenous sources.

The organisms that usually infect burns are *Staphylococcus aureus, Pseudomonas aeruginosa,* and the coliform bacilli. In the past few years, there has been a high incidence of fungal infections resulting from the use of broad-spectrum antibiotics. *Candida albicans,* which normally is found in the gastrointestinal tract, accounts for the majority of the fungal infections. Cultures of the patient's nose, throat, wound, and unburned skin and a punch biopsy may be taken on admission and at biweekly intervals to determine the presence of bacteria and their sensitivity to antibiotics.

Weakened pulmonary function and necrotic lung tissue coupled with the airborne bacteria place the patient at risk for bronchopneumonia. Klebsiella or psuedomonas are generally identified as the causative agents. Pneumonia may also develop as a result of systemic infection, i.e., infection in the burn wound, central venous line, or indwelling urinary catheter. Organisms usually implicated in these infections are pseudomonas or staphylococcus. Antibiotic therapy is aimed at the primary site of infection.

The increased risk of infection after burn injury is not due only to the loss of the protective skin barrier but also to the subsequent immune dysfunction that occurs. Defects of immune function involving cellular and humoral components have been documented. These include altered lymphocytes, increased suppressor cells, depressed monocyte and leukocyte mobility, depressed bactericidal activity, and impaired and depressed antibody, complement, and opsonic protein activity. The immune system is also affected by other physiologic effects of the burn injury, including endocrine, nutritional, and hematologic changes. The reverse is also true, making the treatment of these patients more difficult.

Infection is usually the cause of any deterioration of a burn patient. Signs of infection in the burn patient include increased anxiety, purulent wound drainage, leukocytosis, edema, and pallor of healthy viable tissue. Signs of sepsis in the burn patient are outlined in Table 22–8.

Prevention of infection in the burn patient is difficult. Any person or object coming into contact with the patient is a potential source of infection. To prevent the introduction of organisms into the wound, protective isolation is used and all persons who approach the patient should wear gowns, masks, caps, and gloves. Persons with upper respiratory infections should not be permitted near the patient. Aseptic technique and sterile gloves are used

Table 22–8 Signs of Sepsis in the Burn Patient

Change in sensorium

Fever

Tachycardia

Tachypnea

Paralytic ileus

Abdominal distention

Oliguria

From *Medical-Surgical Nursing: Concepts and Clinical Practice,* 3rd ed., edited by W. Phipps, B. Long, and N. F. Woods, 1987, St. Louis: The C. V. Mosby Co.

during wound care, dressing changes, suctioning, and catheter care. Hydrotherapy tanks and spray tables are used for cleansing of burn wounds and can be a source of infection when used by different patients, so they will require special attention. Care of the severely burned patient in special burn units can contribute to decreased infection because the environment is specifically geared to infection control. If the patient is cared for on a general hospital unit, a private room is essential and all equipment needed by the patient remains in the room. Protective (reverse) isolation precautions are initiated.

The application of topical antimicrobial agents to the burn helps to decrease infection and hasten healing. They are effective because damage to blood vessels in the burn area prevents systemic antibiotics from reaching the burn wound. The currently used topical agents are described more completely in Table 22–9. Antibiotics may be given prophylactically or may be withheld until an infection occurs.

Impaired Skin and Tissue Integrity Eschar is the leather-like covering of dead tissue and exudate that forms after the burn injury. It is conducive to bacterial growth because it contains dead tissue, moisture, and warmth. Cleansing and mechanical debridement are done daily to remove eschar. Washing and friction remove any build-up of debris and support healthy tissue regeneration. Hydrotherapy facilitates the removal of dressings and medications and loosens debris, sloughing eschar, and exudate. It is a more comfortable method for removal of dressings and facilitates range of motion exercise with minimal energy expenditure and discomfort. The solution used in a hydrotherapy tank may be plain water, normal saline, or an electrolytically balanced solution. To minimize the chance of infection, the nurse should keep the procedure as clean as possible. The use of gown, mask, gloves, and a plastic, disposable tub liner will decrease the chance of contamination between patients. Hydrotherapy is usually performed once or twice daily and should not exceed 30 minutes in order to prevent exposure and chilling. It is started after the patient's vital signs and fluid balance have stabi-

Table 22–9   Topical Medications Used in Burn Therapy

Topical Medication	Action	Side Effects
Mafenide acetate (Sulfamylon)	Bacteriostatic against gram-negative and gram-positive organisms (contains sulfonamide) Penetrates thick eschar	Metabolic acidosis Pain on application Allergic rash
Silver sulfadiazine (Silvadene)	Broad antimicrobial activity against gram-negative, gram-positive, and candida organisms No electrolyte imbalances Painless and somewhat soothing Not nephrotoxic	Repeated application may develop slimy, grayish appearance simulating an infection despite negative cultures (Jacoby, 1977) Prolonged use may cause skin rash and depress granulocyte formation Does not penetrate as readily as Sulfamylon
Povodine-iodine (Betadine)	Broad antimicrobial activity against bacteria, fungi, viruses, yeasts and protozoa	Metabolic acidosis due to elevated serum iodine levels Stains clothing and linen Dry, crusting, scabbing wound Skin rash in unaffected area
Silver nitrate	Bacteriostatic effect Lessens pain and eliminates odor Reduces evaporative water loss from burns	Electrolyte imbalances Stains everything it comes in contact with Does not penetrate eschar Pain on application Dressings must be kept wet
Nitrofurazone (Furacin)	Inhibits enzymes necessary for bacterial metabolism Broad spectrum of activity Effective against *Staphylococcus aureus* Not absorbed systemically Low incidence of sensitivity	Contact dermatitis in unaffected skin Urine turns a reddish color

Table 22–9 *(Continued)*

Topical Medication	Action	Side Effects
Gentamicin sulfate (Garamycin)	Broad antimicrobial activity Painless	Ototoxicity Nephrotoxicity Development of resistant bacterial strains
Neomycin	Broad antimicrobial activity Causes miscoding in the messenger RNA of bacterial cells	Serious toxic effects Ototoxicity Nephrotoxicity
Scarlet red	Nonantiseptic (applied to gauze soaked with oil-base red dye) Drying agent Applied to donor site Promotes epithelialization	No antimicrobial effects Stains and irritates skin Infection may develop beneath scarlet red gauze, which may have systemic effects
Xeroform	Nonantiseptic Debrides and protects donor site Protects graft	Removal may be painful because it sometimes adheres to wound Neither antiseptic nor antimicrobial
Sodium hypochlorite (Dakin's solution)	Chlorine-based solution that is bacteriocidal Aids in debriding wounds Aids cleaning and draining "soupy" wounds	Dissolves blood clot May inhibit clotting May irritate the skin
Sutilains ointment (Travase)	Topical enzymatic agent Dissolves necrotic tissue by proteolytic action Facilitates removal of eschar and purulent drainage	Mild, transient pain on application Paresthesia, bleeding, dermatitis Dressing must be kept moist at all times

lized. Hydrotherapy is contraindicated if the patient experiences any sudden changes in temperature, heart rate, blood pressure, or respiratory rate.

The current trend in wound cleansing is to use a spray table. The patient is placed on a special stretcher with a drain and is showered with a hose. Patient comfort is enhanced because areas that are not being debrided can be kept covered.

Different methods of treating the burned area may be used depending on the location of the burn, its size and depth, the facilities available, and the patient's response to therapy. One method may be replaced with another during the course of treatment. Those commonly used today include the open or exposure method, the semi-open method, and the closed or occlusive method.

The open or exposure method of treatment was accidently discovered to be effective in 1888 when, during a serious steamboat fire on the Mississippi River, those in attendance ran out of bandages and later observed that the neglected persons fared better than those who received more intensive local treatment (Cockshott, 1956). Today, the exposure method is used most often in the treatment of burns involving the face, neck, perineum, and broad areas of the trunk. The burned area is cleansed and exposed to air. The exudate of a partial-thickness burn dries in 48 to 72 hours and forms a hard crust that protects the wound. Epithialization occurs beneath this crust and may be complete in 14 to 21 days. The crust then falls off spontaneously leaving a healed, unscarred surface. The dead skin of a full-thickness burn is dehydrated and converted to black, leathery eschar in 48 to 72 hours. Loose eschar may be gradually removed through the use of hydrotherapy and/or debridement. Uninfected eschar acts as a protective covering. The danger of infection exists, however, as bacteria can proliferate beneath the eschar. Spontaneous separation, produced by bacterial action, occurs unless surgical debridement is performed first.

Isolation technique is essential when the exposure method is used. The nurse caring for the patient should wear a sterile gown and mask, and sterile linen should be used on the patient's bed. A cradle may be used on the patient's bed since no clothing or bed clothes are allowed directly over burned areas. Lights or heat lamps may be used with caution to provide warmth. Advantages of the open method are that the wound is easily inspected and the patient has maximal freedom to perform exercises for the prevention of contracture and the improvement of circulation.

Patients having exposure treatment complain of pain and chilling. Pain may be controlled by administering morphine sulfate, meperidine hydrochloride (Demerol), or salicylates as ordered. Discomfort can be decreased if drafts are avoided and the temperature of the room is kept at 24.4°C (85°F). Patients lose more heat from burned surfaces than from normal skin surfaces because the vascular bed that normally contracts and retains heat in the body is lost. The humidity of the room also should be controlled. A humidity level of 40 to 50% is usually considered satisfactory. Portable electric humidifiers and dehumidifiers can be used to achieve and maintain this level.

The semi-open wound care method consists of covering the wound with topical antimicrobial agents and a thin layer of gauze to help keep the agent in contact with the wound. This method permits the passage of wound exudate through the dressing without the loss of antimicrobial cream. The success of semi-open care depends on cleaning the wound once or twice a day, either at the bedside or in the hydrotherapy tank. Meticulous semi-open wound care speeds debridement, enhances the development of granulation tissue, and enables grafting sooner.

In the closed or occlusive method of burn treatment, dressings remain in place over the burn wound. The wounds are washed and dressings changed at least once a day or, in some instances, once each 8-hour period. Commonly, the dressing consists of gauze impregnated with topical ointments and a gauze wrap. Counterpressure wrappings (Ace bandages) may be applied. Large bulky dressings are rarely used today except in selected instances, because they make infection control more difficult. The type of dressing that is usually applied consists of a single layer of fine mesh gauze impregnated with a topical medication and held in place by a wrapping of a coarse gauze such as Kerlix. The purposes of applying some type of light covering include prevention of infection from exogenous sources, facilitation of debridement, promotion of maximal contact by topical agents, and prevention of fluid evaporation with loss of body heat. When a dressing is in place, nursing observation includes monitoring for signs of impaired circulation (numbness, pain, and tingling) and being alert for signs of infection (odor on dressings, elevated temperature, and elevated pulse rate).

The dressing change is usually a painful procedure, requiring administration of analgesics. Analgesics should be given 30 minutes before the procedure for maximal effectiveness. Most dressing changes are performed after hydrotherapy, in order to facilitate dressing removal and lessen pain. Additional debridement of eschar and dead tissue may be performed before the new dressing is applied.

Wet dressings may be used with silver nitrate or normal saline applications. Normal saline is applied to clean granulation tissue or to new grafts to maintain moisture or is used with fine mesh gauze to provide for slight debridement. A single layer of fine mesh gauze is usually placed over the wound, covered with thick gauze pads to maintain moisture, and held in place with a gauze wrapping. The dressings must be kept wet. Plastic wrap should *not* be used to cover the dressings. This prevents fluid evaporation, causes increased heat at the wound site, and results in patient discomfort and increased tissue destruction and risk of infection.

Skin grafts can be applied to cover the burn wound and speed healing, prevent contractures, and shorten convalescence. Successful grafting reduces the patient's vulnerability to infection and prevents the loss of body heat and water vapor from the open wound. Grafting can also be done for cosmetic or functional purposes during the rehabilitative period. Most skin grafts are applied between the third and twenty-first day after the initial injury, depending on the depth and extent of the burn and the condition of the base.

Grafts can be obtained from various sources. An autograft is a graft of skin obtained from the patient's own body and is intended to provide permanent coverage. A homograft is a graft of skin obtained from a cadaver 6 to 24 hours after death. A heterograft is a graft of skin obtained from another species, such as a pig. Synthetic substitutes for skin as well as growing the patient's own skin from skin biopsies (cultured skin) may also be utilized. Homografts, heterografts, and synthetic substitutes are intended to provide temporary coverage while the burn wound heals. A homograft may grow or "take" but, in a matter of weeks, it will be rejected by the body and sloughed. The advantage of a temporary graft is to reduce water, electrolyte, and protein loss at the burn surface. The covered would is less painful and allows the patient freedom of movement. Temporary grafts are used until the patient is ready for autografts. Often, autografting is delayed because of complications, such as pneumonia or gastric hemorrhage.

Split-thickness skin grafts are used most frequently in early stages of wound treatment. The grafts include two upper layers of skin (epidermis) and part of the middle layer (dermis) but are not taken so deep as to prevent regeneration of the skin at the site from which they are taken (donor site). The grafts are removed with a dermatone blade from almost any unburned part of the body. The size of these grafts is determined by the sites available and the area to be covered. Grafts may be placed on the recipient bed by two methods: stamping and meshing. Stamping uses "postage stamp" grafts—stamp-sized pieces of donor skin applied over the recipient bed. This technique is generally used with a wound that is unclean because it allows for drainage of excess debris. Meshing involves taking the sheet of skin after it is removed from the donor and feeding it into a meshing instrument that perforates the sheet with tiny slits (Figure 22–5). The meshing of the graft makes it more distensible so it can be stretched to cover wider areas of the body surface.

Full-thickness grafts are composed of layers of skin down to the subcutaneous tissue. They give a better cosmetic appearance than split-thickness

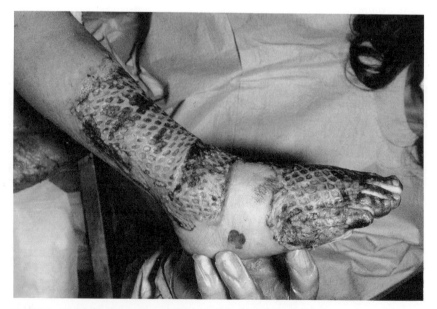

Figure 22–5. Mesh graft covering a full-thickness burn 14 days after placement.
Courtesy of Burn Center, MetroHealth Medical Center, Cleveland, Ohio.

grafts when healed and are used early in wound management and if there is a well-defined area of full-thickness burn. Areas that benefit from full-thickness grafts are hands, neck, and face. Full-thickness grafts can also be used in the rehabilitative stage to restore body function and to repair areas of released skin contractures.

Tangential excision and grafting is a surgical procedure in which the necrotic tissue or eschar is excised down to viable tissue or fascia and immediately covered with an autograft or skin substitute. The procedure is best performed between the second and fifth burn day. This technique is used with a well-defined partial-thickness injury in which deep epidermal cells remain intact for primary healing. Advantages of tangential excision and grafting are outlined in Table 22–10. After surgery, the grafted area may be covered with a large occlusive, bulky dressing to hold new skin securely in place. Splints may be applied in the operating room to provide immobilization and maintain position. The dressing should remain intact for 48 to 72 hours unless it is found to be purulent with a strong odor. Dressing removal is done slowly and carefully so as not to disturb the graft.

The donor site represents a wound similar to that of a partial-thickness injury. Care of the donor site is as important as care of the graft itself, for donor sites that fail to heal result in a net enlargement of the patient's open wound surface. Donor sites may be treated by a variety of methods. One method is covering the exposed surface with fine mesh gauze, Xeroform, or a synthetic dressing and leaving it exposed to the air. Exposing the donor site to a heat lamp also promotes healing, because as the drainage from the wound dries it serves as a protective covering. Another method is to cover the site with sterile gauze and apply a pressure dressing. The site usually heals in 2 weeks.

Many patients complain of severe pain in the donor site, and the nurse should not hesitate to give medications for pain. The pain should subside in 24 to 48 hours as the wound dries. The would should be inspected daily for any signs of infection (erythema, purulent drainage, foul odor). If infection develops, antibiotics may be administered and the wound treated with wet dressings.

Table 22–10 Advantages of Tangential Excision and Grafting

Shortened hospitalization

Prevents potential conversion of burn to full thickness by removing necrotic tissue before infection occurs

Definitive healing diminishes anxiety and lessens trauma to multiple graftings

Allows early grafting and early restoration of function

Scar formation reduced because of use of full-thickness graft

From *Medical-Surgical Nursing: Concepts and Clinical Practice,* 3rd ed., edited by W. Phipps, B. Long, and N. F. Woods, 1987, St. Louis: The C. V. Mosby Co.

Alteration in Nutrition   Metabolism is increased after moderate to severe burns as a result of stress, fluid loss, fever, infection, hypercatabolism, and immobility. Shivering and the elevated levels of catecholamines (cortisol and glucagon) found shortly after thermal injury increase tissue oxygen consumption and heat production, deplete liver and muscle glycogen stores and fat deposits, and lead to a negative nitrogen balance and weight loss. Protein is broken down, providing amino acids for gluconeogenesis, and amino acids are prevented from incorporating into protein. The diminished rate of protein production prolongs wound healing and increases the patient's susceptibility to infection.

A burn patient remains catabolic until the caloric intake exceeds caloric expenditure. Hypermetabolism continues until the wounds are 90% healed and homeostasis is restored (Wachtel, Yen, Fortune, Long & Brimm, 1983). The patient's total energy and protein requirements become those needed for normal homeostasis plus those required to offset the catabolic state and repair the injury.

The protein and caloric needs of the burned person are highly variable, depending on the extent and depth of injury and the patient's age, sex, preburn nutritional status, and preexisting diseases. The daily protein requirement is greater than normal because of the negative nitrogen balance. The normal daily protein requirement is 0.8 g/kg of body weight for the adult. The massive mobilization of protein after the burn injury increases the daily requirement by two to four times the amount required before the injury: approximately 1.5 to 3.2 g/kg of body weight. Protein must be used for tissue repair and healing, not as a source of energy. Therefore, it is important to provide adequate carbohydrate and fat calories to satisfy energy needs. An appreciable loss of zinc generally accompanies a protein and weight loss. Studies demonstrate that zinc deficiency impairs wound healing and recent data indicate that a zinc deficiency will impair cellular immunity (Larson et al., 1970; Pasulka and Wachtel, 1987).

The daily caloric requirement increases from a normal 1,700 to 3,000 calories to 3,500 to 50,000 calories. Because the demand for calories increases with a major burn, appropriate vitamin therapy is essential. Vitamins and minerals are given at two to three times the recommended daily allowances established for normal healthy adults. Vitamin C promotes healing and the daily requirement in the burn patient increases from a normal of 45 mg to 1 to 2 g. The B complex vitamins are necessary for the metabolism of the increased protein and carbohydrate intake. Vitamins A, E, and K and folic acid are monitored and supplemented as indicated. Serum levels of calcium, phosphate, and potassium are also monitored. Therapeutic levels of iron must be maintained to prevent the ongoing threat of anemia associated with burn injury.

Weight loss and gain are monitored for evaluation of nutritional status. Weight gain occurs initially because of fluid retention, however, after diuresis there is a marked loss of weight. Severe weight loss is closely related to protein loss or the loss of body cell mass and the enormous amount of body fluid lost through the burn wound itself. As in other metabolic responses, weight loss is dependent on the extent of injury: the greater the burn, the greater the weight loss.

Paralytic ileus or gastric dilation is frequently seen in severely burned patients because of the neuroendocrine response to stress, hypovolemia, or septicemia. This prevents enteral feeding until gastrointestinal tract motility is restored. Total parenteral nutrition (TPN) is indicated once fluid resuscitation is completed. TPN with supplemental fat solutions is used to provide calories.

Oral or tube feeding is the preferred method of providing adequate nutrition, and should be used as soon as possible. The enteral route is the most natural and convenient means of nutritional support and is discussed in detail in chapter 8. The burn patient will seldom consume more food after injury than before injury. Therefore, combination of the parenteral and enteral modes may be necessary to meet the enormous nutritional requirements. Dietary supplements that contain additional calorie and protein can be provided by milkshakes that can be specially made by the hospital dietary department. Patients should be encouraged to drink supplements between meals.

Postburn lactose intolerance may occur in patients being tube fed. Signs of bloating, flatulence, cramps, and diarrhea may be seen. A modification of the strength and type of supplement may be necessary; starting the supplement at one-half or one-quarter strength, diluted with water, will often alleviate gastrointestinal complications.

The patient should advance to a regular diet as quickly as possible. However, ingenuity by the nurses and dietitian are often needed in order to motivate the patient to eat the food necessary to meet nutritional requirements. Relatives can suggest favorite foods. The nurse should time all dressing changes and treatments so they do not immediately precede meals.

Fecal impaction is a common problem in burn patients. Bulk foods and fruit juices should be provided in the diet. Bulk-forming laxatives such as preparations of the psyllium seed (Metamucil) or a fecal softener such as docusate sodium (Colace) may be ordered by the physician.

Maintenance of a nutritional support program is critical to the survival of a thermally injury patient. The goals of the nutritional support program are to establish eating by the traditional route as soon as possible and to maintain sufficient caloric and protein intake to restore tissue loss. A team approach provides comprehensive input and integrates the efforts of the patient and family, physician, nurse, pharmacist, dietitian, and occupational and physical therapists.

Fear and Anxiety   The psychological responses of the patient during the immediate postburn period are in response to a threat to survival. The fear of death is real as the patient senses the acuteness of the situation by experiencing pain, disfigurement, isolation, and dependency. Reactions of patients are determined by their personality, degree of total adjustment to life, and the extent and location of their burns. The nurse should offer support and encouragement to the patient as well as explain all treatments and procedures in order to ease the patient's anxiety. Setting short-term achievable goals will help motivate the patient. Providing the family with an explanation of the patient's needs will not only ease their fears but will also allow them to help the patient. Chapter 3 (Crisis), chapter 4 (Coping), and chapter 5 (Behavioral Responses to the Critical Care Environment) will provide useful adjunct information in recognizing and treating the patient and family in crisis.

Pain   Pain is elicited by specific activities such as wound cleansing and debridement, dressing changes, and physical therapy. Acute pain, with its usually abrupt onset and finite period of time to resolution, is most successfully treated with analgesics. Analgesics should also be used to prevent pain from recurring after it is initially decreased as it takes less medication to prevent pain than to abolish it. Most patients are undermedicated for severe burn pain, perhaps from a fear that they will become addicted to the narcotic analgesics. Dosages can be adjusted to the individual needs of each patient.

Anxiety over anticipated procedures may cause a progressive increase in the degree of pain experienced by the patient (Wingate, 1983). Muscle tension related to fear and apprehension is known to lower pain threshold. Sleep deprivation, a common occurrence in critical care units, can also make the patient less tolerant of pain. Self-hypnosis or relaxation exercises can be effective in altering the perception of either actual or anticipated discomfort and should be consistently reinforced by the team (Bernstein, 1976). Outlined in Table 22–11 are nursing interventions that can aid in minimizing pain during dressing changes and other procedures.

Rehabilitation Period

The rehabilitation process begins at the time of admission. However, rehabilitation as the third stage of treatment begins when the patient's burn is reduced to less than 20% of the body-surface area and the patient is capable of

Table 22–11   Nursing Interventions for Minimizing Pain in the Burn Patient

Provide analgesic medications 30 min before dressing change.

Provide clear explanations to gain patient's cooperation.

Handle burned areas gently.

Use sterile technique (infection causes increased pain).

Encourage patient to participate in treatment whenever possible.

Use distracting techniques (radio, conversation) and relaxation techniques when appropriate.

assuming some self-care activity. The principles of management are to return the patient to a productive place in society and to accomplish functional and cosmetic reconstruction. It is important to remember that rehabilitation begins on admission and does not end when the patient is discharged. It may take from 2 to 5 years after discharge for the patient to reach a maximum level of emotional and physical adjustment.

The nursing diagnoses relevant to the rehabilitation phase of caring for a patient who has sustained a thermal injury are summarized in Table 22–12. Related factors and desired patient outcomes are included. Interventions related to each diagnosis are discussed below.

Intervention

Impaired Physical Mobility   A comprehensive program of positioning, splinting, exercise, ambulation, and activities of daily living must begin on the first or second day after the burn and be carried through until after discharge. Any delays in initiating treatment will be detrimental to the patient's ultimate functional outcome. Contractures are among the most serious long-term complications of burns today. They result from muscle and joint stiffening, skin grafting, and prolonged bed rest. While the occupational and physical therapists address the patient's rehabilitation needs during all phases of the patient's recovery, the nurse is responsible for ensuring that all interventions are followed.

The nurse is responsible for assessing the patient's response to positioning, splinting, exercise, and the ability of the patient and family to perform daily wound care after discharge. Correct positioning must be maintained to avoid the development of contractures. The splinted limb must be assessed for adequate circulation, cyanosis, temperature, and the presence of pulses. The ability to exercise, perform activities of daily living, and ambulate must be continually assessed for both physical and emotional tolerance. Complete and comprehensive instructions followed by demonstration of ability to care for wounds and dressings are necessary prior to discharge.

Therapeutic positioning, the act of placing body parts in antideformity (anatomical) positions, is vital to the prevention of burn contractures. Frequent repositioning of the patient in bed (lying on the side, supine, prone) must be done regularly during the day and night. Correct positioning varies depending on the area of the body burned and is summarized in Table 22–13.

Positioning can be enhanced by placing the patient on a Stryker frame, Foster bed, or one of the many different types of flotation/low air loss beds/mattresses currently available. These beds facilitate the use of the bedpan and urinal, permit change of position with a minimum of handling, and permit larger skin surfaces to remain free from body pressure than is possible when the patient lies on a regular mattress/bed. Because they allow turning of the

Table 22–12   Relevant Diagnoses During the Rehabilitation Phase

Nursing Diagnoses	Related Factors	Expected Outcomes
Activity intolerance	Immobilization from splinting, generalized weakness, bedrest, pain	*The patient will:* Achieve activity tolerance consistent with desired levels
Anxiety	Change in health status, role functioning/socio-economic status	Exhibit decreased anxiety
Impaired skin integrity and body image disturbance	Scarring, contractures, discoloration	Demonstrate a realistic concept of changes in body image and alterations required in daily activities
Comfort, alteration in: pain	Increasing activity, (exercise, ambulation, activities of daily living)	Verbalize no pain
Coping, ineffective family: compromised	Inadequate or incorrect information or understanding, prolonged disability of significant person	Demonstrate appropriate coping skills (patient and family)
Coping, ineffective individual	Burn injury, personal vulnerability	
Diversional activity deficit	Long-term hospitalization, away from work, friends, and usual recreational activities	Participate in diversional activities
Fear	Long-term illness, surgery, treatments, changes in lifestyle, pain, disfigurement, job security	Verbalize fears and participate in planned interventions that will decrease fears
Knowlege deficit	Wound/skin care, positioning, exercises, use of adaptive devices	Demonstrate correct understanding of self-care and follow-up (patient and family)
Mobility, impaired physical	Intolerance to activity, decreased strength and endurance, pain, severe anxiety, contracture formation	Achieve optimal joint mobility
Self-care deficit	Intolerance to activity, fatigue, pain, discomfort, severe anxiety	Demonstrate ability to perform activities of daily living

Table 22–13 Therapeutic Positioning for the Burn Patient

Area Burned	Description of Position
Neck	No pillow Towel roll under cervical spine Neck splint
Shoulder	90-degree abduction, neutral rotation Elbow splint may be used to aid in maintaining position
Axilla	Abduction with 10–15 degree forward flexion and external rotation Support abducted arm with suspension from IV pole or with beside table Axilla splint
Elbow	Extension Support extended arm on beside table or foam trough Elbow splint

Hand
  Dorsal surface
  Palmar surface
	Hand splint
	  Flexion
	  Hyperextension

Hip	Extension with neutral rotation Supine with lower extremity extended Lying prone (if medically appropriate) Trochanter roll Foam wedge along lateral aspect of thigh Knee or long leg splint
Knee	Extension Lying prone (if medically appropriate) Patient out of bed with lower extremities extended and elevated Knee splint
Ankle	Dorsiflexion Padded footboard with heels free of pressure Ankle splint

From *Medical-Surgical Nursing: Concepts and Clinical Practice,* 3rd ed., edited by W. Phipps, B. Long, and N. F. Woods, 1987, St. Louis: The C. V. Mosby Co.

patient with minimum of handling they also help decrease pain. These special beds are particularly useful when both the back and front of the trunk, thighs, and legs have been burned.

Prolonged rest in semi-Fowler's position or with a pillow pushing the head forward must be avoided (see chapter 14). Many patients like this position because it enables them to see around the room better. Often, the bed can be turned so that the patient can look around without having to assume positions that may lead to the formation of contractures.

Splints are used to prevent or correct contractures and to immobilize joints after grafting. They are custom-made and often molded directly on the patient to ensure optimal conformity to the limb or body part (Figure 22–6). It is the responsibility of the nurse to apply the splint properly and according to an established schedule. An improperly applied splint can promote contractures and lead to additional complications.

Exercises for the prevention and correction of contractures are begun as soon as the patient is stable. Active exercises are preferred although active assistance and gentle pressure exercises may be more realistic. Supervision by a physical or occupational therapist is desirable. Exercises may be performed more easily in water and may be done along with dressing changes if the patient is able to tolerate the activity. When burns are completely covered (by healing or by graft), exercises may be performed more easily in an occupational therapy or physical therapy department where the patient may benefit from a change of environment. In order to prevent scar contracture formation, daily therapy sessions may be necessary for several weeks or months. A plan for continued exercise and splinting must be established prior to discharge.

Ambulation decreases the risk of thromboemboli, promotes optimal ventilation, helps maintain range of motion and strength in the lower extrem-

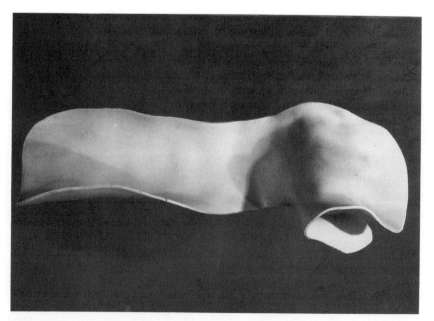

Figure 22–6. Orthoplast hand splint. Courtesy of Burn Center, MetroHealth Medical Center, Cleveland, Ohio.

ities, orients the patient to the environment, and provides a sense of functional independence. Mobilizing the patient requires a progressive approach in patients with large burns who have less ability to tolerate activity. Initially, the patient may need to be transferred with maximum assistance onto a stretcher chair and progress to a sitting position. Gradually, the patient may progress to a standing pivot transfer into a nearby chair and eventually may ambulate with minimal assistance. Prior to getting out of bed, an elastic bandage support must be applied to lower extremities to prevent venous stasis, edema, and orthostatic hypotension.

Self-Care Deficit   One of the ultimate goals in the rehabilitation of the burned patient is to maintain or restore the patient's independence in performing the activities of daily living. The occupational therapist aids in this process by selecting activities that are appropriate to the patient's medical, physical, and mental status. Activities that the nurse can encourage are self-feeding, telephoning, reading mail, and assisting with grooming or burn-wound management. The nurse must know what the patient is being taught by the physical and occupational therapists so that progress can be continued on the nursing unit. Aids can be developed by the occupational therapist to help the patient perform activities of daily living.

Ineffective Coping   After the initial period, the long healing process begins, accompanied by the realization of endless implications for the future. Burns on the face make adjustment particularly difficult. Different kinds of fears develop, including those related to pain, disfigurement, prolonged hospitalization, job security, change in lifestyle, and reaction of family and friends to the burn injury. To some, the thought of being different or conspicuous may be unbearable. If possible, the patient should see facial burns only after being prepared for the experience. Support and understanding will be needed in order for the patient to cope with what will be seen in the mirror. The patient will exhibit readiness by asking to look in the mirror. Interaction with other burn patients who are further along in their healing process may help the patient feel that recovery is possible. In some instances, the recovery is incredible, and although differences in skin pigmentation remain, the redness that accompanies healed burn wounds often fades considerably within a few months. Pigmentation problems are more acute for persons with brown or black skin. Their healed skin may be a different shade, freckled, or whitish in color.

After discharge, the patient will have to adjust to temporary or permanent function loss, cosmetic disfigurement, and the reaction of others. The ability to make these adjustments will depend on coping mechanisms developed before the injury, the severity and site of the burn, and the reactions of others that the patient has already experienced. How well the patient is able to adapt to these changes can be evaluated during outpatient visits.

The patient should have the opportunity to talk about any concerns or fears. Some patients may discuss these with the nurse when they cannot express them to relatives, and the nurse must be prepared to listen and help the individual accept necessary changes in lifestyle. Almost every burned patient and family need the help of a social worker. The nurse should recognize this need and initiate the referral. Visiting hours can be used to talk with relatives who may be able to give information that will clarify the patient's needs and resources. This time also provides an opportunity for the nurse to help relatives accept their loved one's change in appearance and to help them plan for the return of the loved one to the community.

Impaired Skin Integrity and Body Image Disturbance   Anytime a wound of connective tissue heals, hypertrophic scarring will occur unless the skin is adherent to the underlying structure. Hypertrophic scarring results from the overgrowth and overproduction of tissue. This occurs especially in areas of stress and movement, such as the hands, legs, and chest (Figure 22–7). The thickened rigid scar that results may later cause contractures, especially when over a joint.

The application of controlled constant pressure to the surface of an immature scar will reduce the scar and leave a smooth pliable tissue (Larson et al., 1971). If this pressure is applied to new, healthy tissue, hypertrophic

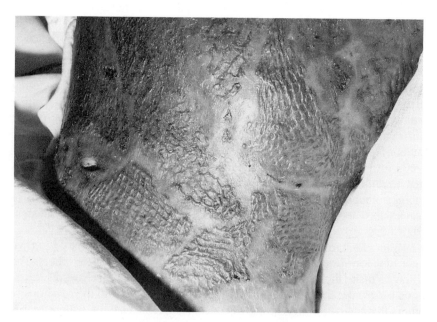

Figure 22–7.   Hypertrophic scarring over chest and abdomen. Courtesy of Burn Center, MetroHealth Medical Center, Cleveland, Ohio.

scarring can be prevented. The Jobst garment, which is specially designed using an elastic woven material, provides tridimensional control. It must be tight enough to produce the 24 mm Hg of pressure required to exceed capillary pressure and thus reduce edema and scar formation. It is fitted to each patient individually and then custom made (Figure 22–8). Until the garment is completed, Ace bandages can be used for a pressure dressing. Even though pressure garments help decrease the formation of thick, disfiguring scars, patient acceptance is a problem. The garments are uncomfortable and make the patient warm, especially during hot weather. The patient must wear the garment 23 hours a day for 6 months to a year.

Knowledge Deficit   Prior to discharge, burned patients and their families have a great need for education so that they may assume the increased re-

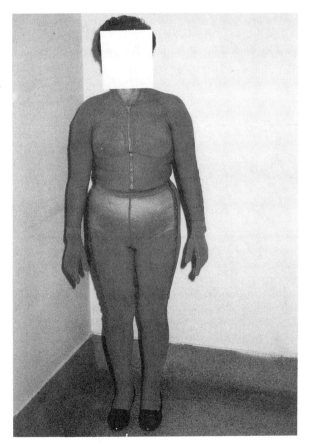

Figure 22–8.   Total body Jobst garment consisting of three separate pieces: jacket, pants, and gloves. Courtesy of Burn Center, MetroHealth Medical Center, Cleveland, Ohio.

sponsibility for their own care. Discharge teaching involves the entire burn team, and since rehabilitation is a gradual process, there should be ample time to plan the return home in every detail.

Early discharge planning accomplishes two goals. First, it helps solve problems early; e.g., if the patient's house burned and needs to be repaired, the family may need to relocate. This could be done prior to discharge, thus preventing the added stress of moving after discharge. Second, early discharge planning emphasizes the future. If discharge is continually discussed, the patient and family may realize more quickly that recovery and return to a fulfilling and productive life are achievable.

Complete and comprehensive instructions followed by demonstrations of understanding contribute to learning the necessary skills to be independent in self-care activities after discharge. Patients should not be discharged from the hospital until they can care for themselves physically, with assistance if necessary, and are prepared to meet the stresses involved in returning to their former living patterns.

Teaching should include the following content areas: wound management and skin care, signs and symptoms of complications, use of pressure dressings, exercises, splinting techniques, activities of daily living, and methods of coping with resocialization. Wound management instructions should include how to care for the healed grafted and nongrafted areas. Signs and symptoms of complications, including areas that may blister and breakdown, and signs of infection should also be addressed. Instructions should be written so that the patient has reference material should he or she get home and have questions. An example of written discharge instructions is provided in Table 22–14. The patient and family should also be given the name and phone number of a doctor or nurse who can be contacted with questions or

Table 22–14   Discharge Instructions for Burn Patient

We on the burn team are happy to see that you are able to go home. To ensure you the speediest possible recovery, it is important that you are able to care for yourself and recognize problems that may interfere with your complete recovery.

If any of the following occur, please call the hospital and ask for the burn clinic. The nurse will be able to assist you.
1. Healed area breaking open. Cover with clean dressing.
2. Formation of blisters.
3. Signs of infection:
   a. Fever, temperature over 37.2°C (99°F).
   b. Redness, pain, swelling, hardness, or warmth in or around wound or any other part of body.
   c. Increased or foul-smelling drainage from wound.
4. Problems with your Ace bandages or Jobst garment, such as improper fit, formation of blisters, or opening of healed area underneath.

Your first clinic appointment will be on _____. If a family member can come with you they can register for you and you may go to the burn clinic waiting room.

Table 22–14 *(Continued)*

Skin Care for Healed Burn

These are your guidelines for your daily skin care of a healed burn. When you do your skin care, this is the time to look at the involved areas and note if there are any changes that need to be reported.

1. Wash healed area every day with solution of 2 tbsp Dreft (or Ivory Snow) and water.
2. Wash gently with washcloth to remove dead skin.
3. Rinse skin well after washing.
4. Dry thoroughly.
5. Apply Nivea lightly twice a day and more frequently if the skin is dry and flaked.
6. Do not put Nivea on open areas.
7. You can purchase Nivea at your local drugstore.

Care For Burn Wound

These are your guidelines for the care of your burn wound. When you do your care, this is the time to look at the involved areas and note if there are any changes that need to be reported.

Procedure for burn wound care:

1. Wash hands.
2. Remove dressing and dispose of in paper bag or wrap in newspaper.
3. Wash hands.
4. Wash open area with gauze using solution of Dreft (or Ivory Snow) and water. Add 1 tbsp Dreft to a basin of water; 2 tbsp Dreft, if you use the bathtub. Use a clean towel and washcloth with each dressing change.
5. Rinse skin well.
6. Wash hands.
7. Apply dressing as described below.
8. Wear gloves. Wash basin or bathtub with a disinfectant such as Lysol.
9. Wash hands.

Care of Clothing

When you are discharged, you may find that healed burn areas are sensitive to harsh detergents, fabric softeners, and clothing dyes. If you are sensitive, we suggest the following:

1. Launder new clothing before use by machine or hand with Dreft or Ivory Snow.
2. Rinse clothes twice.
3. Do not use fabric softeners.
4. If you have open burns or a healed area that opens, wash all clothes separately from other family members'.
5. Scarlet red ointment will permanently stain clothing.
6. If dyes used in clothing cause irritation, wear white articles.

Ace Bandages

You have been taught to put on your own Ace bandages while in the hospital; but if you have a problem with this, please notify the burn clinic. It is also important that you know how to care for them and understand problems that occur.

Table 22–14   *(Continued)*

1. If they are too loose, they will be ineffective and must be rewrapped.
2. If they are too tight, they will cause discomfort, numbness, tingling, and puffiness and must be rewrapped.
3. They must be worn for a long period of time, probably 6–12 months to be effective, so please do not stop wearing them until your doctor tells you to.
4. To care for your Ace bandages:
   a. Hand wash with Dreft or Ivory Snow in cold water.
   b. Towel dry.
   c. Lay flat or place over rod or clothesline.
   d. Do not use clothespins.

Jobst Garment

You have been taught to put on your Jobst garment while in the hospital; but if you have a problem with this, please notify the burn clinic. It is also important that you know how to care for it and understand problems that can occur.

1. If it is too loose, it will be ineffective and you will require a new garment.
2. If it is too tight, it will cause discomfort, numbness, and tingling. Do not wear it if this occurs, but notify the burn clinic as soon as possible.
3. To care for your Jobst garment:
   a. Hand wash with Dreft or Ivory Snow in cold water.
   b. Towel dry.
   c. Lay flat or place over rod or clothesline.
   d. Do not use clothespins.

Courtesy of Metro Health Medical Center, Cleveland, Ohio, Department of Nursing Service.

problems. A home health nurse may be of assistance in dressing the patient's wounds.

Follow-up care may not take place at the institution where the patient was hospitalized, especially if the patient lives some distance away. The burn team members may need to contact their counterparts in the patient's community to plan follow-up care. If possible, a member of the follow-up team should visit the patient in the hospital before discharge.

Job retraining may be necessary if the burn injury caused loss of joint function or other physical limitations that may prevent the patient from doing his or her former job. The local office of the State Labor and Industry Board can assign a vocational counselor to help the patient return to the work force. Even if retraining cannot begin for several months, the contact with the vocational counselor and anticipation of retraining may help the patient look beyond his or her immediate problems and think of the future.

SUMMARY

Burns are the most common and profound trauma to skin. With a major burn, there is an overwhelming insult to the patient both physically and psychologically. A complication such as pneumonia, infection, or shock can be as serious a threat to the patient as is the burn injury itself. The care of these patients is multidimensional and provides an ongoing challenge to critical care nurses in directing the patient back to health.

BIBLIOGRAPHY

Achauer, B. M., & Martinez S. E. (1985). Burn wound pathophysiology and care. *Critical Care Clinics, 1,* 47–58.

American Burn Association (1984). Guidelines for service standards and severity classifications in the treatment of burn injury. *American College of Surgeons Bulletin, 69,* 24–28.

Bernstein, N. R. (1976). *Emotional care of the facially burned and disfigured.* Boston: Little, Brown.

Cockshott, W. P. (1956). The history of the treatment of burns. *Surgery, Gynecology and Obstetrics, 102,* 116–124.

Jackson, D. M. (1953). The diagnosis of the depth of burning. *British Journal of Surgery, 40,* 588.

Jacoby, F. J. (1977). Individualized burn wound dressings. *Nursing '77, 7*(6), 62–63.

Jelenko, C. (1981). Burn shock, *Topics in Emergency Medicine, 3,* 69–74.

Larson, D. L., Abston, S., Evans, E. B., Dobrkovsky, M., & Linares, H. A. (1971). Techniques for decreasing scar formation and contracture in the burned patient. *Journal of Trauma, 11,* 807.

Larson, D. L. Maxwell, R., Abston, S., Dobrkovsky, M. (1970). Zinc deficiency in burned children. *Plastic and Reconstructive Surgery, 46,* 13–21.

Maley, M. P. (1982). Burn education and prevention. In R. P. Hummel (Ed.). *Clinical burn therapy,* Boston: John Wright.

Pasulka, P. S., & Wachtel, T. L. (1987). Nutritional considerations for the burned patient. *Surgical Clinics of North America, 67*(1), 109–132.

Pruitt, B. A. Jr., & Goodwin, C. W., Jr. (1981). Stress ulcer disease in the burned patient. *World Journal of Surgery, 5,* 209.

Trunkey, D. D. (1983). Transporting the critically burned patient. In T. L. Wachtel, V. Kahn, H. A. Frank (Eds.), *Current concepts in burn care.* Rockville, MD: Aspen Systems.

Wachtel, T. L., Yen, M., Fortune, J. B., Long, W. B., & Brimm, J. E. (1983). Nutritional support for burned patients. In T. L. Wachtel, V. Kahn, & H. A. Frank (Eds.), *Current concepts in burn care.* Rockville, MD: Aspen Systems.

Wingate, E. (1983). Emergent burn care: A time for life-saving measures. *Critical Care Update, 10,* 49–54.

ADDITIONAL READINGS

Abshagen, D. (1984). Topical agents and emergency care for minor burn injuries. *Journal of Emergency Nursing, 10,* 325–331.

Achauer, B. M. (Ed.) (1987). *Management of the burned patient.* Norwalk, CT: Appleton & Lange.

Andreason, N. J. C., Nayes, R., Jr., Hartford, C. E., Brodland, G., & Proctor, S. (1972). Management of emotional reactions in seriously burn adults. *New England Journal of Medicine, 286,* 65–69.

Artz, C. P., Moncrief, J. A., & Pruitt, B. A. (1979). *Burns: A team approach.* Philadelphia: W. B. Saunders.

Busby, H. D. (1979). Nursing management of the acute burn patient and nursing management of optimal burn recovery. *Journal of Continuing Education in Nursing, 10,* 16–30.

Charnock, E. L., & Meehan, J. J. (1980). Postburn respiratory injuries in children, *Pediatric Clinics of North America, 27,* 661–676.

Curreri, P. W., & Luterman, A. (1978). Nutritional support of the burned patient. *Surgical Clinics of North America, 58,* 1151–1156.

Demling, R. H. (1987). Fluid replacement in burned patients. *Surgical Clinics of North America., 67,* 15–30.

Dobbs, E. R., & Curreri, W. P. (1974). Burns: Analysis of results of physical therapy in 681 patients. *Journal of Trauma, 12,* 242–248.

Dyer, C. (1980). Burn care in the emergent period. *Journal of Emergency Nursing, 6,* 9–16.

Feller, I., & Archanbeault, C. (1973). *Nursing the burned patient.* Ann Arbor, MI: Institute for Burn Medicine Press.

Feller, I., Jones, C. A., & Richards, K. (1977). *Emergent care of the burn victim.* Ann Arbor, MI: Institute for Burn Medicine Press.

Finlayson, L. (1980). Emergent care of the burn patient. *Critical Care Update, 7,* 18–19, 22–23.

Freeman, J. W. (1984). Nursing care of the patient with a burn injury. *Critical Care Nurse, November/December,* 52–68.

Gatson, S. F., & Schumann, L. L. (1980). Burn wound management. *Critical Care Update, 7,* 5–17.

Gordon, M. (1985). *Manual of nursing diagnosis.* New York: McGraw-Hill.

Hardy, J. D. (Ed.) (1977). *Textbook of surgery: Principles and practice* (5th ed.). Philadelphia: J. B. Lippincott.

Heidrich, B., Perry, S., & Amand, R. (1981). Nursing staff attitudes about burn pain. *Journal of Burn Care Rehabilitation, 2,* 259–261.

Hills, S. W., & Birmingham, J. J. (1981). *Burn Care.* Bethany, CT: Flescher.

Hummel, R. P. (Ed.) (1982). *Clinical burn therapy: A management and prevention guide.* Littleton, MA: John Wright.

Jacoby, F. J. (1984). Care of the massive burn wound. *Critical Care Quarterly, 7*(3), 44–53.

Jacoby, F. G. (1976). *Nursing care of the patient with burns* (2nd ed.). St. Louis: C. V. Mosby.

Jelenko, C. (1974). Chemicals that "burn." *Journal of Trauma, 14,* 65–72.

Jones, C. A., & Feller, I. (1977a). Burns: Avoiding and coping with complications before and after grafting. *Nursing '77, 7,* 72–81.

Jones, C. A., & Feller, I. (1977b). Burns: The home stretch . . . rehabilitation. *Nursing '77, 7,* 54–57.

Jones, C. A., & Feller, I. (1977c). Burns: What to do during the first crucial hours. *Nursing '77, 7,* 22–31.

Kenner, C. V. (1981). Burn injury. In C. V. Kenner, C. E. Guzzetta, & B. M. Dossey (Eds.), *Critical care nursing: Body–mind–spirit.* Boston: Little, Brown.

Kenner, C., & Manning, S. (1980). Emergency care of the burn patient. *Critical Care Update, 7,* 24–27, 30–33.

Kilbee, E. (1984). Burn pain management. *Critical Care Quarterly, 7*(3), 54–62.

King, M. W. (1982). Nursing considerations of the burned patient during the emergent period. *Heart and Lung, 11,* 353–363.

Kinzie, Y., & Lau, C. (1980). What to do for the severely burned. *RN, 43*(4), 46–51, 104–110.

Klein, D. G., & O'Malley, P. (1987). Interventions for persons with burns. In W. J. Phipps, B. C. Long, & N. F. Woods (Eds.), *Medical–surgical nursing: Concepts and clinical practice.* 3rd ed. St. Louis: C. V. Mosby.

Klein, D. G., & O'Malley P. (1987). Topical injury from chemical agents: Initial treatment. *Heart and Lung, 16*(1), 49–54.

LeMaster, J. E. (1983). Rehabilitation of the burn-injured patient. In T. L. Wachtel, V. Kahn, & H. A. Frank (Eds.), *Current concepts in burn care.* Rockville, MD: Aspen Systems.

Luterman, A., Adams, A., & Curreri, P. W. (1984). Nutritional management of the burn patient. *Critical Care Quarterly, 7*(3), 34–43.

Marvin, J. A. (1983). Planning home care for burn patients. *Nursing '83, 13*(8), 65–67.

Marvin, J. (1978). Acute care of the burn patient. *Critical Care Quarterly, 1,* 25–35.

Moritz, A. R., & Henriques, F. C., Jr. (1947). Studies of thermal injury, II. The relative importance of time and surface temperatures in the causation of cutaneous burns. *American Journal of Pathology, 23,* 531.

Mosley, S. (1988). Inhalation injury: A review of the literature. *Heart and Lung, 17,* 3–9.

Moylan, J. A., Inge, W. W., & Pruitt, W. A. (1971). Circulatory changes following circumferential extremity burns evaluated by the ultrasonic flowmeter: An analysis of 60 thermally injured limbs. *Journal of Trauma, 11,* 763.

Nadel, E., & Kozerefski, P. M. (1984). Rehabilitation of the critically ill burn patient. *Critical Care Quarterly, 7*(3), 19–33.

Nursing grand rounds (1980). Severely burned patients: Anticipating their emotional needs. *Nursing '80, 12*(9), 47–50.

Ragiel, C. A. (1984). The impact of critical injury on patient, family, and clinical systems. *Critical Care Quarterly, 8*(3), 73–78.

Rauscher, L. A., & Ochs, G. M. (1983). Prehospital care of the seriously burned patient. In T. L. Wachtel, V. Kahn, & H. A. Frank (Eds.), *Current topics in burn care.* Rockville, MD: Aspen Systems.

Robertson, K. E., Cross, P. J., & Terry, J. C. (1985). Burn care: The crucial first days. *American Journal of Nursing, 85*(1), 30–45.

Salisbury, R. E., Newman, N. M., & Dingeldein, G. D. (Eds.) (1983). *Manual of burn therapeutics.* Boston: Little, Brown.

Schumann, L., & Gatson, S. (1979). Common sense guide to topical burn therapy. *Nursing '79, 9*(3), 34–39.

Shenkman, B., & Stechmiller, J. (1987). Patient and family perception of projected functioning after discharge from a burn unit. *Heart and Lung, 16*(5), 490–495.

Surveyer, J. A. (1980). Smoke inhalation injuries. *Heart and Lung, 9*(5), 825–832.

Trunkey, D. D. (1981). Transporting the critically burned patient. *Topics in Emergency Medicine, 3,* 21–24.

Wachtel, T. L., Frank, H. A., Fortune, J. B., & Inancsi, W. (1983). Initial management of major burns. In T. L. Wachtel, V. Kahn, & H. A. Frank (Eds.), *Current concepts in burn care*. Rockville, MD: Aspen Systems.

Wachtel, T. L., & Fortune, J. B. (1983). Fluid resuscitation for burn shock. In T. L. Wachtel, V. Kahn, & H. A. Frank (Eds.), *Current concepts in burn care*. Rockville, MD: Aspen Systems.

Walkenstein, M.D. (1982). Comparison of burned patients' perception of pain with nurses' perception of patients' pain. *Journal of Burn Care Rehabilitation, 3,* 233–236.

Williams, B. P. (1969). The problems and life-style of a severely burned man. In B. Bergersen, E. H. Anderson, M. Duffy, M. Lohr, & M. H. Rose (Eds.), *Current concepts in clinical nursing* (Vol. 2). St. Louis: C. V. Mosby.

Index